Fiber Pathways of the Brain

Fiber Pathways of the Brain

Jeremy D. Schmahmann, MD

Associate Professor of Neurology
Harvard Medical School
Boston, Massachusetts

Director, Ataxia Unit
Cognitive/Behavioral Neurology Unit
Geriatric Neurobehavior Clinic
Department of Neurology
Massachusetts General Hospital
Boston, Massachusetts

Deepak N. Pandya, MD

Professor of Anatomy and Neurobiology
Boston University School of Medicine
Boston, Massachusetts

Harvard Neurological Unit
Beth Israel Deaconess Medical Center
Boston, Massachusetts

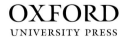
OXFORD
UNIVERSITY PRESS

2006

OXFORD
UNIVERSITY PRESS

Oxford University Press, Inc., publishes works that further
Oxford University's objective of excellence
in research, scholarship, and education.

Oxford   New York
Auckland   Cape Town   Dar es Salaam   Hong Kong   Karachi
Kuala Lumpur   Madrid   Melbourne   Mexico City   Nairobi
New Delhi   Shanghai   Taipei   Toronto

With offices in
Argentina   Austria   Brazil   Chile   Czech Republic   France   Greece
Guatemala   Hungary   Italy   Japan   Poland   Portugal   Singapore
South Korea   Switzerland   Thailand   Turkey   Ukraine   Vietnam

Published by Oxford University Press, Inc.
198 Madison Avenue, New York, New York 10016

www.oup.com

Oxford is a registered trademark of Oxford University Press.

Library of Congress Cataloging-in-Publication Data
Schmahmann, Jeremy D.
Fiber pathways of the brain/Jeremy D. Schmahmann, Deepak N. Pandya.
p. cm.
Includes bibliographical references and index.
ISBN-13 978-0-19-510423-3
ISBN 0-19-510423-4
1. Cerebral cortex. 2. Myelinated neurofibrils. I. Pandya, Deepak N. II. Title.
QP383.S36 2006
612.8'25—dc22   2005011108

9 8 7 6 5 4 3 2 1
Printed in China
on acid-free paper

To the memory of Henricus (Hans) G. J. M. Kuypers (1925–1989), whose original ideas concerning corticocortical organization had a fundamental impact on the thinking and career path of D. N. P., and through him to J. D. S. Dr. Kuypers encouraged both of us to study the anatomic basis of behavior and to seek functional relevance in anatomic circuits.

To the memory of Norman Geschwind (1926–1984), mentor and friend to D. N. P., teacher and source of inspiration to both of us in basic as well as clinical neuroscience. Dr. Geschwind revitalized behavioral neurology as an integrated discipline in which innovative clinical ideas are fundamentally dependent upon a detailed understanding of the structure and organization of the nervous system.

To Jinny and Adin, whose love sustains me,
to the memory of my parents, Bella and Oscar,
and to my family, friends, patients, and colleagues.
—J. D. S.

To my dear wife, Bonnie, and children, Jay, Dina, and Sunita,
and to all my colleagues with whom I have had the great opportunity
to navigate through the intricacies of the cerebral cortex.
—D. N. P.

"To say that the white matter is but a uniform substance like wax in which there is no hidden contrivance, would be too low an opinion of nature's finest masterpiece. We are assured that wherever in the body there are fibers, they everywhere adopt a certain arrangement among themselves, created more or less according to the functions for which they are intended . . . all the diversity of our sensation and our movements depends upon this. We admire the skillful construction . . . where each of these fibers, confined in a small space, functions without confusion and without disorder."

—Nicolaus Steno, 1669

"The work which I have now the honour to present . . . calls the attention of the reader to those laws of Divine order by which the universe is governed and supported; in it we find that the minutest beings share in the protection, and triumph in the bounty of the Sovereign of all things: that the infinitely small, manifest to the astonished eye the same proportion, regularity and design, which are conspicuous to the unassisted sight in the largest parts of creation. By finding all things formed in beauty, and produced for use, the mind is raised from the fleeting and evanescent appearances of matter, to contemplate the permanent principles of truth . . ."

—George Adams, 1798

Foreword

Nothing defines the function of a neuron better than its connections. Information flows along connections; growth factors are transported along connections; viruses move along connections; epileptic discharges spread through connections. When deprived of connections, neurons pine away and eventually expire through retrograde and transsynaptic degeneration. The neuronal death in amyotrophic lateral sclerosis, neurofibrillary tangles in Alzheimer's disease, atrophy in olivopontocerebellar degeneration progress through neural connections. Once the adult stage of development is reached, connections become more important than even genes or molecules. Despite their vastly different functions, for example, it is quite likely that the genes and proteins of visual and auditory neurons in the cerebral cortex are nearly identical. What ultimately determines the vast differences in their function is not the molecular profile but connectivity.

But why should we bother about connectivity in the age of functional imaging, at a time when magnets of ever increasing strength promise to detect the location of even the faintest thought? Isn't it enough to locate cortical areas engaged in deception, wrath, introspection, empathy? Do we really have to worry about their connections? The answer is "yes," principally because the function of a complex system cannot be deduced from an inventory of its components. The relation among components introduces attributes that are not contained in the list of constituent elements. This is why a chemical analysis of the ink does not allow the differentiation of a sublime statement from a ridiculous one. In the case of the nervous system, the unit of relational architecture that allows the whole to exceed the sum of the parts is known as a large-scale network. Its elucidation requires an elaborate understanding of connectivity patterns.

If the cerebral cortex had been organized in the form of an assembly line, where each station adds a new ingredient and hands its product to the next, connections might well have been inferred from judiciously designed functional imaging experiments. But reality is more complex. Connections in association cortex do not follow strict hierarchies. There are feed-forward and feedback connections, reentrant and corollary discharges, nodes of convergence and divergence, and a tremendous capacity for parallel processing whereby two cortical areas can communicate with each other through dozens of alternate pathways, some direct and some through intermediaries that place their own spins on the message that is being transmitted. Through this architecture, the same area can serve as the beginning, the middle and the end of a cognitive process.

The distribution of connections is complex but not chaotic. The choices are many but they obey phylogenetically established constraints. For example, unimodal association areas in different modalities are not interconnected monosynaptically to each other; the hypothalamus establishes its heaviest connections with limbic and paralimbic areas; peristriate areas are connected to visual cortex in parallel rather than serially. Understanding these patterns of cortical connectivity is absolutely essential for understanding the relational architecture, and therefore function, of large-scale neurocognitive networks.

This book is all about tracing the white matter trajectories of axonal pathways emanating from the cerebral cortex of the monkey brain. It is a splendid volume that reflects a labor of love from a team that combines great experience with great enthusiasm. In my opinion, this is the most important single-volume contribution to primate neuroanatomy since the 1947 publication of Von Bonin and Bailey's *The Neocortex of Macaca Mulatta*. The book has three major components: an erudite historical account of relevant neuroanatomical themes, a comprehensive cytoarchitectonic map, and an unparalleled account of white matter pathways emanating from cortical tracer injection sites in 36 monkeys. In this third and most important component of the book, the connections of the injection sites and their white matter trajectories are beautifully illustrated. Not only does this volume provide a compact compendium of region-specific connections, but it also provides something entirely unique, the ability to determine the disconnections that a focal white matter lesion would cause.

But why should we bother about connections in the monkey when the goal is to understand the functions of the human brain? The reasons are simple and sobering. There is currently no method that can come close to tracing connections in the human brain with the sort of precision described in this book. To be sure, developments based on diffusion tensor imaging and the computational analysis of effective connectivity do appear promising, but they have a long way to go before they can tell us the cells of origin, white matter trajectories, and termination fields of pathways emanating from cortical areas no larger than a few millimeters in size. I have little doubt that breakthroughs will occur and that we will eventually be able to understand human brain connectivity. Until then, however, this book will remain the standard reference source for the connection pathways of the primate cerebral cortex.

M-Marsel Mesulam, MD
Chicago, Illinois

Preface

Fiber Pathways of the Brain was conceived in an attempt to address a fundamental gap in our knowledge of the organization of the brain. The investigation by Joseph Jules Dejerine (1849–1917) in 1895 of the fiber systems of the human brain remains the only comprehensive account of the anatomy of the cerebral white matter pathways. In the material available to him and other early investigators, however, it was not possible to ascertain the origins and terminations of the fiber pathways and thus to determine what information these systems convey. This remains a central problem. Whereas there is a considerable literature on the connections of the cerebral cortical and subcortical regions in the nonhuman primate, there is presently no comprehensive account of the fiber bundles that link them.

In our studies of the cortical and subcortical connections of cerebral association areas, we have been impressed by the ability of the radioisotope technique to delineate not only the projections arising from the cortical areas but also the fiber systems that convey these connections. In this monograph we rely on the technique of radioisotope tract tracing to provide an analysis of the fiber systems in the nonhuman primate brain. Throughout this project, the descriptions and depictions by the early anatomists of the fiber pathways in the human brain have served as a beacon, an invitation to match and update their work with contemporary techniques in the experimental animal.

We were also motivated throughout this endeavor by the clinical mandate set forth by Norman Geschwind, who emphasized the phenomenon of cerebral disconnection as a critical element in the disruption of higher-order behavior. Geschwind's conception presaged the notion that brain function is the result of effective communication between structures geographically distributed around the nervous system. This idea places the means of communication, namely the white matter fiber systems, squarely at the core of the distributed neural circuitry hypothesis. In so doing, it underscores the relevance of this anatomical investigation as much for clinical purposes as for the broader need to explore the neural substrates of behavior.

This work is presented in monograph form in an attempt to provide a single coherent reference that will permit the comparison, analysis, and discussion of brain fiber systems. An overarching view of the cortical and subcortical pathways could not adequately be achieved in a series of papers devoted to each fiber bundle. We wanted to explore the historical evolution of ideas about the white matter, analyze the fibers that subserve each brain region, and develop hypotheses regarding their possible functional roles. The knowledge gained in the past few decades concerning the anatomy, connections, and functional attributes of the cerebral cortex, and the association cortices in particular, has made it possible to speculate on the functions of the white matter bundles by recognizing the cortical and subcortical areas that they link.

Since we began this project in 1994, studies of cerebral white matter have risen to the forefront of contemporary clinical and basic neuroscience research. The development of diffusion tensor and diffusion spectrum magnetic resonance imaging and white matter tractography permits the visualization of the fiber pathways with a precision that had previously been unattainable *in vivo*. These emerging techniques rely on knowledge of anatomical pathways that was derived from methodologies constrained by the limitations inherent in the earlier experimental approaches. In addition, the evolution of the notion that cognitive and behavioral changes, including dementia, may result directly from damage to cerebral white matter has added a clinical urgency to the need to better understand the cerebral white matter and the fiber tracts it contains. The new information stemming from the analysis of the constituents and topography of white matter tracts in the monkey therefore has significance for understanding both brain anatomy and organization, and the clinical disorders that affect white matter. We hope that this work will facilitate a more sophisticated and detailed understanding of the fiber systems, prove useful in future investigations, and contribute to achieving the goal of improving diagnosis and management of brain-based disorders in humans.

The process of learning about the fiber systems of the brain has at times been arduous, but it has been deeply satisfying for us to work in a collaborative manner, rendering the task not only manageable but also thoroughly enjoyable. The many years that we have worked together on this and other projects have been mutually rewarding and beneficial. Our journey through this project has been like the course of the fiber systems through the hemispheres: it had an origin and an intended termination, but the course taken held a wonder of its own. We are pleased now to be able to share the results of these investigations with the larger community.

Acknowledgments

This project could not have been completed without the superb assistance of a number of individuals and institutions whom we acknowledge here with deep gratitude. Together, J. D. S. and D. N. P. generated hand-drawn images of the fiber systems on template images of the brain. J. D. S. then transformed these into the line art seen throughout the monograph. These line drawings, however, had to be scanned and manipulated using contemporary computer graphics. Similarly, the photomicrographs were often photomontages, even using a 0.5× lens and stage, and this too required close attention to detail. This exhaustive work was performed by Charlene DeMong, and we are grateful to Charlene for her commitment to this project. Amy Hurwitz and Lisa Patterson provided much-needed assistance during the earliest phases of the project. The valuable efforts of Jason MacMore have also been indispensable throughout the completion of the final stages of this work.

Historical accounts from medical antiquity until the latter part of the 17th century were derived from secondary sources, including Todd (1845), Neuberger edited by Clarke (1897/1981), Polyak (1957), Garrison/McHenry (1969), Meyer (1971), and Clarke and O'Malley (1996). Large sections of the text dealing with the era of gross dissection forward, commencing with Vicq d'Azyr, consist of primary historical research, except where specifically quoted and referenced from other sources. We gratefully acknowledge the assistance of librarians in the Countway Library of Medicine housing the Boston Medical Library, the library of Harvard Medical School, and the Rare Books and Special Collections Department.

The translation of papers by earlier investigators made it possible to understand the contributions of pioneers in this field and helped resolve the confusion that has abounded in the discussion of many of the white matter pathways. We are indebted to Jan Drappatz, who during his neurology residency at Massachusetts General Hospital engaged enthusiastically in this project, translating with us the German texts of Reil, Burdach, Onufrowicz, Kaufmann, Muratoff, Obersteiner and Redlich, Sachs, and others. It was a pleasure working with Jan to interpret the sometimes-arcane linguistic style of the early writers in order to develop a readable text true to the original intention of the authors. Similarly, Jean-Jacques Soghomonian, Associate Professor of Anatomy and Neurobiology at Boston University School of Medicine (BUSM), worked with us to translate relevant sections of the work by Dejerine that proved invaluable in our analysis. We were mindful of Macdonald Critchley's cautionary note (1979, p. 35) about "the exceeding difficulty, if not impossibility, of rendering a faithful translation from one language to another . . . (and that) every language has its little stock of subtle words which baffle an interpreter." The translations of Drs. Drappatz and Soghomonian made it possible for us to listen to the scholarly deliberations that characterized the early literature. Many of the seminal observations from these pioneers are presented in unabridged form in footnotes to the text, as they are either not available at all or can be found only in précis form or as limited direct quotes in a small number of other sources devoted to the history of neuroscience. To our knowledge no comprehensive compilation of these historical accounts of the anatomy of the white matter systems in the words of the original investigators is currently available in the English language.

J. D. S. takes this opportunity to gratefully acknowledge the deep clinical grounding imparted at the University of Cape Town Medical School by my teachers, including Francis Ames, Solly Benatar, Ralph Kirsch, Stuart Saunders, and J. C. de Villiers, and the mentoring and inspiration of my teachers in the Neurological Unit of Boston City Hospital, including Thomas D. Sabin, Simeon Locke, H. Royden Jones, Jr., and Thomas Kemper. Alan Peters gave me the opportunity to train in his department of anatomy and neurobiology at BUSM, and this made it possible to embark on the journey with my mentor, friend, and co-author D. N. P. Joseph P. Martin and Allan Ropper invited me to join the Massachusetts General Hospital (MGH) and Harvard Medical School, which have been my intellectual home and source of inspiration since 1989. I am grateful to Anne B. Young, chair of the Department of Neurology at the MGH, for fostering and encouraging an atmosphere of independent scholarship. This has allowed me to explore these questions of neuroanatomy while pursuing active clinical and teaching interests. The Department of Anatomy and Neurobiology at BUSM has continued to be a supportive and scientific home for D. N. P. and a gracious host to me. I would also like to express my gratitude to my other teachers and colleagues at the Boston City Hospital (Milton Jay, Harold Schiff, Fereydoun Sharokhi, and Nagagopal Venna); Lahey Clinic Medical Center (Paul T. Gross, José Gutrecht, Steven Kott, Simmons Lessell, Irma Lessell, and Prather Palmer); New England Deaconess Medical Center (Roy Freeman and Daniel Tarsy); and the BUSM Department of Anatomy and Neurobiology (Mark Moss and Douglas Rosene). I have also learned from my clinical interactions with many colleagues at the Massachusetts General Hospital, including Raymond D. Adams, Marilyn Albert, Bob Brown, Ferdy Buonanno, David Caplan, Verne Caviness, Bill Falk, C. Miller Fisher, Tessa Hedley-Whyte, Phil Kistler, Walter Koroshetz, Neil Kowall, Nikos Makris, Bruce Price, the late E.P. Richardson, Martin Samuels, Janet Sherman, and Mark Tramo.

D. N. P. would like to express deep gratitude to the late Walle J. Nauta, who inspired me to enter the field of neuroanatomy and provided continued encouragement and friendship for many years. I am indebted to the late Hans Kuypers, under whom I received training in neuroanatomy in the mid-1960s. Dr. Kuypers was a perfect teacher to many of us. I have tried to follow his thinking in my approach to neurological investigation. I am grateful also to the late Dr. Friedrich Sanides for introducing me to the intricacies of cortical architecture. My research was greatly supported by the late Norman Geschwind, who was always ready to accommodate my needs and who provided much-needed mentoring during my early career in Boston. I am grateful to Alan Peters and Mark Moss for providing me with generous support and inspiration. Most of my research studies were conducted in the department of anatomy and neurobiology at BUSM. In the 1970s, while working as a full-time internist at the Bedford Veterans Administration Hospital, I was able to continue my research and teaching through the kind generosity of the department of medicine. Many of our concepts regarding cortical connections and pathways have evolved over the course of several years. I would therefore like to express my sincere thanks to all our colleagues with whom I have had the opportunity to work: Helen Barbas, Clifford Barnes, Gene Blatt, Nelson Butters, Doug Chavis, Ben Cipolloni, Patricia Dye, Barbara Fullerton, Albert Galaburda, Mark Hallett, David Heilbronn, Ken Heilman, Eduardo Karol, Pat Lele, Nikos Makris, Marsel Mesulam, Robert Morecraft, Elliot Mufson, Sanat Mukherjee, Michael Petrides, Kathy Rockland, Doug Rosene, Monalisa Schultz, Benjamin Seltzer, Don Siwek, Gary Van Hoesen, Luigi Vignolo, Brent Vogt, and Edward Yeterian.

The case material that we have analyzed here has been generated over a number of years. Many individuals have been involved in preparing these materials with great dedication and enthusiasm. We therefore would like to acknowledge their valuable technical assistance: Deborah Burke, Brian Butler, Mary Chiavarras, Andrew Doolittle, Valerie Killgreen, John C. Klick, Valerie Knowlton, Ann Mahoney, David Moser, Tim Murphy, and Michael Schorr. Without the efforts of these individuals, many of whom have gone on to their own careers in neuroscience, this work would not have been possible. The meticulous artist's renditions of the fiber tracts depicted in chapters 13 through 19 were prepared by Marcia Williams.

For both of us, our colleagues, students, residents, and fellows teach us constantly and remind us of the wonder and humility inherent in this field. Our patients, who exemplify courage and the human spirit in the face of adversity, are our driving force to increase knowledge of the brain so that we may more effectively answer their call. It would have been inconceivable to have completed this project without the support of our families, and we would like particularly to thank our wives Jinny (J. D. S.) and Bonnie (D. N. P.) for their nurturing and patience. The untiring assistance of Marygrace Neal over the years has been of inestimable value in facilitating the completion of this project.

Oxford University Press, personified for us first by Jeffrey House and then by Fiona Stevens, has been patient beyond measure. Expecting a completed work in 1998, Fiona stayed with us as the project stretched from 4 years to 12, and the encouragement, support, and editorial counsel offered by her and other members of the Oxford University Press staff have been valued and crucial.

Financial support that has helped this work come to fruition was provided in part by the National Institutes of Health, the Veterans Administration, and the Boston University School of Medicine Alzheimer's Disease Center (J. D. S. and D. N. P.) and by the McDonnell-Pew Program in Cognitive Neuroscience and the Birmingham Foundation (J. D. S.).

Contents

Relevance of the Cerebral
White Matter Fiber Pathways

PART I

Introduction

The cerebral cortex has long been recognized as the essential neural correlate of human experience. Its approximately 20 billion neurons (Pakkenberg and Gundersen, 1997) are arranged in multiple distinct areas that have been characterized extensively with respect to their morphological and cellular specialization. The architecture of each of these cortical areas subserves functionally distinct domains of sensorimotor perception and action, emotional experience, and complex reasoning. The cerebral cortex does not support nervous system function in isolation, however. It has become apparent that all behaviors are subserved by distributed neural systems that comprise anatomic regions, or nodes, each displaying unique architectural properties, distributed geographically throughout cortical and subcortical areas of the nervous system, and linked anatomically and functionally in a precise and unique manner (Geschwind 1965a,b; Goldman-Rakic, 1988; Goldman-Rakic and Selemon, 1990; Jones and Powell, 1970; Luria, 1966; Mesulam, 1981, 1990, 1998, 2000; Nauta, 1964; Pandya and Kuypers, 1969; Pandya and Yeterian, 1985; Ungerleider and Mishkin, 1982).

In contrast to the detailed understanding of the cerebral cortex, there is a dearth of information on the fiber pathways that link the different components of the distributed neural system. Descriptive terms such as centrum semiovale and corona radiata were initially applied to the cerebral white matter because of its seemingly amorphous appearance on naked eye inspection. Investigators in the 1800s used gross dissection and, later, myelin-stained material to evaluate the fiber bundles, and degeneration techniques were used in clinical cases to examine connectivity among cortical areas. These studies identified and named some of the major association tracts, including the cingulum bundle and uncinate fasciculus. Descriptions of other systems, including the arcuate fasciculus/superior longitudinal fasciculus and the inferior longitudinal fasciculus, have remained in use despite unresolved controversies in the literature. Some information concerning the fibers leading from the cerebral cortex to subcortical structures (the projection systems) was also available from earlier studies. It was not known, however, how the subcortical fibers differentiate from the association systems as they emanate from the cerebral cortex, and details regarding the trajectories of the fibers within the internal capsule and sagittal stratum remained to be established. The limitations of the techniques used by the early investigators also made it impossible to determine the precise organization of these pathways, or their origins and terminations.

There is a considerable literature on the biology and pathology of myelinated axons, but little is known about the way these axons form the connecting links of the distributed neural systems or the kind of information that these fiber bundles convey. Understanding the white matter tracts is a pivotal step in the further elaboration of knowledge of brain structure and function, particularly with regard to the anatomic substrates of higher-order behavior. Fundamental questions concerning their organization remain unresolved, however. Which fiber pathways do the different cortical areas use to convey information to the other cortical and subcortical nodes? Are fiber bundles specific to certain cortical areas? Is there intrabundle topography of axons arising from adjacent cortical areas?

A deeper understanding of the white matter pathways is relevant also for clinical purposes. A number of diseases are characterized predominantly by affliction of the white matter, such as multiple sclerosis, and in other conditions white matter abnormalities exist but have been underappreciated, such as in Alzheimer's disease and normal aging. Selected disconnection syndromes have received prominent attention through the clinical efforts of such investigators as Dejerine, Geschwind, and Gazzaniga, but the cognitive failure that accompanies white matter destruction following ischemia, radiation damage, and human immunodeficiency virus infection, among many others, underscores the recognition that these classic syndromes represent examples of a substantially larger clinical problem. Information about damaged pathways in clinical studies would be enhanced by knowledge of the entire trajectory of the affected pathways derived from experimental investigations in the non-human primate.

The recent development of diffusion tensor magnetic resonance imaging (DTI) has made it possible to identify *in vivo* some details of organization within the major white matter pathways (Basser et al., 1994; LeBihan et al., 2001; Pierpaoli et al., 1996), both in normal brains and in clinical situations in which the pathways are damaged (Cellerini et al., 1997; Jones et al., 1999; Makris et al., 1997). This promising technology was initially limited by the visualization only of the major tributaries of the pathways and the inability to determine their origins or terminations or the nature of the information they convey. The imaging techniques and mathematical models have become increasingly sophisticated with the development of MR tractography (e.g., Bammer et al., 2003; Catani et al., 2002) and diffusion spectrum imaging (Lin et al., 2003), and it is likely that the field of *in vivo* white matter tractography in humans will acquire a greater degree of technical precision, useful for understanding normal brain anatomy and relevant for clinical studies as well.

There are some important constraints upon tractography, however. The calculated trajectory of the fiber tract may fail to follow the true fiber tract trajectory because of the ability of trajectories to jump to adjacent structures via noisy or partially volumed voxels (Basser et al., 2000), and because tractography is particularly prone to noise due to cumulative error along the length of the trajectory path (Tench et al., 2002). Tractography therefore has the potential to introduce fiber continuity where there is none, producing anatomically plausible but erroneous trajectories and false connections (Basser et al., 2000), and the reliability of this technique is receiving active scrutiny (e.g., Ciccarelli et al., 2003). These new imaging techniques also rely on *a priori* hypotheses derived from earlier anatomical conclusions regarding the course of the fiber bundles (Basser et al., 2000; Catani et al., 2003), particularly for the association fiber pathways. Misinterpretations of postmortem histologic and gross dissection preparations, as well as the terminological confusion that developed as a consequence of early uncertainty, have become traditional teaching in anatomical texts, and these erroneous conclusions are now being replicated in the DTI literature. These include descriptions of probably nonexistent bundles such as an "inferior fronto-occipital fasciculus," the conflation of the actual fronto-occipital fasciculus with the subcallosal fasciculus of Muratoff, and the bundling together of all three components of the superior longitudinal fasciculus and their merger with the anatomically separate and functionally distinct arcuate fasciculus, among others.

The central problem is that there has been no "gold standard" for *in vivo* fiber tractography (Basser et al., 2000; Crick and Jones, 1993), and postmortem dissection, sometimes regarded as the "definitive standard" (e.g., Catani et al., 2003), is anything but definitive, as a century of anatomical and terminological confusion will attest. It should be possible to identify fibers more precisely using MRI once it is known from tract-tracing studies in the experimental animal where they are situated, and what brain regions they link. Whereas the monkey and human brains display considerable differences in detail, the overall structural similarities down to the level of architectonic differentiation are well established (Brodmann, 1909; Macchi and Jones, 1997; Pandya and Barnes, 1987; Petrides and Pandya, 1999; Rajkowska and Goldman-Rakic, 1995a,b). Extrapolation of data concerning white matter pathways from monkey to human has a number of limitations but may be permissible with the understanding that areas in the human brain that are greatly expanded are likely to have more elaborate and complex connections and functions. The analysis of the origins and terminations of the white matter fibers in the experimental animal may thus be useful in the development of a more comprehensive understanding of the data obtained from these imaging studies in humans.

There is a considerable body of literature dealing with corticocortical and corticosubcortical connections in the nonhuman primate, and there are selected studies of white matter pathways using contemporary anatomical techniques. There has been no comprehensive attempt, however, to delineate all the white matter pathways arising from the different areas of the cerebral cortex, together with the termination patterns of projections conveyed by these pathways. In our earlier analyses of corticocortical and corticosubcortical connections in the rhesus monkey we were impressed by the ability of the autoradiographic tract-tracing technique that uses isotope-labeled amino acids to demonstrate the high degree of organization of axons in the white matter. This technique reveals the origins, terminations, and trajectories of the association fibers, as well as of the callosal, striatal, thalamic, pontine, and other subcortical fiber systems. We therefore embarked upon this study to outline the different white matter pathways of the cerebral hemispheres using the autoradiographic technique in the animal model, in order to understand the organization of the fibers that emanate from the cerebral cortex, the "parent" node in the distributed system. Along with the trajectories of the pathways, we documented their termination patterns, enabling the simultaneous determination of the cortical and subcortical relations of each cerebral cortical architectonic region and the fiber bundles that link them. We hope that this anatomical investigation of the fiber pathways in the nonhuman primate will provide the exposition necessary for the more accurate analysis and interpretation of major white matter tracts in the human brain and the further delineation of the distributed systems subserving brain function.

The monograph begins with an historical account of the evolution of ideas about the structure and organization of white matter. This synthesis provides a framework for understanding early notions about the organization of cerebral white matter, it underscores the realization by early neuroscientists of the importance of fiber pathways for a variety of neurological disorders, and it describes the limitations encountered in these earlier studies. As a result of our analysis, we have presented revised notions of some of the fiber bundles described and discussed in the literature over almost two centuries. In this historical review, we pay homage to the investigations of the pioneers in this field. The technical details of our experimental approach are presented in the methods section, including a description of the isotope technique, our novel approach of identifying the fibers in Nissl-stained sections, and the use of computer technology to permit *de novo* charting of fiber systems from all regions of the cerebral cortex onto a single template brain. This is followed by photomicrographs of the representative sections from the template brain used in this work, with architectonic designations identified. The fiber bundles emanating from all cortical areas share certain features, and these are outlined in the section on organizing principles. A case-by-case description of the results follows in the section on organization of cerebral white matter by region of origin. The chapters in this section present detailed descriptions, illustrations, summary diagrams, and synthesis of the cortical and subcortical fiber pathways emerging from the parietal, superior temporal, inferior temporal, occipital, precentral motor, prefrontal, and cingulate areas. In the next section anatomical details of individual fiber bundles are presented, followed by discussion of their putative functional attributes. The composite summary of cerebral white matter fiber pathways is a series of composite summary diagrams in the coronal plane that depicts the location and constituents of the various white matter tracts. Neurobehavioral manifestations in patients with white matter lesions are addressed in the section on clinical relevance to emphasize the importance of these pathways in the human brain. In the conclusion, we draw upon the anatomy of the cerebral hemisphere fiber pathways to develop hypotheses about their putative functional properties and their roles in a more general view of brain organization. The final chapter, Notes, contains comments and discussion relevant to the text and includes translations of the work of some of the early investigators.

White Matter Pathways in Early Neuroscience

Our study of the fiber tracts of the rhesus monkey brain using the anterograde autoradiographic tract-tracing technique follows a long and honored tradition of using contemporary methods to investigate the cerebral white matter. We begin with a comprehensive historical review of the evolution of ideas and observations about the structure and function of the white matter to the present. We undertake this historical review in the light of historian Max Neuburger's (1868–1955) statement that understanding the achievements of modern science "is inconceivable without a knowledge of the history of its development and growth, its origins and sources" (Neuburger/Clarke, 1897/1981, p. 4). In Neuburger's words, "truth is no longer sought in the yellowing pages of old manuscripts, [but] ignorance of the past necessarily leads to an overestimation of the heights achieved by present knowledge" (ibid., pp. 2–4). Like the Italian anatomist Caecilius Folius (1615–1650), we "know quite well that knowledge is acquired by adding one piece of it to another, and that all of us, like children sitting on the shoulders of giants, can see far more than our predecessors could" (ibid., p. 285).

Medical Antiquity

Neurological science traces its recorded origins to the Edwin Smith papyrus of the 17th century BC, a hieroglyphic copy of a manuscript from the Egyptian Pyramid Age composed around 3000 to 2500 BC. In this document, the "brain" is named, its most overt features, including the convolutions and the presence of cerebrospinal fluid, are recognized, and individuals with neurological disorders are described. Conceptual approaches to brain organization and function during classical Greek antiquity were as systematic and detailed as the techniques and known facts would allow, and they were heavily influenced by spiritual and theological notions and by the attempt to identify a locus in the body for the *hegemonikon*, or the ruling soul. The art and science of medicine flourished in antiquity also in the Indian and Chinese subcontinents, similarly influenced by prevailing philosophical and spiritual notions. Detailed accounts of the Ayurvedic approach of Indian medicine (see, for example, Bagchi, 1979; Narayana, 1995) and traditional Chinese notions (as embodied in "The Yellow Emperor's Classic of Internal Medicine," Yellow Emperor, Huang Dynasty [2697–2595 BC], and Shen Nong's "Canon of Herbs" [2700 BC]) are beyond the scope of the present monograph; suffice it to say that the evolution of medical knowledge was not confined to Western medicine, and there appears to have been mutual exchange of ideas in the medical sciences between these ancient societies.

Pythagoras (c. 572–c. 490 BC) is credited with introducing the notion that the brain is concerned with reasoning. The precedent for the influence of teachers on their students and the course of subsequent scientific inquiry was established early, in that Pythagoras' student, the physician Alcmaeon (Alkmaion) of Athens, performed human dissections and recognized the role of the brain in sensation, movement, and thinking. Brain dissection was first undertaken systematically by Anaxagoras of Klazomenai (c. 500 BC), who considered the brain to be the organ of the mind, the origin of the nerves, and the seat of the soul. In Hellenized southern Italy, Philolaos of Croton or Tarent (c. 400 BC) also regarded the brain as the seat of intelligence, but he introduced the debate, which would persist for 2,000 years, that the heart, not the brain, was the seat of *hegemonikon*, a fallacy that would receive later support from Aristotle and the ideologists of early Christianity. The Hippocratic school (460 BC–370 BC) recognized the brain as the substrate of nervous action, ascribing to it intelligence, dreams, and thoughts. They introduced the notion of the brain as a gland, secreting phlegm or *pituita,* and acting as a cooling device, a notion that would also persist for two millennia. Vigorous scientific inquiry occurred during the Alexandrine period, when Greek culture was implanted in Egypt (323 BC–212 BC). This included human dissection by Herophilus of Chalcedon (335 BC–280 BC), who described the cerebral ventricles and noted the convoluted character of the cerebrum, and Erasistratus of Chios (c. 310 BC–250 BC), who concluded that cerebral convolutions are related to intelligence because they are more numerous in man than in animals. Other conceptual advances were introduced by Asclepiades of Bithynia (c. 124 BC), who described mania, delirium, and absence of mind (psychosis), and by Rufus of Ephesus (c. AD 100), whose dissections in apes led him to concur with the observations of Erasistratus that nerves of motion are distinguished from those of sensation, and to conclude that nerves originate from the brain.

The Galenic Period

The lasting work of early Greek antiquity that influenced medicine and science for fully 1,500 years was that of Galen of Pergamon/Pergamos/Pergamum (AD 129/130–200/201). In the era in which human dissection was proscribed, he performed vivisections on a variety of animals and examined the bones of humans that were available to him. He named the dura mater, pia mater, corpus callosum, the four ventricles, fornix, corpora quadrigemina, pineal and pituitary glands, and infundibulum. He described the intraventricular foramen (later named for Alexander Monro, Secundus [1733–1817]) and the cerebral aqueduct (later identified by Sylvius, see below) and the cervical, brachial, and lumbosacral plexuses, and he followed nerves from their origins to terminations in muscles and viscera. Galen discarded the Hippocratic notion that the brain is a gland, argued that it was the seat of intelligence, emotion, and sensation, and described it as a structure analogous to the bone marrow and continuous with the spinal cord. He initiated the idea of brain localization by declaring the frontal lobes to be the seat of the soul (*pneuma*) and the source of the "animal spirit." He introduced the concept of anatomical localization in clinical neurological science, holding that the "method of looking for the place chiefly affected is of great importance for all the organs, but particularly in disease of the brain" (Garrison/McHenry, 1969, p. 121).[1] At the center of Galen's physiological conceptions of brain function was the notion that natural spirit, a mysterious substance indispensable for life and originating in the liver, transforms into vital spirit conveyed by the heart to the brain, and this in turn transforms into the more refined animal spirit. A necessary ingredient for this brain process was air inspired into the cerebral ventricles. These fanciful notions seem less ludicrous when terms such as oxyhemoglobin, cerebrovascular system, and propagation of electrical impulses in neural transmission replace the more vaguely conceived "spirituous substances." The comment of Robert Bentley Todd (1809–1860) in his discussion of the work of Thomas Willis is perhaps appropriate for Galen as well: "We may find in the writings of this great man the germs of many a theory which, in our times, has been brought forward with a more plausible aspect, disencumbered of the quaint phraseology and superabundant metaphor so common in his day" (Todd, 1845, p. 135).

The Middle Ages

Galen's voluminous contributions were summarized and disseminated in the *Continens Liber* of Rhazes (864–930 AD), which was translated into Latin in 1279, the *Canon* of Avicenna (980–1037) published in 1500, and the 200-volume work of the Benedictine monk Constantine (12th century). By the Middle Ages, mental faculties were thought to be localized either in the brain substance, as Galen had posited, or in the cerebral ventricles, as suggested by Herophilus of Chalcedon and medieval writers such as Nemesius, Bishop of Emesa (c. AD 390, published manuscript 1512) and St. Augustine (4th century). Little of substance was added to Galen's notions throughout this entire period, however, "with the exception of some therapeutic wrinkles" (Garrison/McHenry, 1966, p. 24).

Albert von Bollstädt (Albertus Magnus, 1193–1280) first depicted the cerebral ventricles in *Philosophia Naturalis* (published in 1496, according to Garrison/McHenry). He localized common sense in the frontal lobes, imagination in the midbrain, and memory in the cerebellum or in the four ventricles. Mondino dei Luzzi (Mundinus, 1275–1326) wrote his *Anothomia* in 1316 (first printed in 1478), which passed through numerous editions over the next 200 years. He summarized the anatomy known to Aristotle, Galen, and Avicenna, and he reintroduced human dissection, which had not been practiced since the time of the early Greeks. He ascribed a variety of qualities and attributes to the different components of the cerebral ventricular system. Fantasy and retention were in the anterior compartment of the lateral ventricle, special senses in the middle compartment, imagination and the ability to combine separate things in the posterior compartment. The third ventricle was endowed with the power of cognition and prognostication, and the fourth ventricle was concerned with the reception of impressions and memory (Clarke and O'Malley, 1996, p. 22). The drawings of Gregor Reisch (c. 1467–1525) in *Margarita Philosophica* (1503) further perpetuated the notion that complex functions reside in the ventricles, with functional specialization according to the different parts of the ventricular system. Diagrams of the brain, cranial nerves, optic chiasm, peripheral nerves, and muscles that began to approximate anatomic precision were those of Leonardo da Vinci (1452–1519), who also made the first successful wax casts of the cerebral ventricles. His anatomical drawings were not made available, however, until 1784. New realism was added to the published accounts of the nervous system in the depictions of the brain by Lorenz Fries (Laurentius Phryesen, c. 1480–1532) in 1519, Jacopo Berengario da Carpi (Berengarius, c. 1470–1550) in 1523, Johann Eichman (Dryander) (d. 1560) in *Anatomia Capitis Humani* (the first anatomical work devoted to the head and brain) in 1536, and Charles Estienne (Stephanus, 1503–1564) in 1546. The major advance in neurological anatomy, however, awaited the work of Vesalius.

The Era of Vesalius

Whereas Galen had described the corpus callosum and the fornix in animals, the white matter and the gray matter of the brain were not differentiated from each other in antiquity, and the early Renaissance anatomists paid more attention to the ventricular system than to the brain parenchyma because the prevalent doctrine was that mental function resided in the ventricles.

With the publication in 1543 of Andreas Vesalius' (1514–1564) *De Humani Corporis Fabrica* (On the Structure of the Human Body), a new era of anatomical and scientific investigation and thought was introduced. "(T)he first period of Postclassical European anatomy, characterized by a helpless dependence upon the written word of Greek and Arab authorities, often erroneous, and based upon animal rather than human sources, was at an end" (Polyak, 1957, p. 92). In the seventh book of *Fabrica*, illustrated by the artist Jan Stephan Kalkar, a student of Titian, Vesalius was the first to distinguish the softer and yellowish cerebrum from the harder and whiter deeper substance below it that was continuous with the corpus callosum. He provided a comprehensive account of the corpus callosum, the first description of it in man, and he recognized that it linked the two halves of the brain. He also depicted the internal capsule, caudate nucleus, putamen, and globus pallidus, as well as the midbrain, pulvinar, corpora quadrigemina, pineal gland, pituitary gland, and superior and middle cerebellar peduncles.

Volcher Coiter (1534–1576) distinguished between the gray and white matter of the spinal cord in 1572, but this was not illustrated until 1666 by Gerard Blasius (1625–1692) in the first separate treatise of the spinal cord, *Anatome Medullae Spinalis et Nervorum*. Gross dissection of the white matter of the brain was performed in 1586 by Arcangelo Piccolhomini (1526–1605), who introduced the terms "cerebrum" for the cerebral cortex and "medulla" for the white matter. In 1573, Co(n)stanzo Varolio (or Variolus, 1543–1575), who examined the brain from its base up for the first time (as opposed to from the top down), described the lobes of the brain related to the different cranial fossae and described in detail the hippocampus, optic nerve, cerebral peduncle, and the "pons Varolii" that bears his name.

The Scientific Method from Willis to Vicq D'Azyr

When Thomas Willis (1621–1675) published *Cerebri Anatome* in 1664, he introduced a new level of anatomic accuracy to the understanding of the inner structures of the brain. His monograph provided the first reclassification of cranial nerves since Galen and contributed the word "neurology" (the doctrine of the nerves) to the lexicon. As stated by Polyak (1957, p. 105), Willis' functional interpretations were still based on

Galenic ideas of the production and distribution of "animal spirit." Unlike Galen, however, Willis thought these spirits were produced not in the white matter, but in the cerebral cortex. He endorsed the notion proposed by Erasistratus (3rd century BC) that convolutional complexity in humans is reflected in intelligence, and the cortex not only stored memories but was also the originator of memories and the organ of thought. Willis observed the corona radiata and the capsular striations through the corpus striatum. His notion of the "medulla oblongata" was that it comprised all the deep white matter, the ventricles, basal ganglia, thalamus, and brainstem, and he viewed it as a bifurcate structure resembling the letter Y with a limb in each cerebral hemisphere and the stem corresponding to the brainstem. He thought of it as a "royal highway" into which animal spirits constantly flow from their twin sources, the cerebrum and cerebellum, and are then carried into all parts of the nervous system. Spirits directed outward served a locomotor function, whereas spirits were directed inward in response to sensation.[2]

In 1664 Marcello Malpighi (1628–1694) used a primitive microscope to provide the first proof that the white matter was composed of "fibers." After boiling the brain in water, he traced the white matter fibers of the brain and cerebellum and observed that they take their origin from the top of the spinal marrow contained within the cranium ("medulla oblongata"). These fibers "ramify from four reflected crura of this medulla in all directions, until they end by their branched extremities in the cortex," where they were embedded like the roots of a plant (translated and quoted on p. 136 of Todd, 1845, derived from Malpighi, *Exercitatio Epistolica de Cerebro*, 1664. These ideas are further expanded in Malpighi, 1669).

In an essay in 1665 (published in 1671), Nicolaus Steno (Niels Stensen, 1638–1686) suggested that one way to study the white matter of the brain was to follow "the nerve threads through the substance of the brain to find out where they go and where they end" (translated in Clarke and O'Malley, 1996, p. 584). He concluded: "To say that the white matter is but a uniform substance like wax in which there is no hidden contrivance, would be too low an opinion of nature's finest masterpiece. We are assured that wherever in the body there are fibers, they everywhere adopt a certain arrangement among themselves, created more or less according to the functions for which they are intended. If the substance is everywhere of fibers, as, in fact, it appears to be in several places, you must admit that these fibers have been arranged with great skill, since all the diversity of our sensation and our movements depends upon this. We admire the skillful construction of the fibers in each muscle; how much more then ought we to admire it in the brain, where each of these fibers, confined in a small space, functions without confusion and without disorder."

Using a technique of scraping the white matter to display its fiber bundles, in 1672 Willis demonstrated an intricate arrangement of the medullary tracts, pathways, or cords within the substance of what was then termed the medulla oblongata. He was "astonished at the innumerable arrangements of nerve fibers distributed in wonderful order into the different parts of the entire body." These fibers conveyed animal spirits, "confined by certain bounds and limits, so to speak, within the compressed space of a single chamber, [that] attend to the infinite varieties of actions and passions" (quoted in Clarke and O'Malley, 1996, p. 584).

The scraping method of dissection that was suggested by Steno and performed by Willis to carry out detailed studies of the cerebral white matter was used by Raymond

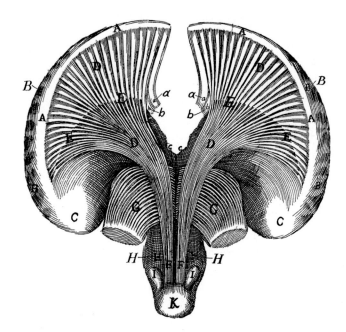

Figure 2-1

The illustration by Raymond Vieussens, figure 16 in *Neurographia* (1684), depicting "the base of the cerebrum, after the removal of the cerebellum and all the vessels, freed from nearly all its outer cineritious substance and shaved down" to show the fibers of the white matter.

de Vieussens (c. 1635–1715), who amended Malpighi's approach of boiling the brain in water. In his *Neurographia universalis* (1684), Vieussens readily distinguished the medullary white substance from the gray matter and showed that it "is composed of innumerable fibrils connected together and arranged into various fasciculi, which become very obvious when it is boiled in oil" (Todd, 1845, p. 136) (figure 2-1). Vieussens first observed the oval shape of the medullary white matter, introduced the term "centrum ovale," and demonstrated its continuity with the internal capsule, cerebral peduncle, and pyramidal fasciculi of the pons and medulla oblongata. He viewed the medullary fibers within the context of Galenic ideology. They "give the appearance of a spongy body which the animal spirit may permeate in many different and rather inexplicable ways, so that within it the spirit undergoes many different and inexplicable motions; because of their different arrangements different thoughts are aroused in the mind" (Clarke and O'Malley, 1996, p. 586).

The crossing of the pyramidal fibers below the pons was described by Domenico Mistichelli (1675–1715) in his 1709 treatise on apoplexy. In 1710 François Pourfoir de Petit (1664–1741) observed the same phenomenon in his *Lettres d'un medicine*. Based on clinical and experimental studies in dogs, he confirmed the observations of Hippocrates and Arateaeus that brain lesions are on the side opposite to the paralysis of the limbs. Pourfoir de Petit also noted that paralysis was complete and lasting only when the corpus striatum was damaged, whereas injury of the cerebral cortex alone produced only weakness. This led to the conclusion that animal spirits issued from the cortex, streamed through the fibers of the white matter, and crossed the corpora striata, made up of medullary (white matter) fibers, to form places where they could collect together.

Great importance was placed on the corpus callosum by Giovanni Maria Lancisi (1654–1720). In 1718 he stated that "it is quite clear that the part formed by the weaving together of innumerable nerves is both unique and situated in the middle [of the brain]; and so it can be said it is like a common marketplace of the senses, in which the external impressions of the nerves meet. But we must not think of it as merely a store-house for receiving the movement of structures: we must locate in it the seat of the soul, which imagines, deliberates, and judges" (quoted in Neuburger/Clarke, 1897/1981, p. 50, footnote 12).[3]

François Gigot de La Peyronie (1678–1747), too, concluded that the corpus callosum must be of the greatest importance for the support of life. Further, by relating cause and effect, he concluded that mental changes were observed only when the corpus callosum was diseased, and thus it was the seat of the intellectual faculties.

The work of Albrecht von Haller (1708–1777) is credited by Neuburger as having paved the way for future brain and spinal cord physiology. He differentiated between irritability and sensitivity in the nervous system, localized sensation to nerves and movement to muscles, and demonstrated the autonomous contractility of heart muscle. Haller believed that both the cerebral cortex and the dura mater lacked sensitivity, whereas the white matter of the brain was sensitive in all his experiments (Neuburger/Clarke, 1897/1981). He refuted the notion that the soul was located or distributed in the nervous system and introduced the idea of functional omnivalence—that any part of the brain (cerebrum and cerebellum) could function vicariously for another. There was, however, a distinction between the less significant cortex and the more important white matter that contained the "sensorium commune."[4]

On Feb. 2, 1776, Francesco Gennari (1752–1797) discovered the white matter streak in the occipital cortex; he designated it lineola albidior in 1782, and Heinrich Obersteiner (1847–1922) later named it the line of Gennari. This was the first anatomic underpinning of cortical heterogeneity and provided a rational basis for the ensuing notions of cortical localization.

Félix Vicq d'Azyr (1748–1794) independently confirmed Gennari's white line in 1781. In his 1786 *Traité d'anatomie et de physiologie*, one of the most extraordinary anatomical folios that had yet appeared, Vicq d'Azyr displayed the results of his dissections, which were facilitated by hardening the brain in alcohol—an innovation in the study of nervous system anatomy (figure 2-2). He identified the cerebral convolutions and internal structures of the brain. He described the mamillothalamic tract that bears his name, as well as the central sulcus (which François Leuret [1797–1851] in 1839 named for Luigi Rolando [1773–1831], who described it in 1809), the postcentral and precentral convolutions, and the insula (25 years before Reil). On horizontal sections of brain, he recognized the continuity of the white matter of the corpus callosum, the centrum ovale, and the white matter medial and lateral to the corpora striata. He described the anterior and posterior commissures that "are intended to establish sympathetic communications between the different parts of the brain, just as the nerves do between the different organs and the brain itself" (quoted in Clarke and O'Malley, 1996, p. 592). He differentiated for the first time the notion of commissural connections between the hemispheres as opposed to association pathways that run between the different regions of the same hemisphere. He included in the commissural category not only the corpus callosum and anterior and posterior commissures but also the quadrigeminal bodies, cerebral peduncles, pons, anterior medullary velum, interthalamic adhesion, infundibulum, and tuber cinereum. In the association system he considered the stria terminalis ("taenia semi-circularis"), fornix, peduncles of the pineal gland, and mamillothalamic tract. Vicq d'Azyr concluded that "everything is arranged in the system to multiply the connections

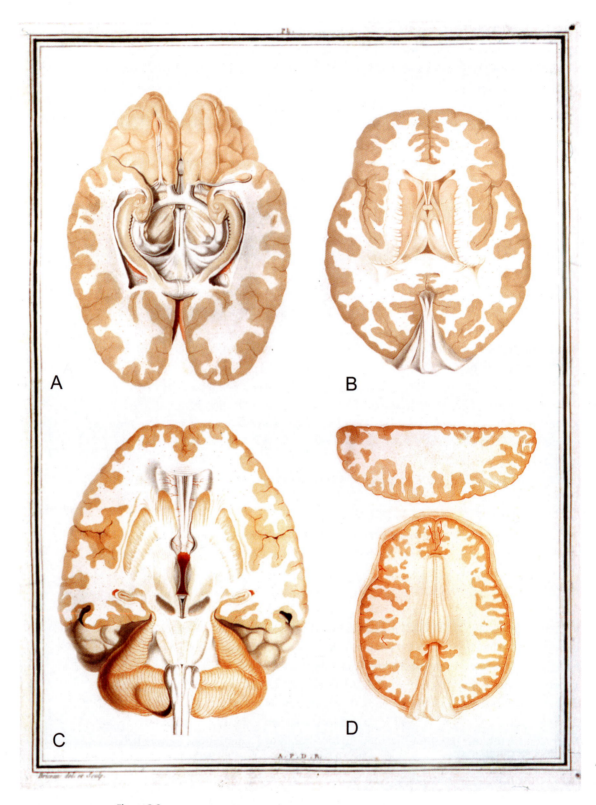

Figure 2-2
Images adapted from the atlas of Félix Vicq D'Azyr (*Traité d'anatomie et de physiologie,* 1786). Each of these four images occupies an entire page, and the decorative boundary that adorns each page is reproduced here. A, plate XX; B, plate XXII; C, plate IV; D, plate IX. The images in B through D are flipped vertically to show the frontal lobe at the top.

of different parts of the brain so that inconveniences which could result from difficulty occasioned in any part of the brain, are prevented" (ibid., p. 593). This concept presaged the role of synaptic plasticity in functional recovery.

The Era of Gross Dissection

The investigations of Willis, Steno, Malpighi, Vieussens, and others resulted in the initial recognition that the cerebral white matter was heterogeneous and complex. A completely new understanding of the organization of the white matter became possible, however, with the evolution of new brain-fixation techniques and the novel approaches to gross dissection of its internal structure that these techniques facilitated. In 1809 Johann Christian Reil (1759–1813) realized that using fresh unfixed tissue resulted in decaying material in which many original structures and relationships were lost. After soaking the brain in alcohol with potash or ammonia added, he investigated the white matter of the cerebral hemispheres (figure 2-3) and introduced the term "corona radi-

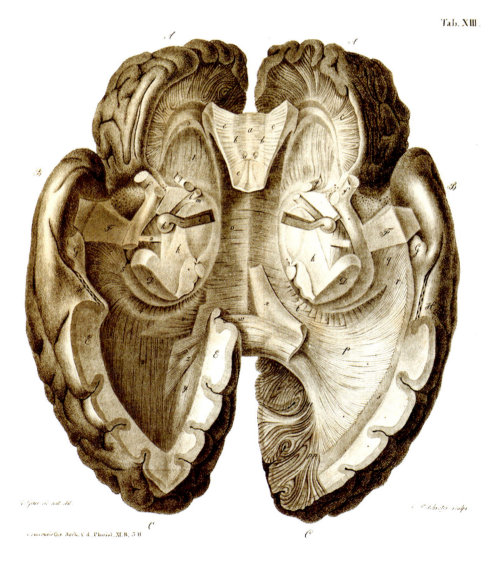

Tab. XIII.

Figure 2-3
Tafel XIII of Johann Christian Reil (*Archiv für die Physiologie*, 1812, volume XI) to show his gross dissection of the human brain viewed from below.

ata" to describe the radiation of fibers in Vieussens' centrum ovale.[5] He emphasized the close relation between these fibers, the internal capsule, and the cerebral peduncles, described the corpus callosum, anterior commissure, and uncinate fasciculus, and recognized the external capsule. He regarded the fibers that lead toward the occipital pole as being a caudal extension of the corona radiata, described the insular cortex that bears his name, and suggested that the cerebral convolutions were the seat of mental processes: "Around these centers [the basal gray masses] are all the convolutions of the hemispheres like the rays of the sun, or like rivulets that absorb their life spirits from the ocean; around these [centers] lie the main instruments of the soul; around them originate the organs of artistic perception, of the ability for induction and representation" (Reil, 1809d, p. 207; also quoted in Clarke and O'Malley, 1996, p. 391).

Haller's notions of equipotentiality survived into the 19th century, supported, for example, by Reil, Jean Marie Pierre Flourens (1794–1867), and others, despite Robert Boyle's (1627–1691) earlier conclusion that there was a motor area in the brain. Boyle had demonstrated the presence of a motor area in a patient with a palsy of the arm from a depressed skull fracture that resolved when the depressed bone was raised. Similarly, in his writings between 1738 and 1744, Emanuel Swedenborg (1688–1772), who recognized that fibers descend from the brainstem to the spinal cord and proposed the concept of an upper-motor and lower-motor neuron, defined the location of the motor area in the cerebral cortex. According to Garrison/McHenry (1969, p. 108), Swedenborg placed the representation of the extremities in the upper frontal convolutions, the abdomen and thorax in the middle frontal convolutions, and the head and neck in the lower frontal convolutions.

Against this background, the genius of Franz Joseph Gall (1758–1828), in collaboration with Johann Kaspar Spurzheim (1776–1832), led to a fundamental shift in the concept of brain structure and function. Best known for the spurious field of phrenology that Gall and Spurzheim promoted, their anatomy and conceptions of the nervous system represented a completely new direction that would prove to be validated repeatedly. Contemporary systems neuroscience has its origins in Gall's work.

Gall and Spurzheim initiated the concept that brain function is based on the preeminent importance of cerebral cortex ("the convolutions are of an essential nature and necessary for intellectual functions" [quoted in Clarke and O'Malley, p. 394]), that there is functional specialization of different parts of the cortex, that the cortex is the originator of the connecting fibers of the white matter, and that there is specificity of the connections of the different regions of the cortex. The publication in 1810 of *Anatomie et physiologie du systeme nerveux* also provided a fundamentally novel understanding of the organization of the white matter pathways in the cerebral hemispheres (figure 2-4). This work on the intracerebral white matter was designed to elucidate the connections between the postulated surface organs of the cortex, and it provided anatomical support for their notion that functional differences of the cortical organs were the result of different peripheral connections as well as discrete central relationships. Their diagrams of blunt dissection of fiber bundles established that white matter consists of tracts connecting cortical gray matter regions that they considered to be the organ of mental activity. Whereas callosal and association systems had been proposed by Vicq d'Azyr, Gall and Spurzheim proposed the existence of projection systems as opposed to association systems. The projection system ("divergent, or sortant") was equivalent to the afferent and efferent projection fibers that link the cortex with subcortical regions, brainstem, and spinal cord. Association fibers

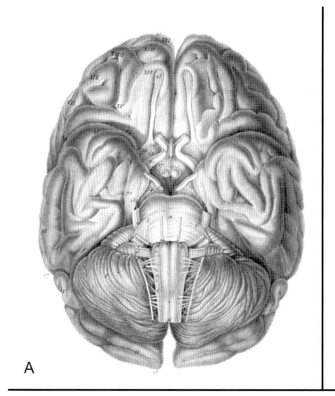
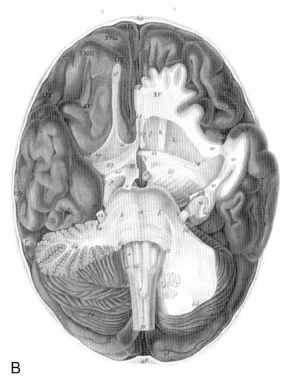

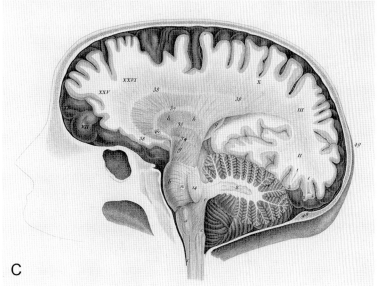

Figure 2-4

Images from the atlas of Franz Joseph Gall and Johann Kaspar Spurzheim (*Anatomie et physiologie du systeme nerveux*, 1810) showing cerebral convolutions and dissections revealing differentiating features of cerebral cortex and white matter. A, plate IV; B, plate XIII; C, plate X.

("convergent, or retrant"), were an entirely intracerebral system greatly developed in humans, being more numerous and containing larger bundles of fibers than the projection system. Further, these association fibers were of two kinds: short or arcuate fibers, and long fibers that connect parts of the different cerebral lobes. Commissural fibers that link the two hemispheres were considered by Gall to be part of the association system.

The importance of the anatomical studies of Gall and Spurzheim was recognized by their contemporary Alexander Monro, Tertius (1773–1859), professor of anatomy at the University of Edinburgh, like his father and grandfather before him. Monro wrote that "(t)he Plates of the brain of DRS GALL and SPURZEIN, are, taken as a whole, far superior to any that have been published; and by their method of exhibiting the brain, they have thrown much light upon the relative situation of parts" (Monro, 1813, p. 135).

John Gordon (1786–1818) published a scathing critique of the anatomical work of Gall and Spurzheim, quoting their work liberally in order to belittle it. As Gordon (1817, pp. 126–135) points out, Gall and Spurzheim noted that all white matter comprises fibers (although this was not a new observation); that all white matter originates and ends in the cerebral cortex; and that the cerebral convolutions contain both converging (association) and diverging (projection) fibers. Gordon was incensed by the statement of Gall and Spurzheim that the corpus callosum fibers are topographically arranged—frontal lobe fibers in the genu, fibers from the pericentral region in the body of the corpus callosum, and parietal and occipital lobe fibers in the caudal part of the corpus callosum, including the splenium. Further, Gall and Spurzheim concluded that the anterior commissure contains fibers that have their origins in the rostral part of the temporal lobe and in the ventral part of the frontal lobe. The anatomical conclusions of Gall and Spurzheim that Gordon enumerated have subsequently been validated repeatedly, as the results of our monograph also confirm. In hindsight, and perhaps to Gordon's chagrin, it transpires that the principles of cerebral white matter organization that were postulated by Gall and Spurzheim were prescient and accurate.

Neuburger also acknowledged that "Gall, who, as no one before him, succeeded in analyzing the structure of the white matter . . . was the first to claim that mental activities were localized in the cortex alone, (and) the white matter he relegated to the role of a system of conduction and projection" (Neuburger/Clarke, 1897/1981, p. 277). It took some time for the new ideas about white matter to become accepted, as reflected in the 1823 statement of François Magendie (1783–1855), who recognized the central role in locomotion played by "the white matter fibers that radiate from the pyramids to the cerebral hemispheres" but considered "that properties relating to movements reside chiefly in this (white matter) part of the brain" (Neuburger/Clarke, 1897/1981, p. 275).

Gall's "doctrine of plurality of cerebral organs" was favorably looked upon by Karl Friedrich Burdach (1776–1847), whose three-volume work between 1819 and 1826 defined and designated fiber bundles through gross dissection (figure 2-5). Burdach identified the tapetum, cingulum, uncinate fasciculus, and arcuate or superior longitudinal fasciculus, as well as other systems that he termed the inferior longitudinal fasciculus, and the "baseos internus" (Burdach, 1826, vol. 3, p. 959). The existence of intracerebral association fibers was proposed by Vicq d'Azyr and Gall and Spurzheim, and a preliminary characterization was attempted by Reil, but Burdach was the first to identify, characterize, and name these association fiber bundles in more detail.[6]

Intricate gross dissections of white matter were pursued subsequent to these early works and illustrated magnificently. Herbert Mayo (1796–1852) illustrated the fiber bundles in his engravings in 1827 (figure 2-6). Friedrich Arnold (1803–1890) depicted the fiber systems in his atlas (Arnold, 1838a) and described them (Arnold, 1838b), including bundles later to be named for him (the frontopontine tract [Arnold's bundle]

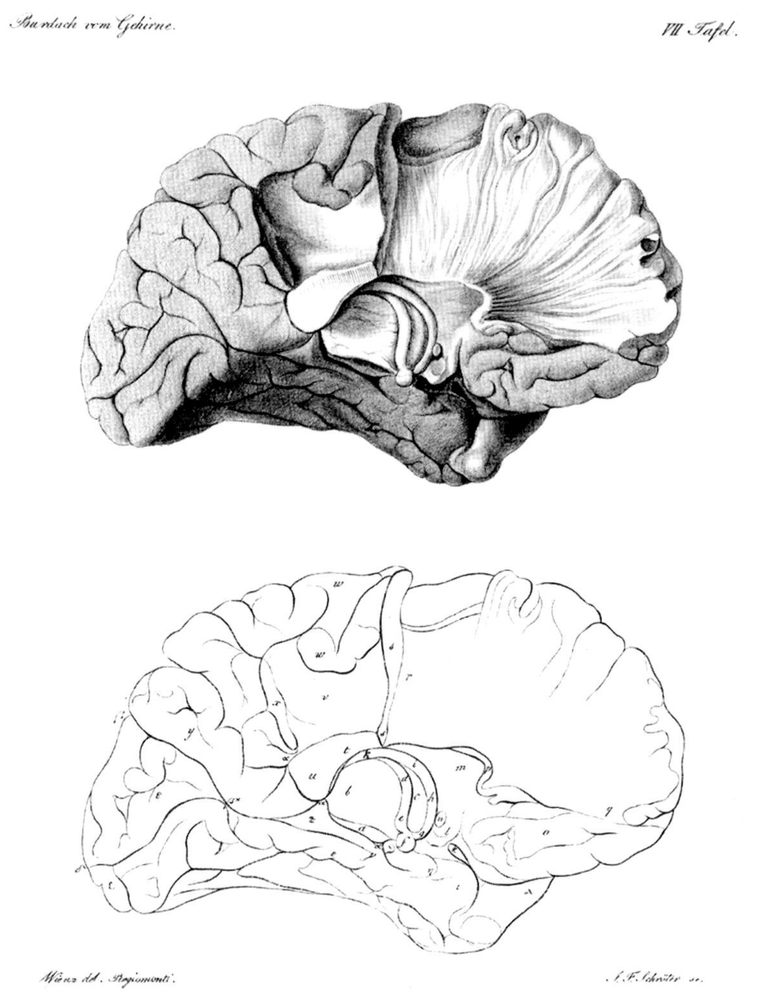

Würz del. Regiomonti.

J. F. Schröter sc.

Figure 2-5

Tafel VII from Karl Friedrich Burdach (*Vom Baue und Leben des Gehirns, Zweyter Band*, 1822) showing gross fiber dissection in the white matter of the frontal lobe.

and the temporothalamic fasciculus [Arnold's tract]; Arnold, 1851). He also observed the arcuate fibers linking adjacent gyri (figure 2-7) that had been described by Gall and Spurzheim (later called the fibrae arcuateae of Arnold). Achille-Louis Foville (1799–1878) diagrammed his gross fiber dissections in 1844, focusing on the corpus callosum (figure 2-8). He showed longitudinal fibers from the occipital lobe progressing rostrally, but he was not able to discern their destination.

Louis-Pierre Gratiolet (1815–1865) was the first to parcellate the cerebral hemisphere into lobes. The names he gave them remain in use today, including the Sylvian fissure, after Franciscus de le Boë, or Sylvius (1614–1672) who described it (as acknowledged by Caspar Bartholin the Younger [1655–1738] in 1641) and published his description in 1663 (Clarke and O'Malley, 1996, p. 390). Gratiolet also made a systematic study of the white matter in monkeys using the technique of gross dissection. He observed the anterior commissure, corpus callosum, and U-shaped association fibers connecting adjoining gyri of the same hemisphere. His notable additions to the description of white matter systems were the fibers that originated from Reil's corona radiata, the radiations from the quadrigeminal body, medial geniculate nucleus, and cerebellum, and most particularly the optic radiations (of Gratiolet), a fiber system coming via the optic

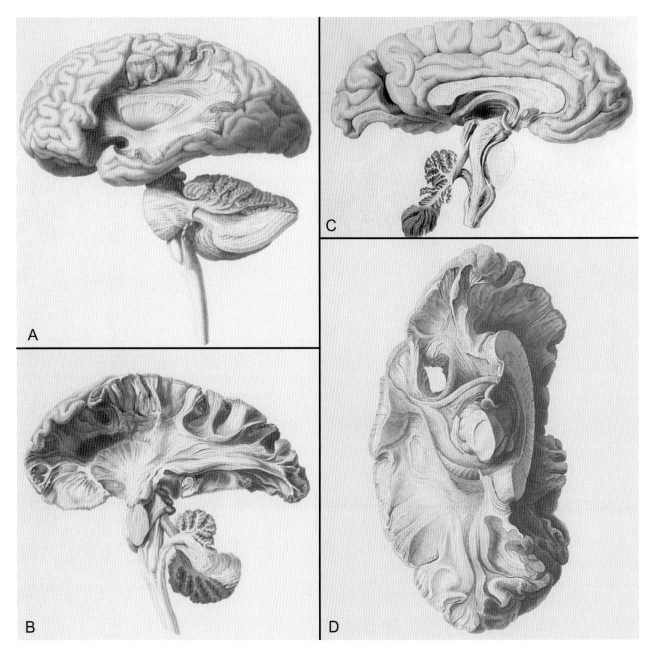

Figure 2-6
Depictions of white matter dissections of the cerebral hemisphere, cerebellum, and brainstem by Herbert Mayo (1827) in his *A Series of Engravings Intended to Illustrate the Structure of the Brain and Spinal Cord in Man*. A, plate III; B, plate IV; C, plate V; D, plate VI. The uncinate fasciculus and superior longitudinal fasciculus are seen in A, and the arcuate or U-fibers are shown in B and D. The medial hemisphere in C is dissected in D and shown from the ventral aspect.

tract and leading to the posterior part of the cerebral cortex, including the parietal and occipital lobes (figure 2-9). Gratiolet's observation that a fiber system of a sensory (visual) modality leading all the way to the cortex, and terminating in only a restricted part of the cortex, had far-reaching significance: it was the first confirmation of a special sensory tract above the level of the brainstem. Flourens, a figure of great stature and in-

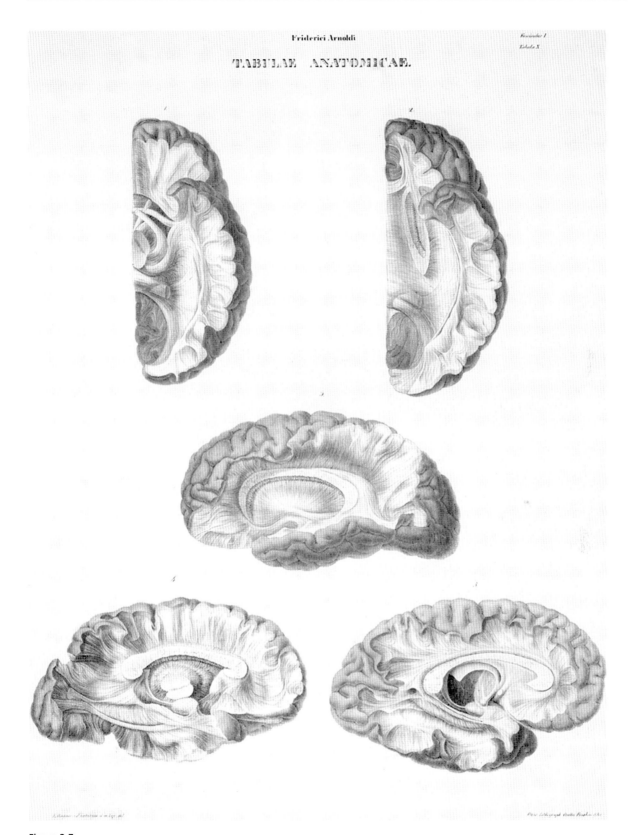

Figure 2-7

Images from the *Tabulae Anatomicae* of Friedrich Arnold (1838), Tafel X, in which his gross dissections of the white matter reveal the arcuate fibers that were named for him.

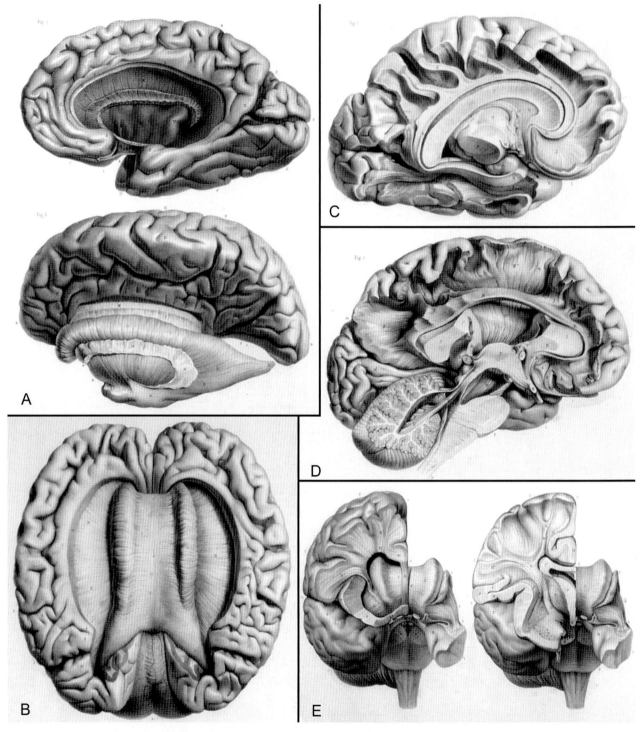

Figure 2-8

Selected illustrations from Achille-Louis Foville's (1844) *Traité complet de l'anatomie*. A, Plate 16 shows the gyral surface of the medial hemisphere and a schema of the ventricular system. B, Plate 15 depicts a dorsal view of the dissected corpus callosum linking the two hemispheres. C, Plate 14 shows Foville's notion of the transected corpus callosum and the cingulum bundle. D, Plate 18 shows corona radiata fibers, the cingulum bundle, and the superior cerebellar peduncle. E, Plate 19 is an anterior view of the dissected hemispheres showing the corpus callosum, corona radiata, and internal capsule.

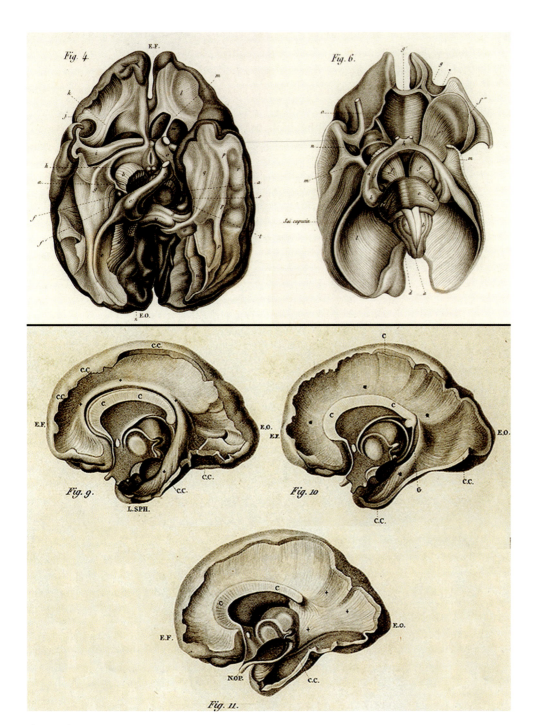

Figure 2-9

Gross dissections by Louis-Pierre Gratiolet (adapted from Leuret and Gratiolet, 1839, *Anatomir comparée du système nerveux*) depicting the fiber bundle that came to be known as the optic radiation. Fig. 4 and Fig. 6 (top) are monkey brain dissections, from Plate XXVII. Label "e" in Fig. 4 (adjacent to "d" and caudal to "c'") refers to the roots of the optic nerve. Label "l" in figure 6 refers to the radiation ("expansion") of the optic nerve into the right hemisphere. Fig. 9, Fig. 10, and Fig. 11 (bottom) are from Plate XXX, depicting the fetal human brain. *Fig.9 labels*: +, ring formed by the white matter fibers of the medial edge of the hemisphere ("l'ourlet"– literally, hem); CC, cerebral cortex; C, corpus callosum. *Fig. 10 labels* *, radiation of the corpus callosum into the hemisphere. *Fig 11 labels:* +, radiation of the optic nerve into the hemisphere.

fluence at the time, strongly opposed Gall's cortical localization theory and phrenology and believed in the functional omnivalence (equivalence) of the cerebrum and cerebellum. He did, however, propose that vision is localized in the cerebral cortex and argued against the notion that the cerebral cortex in some way presides over sensory functions without being able to see, hear, or feel. Gratiolet's observations provided support for Flourens' view that the cerebral hemisphere is indeed directly related to the sense organs, and therefore the brain could not be exclusively a substratum of so-called psychic function above the level of sensory experience. "(T)he cerebral cortex had to be recognized not as a kind of anatomical abstraction outside the so-called somatic sphere, but as the highest level of nervous system whose roots reach to the very confines of bodily organization" (Polyak, 1957, p. 137). However, in contrast to Flourens' omnivalence theory that the entire cerebral hemisphere was a uniformly organized substratum with homogeneous function, Gratiolet had determined that the visual pathways terminated in a distinct area of the cortex, and there were large parts of cortex outside the reach of these fibers.

Gross dissections of the fiber systems of the brain have continued sporadically into the present era. The results of some of these efforts, and the differing interpretations surrounding the published observations, are considered in more detail in chapters that deal with the individual bundles. In the early 20th century attempts were made to delineate association fiber systems using what were considered to be enhanced techniques of gross or blunt white matter bundle dissection (see, e.g., Hoeve, 1909; Jamieson, 1908–9; Johnston, 1908). Investigators at that time confirmed many of the findings of a century earlier, but they continued to debate the nomenclature and the possible origins and terminations of the tracts identified with these techniques. Thus, Trolard dissected the fiber systems around the claustrum (1905) and the inferior longitudinal and arcuate fasciculi (1906); Curran (1909) believed he had identified an inferior fronto-occipital fasciculus as well as the uncinate, arcuate, and transverse occipital fasciculi; Davis (1921) dissected the inferior longitudinal and uncinate fasciculi and the geniculocalcarine tract and Curran's (probably spurious) inferior fronto-occipital fasciculus; Ranson (1921) described subcortical fiber systems, including the temporothalamic fibers that bear the name Arnold's tract (the temporopulvinar bundle of Arnold, according to Ludwig and Klingler [1956] and Klingler and Gloor [1960], as opposed to the frontopontine system [Arnold's bundle]); and Rosett (1933) unsuccessfully attempted to clarify the nature of the subcallosal bundle. Klingler amended the technique of gross dissection by freezing the brain after fixation in formaldehyde. This facilitated his meticulous dissections of the white matter and made it possible to delineate fiber bundles with greater clarity (Ludwig and Klingler, 1956), albeit, so contemporary findings indicate, without necessarily resulting in greater anatomic accuracy. Gross dissections have also been performed more recently by Kertez and Geschwind (1971), Gluhbegovic and Williams (1980), Ross (1980), Heimer (1983, 1995), Ebeling and von Cramon (1992), and Türe with Yasargil et al. (1997, 2000). Wendell Krieg (1906–1997) provided schematic representations of the fiber systems in three-dimensional format in the rat (Krieg, 1947) and monkey (Krieg, 1954, 1975), as derived from myelin-stained material.

Controversy has surrounded this method from its earliest days in the 1500s.[7] The gross dissection method left many questions unanswered. The course and arrangement of the fiber bundles could not be determined, and it was not clear whether fibers terminated in the cortex, originated in it, or simply turned around and passed back again to the brainstem. Todd (1845) encapsulated the problem thus (pp. 133–137): "The problem which the anatomist has to solve is, Given certain columns or bundles of fibers in the medulla oblongata, to determine how they connect themselves with the other segments of the brain. (I)n the statements of all anatomists, who avail themselves of no other aid than that which the naked eye affords, there is much that must necessarily be uncertain or doubtful. (I)t will not suffice to display the direction of all the fibres, nor indeed is any mode of preparation adequate for that purpose. Nor is there any other mode of removing these uncertainties than by the successful application of extensive and patient microscopic analysis to the whole cerebral structure." Advances in the understanding of the cerebral white matter had to wait for the development of the compound achromatic microscope in the 1820s,[8] the new understanding in the 1840s that white matter fiber bundles were comprised of axons derived from nerve cells, and the progressive elaboration of fixation and staining techniques.

Todd's conclusion that gross fiber dissection had inherent limitations was echoed by Charles Edward Beevor (1854–1908) in 1891 (p. 135): "The method by dissection of the brain with the scalpel has been much employed, and though it is doubtless of value in tracing out the coarser strands, it is open to the objection that the parts are very much displaced by the operation necessary to follow out the fibres, and also that relations may be artificially produced which do not actually exist. Moreover it is quite impossible to trace the fibres to their ultimate ending, as this can only be accomplished by the use of the microscope." These concerns were supported by subsequent events. The study of white matter fiber systems by gross fiber dissection was marked by confusion and uncertainty, as described in detail in the relevant sections of our text. This development notwithstanding, some contemporary authors (e.g., Türe et al., 1997, 2000) have taken to resurrecting this approach.

The Neuron Theory

The early tractographers performed their gross dissection of cerebral white matter unaware that the neuron was an independent entity and that the fibers were composed of axons derived from nerve cells. The more detailed understanding of the cerebral white matter was therefore dependent upon the discovery of the neuron and the microscopic and staining techniques that would facilitate the finer analysis of the fiber bundles. A brief synopsis is relevant here, given the central importance of this concept to the technique used in the current investigation.

The existence of the nerve fiber was discovered before the nerve cell body. Using the crude microscope that he had invented, in 1674 Antoni van Leeuwenhoek (1632–1723) examined the optic nerve of a cow and saw filamentous particles. In a letter written in 1677, he provided the first account of the peripheral nerve fiber, reporting that the nervous system "consisted of diverse, very small threads or vessels lying by one another" (translated and quoted in Clarke and O'Malley, 1996, p. 32). The Galenic view was that spirituous substances were conveyed by hollow nerve passages, and Leeuwenhoek wondered whether the vessels that he had seen "might not be those that conveyed the animal spirits through the spinal marrow." Malpighi determined in 1681 that gray matter was made up of cellular follicles, white matter of fine excretory ducts. Giovanni Alfonso Borelli (1608–1679) challenged the concept of nerves as hollow tubes, believing instead that they "are channels filled with a certain spongy substance, like the pith of the elder tree. This spongy pith of the fibres is easily moistened by the spirituous juice of the brain, to which they are directly attached . . ." (*De motu animalium*, Rome, 1680–1681, 2 volumes, translated and quoted in Clarke and O'Malley, 1996, p. 164).

The nerve fiber was identified as the ultimate structure of peripheral nerve in 1781 by Felice Gaspar Ferdinand Fontana (1730–1805), who termed it the primitive nerve cylinder. Using the new achromatic compound microscope, Christian Gottfried Ehrenberg (1795–1876) demonstrated the existence of nerve fibers within the medullary substance of the cerebral white matter in 1833. Gabriel Gustave Valentin (1810–1883) documented the existence of the nerve cell in 1836 and identified the nerve cell body, including the nucleus, nucleolus, and parenchyma. He believed, however, that the nerve cell and the nerve fiber were not connected but merely juxtaposed. In 1838, for the first time, Robert Remak (1815–1865) described both myelinated and unmyelinated nerve fibers and suggested that the nerve fiber and nerve cell, which had previously been described separately by a number of observers, were in fact joined. Knowledge of the anatomy of nerve cells and fibers was further advanced by Jan Evangelista Purkyně (Purkinje) (1787–1869), who also identified the cerebellar cortical neuron that bears his name (Purkyně, 1837). Theodor Schwann (1810–1882) described the myelin sheath investing the axon and in 1839 enunciated the cell theory that "there is one common principle of development for the most diverse elementary parts of the organism, and this principle is the formation of cells."[9] Adolph Hannover (1814–1894) developed a fixation technique using chromic acid and illustrated its results describing myelinated fibers (Hannover, 1840). He observed axons lining the floor of the fourth ventricle, extending down into the spinal cord, and being as thick as peripheral nerve fibers, with a very similar appearance. He observed there were transverse fibers in the spinal cord of animals, running individually as well as in bundles, and he substantiated Remak's assertion by being the first to observe that fibers in the brain originate from brain cells and retain a lifelong, permanent connection with these central structures. The origin of myelinated fibers from nerve cells in the central nervous system as well as in peripheral ganglia was further established by Rudolf Albert von Koelliker (1817–1905), who also concluded that all nerve fibers are connected with nerve cells (von Koelliker, 1849), and by Otto Friedrich Karl Deiters (1834–1863), whose name is eponymously linked with the lateral vestibular nucleus. Augustus Volney Waller (1816–1870) sectioned the glossopharyngeal and hypoglossal nerves of frogs in 1850 and observed degeneration of the distal portions of these nerves. This observation led to the idea that the cell body is a nutritional and trophic center and that the nerve fiber is dependent upon it. It also formed the basis of later tract-tracing and connectivity studies using the principle of degeneration.

The evolution of the concept of the neuron and the improvements in the available microscopes prompted the development of better staining techniques to enhance the visualization of neural structures. Louis-Antoine Ranvier (1835–1922) used a new silver impregnation method to describe the node that bears his name in 1871. Franz Nissl (1860–1919) first described the constituents of the nerve cell body using basic aniline dyes (Nissl, 1892). Joseph von Gerlach (1820–1896) used the carmine stain to develop his nerve net theory in 1872 based on observations in the spider and started a controversy (nerve net vs. neuron theory) that continued until the turn of the 20th century. Camillo Golgi (1843–1926) published in 1883 a new staining technique that combined potassium bichromate and silver nitrate and that was considerably better than any previous technique; it permitted visualization of the nerve cell, its axon (nerve extension), and dendrites (protoplasmic extensions). He described neurons with long axons (Golgi type I cells) and those with short axons (Golgi type II cells.) His observations led him to a firm belief in the nerve net theory. Paul Ehrlich (1854–1915) developed the methylene blue stain that outlined the nerve cell and all its processes, including nerve endings and myelinated nerve fibers. The neuron doctrine was introduced by Wilhelm His (1831–1904) in 1887. Using the approach of developmental histology, he determined that "each nerve fiber originates as a process from a single cell. This is its genetic, nutritive and functional center; all other connections of the fiber are either indirect or secondary" (His, 1887, translated in Clarke and O'Malley, 1996, p. 102). Auguste-Henri Forel (1848–1931) used Golgi staining and the retrograde degeneration technique of Johann Bernhard Aloys von Gudden (1823–1886) to demonstrate that a nerve network does not exist. Forel also showed that each nerve cell is in contact with but not in continuity with its neighbor (the contact theory of Forel) and that nerve fibers originate only from nerve cells. Further, whereas a fiber will degenerate if the nerve cell is damaged, as Waller had shown, the nerve cell itself will degenerate if its axon is damaged.

Santiago Ramón y Cajal (1852–1934) provided independent histological confirmation in 1888 of the contiguity of nerve cell elements. Cajal's study of basket cells and Purkinje neurons in the cerebellar cortex, and then of neurons in the cerebral cortex, laid to rest the neural net theory of Golgi and established the neuron doctrine. (Heinrich Wilhelm Gottfried von Waldeyer-Hartz [1836–1921]) introduced the term "neuron" [Waldeyer, 1891], and the term "neuron doctrine" evolved thereafter.) In his Croonian lecture, Cajal (1894) summarized the understanding of the nerve cell and the fibers that make up the white matter systems. "In a synthetic manner one can say that the whole nerve center is the result of association of the four following paths: the nerve cells with short axis cylinders, that is, branching in the very thickness of the gray matter; the terminal nerve fibers which come from other centers or distant regions of the same center; nerve cells with a long axis cylinder, that is, extending as far as the white matter; the collaterals which originate either during the passage of axis cylinder extensions of the cells with long processes [axons] across the gray matter, or during the course of the tubes [*bundles*] of white matter." (Proc. R. Soc. 1894;55:444–468. Translated in Clarke and O'Malley, 1996, p. 123). The development of *in vitro* neuronal cell culture in 1907 by Ross Granville Harrison (1870–1959) initiated a new field of cytology and provided decisive confirmation of the neuron doctrine.

Rudolf Virchow (1821–1902) described and named the neuroglia (nerve glue) in 1856. The role of neuroglia in neural transmission and maintenance of neuronal integrity has been recognized in recent years. The glia are relevant to our study of the fiber pathways because their morphology, including the size, orientation, and cell packing density, serves as a guide to the orientation of the fiber bundles and for the comparison of the major fiber bundles between species.

Microscopic Study, Clinicopathologic Correlations

Along with further refinements in the optical physics of the microscope, laboratory techniques improved in the 1800s, permitting thin sections of brain to be made that could be stained for the analysis of normal and degenerated nerve fiber tracts. These new techniques revealed the relationship between the cortical neurons and the axons in the white matter and a previously unimagined level of detailed organization of the cerebral cortex, the subcortical nuclei, and the fiber systems that connect them. Fixation of the brain was a crucial step in the microscopic analysis. It was first hardened in alcohol (Reil, 1809a–d), then in chromic acid (Hannover, 1840) and chromic salts that were used for staining. Formaldehyde was not introduced until 1893 by Ferdinand Blum (1865–1957), and its utility was confirmed by Hermann (1894). The serial sectioning method that Benedict Stilling (1810–1879) introduced (Stilling, 1842) could be applied routinely to the hardened brain, and the use of the microtome (George Adams [1750–1795], 1798) and paraffin (Klebs, 1869) and celloidin embedding (Duval, 1879) facilitated evaluation of the microscopic features of the nerve cells and fibers that were made more visible with the new dyes and techniques. These included carmine (Corti, 1851; Gerlach, 1858; Goeppert and Cohn, 1849; Hartig, 1854; Osborne, 1857), aniline dyes (Perkin, 1861), hematoxylin (e.g., Gage, 1892–3), the "black reaction" of osmic acid that Camillo Golgi described in 1873 (Golgi, 1883) and that was extensively used by Ramón y Cajal in his investigations (1899–1904), and the special stains of Paul Ehrlich as discussed in his encyclopedia of 1903, Vittorio Marchi (1851–1908) in 1885, Franz Nissl in 1892, and Max Bielschowsky (1869–1940) in 1902. The myelin stain was developed by Carl Weigert (1845–1904) in 1882 (Weigert, 1884) and enhanced by Pal (Wethered, 1888).

Ludwig Türck (1810–1868) used Stilling's serial section technique to study degenerated pathways following brain lesions (Neuburger, 1910; Türck 1849, 1850, 1851). He described the anterior corticospinal tract that was named for him by Jean-Martin Charcot (1825–1893) in 1875 (Charcot, 1878). (The temporopontine tract was incorrectly named for Türck, an error that dates from Meynert, 1885. See Schmahmann et al., 1992.) Türck's discovery of this method of tract tracing through degeneration was essentially simultaneous with the well-known work of Waller in 1850. von Gudden further developed the degeneration method of tracing nerve fibers, producing secondary atrophy of nerve centers and their connections by removing sense organs such as the eye or cranial nerves. He defined the decussation of the visual pathway in the optic chiasm of the rabbit, showed that if a cerebral hemisphere is removed and the thalamus left intact, a decrease in the size of the thalamus results (von Gudden, 1870), and observed that degeneration of the proximal end of a divided nerve is directed toward the cell body (Gudden's law). The secondary degeneration technique was adapted by Gudden's student, Constantin von Monakow (1853–1930), to study corticothalamic and other subcortical connections (von Monakow, 1882a,b, 1885, 1895) and by Sir David Ferrier (1843–1928) and Gerald Francis Yeo (1845–1909) to study motor pathways in the internal capsule (Ferrier and Yeo, 1884; Schäfer, 1883); it remained the principal method of neuroanatomical tract-tracing studies for a century.

In a series of papers from 1867 to 1872, Theodore Hermann Meynert (1833–1892) applied the improved histological techniques to study the cerebral white matter systems in the bat (Meynert, 1872; see translated works in Stricker, 1872, and Meynert, 1885, and figure 30.1 A-D). He established with greater clarity the three principal types of white matter systems that had first been suggested in 1786 by Vicq D'Azyr (callosal and association systems) and in 1810 by Gall and Spurzheim (projection systems, and association [including callosal] systems). These systems described by Meynert were (1) the association systems including the short arcuate fibers (the fibrae arcuateae of Arnold, 1838a,b, that Gall and Spurzheim, 1810, had previously identified, or the U-shaped fibers of Meynert) and the long association fibers by means of which various parts of the cerebral cortex are interconnected and communicate with each other; (2) the commissural pathways linking the two hemispheres; and (3) the afferent and efferent projection systems between the cerebral cortex and subcortical structures that facilitate somatotopic representation in the cortex. Meynert also identified the afferent systems entering the cerebral hemispheres from the cerebellum. (These influential ideas and illustrations of Meynert, including the prevailing misconception that the basal ganglia contribute to the cerebral peduncle, are incorporated in his 1872 writings and diagrams, reproduced in the Notes.[10])

Paul Emil Flechsig (1847–1929) used the carmine stain and Weigert's myelin stain to study the evolving patterns of myelination through development in a body of work extending over five decades (from 1872 to 1927). Flechsig's efforts laid the foundation for a number of fundamental concepts of brain organization. He provided a comprehensive and enduring understanding of myelinogenesis in the human brain. He determined that different tracts develop myelin sheaths at different periods of prenatal and postnatal life and that fibers belonging to the same system mature at approximately the same time, whereas those of anatomically and functionally different tracts do so at different periods. He introduced the "fundamental law of myelinogenesis" that the sequence of myelination during individual development repeats their phylogenetic appearance. This was an extension of the "biogenetic law" of Ernst Haeckel (1834–1919) that "ontogeny recapitulates phylogeny" (Haeckel, 1879, 1902).[11] Based on his study of myelination patterns of cerebral white matter, Flechsig described projection[12] and association fibers, developed the concept of cerebral "association areas," and expanded the notion of sensory versus association cortex.[13] He described the course of the pyramidal tracts from the cerebrum through the internal capsule to the spinal cord and showed that the basal ganglia do not contribute anatomically to the pyramidal tract. He demonstrated the auditory radiations and the loop of the visual radiations in the temporal lobe that later came to bear the name of Meyer.

Flechsig believed that the great fiber tracts that myelinate by the end of intrauterine existence and the first few weeks of extrauterine life together constitute Meynert's projection system and make up Reil's corona radiata. He concluded that the association areas are essentially devoid of projection systems, having no or very few direct connections with peripheral receptor organs. Rather, the sensory afferents are conveyed to the association cortices by means of the short "association fibers of Meynert" and by callosal fibers. Further, "lesions involving the sense centers are followed by a train of symptoms of an entirely different character from those which accompany lesions of the association centers" (Barker, 1899, p. 1074). According to Barker (1899, pp. 1081–1082), Flechsig's ideas met with some opposition. Monakow was among "a number of leading neurologists and psychiatrists . . . unwilling to grant that the areas of the cortex to which projection fibers are distributed are as limited as Flechsig would have us believe. Thus, von Monakow asserts that projection fibers go to nearly all parts of the cortex, though certainly some parts of it receive fewer by far than others. Von Monakow bases his objection upon the results of his studies of secondary degenerations. He believes . . . that the sense areas occupy much more extensive fields of the cerebral surface than those indicated by Flechsig in his diagrams. . . . Flechsig responded to these comments by pointing out 'that lesions of the parietal cortex have been followed in a number of instances by degenerations of projection fibers, but in all such instances he believes the cortical nodule had affected bundles of projection fibers belonging to other parts of the cortex, but situated beneath the area diseased. The results of experimental degenerations in animals following extirpation of cortical zones can not properly be directly applied to human beings, for in man there is a development of the association centers not reached in the brain of any other animal.'"

The work of Flechsig had a profound influence on myelination studies later conducted by Paul Ivan Yakovlev (1894–1983), and Flechsig's thinking about the association areas played an important role in Norman Geschwind's reinvigoration and expansion of the ideas about higher-order brain function and disconnection syndromes.

In 1892 and 1893, Heinrich Sachs used histological and degeneration studies to accurately define the sagittal stratum that includes, in part, the optic radiation, and he divided it into external and internal segments. He also identified transverse fibers within the occipital lobe that came to bear his name. Wladimir Muratoff (1893a,b; Muratow, 1893) identified a longitudinally oriented subcallosal fasciculus in dogs. In cases of agenesis of the corpus callosum, Onufrowicz (1887) along with his mentor Forel (1881, 1907) became convinced of a fronto-occipital fiber bundle in their erroneous interpretation of what Sachs (1892) and Moriz Probst (1901a) subsequently identified as misdirected callosal fibers.

Apart from his important contributions in the field of aphasiology and cortical localization, Carl Wernicke (1848–1900) published an atlas of myelin-stained serial sections of the human brain in the coronal (1897), axial (1900), and sagittal planes (1903). Projection systems were darkly stained, whereas long association fibers had poor myelin staining properties, with the exception of the cingulum bundle and the uncinate fasciculus, which were prominent. He identified a fasciculus of the caudate nucleus, the superior longitudinal fasciculus lateral to and more lightly staining than the corona radiata, the uncinate fasciculus, the cingulum bundle including a ventral component, and an inferior longitudinal fasciculus that is anatomically identical to the external aspect of the sagittal stratum. He identified a vertical fiber tract intrinsic to the occipital lobe, later named for him, and a "corona radiata temporalis" in the temporal stem, that was also named Wernicke's bundle. Wernicke used this anatomic knowledge to further understand and explain clinical disorders of higher function.

Joseph Jules Dejerine (1849–1917), like Wernicke, contributed significantly to the field of clinical neurology by describing a number of clinical syndromes. In 1895 he published his enduring anatomical work, *Anatomie de systeme nerveux*, in which he described the association fiber pathways in detail (figures 2-10 and 2-11) and included scholarly accounts of the historical development of notions concerning the fiber systems. He used myelin-stained normal human material and the Marchi technique to study degeneration in clinicopathological cases to understand which areas of cortex these pathways connect. Dejerine's concepts of the white matter systems have been the preeminent authority on this topic for over a century. A brief summary will not suffice; rather, his conclusions are discussed in detail in the sections of our monograph that deal with each of the individual fiber bundles. His historical accounts and descriptions attempted to resolve the discrepancies regarding the various pathways, and we take our cue from Dejerine in the present work, using contemporary tract-tracing methodology (autoradiography) to try to settle unresolved issues regarding the fiber systems in the monkey brain. Dejerine's student Vialet (1893) also used myelin-stained material to define the transverse fiber systems intrinsic to the occipital lobe, one of which bears his name (the ventral occipital transverse fascicle).

Dejerine matched his anatomical investigations with clinical observations in patients, and his description (Dejerine, 1892) of alexia without agraphia resulting from a lesion of the left occipital lobe together with a lesion of the splenium of the corpus callosum is the first account of a disconnection syndrome. Clinical neurology was emerging as a discipline at this time, and many of the seminal observations and interpretations of Charcot and his students in the latter part of the 19th century dealt explicitly with the clinical consequences of white matter lesions as manifested, for example, in multiple sclerosis.

A greater appreciation of the complexity of the white matter fiber pathways had thus become apparent, and their crucial importance was recognized in linking cortical areas with each other and with subcortical sites, peripheral sensory receptors, and motor effector organs. Santiago Ramón y Cajal in 1933 discussed the understanding at that time[14] and recognized the challenges posed by the lack of adequate information concerning the detailed connections of these areas: "In summary, at this very moment the little we know about the kinds of neuro-neuronal connections in the cerebral cortex agrees in principle with the arrangement of the connections made in other parts of the brain. The elucidation of the manner of connection between the innumerable endogenous, exogenous, collateral, and terminal branches originating in thalamic, callosal, and association fibers in every way constitutes at present an overwhelming problem. It will put to the test the sagacity and patience of many generations of future neurologists" (Cajal, 1933). The era of connectional neuroanatomy would begin to address these deficiencies and further elucidate the role of the fiber systems.

Cortical Cytoarchitecture and Connectional Neuroanatomy

The fibers in the cerebral white matter link different cortical and subcortical areas, and so an appreciation of the organization of cerebral cortex with respect to its architecture and connections is relevant. Cortical architectonics and connectional neuroanatomy are both vast disciplines that cannot be summarized here, but it is useful to consider some major milestones in the development of these disciplines, particularly as they relate to a comprehensive understanding of the white matter tracts.

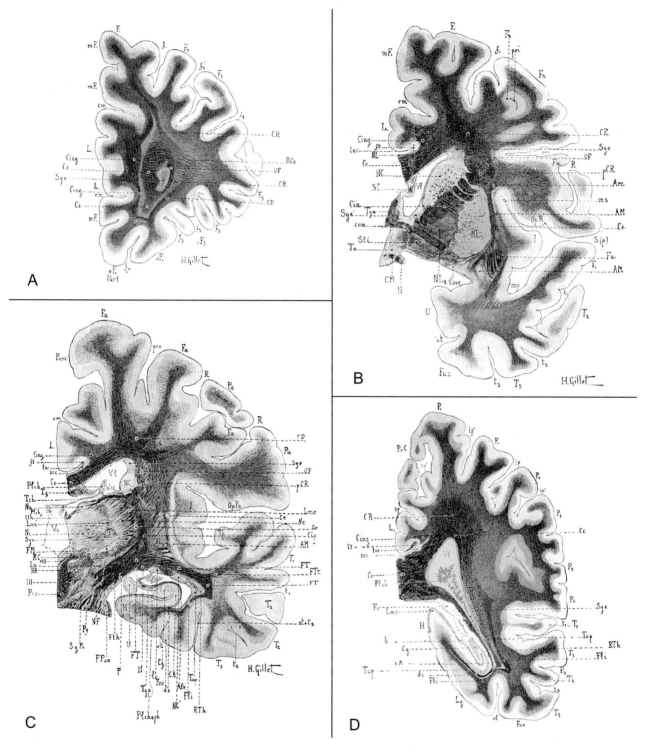

Figure 2-10

Images from Joseph Jules Dejerine's (1895) *Anatomie des centres nerveux* showing coronal sections of human brain stained for myelin. A, Prefrontal region in figure 390, page 785. B, Section through the anterior commissure and rostral temporal lobe in figure 382, page 764. C, Section through the frontoparietal region and thalamus in figure 387, page 774. D, Section through the parieto-occipital region, splenium of the corpus callosum, and the sagittal stratum, figure 383, page 767.

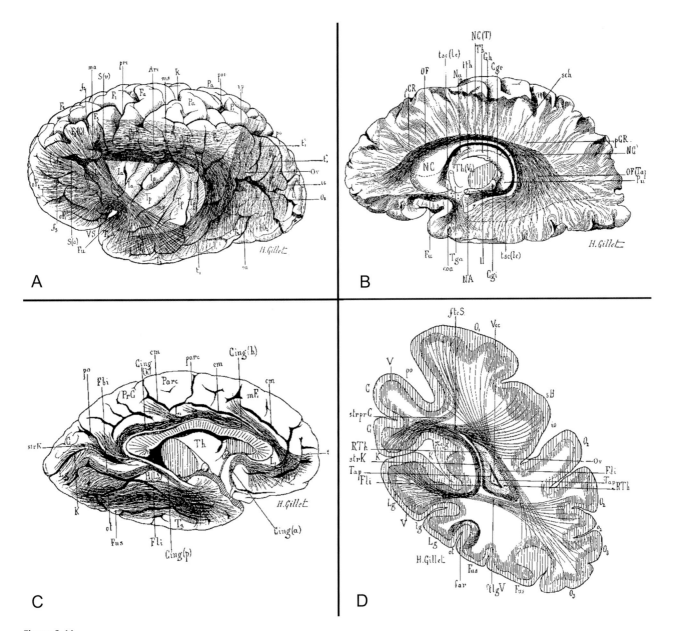

Figure 2-11

Diagrams from Dejerine's (1895) *Anatomie des centres nerveux* summarizing some of the major pathways of the human brain discussed in his work. A, Dejerine's notion of the arcuate and uncinate fasciculi and the vertical occipital fibers in figure 377, page 757. B, The uncinate fasciculus, fronto-occipital fasciculus, and corona radiata are shown in figure 381, page 762. C, The cingulum bundle and inferior longitudinal fasciculus are shown in figure 374, page 752. D, This schematic coronal section depicts the intrinsic fibers of the occipital lobe, including the occipitovertical fascicle, or perpendicular occipital fascicle of Wernicke (Ov), the occipital transverse fascicle of the cuneus of Sachs (ftcS), the occipital transverse fascicle of the lingual lobule of Vialet (ftlgV), the stratum proprium of the cuneus (strprC), and the stratum calcarinum (strK) or U-fiber layer of the calcarine fissure, in figure 389, page 783.

The origins of cortical architectonics were embedded in the notion that the cerebral cortex was functionally heterogeneous, as suggested by Gall and Spurzheim, and anatomically differentiated since the identification by Gennari, Vicq d'Azyr (and Samuel Thomas von Soemmering [1755–1830]; Clarke and O'Malley, 1996, p. 423) of an anatomic difference between the visual area and the remainder of the cerebral cortex. The presence of myelinated fibers within the cerebral cortex was noted in 1840 by Jules-Gabriel-François Baillarger (1815–1890),[15] who mounted thin sections on glass, examined them against the light, and saw lamination in the cerebral cortex for the first time.[16]

The attempts to establish a scientific basis for the system of cortical architecture began with the definitive work using aniline dyes in the monkey by Korbinian Brodmann (1868–1918) in 1905, by Alfred Walter Campbell (1905), Cécile Vogt (1875–1962), and Oskar Vogt (1870–1959) in 1919, and by A. Earl Walker (1938) and Gerhardt von Bonin and Percival Bailey (1947). Architectonic studies in humans were performed by Brodmann in 1909, Constantin von Economo (1876–1931) and Georg N. Koskinas (1925), and Semen Aleksandrovich Sarkisov (1955). These investigators focused on architecture as a specific and defining hallmark of cerebral cortex. Myeloarchitectonic studies of the cortex based on the differential arrangement of the bands of Baillarger were also performed by several investigators (e.g., Hopf, 1954; Vogt and Vogt, 1919). These studies notwithstanding, although architectonic analysis was well accepted for differentiation of subcortical structures in the brainstem, vigorous objections were raised against the architectonic approach being applied to the cerebral cortex during the 1940s and 1950s. These analyses were criticized as being subjective and unreliable, the architectonic differentiation of cortex was considered an isolated anatomic feature of limited value, and the potential significance of this field of inquiry was minimized (e.g., Karl Spencer Lashley [1890–1958]). This type of criticism almost resulted in the premature death of cytoarchitectonics as a discipline. After a lull in the awareness of the relevance of cortical architecture, there was resurgence in the latter part of the 20th century of the appreciation of the importance of this approach (e.g., the work of Friedrich Sanides [1914–1984], Galaburda and Sanides, 1980; Pandya and Sanides, 1973; and Sanides, 1968, 1972; as well as Barbas and Pandya, 1987, 1989; Braak, 1978; Galabura and Pandya, 1983; Hackett et al, 2001; Pandya and Yeterian, 1990; Preuss and Goldman-Rakic, 1991a,b; Rajkowska and Goldman-Rakic, 1995a,b; Seltzer and Pandya, 1978, 1989b; Weller and Kaas, 1987). The relevance of architectonic analysis of the cerebral cortex has subsequently become established in all fields of investigation of the organization and function of the nervous system. In recent years the use of immunocytochemistry and histochemical methods has allowed investigators to further identify subtleties of cortical and subcortical architecture and connections (Huntley and Jones, 1991; Jones, 2003; Morel et al., 1993), and observer-independent methodology has lent further credibility to these approaches (Schleicher et al., 1999). Indeed, cytoarchitectonic analysis is increasingly relevant in the study of structure–function correlations in the human brain when combined with functional imaging data. To this end, Zilles et al. (see Amunts and Zilles, 2001) have suggested that cytoarchitectonic mapping in the human may be based on a definition of areal borders using multivariate statistical analysis, quantitative analysis of similarity and dissimilarity in architecture between cortical areas, and probabilistic mapping of cytoarchitectonic areas in three-dimensional reference space.

Improvements in techniques made it possible to study neural connections in experimental animals with greater precision. This resulted in a vast literature detailing cortical connections in nonhuman primates and other animal models. In the latter part of the 19th and earlier parts of the 20th century, the Marchi method (Marchi and Algeri, 1885) was the principal method used to study neuronal connectivity (e.g., Mettler, Minkowski, Sunderland, Krieg, Crosby, Shower, Hearst, Milch, LeGros Clarke, and Yakovlev). The silver impregnation method of Max Bielschowsky introduced in 1902 represented an improvement upon a similar technique of Cajal. Both the Marchi and Bielschowsky methods were difficult and capricious. The Marchi method was dependent upon degenerating myelin product, and therefore nerve terminals could not be visualized. The Bielschowsky stain did not allow full impregnation of all degenerating fibers. These technical considerations limited the utility of both these methods. The silver impregnation technique introduced by Glees (Glees, 1946; Marsland et al., 1954) was used, for example, by Adey and Meyer (1952), but this method also had limited application because of the difficulty of differentiating intact versus degenerating nerve terminals.

The double silver impregnation technique developed by Walle J.H. Nauta (1916–1994; Nauta and Gygax, 1951, 1954) represented a considerable advance. Unlike the Marchi and Bielschowsky methods, the Nauta-Gygax stain suppressed the distal part of the normal nerve fibers and more readily demonstrated the degenerated nerve fibers. The late 1950s and early 1960s witnessed refinements in this silver impregnation method. The improvements in methodology led to an expansion in the number of anatomical studies being performed; of particular interest here are the corticocortical studies of association areas (e.g., Jones and Powell, 1970; Kuypers et al., 1965; Myers, 1962; Pandya and Kuypers, 1969). This accelerated investigation into cortical connectivity. By the middle and latter part of the 1960s, further improvements in the silver impregnation technique (e.g., Fink-Heimer, 1967; see Heimer, 2003) allowed the visualization of the finer endings of the nerve terminals at the level of the bouton. Several modifications of these methods were used for connectivity studies. These techniques all required the induction of a lesion that would result in focal pathology at a distant site after an appropriate time interval, which could be demonstrated by the silver impregnation. The idiosyncrasies inherent in these methods limited enthusiasm for performing these studies and for the results obtained. Whereas these methods demonstrated the cortical and subcortical areas that were anatomically linked, they could not reliably and consistently demonstrate the fiber pathways that subserve these connections.

The method of strychnine neuronography facilitated the physiological study of cortical connections and was first applied to the study of the sensory cortex in cat and monkey (Dusser de Barenne, 1916, 1924a,b). This approach was further used to examine the visual (McCulloch, 1944), auditory (Bailey et al., 1943a; Petr et al., 1949; Sugar et al., 1948), and somatosensory domains (French, 1948; Sugar et al., 1950), as well as the frontal lobe and limbic system (Pribram et al, 1950; Pribram and MacLean, 1953). In addition, Bailey et al. (1943b) defined physiological connections between remote regions of the cerebral hemispheres in monkey and chimpanzee that suggested they were linked by long association fiber bundles similar to those identified in the human. These studies indicated that area 18 in the dorsal parastriate cortex projected to prefrontal cortex area 8; the inferior temporal region area 20 projected to the parastriate cortex area 18; and area 38 in the rostral inferotemporal region projected to area 47 in the orbitofrontal cortex. The authors concluded that they had identified the origins and terminations of homologues of long association bundles previously recognized in the human, namely the superior longitudinal fasciculus, the inferior longitudinal fasciculus and vertical occipital fascicle of Wernicke, and the uncinate fasciculus, respectively. Thus the strychnine neuronography method enhanced the understanding of the origins and terminations of cortical connections, but its widespread used was hampered by multiple limitations.

A major technological advance in the field of connectional neuroanatomy occurred in the early 1970s. Whereas previous anterograde tract-tracing methods relied upon the ablation–degeneration and subsequent silver impregnation technique, the autoradiographic method developed by Cowan et al. (1972) represented a novel physiological approach to the tracing of neuronal connections. Moreover, in addition to the visualization of the nerve endings, the radioisotope technique also displayed the course of the axons leading from the injection site to their distant terminations. Freed from the unpredictability of the silver degeneration technique, the isotope methodology readily gained acceptance and became widely used as a method to study anterograde connections. Using this approach, a number of studies in the monkey have outlined corticocortical connections (e.g., Amaral et al., 1983; Amaral and Price, 1984; Baleydier and Mauguiere, 1980; Galaburda and Pandya, 1983; Gattas et al, 1997; Jones et al., 1978; Porrino et al., 1981; Preuss and Goldman-Rakic, 1989; Rockland and Pandya, 1979; Seltzer and Pandya, 1978, 1989a; Tranel et al., 1988; Ungerleider et al., 1989; Van Essen et al., 1986; Weller and Kaas, 1983), as well as subcortical connections (e.g., Asanuma et al., 1983; Giguere and Goldman-Rakic, 1988; Jones and Burton, 1976; Schmahmann and Pandya, 1989, 1991, 1993, 1995, 1997a,b; Schmahmann et al., 2004b; Siwek and Pandya, 1991; Tusa and Ungerleider, 1988; Yeterian and Pandya, 1985; Yeterian and Van Hoesen, 1978). Some of these studies have also delineated hemispheric fiber systems (e.g., Mufson and Pandya, 1984; Petrides and Pandya, 1984, 1988, 2002a; Schmahmann and Pandya, 1992, 1994; Ungerleider et al., 1989), but it has been less widely appreciated that this technique is ideally suited for the study of the origins, trajectories, and terminations of the long association pathways in the experimental animal.

The use of retrograde degeneration as a scientific method for studying connections has been known since the 1800s (e.g., Gudden, Monakow, Nissl). This approach suffered the same limitations as the earlier anterograde degeneration techniques. By the early 1970s, physiological retrograde tract tracing became possible with the use of injected horseradish peroxidase (HRP), which results in labeling of neurons in the cortical and subcortical areas that project to the site of the injection (LaVail and LaVail, 1972). Neurons with HRP that had been transported from the injection site in a retrograde manner were rendered visible by the brown reaction product using diaminobenzidine and were enhanced by the blue reaction product using benzidine dihydrochloride (Mesulam, 1976, 1978) and by conjugating HRP with wheat germ agglutinin (Harper et al., 1980). As effective as this method was for determining neurons of origin that project to the injection site, it did not in general provide a satisfactory visualization of fiber tracts.

Similarly, fluorescent retrograde tracers (Keizer et al., 1983; Kuypers et al., 1980) that were easy to use and allowed one to study projections to multiple areas simultaneously in the same animal, and trans-synaptic viral tract tracing techniques (e.g., Ugolini et al., 1987; Middleton and Strick, 1994) that enhanced the ability to analyze connections did not provide adequate visualization of the fiber pathways. Within the past several years, other anterograde tracers and mapping techniques have been introduced, including *Phaseolus vulgaris* leukoagglutinin (PHAL; Gerfen and Sawchenko, 1984; Tourtellotte and Van Hoesen, 1992) and biotinylated dextrans (Veenman et al., 1992). Whereas these approaches demonstrate individual axons with great precision, they are not suitable for tract tracing of fiber systems on a larger scale.

A limitation of the autoradiographic technique is that it can be used only in the experimental animal. Magnetic resonance imaging (MRI) in humans can provide exquisite detail of cerebral anatomy *in vivo*, and the further development of MRI techniques promises to reveal anatomic details at a very high level of resolution. As discussed in chapter 1, diffusion tensor imaging, MR tractography, and diffusion spectrum tractography can visualize white matter pathways *in vivo*, but they do not demonstrate the origins or terminations of the pathways. Further, they rely heavily on *a priori* knowledge of the anatomy of these fiber systems based upon the Talairach atlas (Talairach and Tournoux, 1988) and the understanding of the white matter tracts derived from Dejerine's (1895) epic work. Without a clear and accurate notion of where the fiber tracts are expected to lie in the human as determined by experimental work in the monkey, however, spurious results may be produced and misconceptions regarding these white matter bundles are likely to be created or perpetuated. Cognitive and psychiatric manifestations, as well as motor manifestations, following white matter lesions in patients are being identified with increasing sophistication (see Filley, 2001). We hope that these clinical observations and the evolving *in vivo* white matter tractography, together with the understanding of the fiber pathways that our monograph presents, will facilitate insights into the cerebral white matter in humans.

Approach to the Study
of the Fiber Tracts

PART

Materials Analyzed

The preceding chapter dealt with the attempts by many pioneering investigators to delineate the fiber pathways of the cerebral hemisphere using the techniques available to them, notably gross dissection and lesion-degeneration studies. The current resurgence of interest in the white matter fiber pathways in the normal and diseased states is matched by increasingly accurate methods for the exploration of these tracts, including neuroimaging methods in the human brain, and anterograde tracing techniques in the experimental animal. In this chapter we outline the different methods that we used to study the association, commissural, and projection fiber pathways in the rhesus monkey brain.

Autoradiography

Material was available to us from the brains of 36 adult rhesus monkeys that were used in previous studies. These brains were prepared with the anterograde tract-tracer technique using radiolabeled isotopes.[1] The intensity of the autoradiographic label has remained robust, as the photomicrographs demonstrate. The case numbers and locations of the isotope injections in the brains we have studied are listed in table 3-1 and shown in the diagrams in figure 3-1. The distribution of the isotope-labeled fibers and terminations was charted onto corresponding coronal sections of a standard brain.

Nissl-Stained Template Brain

The brain of a healthy adult rhesus monkey was used to represent the findings in all cases. This brain was embedded in celloidin and prepared with the Nissl stain (cresyl violet).[2]

Cytoarchitecture of Rhesus Brains

Cerebral Cortical Architecture

Cortical architectonic areas were identified on the Nissl-stained sections of the celloidin-embedded template brain. The architectonic features were also verified in each of the experimental cases. The cerebral cortical nomenclature systems used in this work are derived from the maps of Brodmann (1908, 1909) and Bonin and Bailey (1947) and from the following investigators, atlases, and published papers. For visual areas we have followed Gattass and Gross (1981), Ungerleider and Desimone (1986), Colby et al. (1988), Krubitzer and Kaas (1990), and Felleman and Van Essen (1991). For

Table 3-1

Case Numbers by Lobe and Architectonic Area

Parietal Lobe

1. Superior parietal lobule: area PGm, encroaching upon area PEc
2. Superior parietal lobule: medial part of area PEc at the junction of area PE
3. Superior parietal lobule: lateral part of area PEc at the junction of area PE
4. Inferior parietal lobule: caudal part of area PG and in area Opt
5. Inferior parietal lobule: rostral inferior parietal lobule, area PF
6. Inferior parietal lobule: middle part of the parietal operculum

Superior Temporal Region

7. Caudal part of the superior temporal gyrus involving area Tpt
8. Caudal part of the superior temporal gyrus in areas paAlt and Tpt
9. Midportion of area TPO, ventral superior temporal gyrus area TAa, caudal area KA
10. Rostral part of area TS3
11. Areas Pro, TS1 encroaching on TS2

Inferior Temporal Region

12. Ventral part of the temporal lobe, area TE2 and TE3
13. Ventral temporal region, area TF
14. Rostral superior temporal sulcus involving area IPa, lateral border of hippocampus
15. Medial part of the inferior temporal gyrus in area TE1 and TE2
16. Rostral temporal lobe in the midportion of area TE2

Occipital Lobe

17. Medial preoccipital gyrus, medial area 19 (area PO), and area PGm
18. Dorsal preoccipital gyrus, area DP, and upper part of area V4D
19. Dorsal area V4 and adjacent area V4T
20. Ventral preoccipital gyrus above inferior occipital sulcus, in area V4
21. Ventral area V4, with some encroachment in ventral area V3

Cingulate Gyrus

22. Retrosplenial cortex in area 30 and in area 23
23. Rostral cingulate gyrus in area 24

Motor Cortex

24. Frontal operculum in the precentral aspects of areas 1 and 2
25. Ventral area 4, face representation
26. Area 4 behind the arcuate spur, in hand representation
27. Dorsal precentral gyrus area 4, trunk representation
28. Dorsal area 4, foot representation
29. Medial part of the superior frontal gyrus, rostral area MII, face representation

Prefrontal Region

30. Medial surface of the prefrontal cortex involving mainly area 32
31. Above the midportion of the principal sulcus in area 46d
32. Middle part of ventral area 46 in both the sulcal and gyral cortices
33. Orbital frontal cortex in the orbital part of area 47/12

Premotor Region (cases used in chapter 22 only)

34. Area ProM in the frontal operculum
35. Ventral premotor area 6v
36. Dorsal premotor area 6d

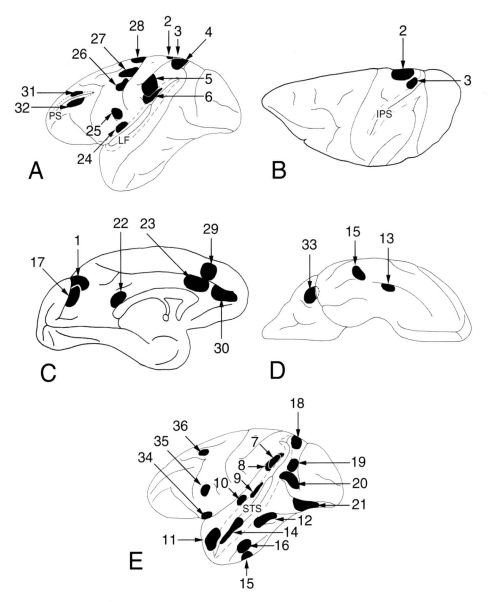

Figure 3-1

Summary diagrams of the cerebral hemisphere of a rhesus monkey showing the locations of the isotope injections in the experimental cases studied. A, Lateral view of the cerebral hemisphere with the principal sulcus (PS) and the Sylvian (lateral) fissure (LF) opened to show the buried cortex. Injections are in the parietal, precentral motor, and prefrontal regions. B, Dorsal view showing the injection sites in the superior parietal lobule. The intraparietal sulcus (IPS) is opened to expose the hidden cortex. C, Medial view of the hemisphere with injections in the medial parietal, medial preoccipital, medial prefrontal, and cingulate cortices. D, Basal surface of the hemisphere, with injections in the ventral temporal and orbitofrontal regions. E, Lateral view of the hemisphere with the superior temporal sulcus (STS) opened to reveal the cortex in its banks, and injections in the superior and inferior temporal regions, parastriate cortices, and premotor region. The numbers correspond to the cases in this series. Cases 1 through 33 were examined in detail throughout the monograph; cases 34 through 36 were used to determine the location of commissural fibers within the corpus callosum, as discussed in chapter 22.

parietal lobe we have followed Pandya and Seltzer (1982) and Seltzer and Pandya (1980), for the superior temporal regions Seltzer and Pandya (1978, 1989b) and Galaburda and Pandya (1983), for the superior temporal sulcus and inferotemporal area Seltzer and Pandya (1978), for the parahippocampal gyrus Rosene and Pandya (1983) and Blatt et al. (2003), for the prefrontal cortex Petrides and Pandya (1994), and for the cingulate gyrus Vogt et al. (1987). *The Rhesus Monkey Brain in Stereotaxic Coordinates* (Paxinos et al., 1999) was also used to assist with the identification of architectonic regions and for comparison with contemporary architectonic nomenclatures.

Subcortical Nuclei and Nuclear Divisions

Standard nomenclature systems are used to designate the major subcortical gray matter structures. Nomenclature used in the text to describe the thalamic nuclear subdivisions is derived from Olszewski (1952), but we also consulted the nomenclatures of Jones (1985) and Ilinsky and Kultas-Ilinsky (1987). Thalamic nuclear subdivisions are not identified in the photomicrographs and diagrams, but the descriptions of the thalamic terminations are included in the text and correspond to published anterograde studies of corticothalamic terminations (e.g., Asanuma et al., 1985; Beck and Kaas, 1998; Fitz-Patrick and Imig, 1978; Graham et al., 1979; Künzle and Akert, 1977; Pandya et al., 1994; Selemon and Goldman-Rakic, 1988; Yeterian and Pandya, 1985, 1988, 1997). Pontine nuclear subdivisions are according to Sunderland (1940a), Nyby and Jansen (1951), and Schmahmann and Pandya (1989).

Many of the cortical areas studied in this work have projections to the nuclei of the basis pontis. These are presented briefly along with the report of the trajectories of the subcortical fiber bundles in the individual case descriptions. A number of investigators have studied these corticopontine pathways, and reference to their work, as well as detailed analyses of the projection patterns in the cases analyzed in the present material, may be found in the previously published reports of Schmahmann and Pandya: posterior parietal cortices (1989), superior temporal region (1991), inferior temporal region (1991, 1993), parastriate and parahippocampal areas (1993), prefrontal cortices (1995, 1997a), and precentral motor and supplementary motor areas (Schmahmann et al., 2004b).

White Matter Architecture

The arrangement of the fibers in the white matter has traditionally been studied using stains that specifically identify myelin. We have used a novel approach, however, that relies on Nissl-stained sections to locate and identify the fiber pathways of the cerebral hemispheres. We studied the Nissl-stained template brain under 40× magnification and evaluated the orientation of the axons within the fiber bundles, including their direction and their position relative to cortical and subcortical landmarks. In addition, the orientation, packing density, and patterns of arrangement of the glia within the white matter were useful for distinguishing the fiber systems. The differential arrangement of fibers using this technique is readily apparent, and the outline of the different fiber pathways is clearer than that seen with conventional myelin stains that mask the fine discriminative detail (figures 3-2 and 3-3). Using this technique we identified major fiber structures, namely the corpus callosum, sagittal stratum, and internal capsule. In addi-

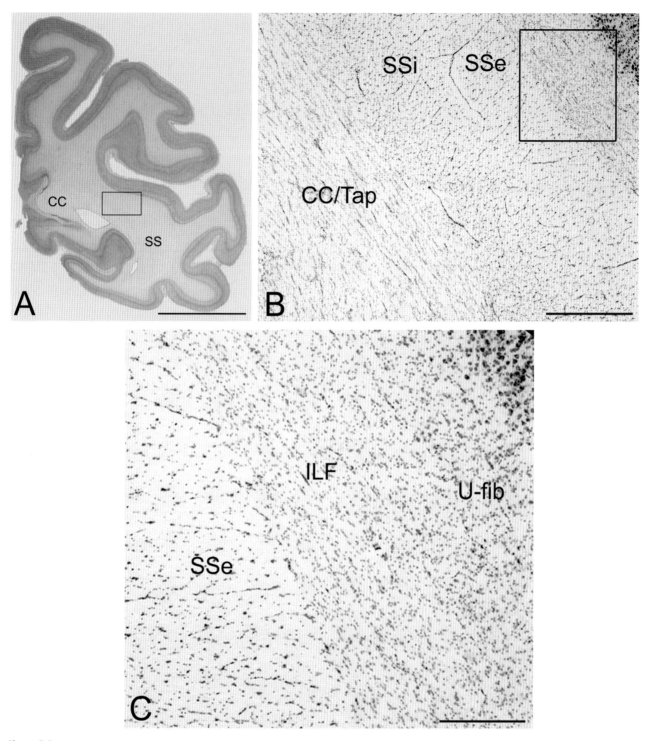

Figure 3-2

Light-field photomicrographs prepared with a Nissl stain. A is a coronal section through the parietal lobe (Mag = 0.5×, bar = 0.5 cm). B is a high power photomicrograph of the rectangular area outlined in A showing the differential distribution of glia in the tapetum of the corpus callosum (CC/Tap), the internal segment of the sagittal stratum (SSi), and the external segment of the sagittal stratum (SSe) (Mag = 2×, bar = 1 mm). C is a higher power magnification of the area outlined in B showing the differential arrangement of the glia in the SSe, the inferior longitudinal fasciculus (ILF) and the local U-fibers (U-fib) (Mag = 4×, bar = 0.5 mm).

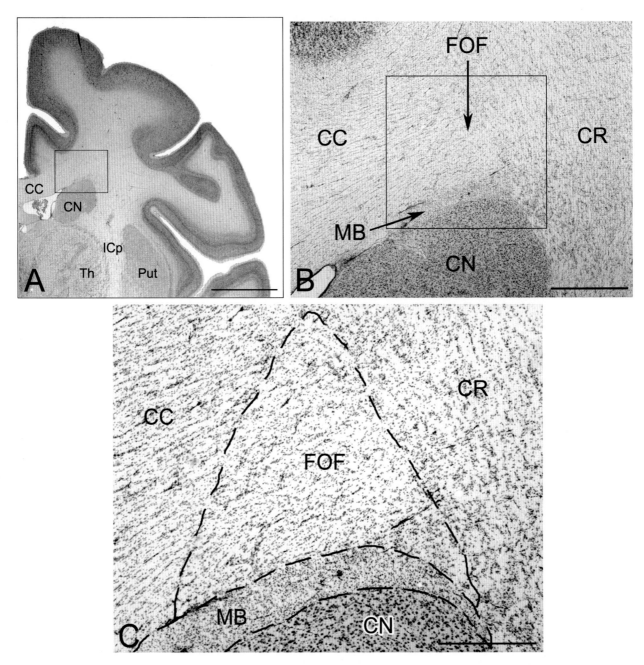

Figure 3-3

Light-field photomicrographs prepared with a Nissl stain. A is a partial view of a coronal section at the fronto-parietal junction (Mag = 0.5×, bar = 1 cm). CC, corpus callosum; CN, caudate nucleus; ICp, posterior limb of the internal capsule; Put, putamen; Th, thalamus. B is a high power photomicrograph of the area outlined in A showing the differential organization of the glia in the corpus callosum, corona radiata (CR) fronto-occipital fasciculus (FOF) and the subcallosal fasciculus of Muratoff (Muratoff bundle, MB) (Mag = 2×, bar = 1 mm). C is a higher magnification view of the area outlined in B demarcating the boundaries of the fronto-occipital fasciculus (FOF) and the subcallosal fasciculus of Muratoff (MB) (Mag = 4×, bar = 0.5 mm).

tion, we could distinguish the subcallosal fasciculus of Muratoff, the fronto-occipital fasciculus, the superior longitudinal fasciculus (SLF) and its three divisions, SLF I, SLF II, and SLF III, the middle longitudinal fasciculus lying in the white matter of the superior temporal gyrus, the inferior longitudinal fasciculus in the parieto-occipital and temporal lobes, and the uncinate fasciculus, extreme capsule, and arcuate fasciculus. The corticosubcortical bundle that divides into corticothalamic and corticopontine/corticospinal systems could also be distinguished using this methodology, having been guided by the experimental isotope cases. This approach helped define the stem portion of the major fiber pathways and allowed the tracts to be distinguished from each other. The anatomical definition of the boundaries of the fiber systems was then able to provide a framework within which the constituents of the fiber pathways could be determined in the different brains.

Rationale for Use of a Standard Template Brain

To understand the organization of the different fiber bundles within the cerebral white matter and to attempt to determine the topographic arrangement of fibers within the fiber bundles, it was necessary to compare the location of the fibers between different experimental cases. This was accomplished by using a single template brain to represent the data. For each experimental case, the autoradiographic data determined by dark-field microscopy were charted directly onto drawings of equivalent coronal sections of the template brain. This method facilitated the comparative analysis of the organization of the fiber pathways in the different experimental cases.

Selection of Template Brain Sections

Twenty-one coronal sections from the normal brain in the rostrocaudal axis were selected to represent the findings for the majority of cases studied. In some instances, notably to represent the motor cases in which most of the fiber pathways dissipate within a short rostrocaudal distance, two additional intervening sections were used. Each section was selected to represent a particular anatomic feature within the coronal level identified. Thus, for example, template brain section 41 is at the genu of the corpus callosum, section 65 contains the anterior commissure as it crosses midline, section 78 reflects the most rostral part of the thalamus, section 89 contains the rostral tip of the intraparietal sulcus and the midpart of the lateral geniculate nucleus, and in section 113 the caudal end of the splenium of the corpus callosum is evident.

Drawing of Template Sections

The selected sections were traced at 9× on an Aus-Jena overhead magnification system. Sections delineated the outlines of the cortex and boundary of the white matter, the ventricular system, and the subcortical nuclei. In addition, the locations of the major fiber tracts such as the corpus callosum and anterior commissure were identified at this low-power magnification, whereas light microscopy was required for identification of less obvious fiber systems.

Selection of Matching Coronal Sections of the Experimental Brains with Reference to the Template Brain

The preliminary step in the analysis of the experimental brains was to determine which rostrocaudal section corresponded with the selected sections in the template brain. Slides for each experimental case were studied, and sections were chosen that corresponded to the anatomical landmarks identified on the template sections. In some cases it was apparent that the plane of coronal section did not match the corresponding section from the template brain exactly. Further, individual variation of sulcal and gyral pattern at this gross morphological level was also observed. In these instances, the sections that corresponded most closely with the essential anatomical features of the template section were chosen. In rare instances, the mismatch between the experimental case and the template were troublesome enough that autoradiographic findings identified on the experimental slide could not be completely represented on the corresponding template section. In these sections, autoradiographic information was transferred to the adjacent template brain section that most closely correlated with the observed finding in the experimental case.

Identification of Autoradiographic Staining, and Transfer of Data onto the Template Brain

The selected sections from the experimental cases were studied under dark-field and light-field microscopy. Labeled fibers were identified under dark-field microscopy at a magnification of 4× and 10×. Light-field microscopy was used to verify the location of the labeled fibers within the identified fiber tracts. Sections adjacent to those selected for charting were studied as well to help understand the details of the fiber systems.

Registration marks were placed on the tracing of each template section previously drawn using the overhead magnification system. These drawings were then photocopied, and these copies were used to chart the labeled fiber pathways and terminations in the experimental cases. Isotope-labeled fibers and terminations in each experimental slide were hand-drawn on the corresponding template section. The precise location, orientation, and extent of the fibers were assessed by visual inspection. The corresponding location on the template of the fibers in the experimental brain was derived from the similarity of the sections of the template brain and the experimental brain, and from the determination by glial pattern of the location of the fiber bundles both within the template brain and in the experimental brain.

Preparation of Line Diagrams

Outlines of the template sections, including the registration crosses, were traced onto vellum using Koh-I-Noor Rapidograph pens and scanned into Adobe Photoshop 5.5. The hand-drawn charting (on the template) of the fibers in each section of the experimental cases was then traced in a similar manner. These depictions of the fibers were then scanned into Adobe Photoshop, and the background was rendered invisible. The fiber tracings with the registration marks were then overlaid onto the template brain, the registration marks were aligned using the "Free Transform" and "Move" tools in Photoshop, and the fiber tracing and template outline were then merged in the final illustration. Labels and arrows were placed on the illustrations using Adobe Photoshop 5.5 or Adobe Illustrator 8.0.

The composite illustrations of the fibers within each of the major cerebral hemispheric lobes were rendered by adding one additional feature to the above method. Fibers in each case were color-coded in Photoshop by selecting the fibers, using the "Fill" tool to give them a chosen color, and then overlaying them onto the template brain using the registration marks as described above. In this manner, the cases within a single lobe could be overlaid onto the same template and the location of the fibers compared from one case to another, as depicted in the summary diagrams for the cases in each lobe (e.g., rostral vs. caudal regions in the parietal lobe). Likewise, the fibers emanating from the different lobes were then color-coded for use in the final summary series of coronal sections (prefrontal region coded red, parietal lobe coded purple, and so forth). In the chapters devoted to individual bundles, the fibers in each experimental case were copied and pasted onto the outlines of the bundle derived from the final composite color figure.

Photomicrography

Dark-field photomicrographs of the fiber pathways and terminations were obtained by using a Nikon Eclipse E800 microscope equipped with a 0.5× stage. Images were captured by a Spot digital camera (Diagnostic Instruments, Inc.) and imported into Photoshop 5.5. Low-power (0.5×) or high-power (4×) magnification images were merged in photomontages, and background artifact in the image was removed using the "Rubber Stamp" tool in Photoshop. Photomicrographs were labeled using Adobe Illustrator 8.0. Light-field microscopic images of the template brain were obtained using the same equipment and computer software.

It may be useful to compare the sections of the template brain used in this work with those in *The Rhesus Monkey Brain in Stereotaxic Coordinates* (Paxinos et al., 1999). Levels of coronal section in our work correspond to those of the Paxinos atlas in the following manner. In this work, sections 20 through 165 are derived from 145 rostral-to-caudal sections, prepared in the coronal stereotaxic plane, at a thickness of 36 to 40 μm, every 10th section processed as described above. In Paxinos et al. there are 135 sections (in figures 7 through 142), prepared in the stereotaxic plane with respect to the interaural line, at a thickness of 45 μm, every 10th section processed. Our section 20 corresponds to Paxinos figure 7 at interaural 37.83 mm, bregma 15.93 mm. Our Section 165 corresponds to Paxinos figure 142, interaural−23.55 mm, bregma−45.45 mm. The most rostral part of the genu of the corpus callosum in our template (section 38, also shown in section 41) corresponds to Paxinos figure 24, interaural 30.00 mm, bregma 8.10 mm. The most caudal part of the splenium of the corpus callosum in our template (section 113) corresponds to Paxinos figure 92, interaural−0.65 mm, bregma−22.55 mm. The anterior commissure in our template (section 65) corresponds to Paxinos figure 50, interaural 18.30 mm, bregma−03.60 mm.

Architecture and Nomenclature
of Rhesus Monkey Cerebral Hemisphere

4

In this chapter we present the photomicrographs of the medial, lateral, and basal surfaces of the rhesus monkey cerebral hemisphere that we used as the template brain, to show the various sulci (figure 4-1). Diagrams representing the medial, lateral and basal surfaces of the cerebral hemisphere (figures 4-2 and 4-3) show the various architectonic areas, and photomicrographs of coronal sections of the template brain taken at the levels depicted on the lateral surface of the hemisphere (figure 4-4) are seen in the series of images in figure 4-5. The sections that outline the trajectories in the coronal plane of the various fiber pathways in the experimental cases 1 through 36 and all the summary diagrams correspond to the images shown in these photomicrographs. The photomicrographs also designate the location of the sulci and demarcate the borders of the architectonic areas referred to throughout this volume. Architectonic areas are according to the authors referenced in chapter 3.

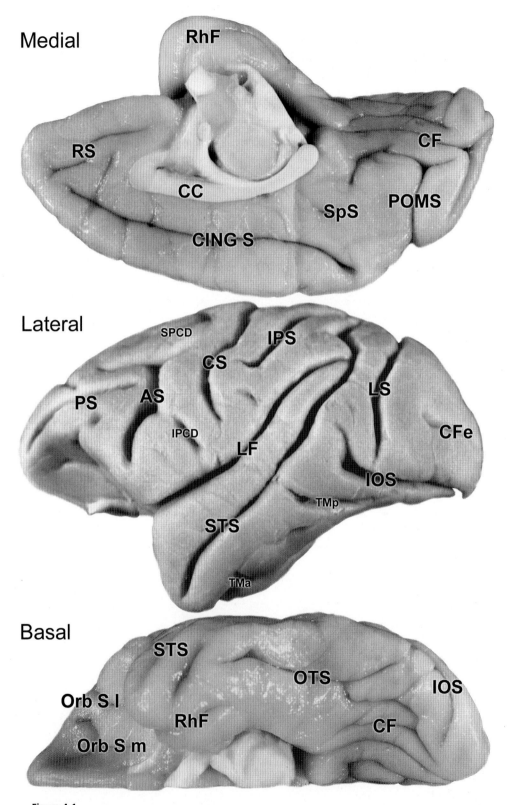

Figure 4-1

Photographs of medial, lateral, and basal views of the cerebral hemisphere of a rhesus monkey show-ing the cerebral sulci. See list of abbreviations, p. 617.

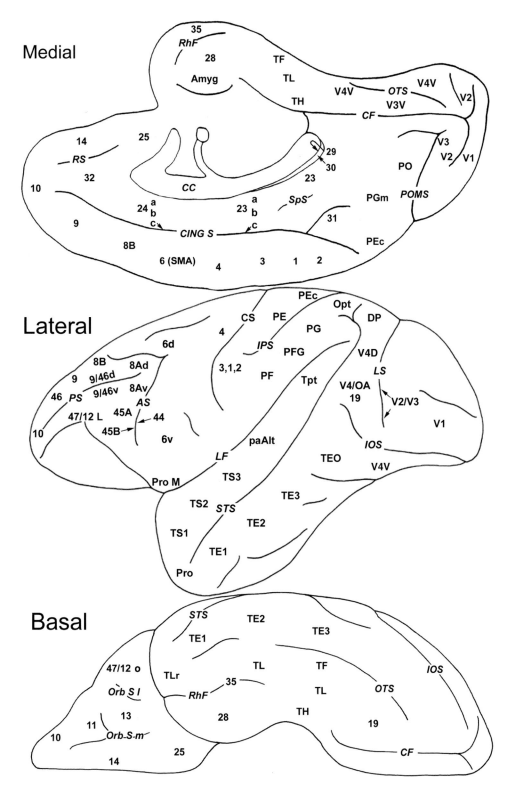

Medial

35
RhF
28
Amyg
TF
TL
TH
V4V
OTS
V4V
V3V
CF
V2
14
25
RS
32
10
24 a b c
CC
23 a b c
29
30
23
SpS
31
PO
PGm
POMS
PEc
V3
V2
V1
9
CING S
8B
6 (SMA)
4
3
1
2

Lateral

PEc
Opt
CS
PE
PG
DP
6d
4
IPS
PFG
V4D
8B
8Ad
3,1,2
PF
Tpt
LS
9
9/46d
8Av
V4/OA
46 PS
9/46v
AS
19
V2/V3
47/12 L
45A
44
V1
10
45B
6v
paAlt
LF
IOS
V4V
TEO
V4V
Pro M
TS3
TS2 STS
TE3
TE2
TS1
TE1
Pro

Basal

STS
TE2
TE1
TE3
47/12 o
TLr
TL
TF
IOS
Orb S l
35
TL
OTS
13
RhF
11
28
TH
19
10
Orb S-m
25
CF
14

Figure 4-2

Schematic diagrams of medial, lateral, and basal views of the cerebral hemisphere of a rhesus monkey to show architectonic designations according to the authors referenced in chapter 3.

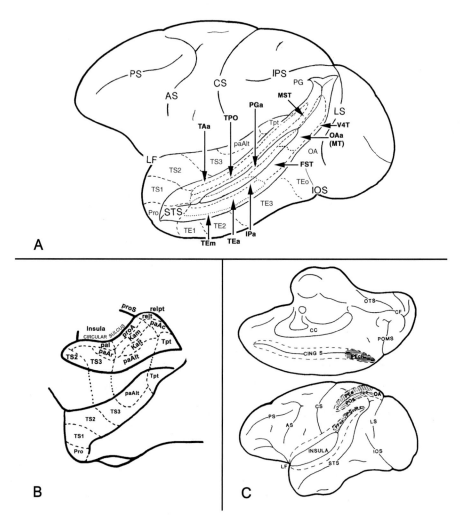

Figure 4-3

Schematic diagrams of rhesus monkey cerebral hemisphere in which the sulci have been opened to show the architectonic areas of the hidden cortices and selected gyral cortices. A, Lateral view of the cerebral hemisphere showing the architectonic parcellation of the superior temporal gyrus (areas TS1, TS2, TS3, paAlt, and Tpt), the inferotemporal region (areas TE1, TE2, TE3, and TEO), and the temporal pole (Pro). Designations of the cortices lying within the superior temporal sulcus (STS) are according to Seltzer and Pandya (1978). Multimodal areas TPO and PGa are located in the upper bank, and the surrounding unimodal association area for the auditory realm (area TAa) is situated in the upper bank of the STS and the superior temporal gyrus. The somatosensory associated area IPa is located at the fundus of the STS. Visual association areas (areas TEa, TEm, V4T and OAa [FST and MT]) occupy the lower bank of the STS and the inferotemporal region, and area MST is in the caudal part of the upper bank of the STS (from Schmahmann and Pandya, 1991). B, Architectonic parcellation of the superior temporal gyrus (as in A) and the supratemporal plane according to Pandya and Sanides (1973). Abbreviations of the architectonic areas according to these authors are Kam, medial koniocortex; Kalt, lateral koniocortex; paAc, caudal parakoniocortex; paAlt, lateral parakoniocortex; paAr, rostral parakoniocortex; proA, prokoniocortex; paI, parainsular cortex; proS, somatic prokoniocortex (SII); reIpt, retroinsular parietal cortex; reIt, retroinsular temporal cortex; Tpt, temporoparietal cortex. C, Architectonic areas within the banks of the intraparietal sulcus and the caudal part of the upper bank of the Sylvian fissure according to Pandya and Seltzer (1982). The intraparietal, lateral (Sylvian), and cingulate sulci are opened to show the location of the architectonic areas lying within the sulci. Within the intraparietal sulcus, area PEa is in the upper bank and area POa in the lower bank, while area IPd lies in the depth of the sulcus. Parietal opercular areas PGop caudally, and PFop rostrally, are seen in the caudal part of the upper bank of the Sylvian fissure.

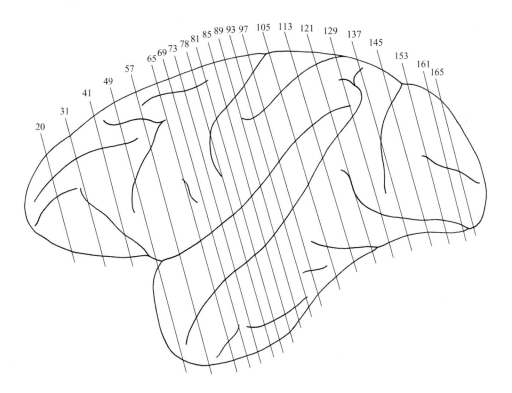

Figure 4-4

Schematic diagram of the lateral view of the rhesus monkey cerebral hemisphere that was used as the template showing the plane of section and the levels from which the coronal sections were taken.

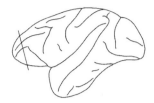

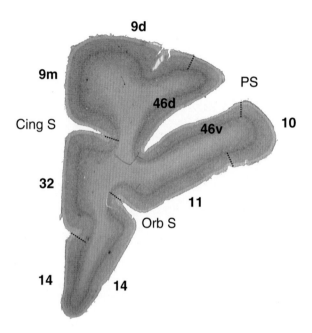

Figure 4-5

Photomicrographs of the 23 coronal sections (numbered 20 through 165) taken from the template brain at the levels indicated on the lateral view of the hemisphere in figure 4-4. Each photomicrograph shows the architectonic areas (in bold font), as well as the designation of the various sulci. Borders of the cortical architectonic areas are shown by the dashed lines. At top right is a schematic view of the lateral surface of the cerebral hemisphere to show the level at which the photomicrograph of each coronal section is taken.

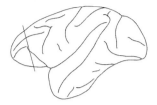

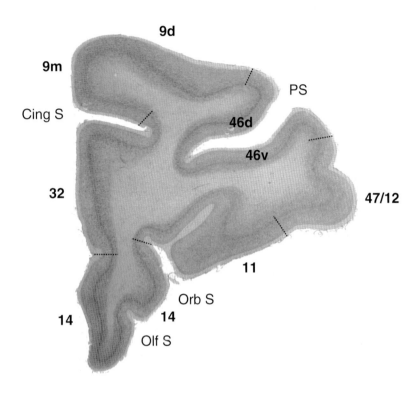

9d

9m

PS

Cing S

46d

46v

32

47/12

11

Orb S

14   14

Olf S

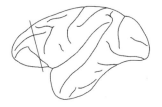

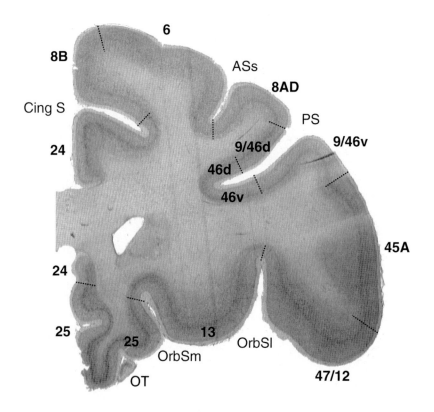

Figure 4-5 (continued)

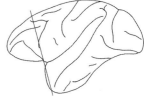

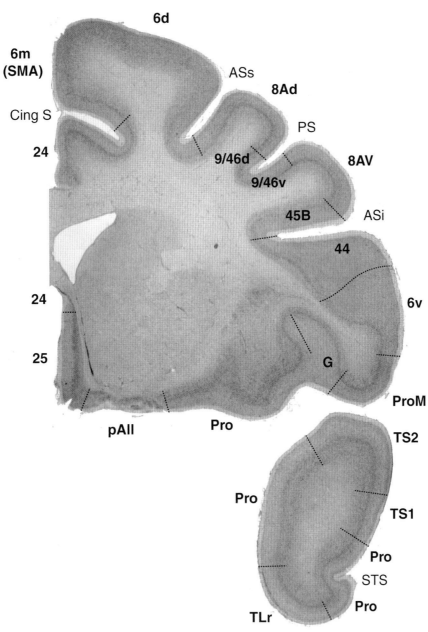

6d

6m
(SMA)

ASs

8Ad

Cing S

PS

24

9/46d

8AV

9/46v

45B

ASi

44

24

6v

25

G

ProM

pAll

Pro

TS2

Pro

TS1

Pro

STS

Pro

TLr

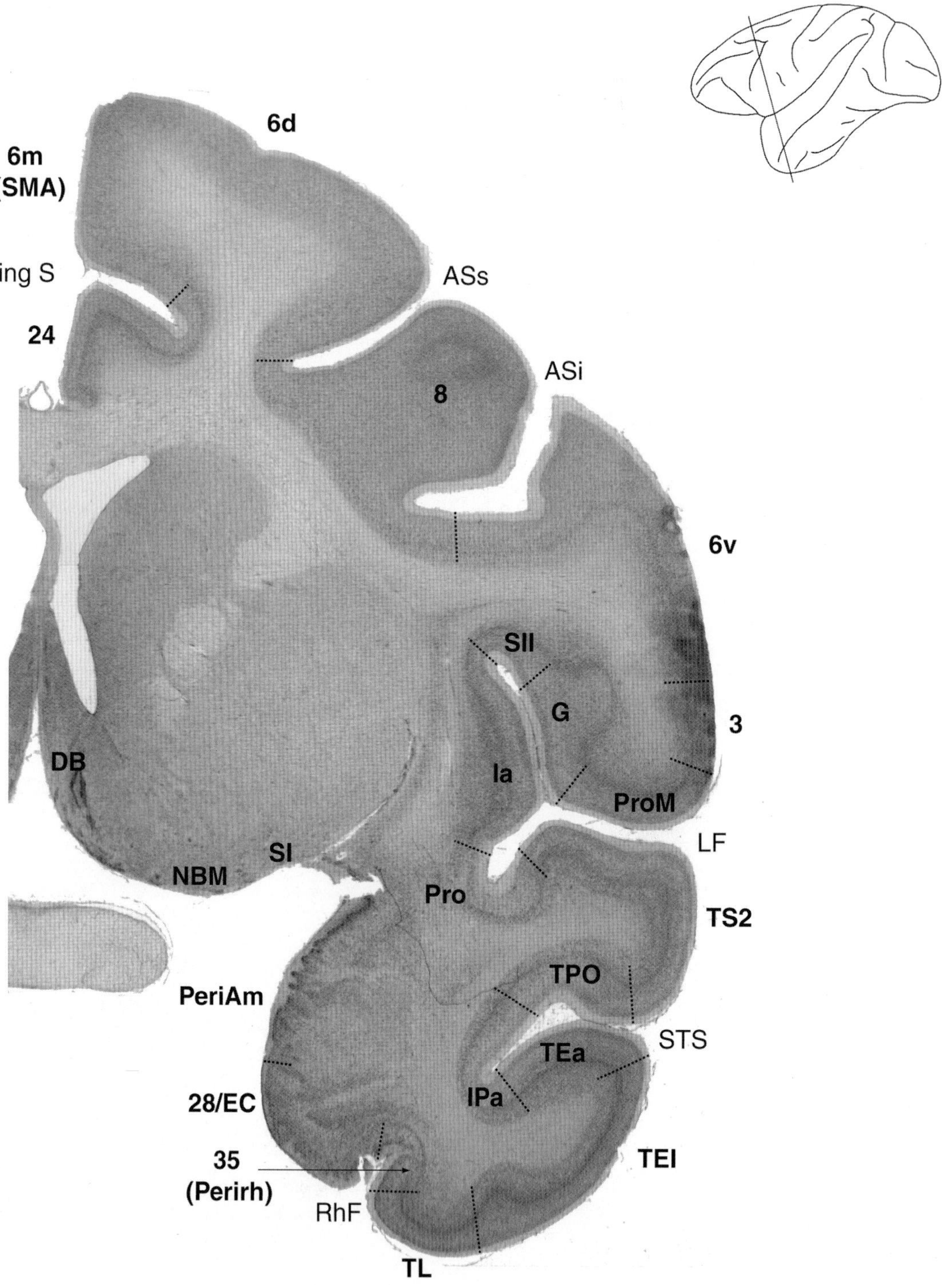

Figure 4-5 (continued)

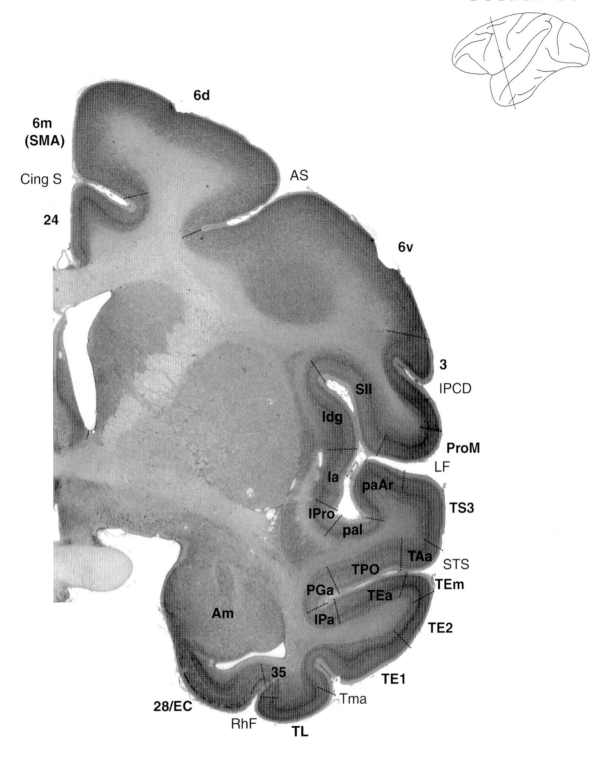

6d

6m
(SMA)

Cing S

24

AS

6v

3

SII

IPCD

Idg

ProM

LF

Ia

paAr

TS3

IPro

pal

TAa

STS

TPO

TEm

PGa

TEa

Am

IPa

TE2

TE1

35

TL

28/EC

Tma

RhF

TL

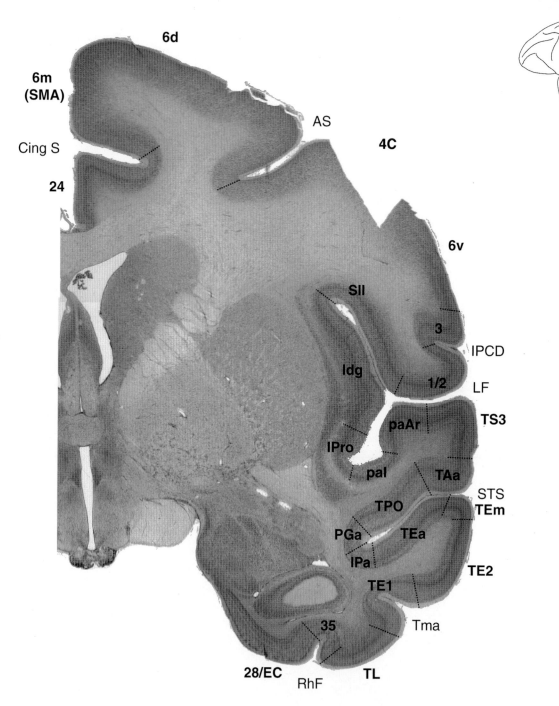

6d

6m (SMA)

Cing S

24

AS

4C

6v

SII

3

Idg

IPCD

1/2

LF

paAr

TS3

IPro

pal

TAa

TPO

STS

TEm

PGa

TEa

IPa

TE2

TE1

Tma

35

28/EC

RhF

TL

Figure 4-5 (continued)

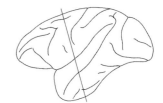

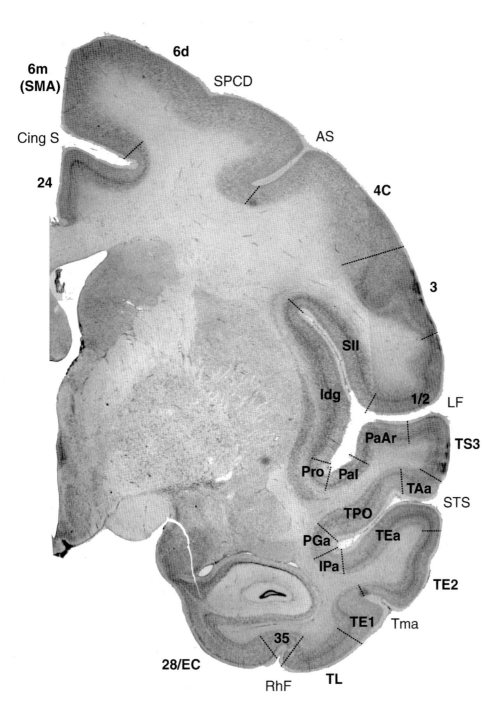

6d

6m
(SMA)

SPCD

Cing S

AS

24

4C

3

SII

Idg

1/2   LF

PaAr

TS3

Pro   PaI

STS

TAa

TPO

PGa

TEa

IPa

TE2

TE1   Tma

35

28/EC

TL

RhF

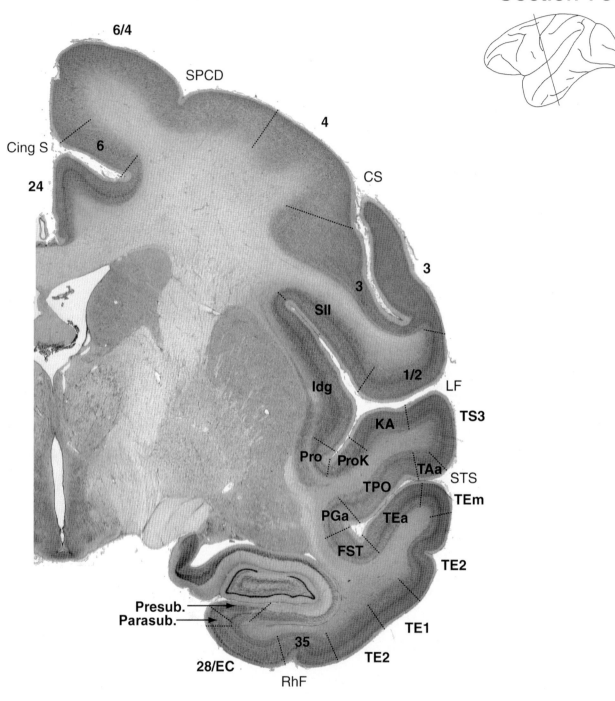

6/4

SPCD

4

Cing S   6

CS

24

3

3

SII

Idg

1/2

LF

TS3

KA

Pro   ProK

TAa

STS

TEm

TPO

PGa   TEa

FST

TE2

Presub.
Parasub.

TE1

35

TE2

28/EC

RhF

Figure 4-5 (continued)

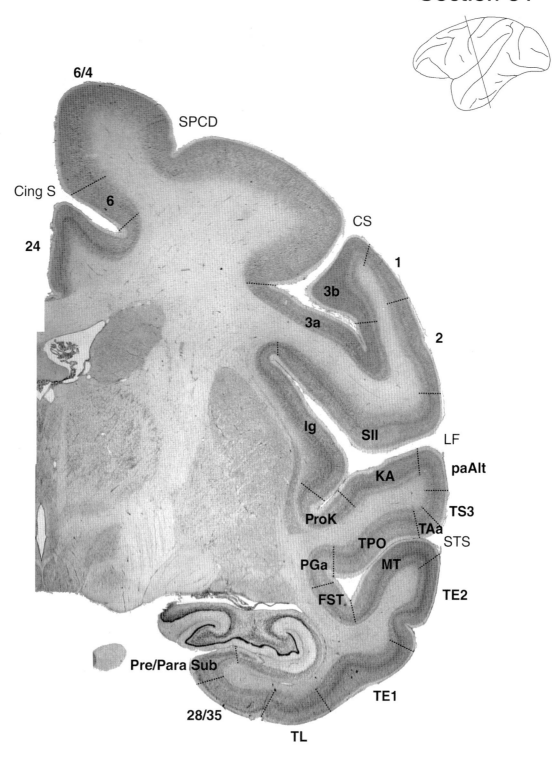

6/4

SPCD

Cing S

6

24

CS

1

3b

3a

2

Ig

SII

LF

KA

paAlt

ProK

TS3

TAa

STS

TPO

PGa

MT

FST

TE2

Pre/Para Sub

TE1

28/35

TL

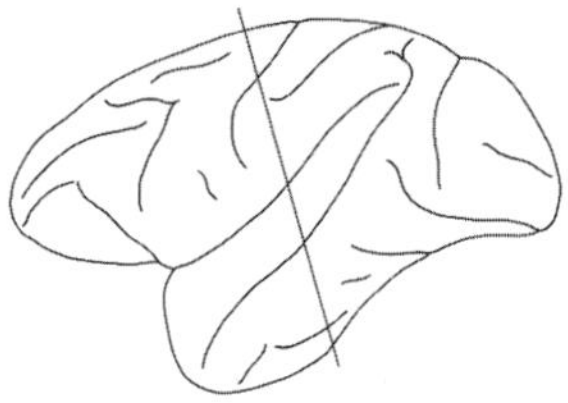

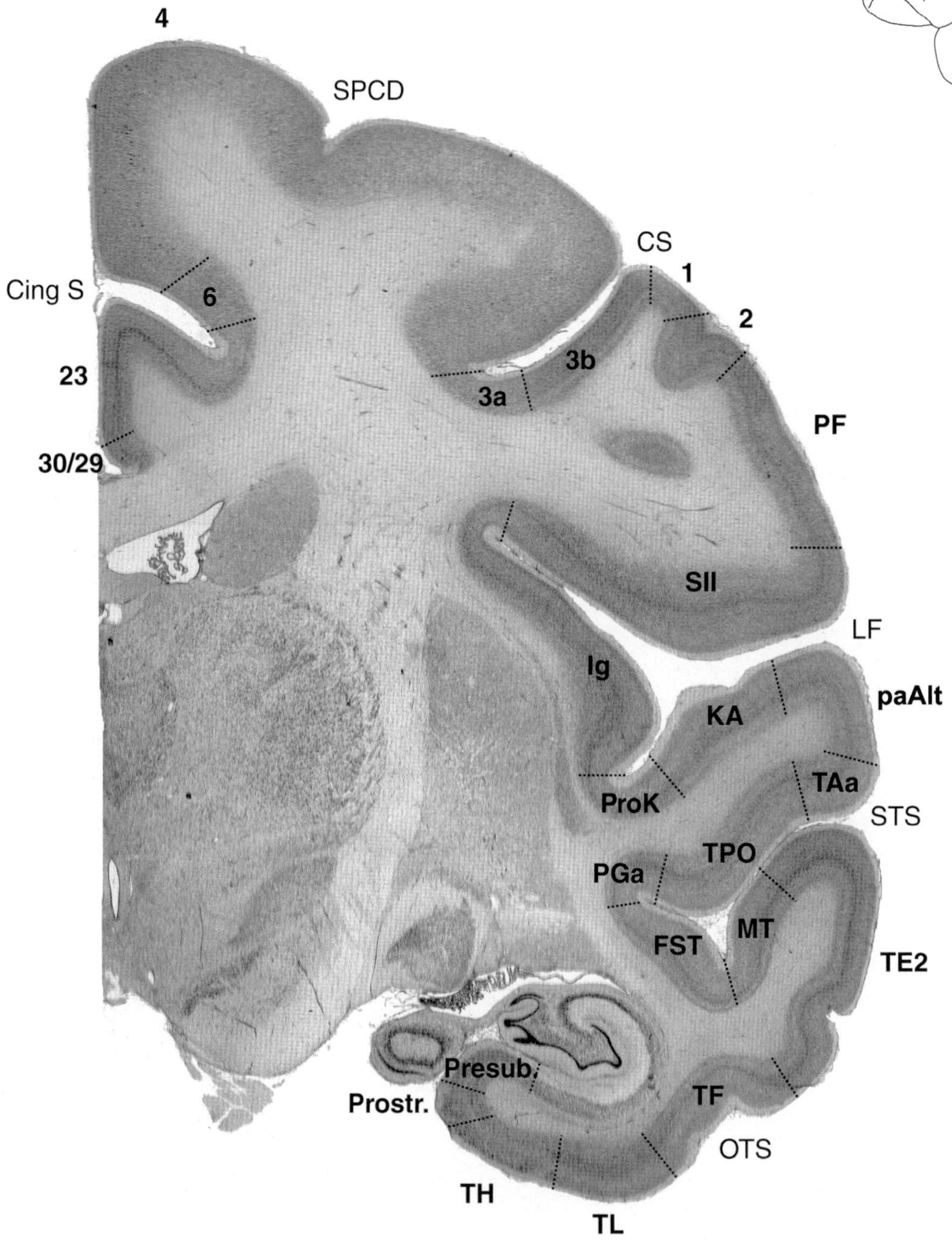

Figure 4-5 (continued)

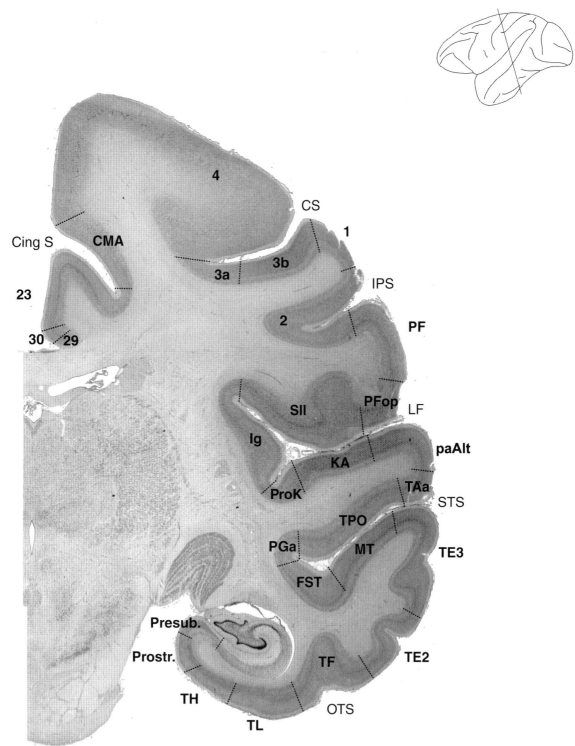

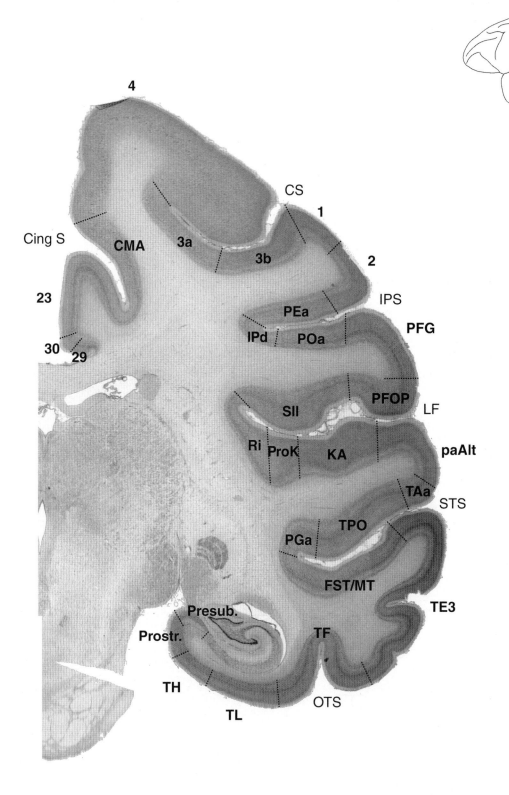

Figure 4-5 (continued)

4

CS

3b

1

3

3a

2

Cing S

CMA

IPS

PEa

POa

PFG

23

IPd

Reipt

PFop

LF

30

29

Reit

paAc

Tpt

TPO

STS

PGa

V4

MT

FST

Presub.

Prostr.

TF

TE3

TH

TL

OTS

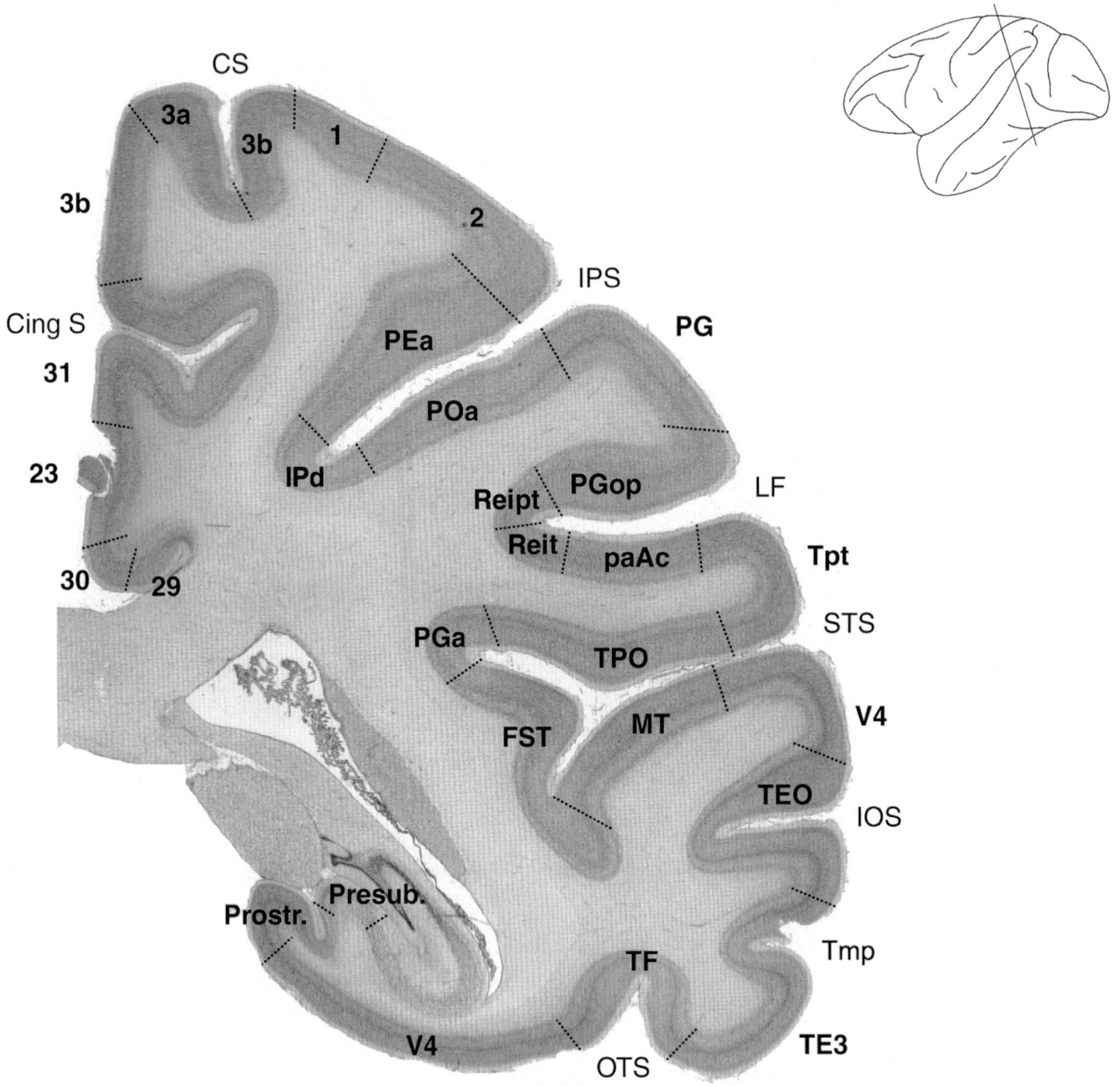

Figure 4-5 (continued)

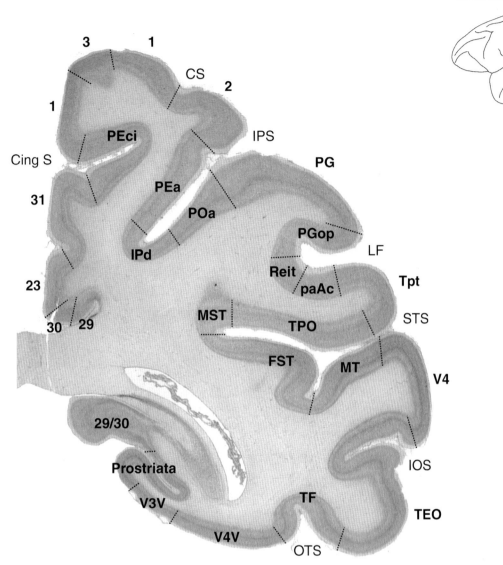

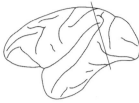

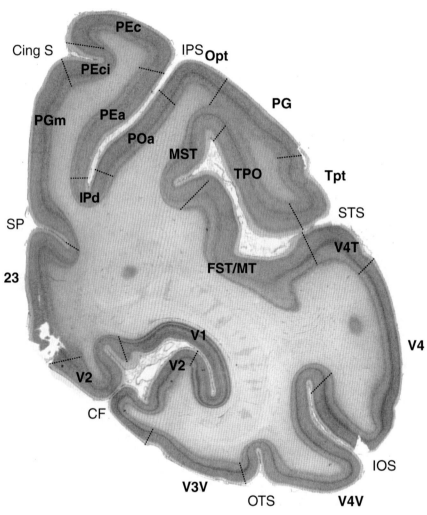

Figure 4-5 (continued)

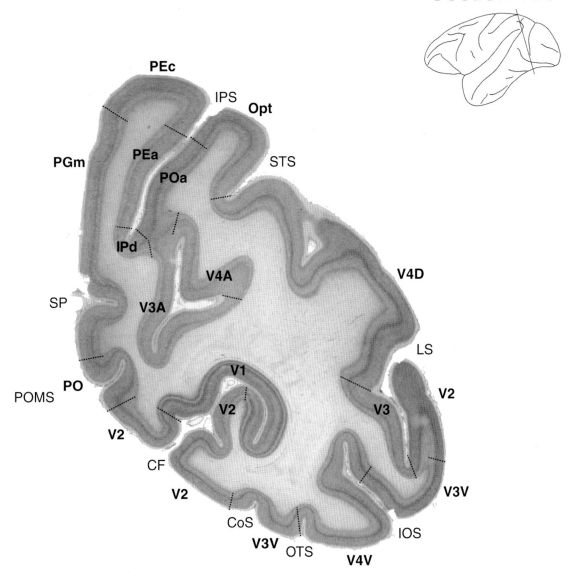

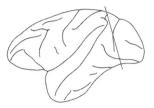

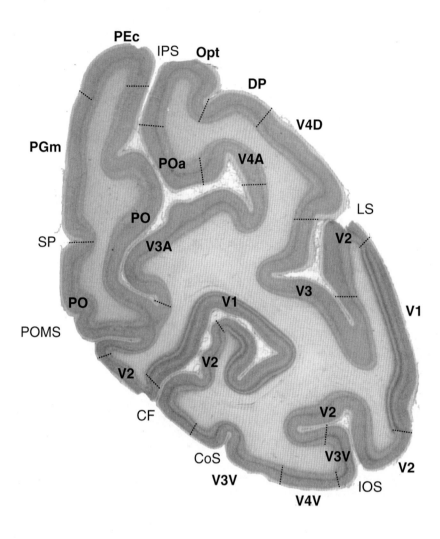

Figure 4-5 (continued)

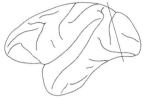

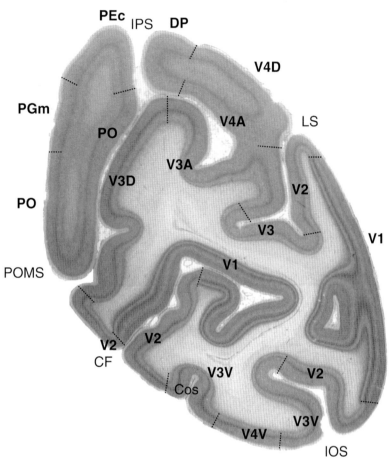

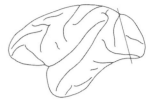

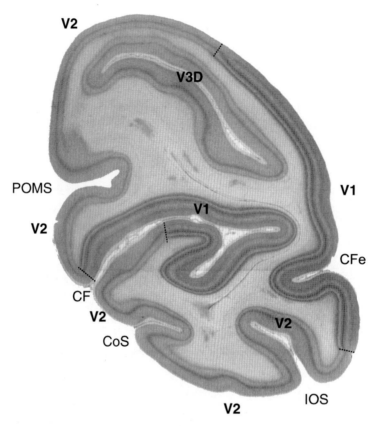

Figure 4-5 (continued)

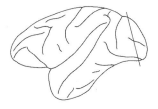

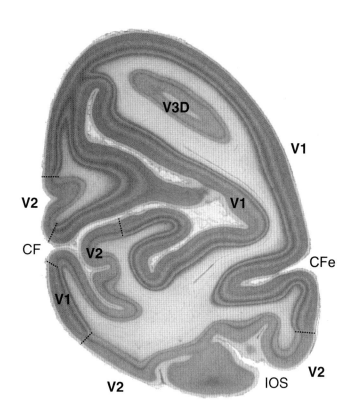

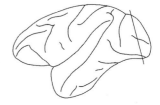

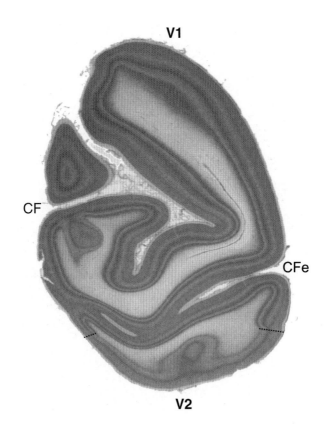

Figure 4-5 (continued)

White Matter Fiber Bundles
by Cortical Region of Origin

In this section we present the results of our investigations. We begin with general principles of organization of the fiber bundles, followed by descriptions of the cortical and subcortical connectional patterns of subdivisions within each lobe. Emphasis is placed upon the organization of fiber pathways emanating from each cortical area, and the cortical termination patterns of the association pathways are considered in detail. A general overview of the termination patterns of subcortical pathways is presented, and comments regarding commissural connections are confined to topographic organization in the midsagittal plane. Case descriptions are complemented by line drawings depicting the fiber tracts and their terminations in successive rostral to caudal template sections in the coronal plane. Following the descriptions of the fiber pathways arising from individual cortical areas, the patterns of cortical and subcortical fibers of each lobe are summarized, accompanied by color-coded diagrams illustrating the topography of the fiber trajectories for each case studied in that lobe.

PART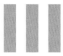

Principles of Organization

5

The cerebral hemisphere is traditionally divided into the lobes named by Gratiolet, with the central sulcus partitioning the hemisphere into pre-Rolandic and post-Rolandic regions. The post-Rolandic cortex contains the parietal, temporal, and occipital lobes; the pre-Rolandic area consists of precentral, premotor, and prefrontal cortices. Neurons in the neocortex are arranged in six laminae, or layers, each with a unique pattern of afferent and efferent connections. The axons of the cortical neurons within these layers constitute the efferent fiber systems, and the laminar location of these neurons determines the target of the efferent fibers. It is therefore pertinent to provide an overview of the organization of the different cortical layers (see Pandya and Yeterian, 2003), the general principles of organization of the fiber tracts, and a conceptual approach to the major functional divisions of the cerebral hemispheres before describing in detail the fibers emanating from individual cortical areas.

Cortical Laminae

In general, the first layer of the cerebral cortex is sparsely populated with neurons and is thought to receive input from intralaminar thalamic nuclei and the reticular formation. This layer also receives feedback from precursor cortical areas. Layers II and IV receive intrinsic connections within the given cortical unit. Layers II, III, and IV receive feedforward input from adjacent cortical regions. Layers III and IV receive thalamic and commissural input. Layers V and VI receive intrinsic connections and some thalamic input.

Information in layer I is transferred to the intrinsic circuitry of the cortical unit by providing afferent contacts with the apical dendrites of supragranular (layers II and III) and infragranular neurons (layers V and VI). Layers II and IV provide information to the supragranular and infragranular neurons within a cortical module. Cells in layer III preferentially provide the long association axons, including commissural fibers. Efferents from layers V and VI participate in a feedback link to the first layer of the adjacent cortical area, and neurons in these layers also project to the thalamus (mostly from layer VI), basal ganglia (predominantly from layer Va), and pons and spinal cord (largely from layer Vb).

While recognizing the laminar specificity of the different fiber systems (layers II and III give rise to association and commissural systems, layers V and VI to subcortical connections), it is not possible to state with certainty from our experimental cases which layer gives rise to which specific fiber pathway, as the entire cortical thickness is labeled

81

by the tracer injection. However, we can discern the various efferent fiber constituents as they emerge from the cortex.

Neurons within a cortical area give rise to three distinct categories of efferent fibers that can be distinguished within the white matter immediately beneath the gyrus. As will be seen, these are (1) the association fibers, (2) the striatal fibers, and (3) the confluence of fibers (the "cord") that carries the commissural and subcortical fibers. Local association fibers, or U-fibers, hug the undersurface of the sixth layer. Neighborhood and long association fibers travel within the central part of the white matter of the core of the gyrus, accompanied in the initial stages by the striatal fibers. Subcortically directed fibers together with the commissural fibers are arranged initially in a "cord" formation and travel centripetally in the central part of the white matter of the gyrus. This general principle of organization of the cortical efferent fibers is valid for the entire neocortex and is exemplified in the photomicrographs in figure 5-1 taken from Case 4, and the diagrammatic representation in figure 5-2A and schema of fibers in figure 5-2B.

Major Subdivisions of Cerebral Fiber Pathways

Association Fibers

Local association fibers, or U-fibers, leave a given area of cortex and travel to an adjacent gyrus, running in a thin, identifiable band immediately beneath the sixth layer.

Neighborhood association fibers arise from a given cortical area and are directed to nearby regions but are distinguishable from the local U-fibers that run immediately beneath the cortex. Neighborhood fibers, for example, connect the inferior parietal lobule to the medial parietal cortex.

Long association fibers emanate from a given cortical region and travel in discrete fiber bundles, leading to other cortical areas in the same hemisphere. These have traditionally been designated association fibers, but to differentiate them from the local and neighborhood association fibers, we refer to these bundles as long association fibers. The following long association fiber pathways can be identified in the cerebral hemispheres.

The superior longitudinal fasciculus (SLF) is a major fiber tract with three distinct subcomponents. SLF I is medially situated in the white matter of the superior parietal lobule and the superior frontal gyrus. SLF II is more laterally situated and occupies a position in the central core of the hemisphere white matter, lateral to the corona radiata and above the Sylvian fissure. SLF III is further lateral and ventral and is located in the white matter of the parietal and frontal operculum.

The arcuate fasciculus runs first in the white matter of the superior temporal gyrus and then in the white matter deep to the upper shoulder of the Sylvian fissure as it courses toward the frontal lobe. It lies ventrally adjacent to SLF II.

The middle longitudinal fasciculus is situated within the white matter of the caudal inferior parietal lobule and extends into the white matter of the superior temporal gyrus.

The extreme capsule is situated between the claustrum and the insular cortex caudally, and between the claustrum and the orbital frontal cortex rostrally.

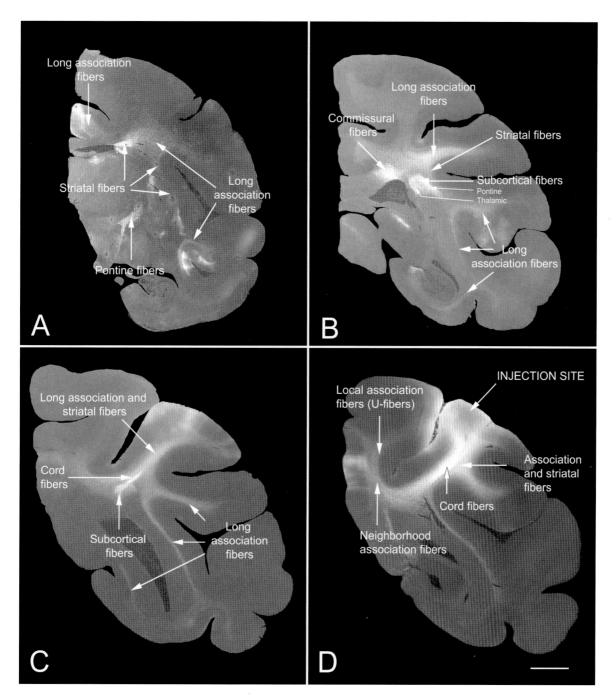

Figure 5-1

Dark-field photomicrographs of rostral to caudal coronal sections, A–D, of a rhesus monkey cerebral hemisphere following injection of isotope tracer into the caudal part of the inferior parietal lobule, area PG/Opt (Case 4). The major fiber bundles that emanate from the injection site are identified by category to illustrate the principle of organization of the white matter pathways common to all cortical areas. Association fibers include local association fibers (U-fibers), neighborhood association fibers, and a number of long association fiber bundles. Striatal fibers travel initially with the association fibers as they leave the cortical area and are more readily identified further along in their course as the external capsule and the subcallosal fasciculus of Muratoff (the Muratoff bundle). The cord of fibers that leaves the cortical area conveys two distinct contingents of fibers: the subcortical bundle of fibers to the thalamus, brainstem (including most notably the pons), and spinal cord; and the commissural fibers that pass to the opposite hemisphere (Mag = 0.5×, bar = 5 mm).

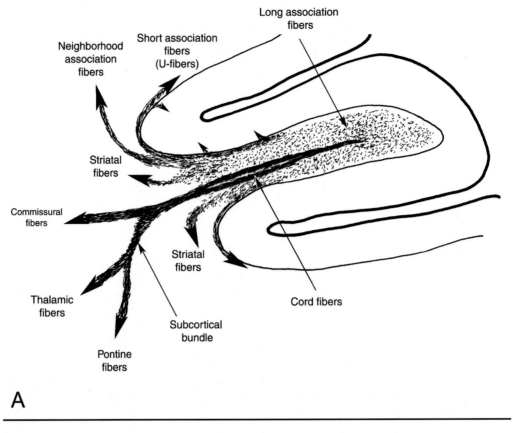

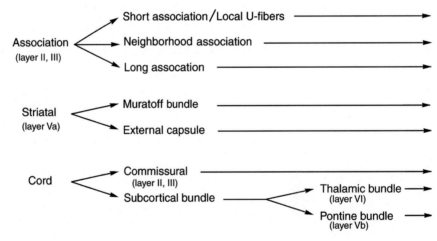

Figure 5-2

A, diagrammatic representation of the organization of white matter fiber pathways emanating from a given area of the cerebral cortex in the coronal plane. Long association fibers are seen end-on as the stippled area within the white matter of the gyrus. In their course, these fibers either remain confined to the white matter of the gyrus, or they travel deeper in the white matter of the hemisphere. Short association fibers, or U-fibers link adjacent gyri. Neighborhood association fibers link nearby regions usually within the same lobe. Striatal fibers intermingle with the association fibers early in their course, and then are identifiable as distinct fiber tracts in the white matter. Cord fibers segregate into commissural fibers and the subcortical bundle, which further divides into fibers destined for thalamus, and those to brainstem and spinal cord in the pontine bundle. B, Schema of the principles of organization of the white matter fiber pathways arising from any given area of the cerebral cortex.

The inferior longitudinal fasciculus is in the white matter between the sagittal stratum medially and the parieto-occipital and temporal cortices laterally. It has a vertical limb in the parietal and occipital lobes and a horizontal component contained within the temporal lobe.

The fronto-occipital fasciculus travels above the body and head of the caudate nucleus and the subcallosal fasciculus of Muratoff (Muratoff bundle, see below), lateral to the corpus callosum and medial to the corona radiata.

The uncinate fasciculus occupies the white matter of the rostral part of the temporal lobe, the limen insula, and the white matter of the orbital and medial frontal cortex.

The cingulum bundle has a dorsal component that occupies the white matter of the cingulate gyrus and a ventral contingent situated in the white matter of the caudal part of the parahippocampal gyrus.

Striatal Fibers

Corticostriatal fibers have two major components. One initially courses with the long association fibers before separating from them and then travels via the subcallosal fasciculus of Muratoff. These fibers lead to the caudate nucleus and putamen. The other striatal fibers enter the external capsule and target the ventral part of the caudate nucleus, the putamen and claustrum.

Cord Fibers

In addition to the association and corticostriatal fibers, every cortical region gives rise to a dense aggregation of fibers, which we have termed the cord, that occupies the central core of the white matter of the gyrus. The fibers in the cord separate into two distinct segments. One segment forms a commissural bundle that travels to the opposite hemisphere via the corpus callosum or the anterior commissure. The other segment continues as a concentration of fibers; we have termed it the subcortical bundle. Depending on its cortical origin, this fiber bundle travels within the internal capsule (anterior or posterior limb) or the sagittal stratum, segregates into a thalamic fiber bundle and a pontine fiber bundle, and gives rise to fibers to other diencephalic and brainstem structures. A distinct group of fibers that we have termed the ventral subcortical bundle (VSB) is one of the thalamic peduncles and occupies the white matter between the stria terminalis and the caudate tail. The cord fibers therefore constitute the precursor from each cortical area of the major white matter fiber pathways other than the association and striatal fibers, namely the corpus callosum, anterior commissure, internal capsule, and sagittal stratum.

Functional Divisions of Cerebral Cortex

Cerebral organization may be conceptualized as comprising five principal areas of function, each subserved by interconnected neural systems with specific anatomical components, including dedicated fiber tracts (see also Mesulam, 2000; Pandya and Yeterian, 1985).

I. *Reticular/arousal/autonomic systems* are critical for the level of alertness of the organism and regulation of the internal milieu. Behaviors that require the participation of an awake behaving organism depend upon the integrity of this system. Structures that subserve this system include the thalamic reticular nucleus, which drives cerebral cortex, and ascending brainstem catecholaminergic nuclei, which provide projections diffusely upon the cerebral cortical and subcortical structures. The hypothalamus is integrally incorporated through neural and hormonal mechanisms into this core level of function and forms an essential part of the motivation/limbic system as well.

II. *Motivation/limbic systems* are crucial for the participation of the organism in both sensory perception and active engagement. These systems are dependent upon the emotional state of the organism and the affective valence of the stimulus. Structures involved in this system include the amygdala, septohippocampal system and basal forebrain (the limbic, or corticoid and allocortical areas), and the cingulate gyrus, parahippocampal gyrus, temporal pole, anterior insular cortex, and caudal orbitofrontal cortex (the paralimbic zone, or mesocortex), as well as the limbic thalamic nuclei.

III. *Sensory-specific systems* include the primary sensory modalities of vision, somatosensory stimuli, and auditory input. These regions, like those in the primary motor area, are characterized by idiotypic cortex. The olfactory cortex is part of the limbic core, the gustatory cortex is in the frontal operculum, and the vestibular area is in the posterior parietotemporal lobe and in the rostral anterior parietal cortex.

IV. *Effector systems* include the idiotypic primary motor cortex, as well as premotor, supplementary motor and cingulate motor cortices, projections from which lead to subcortical structures, brainstem and spinal cord. At the level of higher function, the effector systems also include the feedback from prefrontal cortex to other cortical areas.

V. *Associative systems* transcend specific sensorimotor domains and are characterized by multimodal or supramodal regions that encode high-order behaviors crucial for cognitive operations. (These areas constitute the homotypical association isocortex, including the unimodal, specific association areas and the heteromodal regions concerned with higher-order behavior.)

Mesulam (1998) regards the heteromodal, paralimbic, and limbic cortices as transmodal areas that serve to bind multiple unimodal and other transmodal areas into distributed but integrated multimodal representations. In this view, interconnected sets of transmodal nodes provide anatomical and computational epicenters for large-scale neurocognitive networks, each epicenter displaying relative specialization within specific behavioral domains. These anatomically distinct networks are specialized for spatial awareness (posterior parietal cortex, frontal eye fields); language (Broca and Wernicke areas); explicit learning, memory, and emotion (hippocampus, entorhinal cortex and amygdala); face/object recognition and semantic knowledge (middle temporal region and temporal polar cortex); and working memory/executive functions (lateral prefrontal and possibly posterior parietal cortices). Lesions of the transmodal epicenters lead to global impairments, whereas selective disconnection of the epicenter from relevant unimodal areas results in modality-specific impairments.

In this schema, the cerebral cortex is regarded as the "parent" node in the distributed neural systems that also include subcortical areas such as striatum (e.g., Alexander et al., 1986; Goldman-Rakic and Selemon, 1990; Yeterian and Pandya, 1991) and thalamus (Mesulam, 2000; Schmahmann, 2003). Recent evidence from clinical, anatomical, behavioral, and functional neuroimaging domains implicates the cerebellum also in the distributed neural systems necessary for sensorimotor and cognitive and affective processing (Schmahmann, 1991, 1997; Schmahmann and Sherman, 1998). The cerebellar component is not discussed here, except inasmuch as the substantial corticopontine projections from association areas of cerebral cortex have provided anatomic evidence central to the appreciation of these wider aspects of cerebellar function.

Descriptions of the Experimental Cases

This overview of the neurons from which the fiber bundles arise, and the large-scale connectional networks that they facilitate, serves to introduce the detailed analysis of the fiber trajectories and their terminations. In the following chapters the white matter fiber tracts are described according to their site of origin within the major lobes of the cerebral cortex: parietal lobe (six cases), superior temporal region (five cases), inferior temporal region (five cases), occipital lobe (five cases), cingulate gyrus (two cases), motor cortex (six cases), and prefrontal region (four cases). In each chapter, the experimental cases injected with isotope are analyzed in terms of the injection site and the label that occupies the various fiber pathways and the resulting terminations in coronal sections of the template brain.

Parietal Lobe

6

In this chapter we describe the isotope injection cases in the parietal lobe of six rhesus monkeys, and we analyze the resulting association, striatal, commissural, and subcortical fiber trajectories, as well as the cortical and subcortical terminations. The injections were in the superior parietal lobule in area PGm, encroaching upon area PEc (Case 1), the medial part of area PEc at the junction of area PE (Case 2), and the lateral part of area PEc at the junction of area PE (Case 3). Injections in the inferior parietal lobule were placed in the caudal part of area PG and in area Opt (Case 4), the rostral inferior parietal lobule, area PF (Case 5), and the middle part of the parietal operculum (Case 6).

Cortical terminations are described according to their architectonic designations. These are not labeled on the template sections of each case, and the reader is referred to the template brain atlas in chapter 4 in which the architectonic areas are labeled on external views of the hemisphere as well as in the coronal series. Terminations in thalamus are shown for each case, and the thalamic nuclei are referred to in the text, but the nuclei are not designated on the figures of the coronal sections as this was not the focus of the work. Pontine terminations are described in the text but not illustrated. In most cases the brainstem had been separated from the hemisphere for analysis in prior studies, and the details of the corticopontine projections presented here are derived from these earlier investigations. Striatal terminations are illustrated in the figures, and an overview of their termination patterns is presented in the text.

CASE 1

In this case the isotope injection is located at the medial convexity of the superior parietal lobule in area PGm, encroaching upon area PEc (template sections [Scs.] 129, 137, 145). See figures 6-1 and 6-2.

Association Fibers

Local Association Fibers

Fibers in the white matter of the caudal superior parietal lobule terminate in nearby cortices in a columnar manner with a first-layer preference. These are distributed in the cortex of the superior parietal lobule (SPL) in areas PGm and PEc and in cortex of the upper bank of the intraparietal sulcus (IPS) in area PEa (Scs. 129, 137, 145). Local terminations are also seen in area PO, at the upper banks of the IPS and the parieto-occipital medial sulcus (POMS), and at the medial wall of the hemisphere (Scs. 137, 145).

Long Association Fibers

Rostrally Directed fibers

From the injection site, fibers course rostrally in the medial aspect of the white matter of the SPL, situated immediately subjacent to the cortex of the medial convexity. These fibers terminate in a columnar manner in the medial parietal convexity in area PGm, in the caudal part of the cingulate sulcus in area PEci, and in the caudal part of the medial superior parietal lobule in area PEc (Scs.113, 121). Further rostrally, the fibers terminate in the lower bank of the cingulate sulcus in area 31 in a columnar manner (Sc. 121). Association fibers lying within the ventral/lateral aspect of the white matter of the SPL course rostrally and provide columnar terminations in areas PE and PEa of the SPL (Sc. 113).

The fibers traveling in the lateral part of the SPL white matter curve around the depth of the IPS and then ascend in the white matter of the inferior parietal lobule (IPL). These fibers terminate in a columnar manner in area PG and area PGop of the inferior parietal lobule and in area IPd at the depth of the intraparietal sulcus (Scs. 97, 105, 113). A small contingent of fibers terminates also in the caudal part of area TPO in the upper bank of the superior temporal sulcus (S. 121).

A contingent of fibers travels from the injection site in the SPL white matter and concentrates in a compact bundle around the cingulate sulcus. This bundle then segregates into a dorsal segment that becomes part of the superior longitudinal fasciculus subcomponent I (SLF I) and a ventral segment that becomes a part of the cingulate fasciculus (or cingulum bundle [CB]). The SLF I fibers travel rostrally into the medial aspect of the white matter of the superior frontal gyrus and provide columnar terminations to the upper bank of the cingulate sulcus in area 6 and further rostrally to the supplementary motor area (SMA) and cingulate motor area (CMA) (Scs. 49, 57, 65, 73, 81, 85, 89).

The fibers in the cingulate fasciculus travel rostrally in the dorsal and medial segments of the white matter of the cingulate gyrus and the lower bank of the cingulate sulcus. These fibers terminate in a columnar manner in the depth of the cingulate sulcus in area 24d and in the lower bank of the cingulate sulcus in areas 24b and 24c (Scs. 81, 85).

Fibers enter the fronto-occipital fasciculus (FOF) lying just rostral to the atrium of the lateral ventricle and above the Muratoff bundle (MB). As they proceed rostrally in the frontal lobe, fibers ascend into the middle part of the white matter of the superior frontal gyrus. They terminate dorsally in the dorsal premotor area 6 in a columnar manner and further rostrally in dorsal area 8 (Scs. 49, 57, 65, 73, 81).

Commissural and Subcortical Fibers

From the injection site, a dense cord of intensely labeled fibers descends sharply in the central part of the white matter of the SPL (Scs. 121, 129). Two parallel components can be identified along part of its course.

The medial part of the cord maintains its compact form until its fibers enter the lateral aspect of the splenium of the corpus callosum (CC, Sc. 113), at which stage they promptly fan out before crossing to the opposite hemisphere. The callosal fibers move rostrally and medially (Sc. 105) and occupy a ventral position in the midsagittal plane in corpus callosum sector CC4 (Sc. 97; see chapter 22 for CC subdivisions).

The fibers from the lateral component of the cord enter the superior aspect of the sagittal stratum (SS) in the middle part of sector SS-2 (Sc. 113; see chapter 25 for ss subdivisions) and move rostrally as a subcortical bundle (SB) into the dorsal and medial aspects of rostral SS-2 (Sc. 105). The fibers are first at the dorsal aspect of the sagittal stratum, and then further rostrally they occupy the posterior limb of the internal capsule (ICp) in its retrolenticular component, ICp-5 (Sc. 97; see chapter 24 for internal capsule subdivisions).

As they move rostrally into ICp-4 (Sc. 93), the fibers segregate into a medial and a lateral component. Those in the medial component (the thalamic bundle [ThB]) traverse the dorsal part of the thalamic reticular nucleus and the external medullary lamina (Sc. 93) and provide extensive thalamic terminations, including the lateral posterior (LP), medial pulvinar (PM), and central lateral (CL) nuclei (Scs. 85, 89, 93).

The more laterally placed fibers in the subcortical bundle continue rostrally in the internal capsule into ICp-3 (Sc. 89) and gradually descend to reach ICp-2 (Sc. 85). At this point they descend sharply, medial to the anterior part of the lateral geniculate nucleus and as the pontine bundle (PB) enter the lateral aspect of the cerebral peduncle (Scs. 85, 89). These fibers terminate in the basilar pontine nuclei, concentrated around the traversing corticofugal fibers and the lateral pontine nucleus, as well as in the dorsolateral and the paramedian nuclei.

Some fibers leave the subcortical bundle before the pontine fibers descend into the cerebral peduncle, head medially, and terminate in the zona incerta (ZI, in Sc. 85).

Striatal Fibers

The striatal fibers are conveyed along with the association fibers in SLF I. Fibers start to descend from the SLF I around the level of the caudal pulvinar and enter the fronto-occipital fasciculus, from where some enter the MB. Fibers travel rostrally in the MB and terminate in the head of the caudate nucleus (Scs. 49, 57, 65, 73, 81). In addition, fibers from the MB move laterally through the superior aspect of the posterior limb of the internal capsule as a striatal bundle (StB) and descend to terminate in the dorsal part of the putamen (Put) and to run in the external capsule (EC) before terminating in the ventral part of the claustrum (Scs. 49, 57, 65, 73, 81, 85, 89).

CASE 1

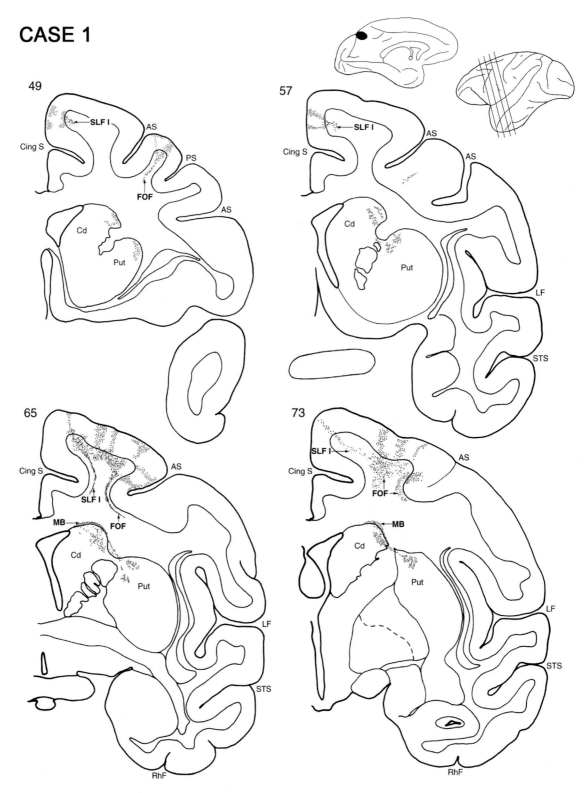

Figure 6-1

Schematic diagrams of 15 rostral–caudal coronal sections in Case 1 taken at the levels shown on the hemispheric diagram above right, to depict the isotope injection site in the medial convexity of the superior parietal lobule in area PGm, encroaching on area PEc (black filled area) and the resulting trajectories of the cortical association, commissural, and subcortical fibers (dashed lines and dots) in

CASE 1

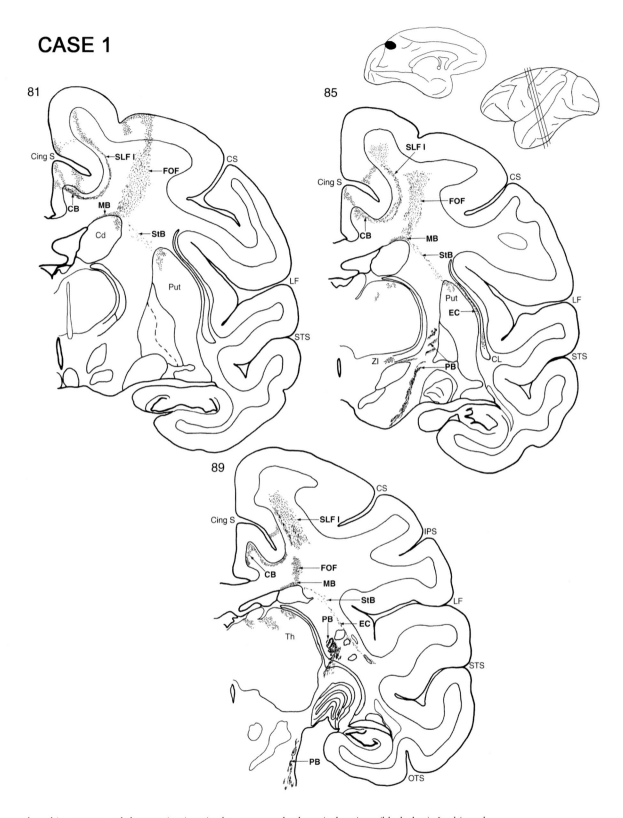

the white matter, and the terminations in the cortex and subcortical regions (black dots). In this and subsequent figures, the association and subcortical fiber pathways are labeled with bold font, and the number at the left upper corner of each coronal section corresponds to the level shown in the photomicrograph of the template brain. See list of abbreviations, p. 617.

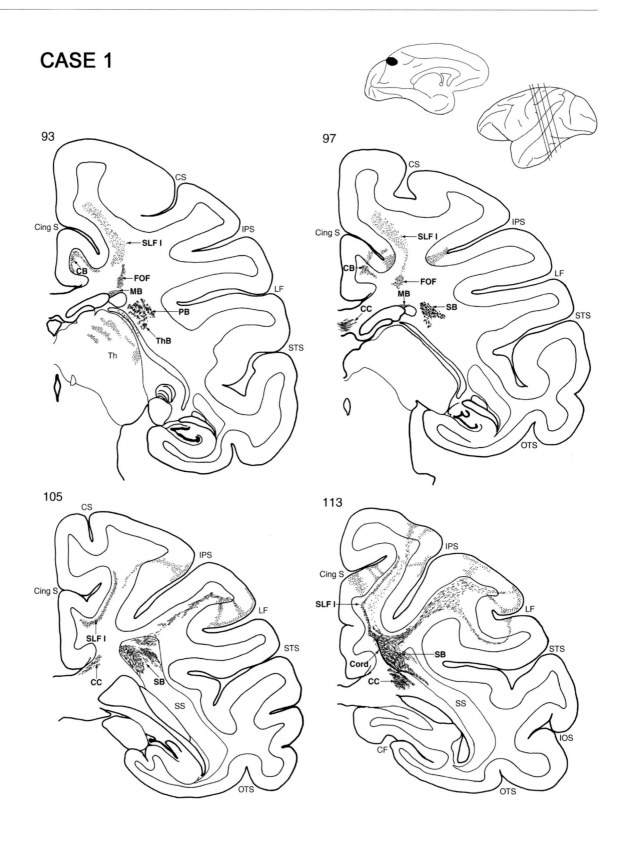

Figure 6-1 (continued)

CASE 1

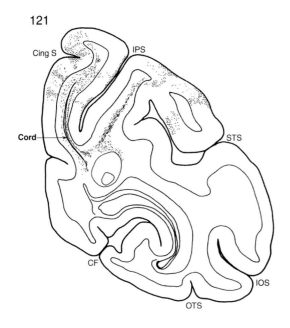

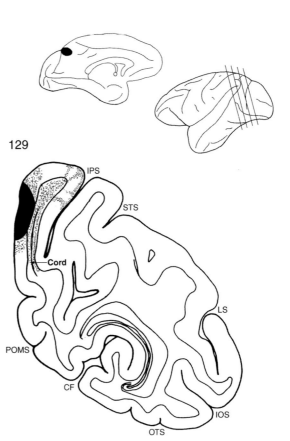

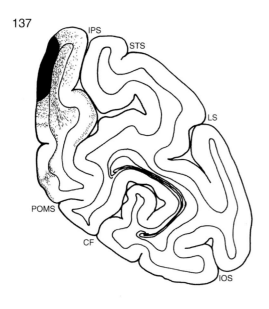

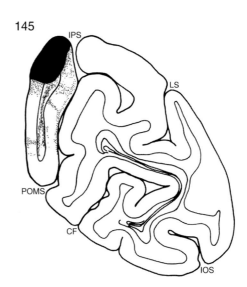

CASE 1

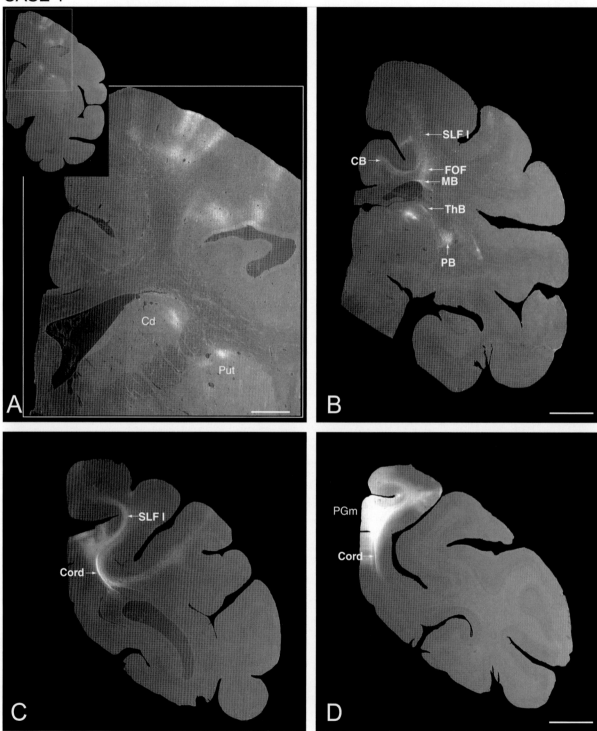

Figure 6-2

Photomicrographs of selected coronal sections of Case 1 to show the injection site in D, as well as the resulting labeled fibers and terminations in A through D. A, High-power photomicrograph (section 65, Mag = 1×, bar = 2.5 mm), taken from the location indicated in the low-power photomicrograph in the inset. Photomicrographs B through D correspond to sections 89, 113, and 129 respectively (Mag = 0.5×, bar = 5 mm).

CASE 2

In Case 2 the isotope injection involved the caudal superior parietal lobule, in the medial part of area PEc at the junction of area PE (Scs. 121, 129). See figures 6-3 and 6-4.

Association Fibers

Local Association Fibers

Local terminations adjacent to the injection site are evident in areas PEc and PGm in a columnar manner (Sc. 129).

Long Association Fibers

Caudally Directed Fibers

A small contingent of fibers travels caudally from the injection site in the SPL white matter and terminates in area PEc with a mixed first-layer and columnar pattern (Scs. 137, 145).

Rostrally Directed Fibers

Fibers leave the injection site and travel rostrally within the white matter of the superior parietal lobule, in the SLF I.

The upper part of SLF I gives rise to terminations in the first layer in area PEa in the upper bank of the IPS, and in areas 2, 1, and 3 as the fibers move rostrally (Scs. 97, 105). Further forward in the frontal lobe, the SLF I fibers course within the white matter of the superior frontal gyrus and give rise to terminations that are mainly columnar in dorsal area 4, and in the dorsal part of area 6 (Scs. 81, 89, 93).

Some of the fibers from the SLF I become concentrated around the depth of the cingulate sulcus, occupying the cingulate fasciculus. These fibers move rostrally in this location and provide columnar terminations in the depth of the cingulate sulcus in area 24d, and in area 24c in the cortex of the lower bank of the cingulate sulcus (Scs. 89, 93).

A collection of fibers streams laterally and ventrally from the dorsal aspect of the SLF I and curves laterally around the depth of the IPS, passing through SLF II, and enters the white matter of the inferior parietal lobule. These fibers terminate in the caudal upper bank of the Sylvian fissure, in the first layer of the second somatosensory area, SII (Scs. 97, 105).

Commissural and Subcortical Fibers

The dense cord of fibers that leaves the injection site makes a steep descent in the central part of the white matter of the superior parietal lobule. It remains as a concentrated bundle until it reaches the depth of the IPS, at which stage it separates into two distinct components (Scs. 97, 105).

The medial component flares out and feeds the lateral aspect of the corpus callosum in sector CC4, as the heavy concentration of fibers heads towards the opposite hemisphere (Scs. 93, 97).

The lateral concentration of fibers (SB) descends obliquely in a vertical and rostral direction into the retrolenticular capsule at level ICp-5 (Sc. 97). As the fibers move rostrally into ICp-4 and ICp-3 (Scs. 93, 89) they are further distinguishable as two separate components, one dorsomedial and one ventrolateral.

The dorsomedial capsular subcortical bundle (the thalamic bundle) penetrates the external medullary lamina, traverses the thalamic reticular nucleus, and terminates in the LP, ventral posterolateral (VPL), and ventral lateral (VL) nuclei, as well as in the pulvinar oralis (PO), PM, and lateral pulvinar (PL) nuclei (Scs. 89, 93).

The ventrolateral subcortical fibers constitute the pontine bundle (PB), and these continue rostrally in the internal capsule as a prominent aggregation of fibers until they reach the ICp-2 above the rostral aspect of the LGN (Sc. 85). At this level, the fibers in the PB descend sharply into the lateral aspect of the cerebral peduncle on their way to the basilar pontine nuclei, where they terminate in the lateral and dorsal parts of the intrapeduncular and peripeduncular nuclei that surround the traversing corticofugal fibers, and to a lesser extent in the dorsal, dorsolateral, lateral, and ventral pontine nuclei. A small contingent of fibers leaves the medial aspect of the pontine bundle to travel around the subthalamic nucleus and terminate in the zona incerta (Sc. 85).

Striatal Fibers

At the level of the rostral tip of the IPS, fibers from the SLF I descend through the fronto-occipital fasciculus (FOF) to enter the MB. From there they descend to enter and terminate in the adjacent part of the body of the caudate nucleus (Scs. 85, 89).

Other fibers derived from the SLF I descend laterally as a striatal bundle (StB), course through the external capsule, and terminate in the caudal part of the claustrum and in the islands of the putamen (Scs. 69, 73, 81, 85, 89).

Some fibers from the MB cross laterally, adjacent to the posterior limb of the internal capsule, and terminate in the form of discrete aggregates in the dorsal aspects of the putamen (Scs. 85, 89).

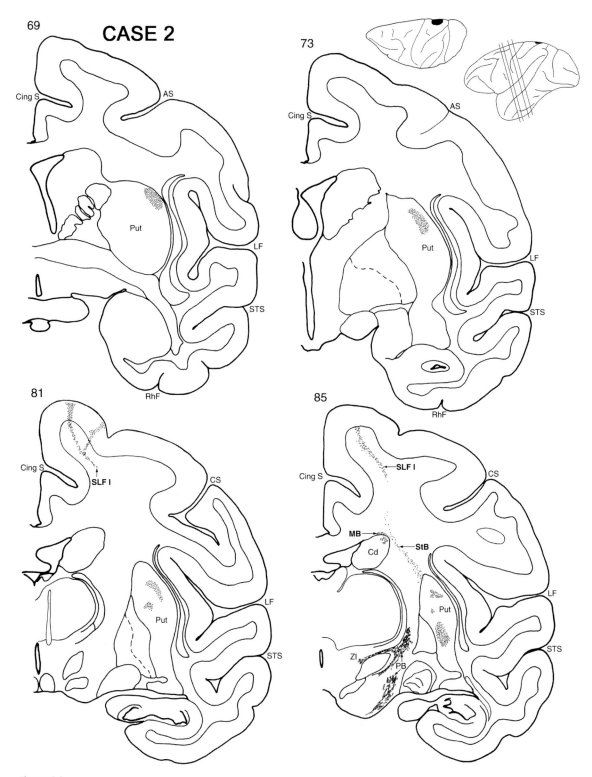

Figure 6-3

Schematic diagrams of 13 rostral–caudal coronal sections in Case 2 taken at the levels shown on the hemispheric diagram above right, to depict the isotope injection site in the caudal superior parietal lobule, in the medial part of area PEc at the junction of area PE (black filled area) and the resulting trajectories of the cortical association, commissural, and subcortical fibers (dashed lines and dots) in the white matter, and the terminations in the cortex and subcortical regions (black dots).

CASE 2

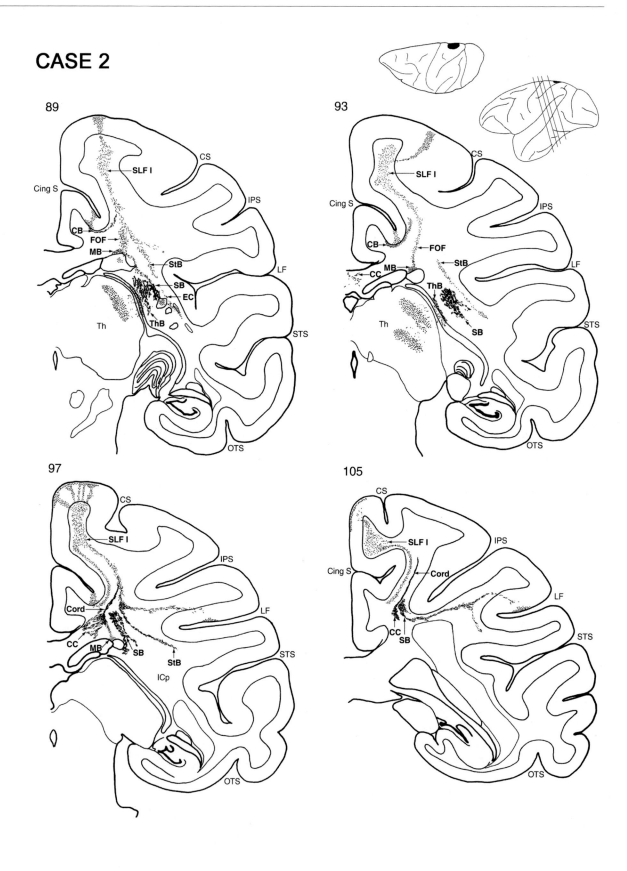

Figure 6-3 (continued)

CASE 2

113

SLF I
Cing S
Cord
IPS
LF
STS
IOS
CF
OTS

121

Cord
IPS
STS
CF
IOS
OTS

129

IPS
STS
Cord
POMS
CF
OTS

137

IPS
STS
LS
POMS
CF

145

IPS
LS
POMS
CF
IOS

CASE 2

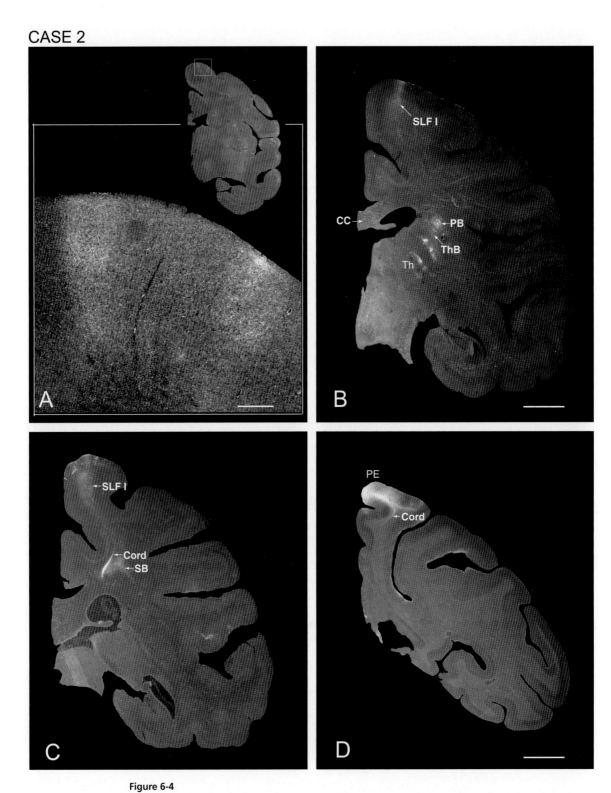

Figure 6-4
Photomicrographs of selected coronal sections of Case 2 to show the injection site in D, as well as the resulting labeled fibers and terminations in A through D. A, High-power photomicrograph (section 81, Mag = 4×, bar = 0.5 mm), taken from the location indicated in the low-power photomicrograph in the inset to show terminations in the junction of areas 4 and 6. Photomicrographs B through D correspond to sections 93, 105, and 129 respectively (Mag = 0.5×, bar = 5 mm).

CASE 3

In this case isotope was injected in the caudal superior parietal lobule, at the lateral part of area PEc (Sc. 129). See figures 6-5 and 6-6.

Association Fibers

Local Association Fibers

Local association fibers terminate near the injection site in a columnar manner in areas PGm, PEc, and PEa (Sc. 129).

Long Association Fibers

Caudally Directed Fibers

Caudal to the injection site, fibers travel in the white matter of the upper part of the superior parietal lobule and terminate in area PEc, first in a columnar manner and then in the first layer. Some fibers also terminate in the upper bank of the IPS in the caudal portion of area PEa (corresponding to area PO) (Scs. 137, 145).

Rostrally Directed Fibers

In the vicinity of the injection site, fibers travel rostrally in the white matter of the SPL and terminate in area PEc and in area PEci (supplementary somatosensory area [SSA]) in the cortex of the cingulate sulcus. On the lateral side of the superior parietal lobule there are terminations in the upper bank of the IPS in area PEa, and further rostrally in area PE. All these terminations are columnar (Scs. 113, 121).

A distinct contingent of fibers courses laterally around the depth of the IPS and moves into the white matter of the inferior parietal lobule before it terminates in a columnar manner in the caudal part of the parietal operculum, in area PGop (Scs. 105, 113).

The long association fibers that constitute the SLF I move rostrally as a loosely arranged system that lies in the crown of the superior parietal lobule. As it moves rostrally, the SLF I occupies the white matter, first of the superior parietal lobule and then of the superior frontal gyrus.

Fibers leave the SLF I medially and form a compact bundle in the cingulate fasciculus that lies immediately beneath the depth of the cingulate sulcus. These fibers terminate in a columnar manner in the depth of the cingulate sulcus in area 24d for a considerable distance along its rostrocaudal extent (Scs. 73, 81, 85, 89, 93). Terminations are also present at the crown of the lower bank of the cingulate sulcus in area 24b, as well as in the upper bank of the cingulate sulcus in the cingulate motor area (Sc. 89).

The remaining fibers of the SLF I constitute the bulk of this bundle. They move forward in the dorsal part of the white matter of the superior frontal gyrus. Fibers leave this bundle and terminate in the dorsal and medial parts of area 4 in a columnar manner but with emphasis in the first layer (Scs. 89, 93). The SLF I fibers continue rostrally and then terminate in dorsal area 6, as well as in the supplementary motor area, in a columnar manner (Scs. 49, 57, 65, 73).

At the rostral end of the fronto-occipital fasciculus (see below), some fibers join the SLF I fibers to terminate in dorsal area 6 (Sc. 73).

Commissural and Subcortical Fibers

From the injection site a dense cord of fibers descends sharply in the central part of the white matter of the superior parietal lobule. During its course this cord is sometimes divisible into two parallel segments. As it reaches the cingulate white matter, the fibers in the cord fan out and divide into two separate systems.

The medial group of fibers descends medial to the fronto-occipital fasciculus and penetrates the corpus callosum in CC5 (Sc. 105) before it moves rostrally and crosses in the midline in CC4 (Scs. 97, 93) to reach the opposite hemisphere (Sc. 93).

The other component, the subcortical bundle, passes lateral to the fronto-occipital fasciculus and occupies the medial and dorsal aspect of the rostral part of sector SS-2 of the sagittal stratum (Sc. 105). These fibers continue forwards into the retrolenticular part of the internal capsule, ICp-5 (Sc. 97), where they divide further into medial (thalamic) and lateral (pontine) bundles.

The thalamic fibers continue rostrally into ICp-4 (Sc. 93), pass through the reticular nucleus and external medullary lamina, and enter the dorsal part of the thalamus. As fibers move rostrally within the lateral thalamic peduncle, they give rise to terminations in intensely labeled lamellae in LP, PL, and VPL nuclei (Scs. 85, 89, 93, 97).

The pontine fiber bundle first evident as a discrete entity in retrolenticular internal capsule level ICp-5 (Sc. 97) comprises parallel lamellae of labeled fibers that continue rostrally in the internal capsule, medial to the putamen, reaching ICp-2 (Sc. 85). As these fibers reach the midpoint of the LGN in ICp-3 (Sc. 89), they descend sharply and course first dorsal to and then medial to the LGN. They then travel in the lateral aspect of the cerebral peduncle (Scs. 93, 89, 85) and terminate in the peripeduncular, lateral, dorsal, and dorsolateral pontine nuclei and to a smaller extent in the intrapeduncular nucleus and the nucleus reticularis tegmenti pontis.

Striatal Fibers

A distinct group of fibers traveling along with the association fibers in the superior frontal gyrus has two discernible components, one traveling laterally and the other medially. The laterally placed striatal bundle (StB) descends and crosses lateral to the ICp through the corona radiata, enters the external capsule (EC), and terminates in the caudal part of the claustrum. More rostrally, these fibers are joined by those arising from the MB to provide considerable terminations in the dorsal and lateral segments of the rostral part of the putamen (Scs. 49, 57, 65, 73, 81, 85, 89).

The medially placed striatal fibers leave the medial component of the SLF I and descend towards the fronto-occipital fasciculus (FOF). They then pass through the FOF and aggregate in the MB. The Muratoff fibers progress rostrally until they reach the head of the caudate nucleus, where they terminate in its dorsal and lateral segments (Scs. 49, 57, 65, 73). Some fibers from the MB cross over the internal capsule to provide terminations in the putamen.

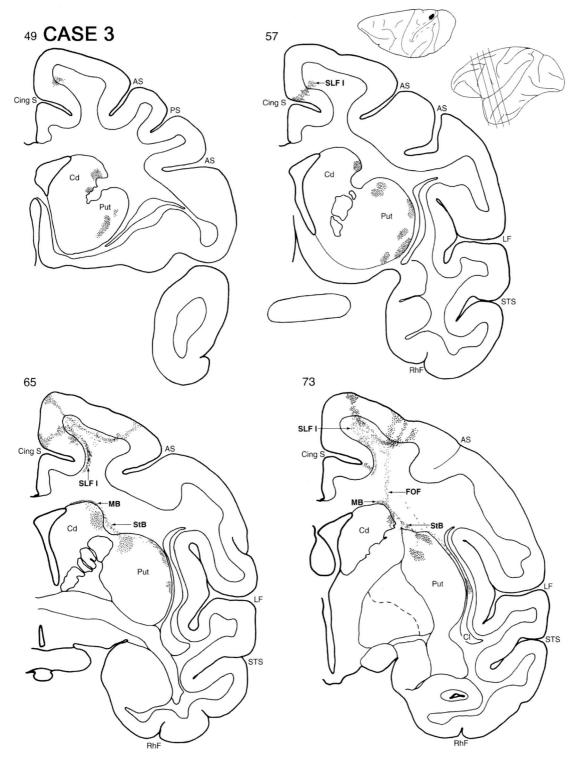

Figure 6-5

Schematic diagrams of 15 rostral–caudal coronal sections in Case 3 taken at the levels shown on the hemispheric diagram above right, to depict the isotope injection site in the caudal superior parietal lobule, at the lateral part of area PEc (black filled area) and the resulting trajectories of the cortical association, commissural, and subcortical fibers (dashed lines and dots) in the white matter, and the terminations in the cortex and subcortical regions (black dots).

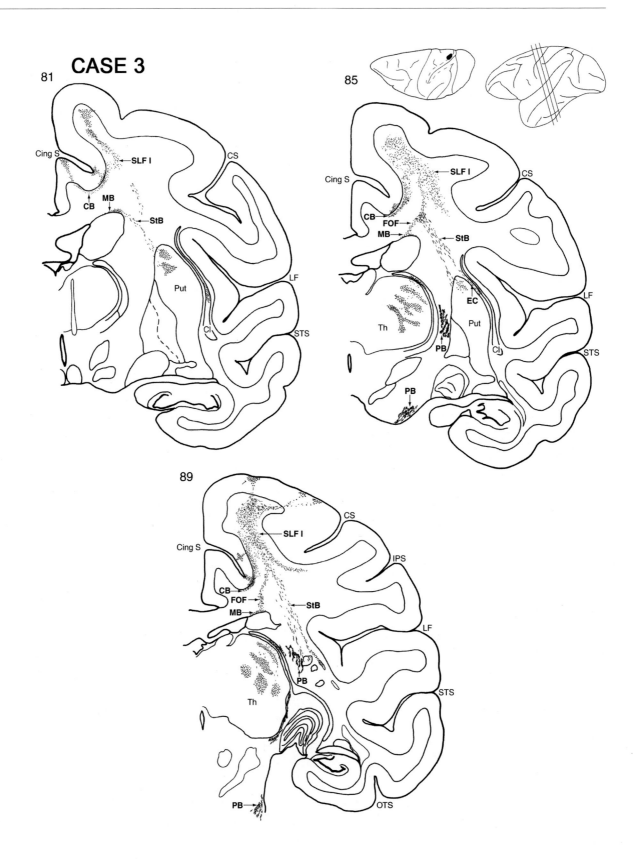

Figure 6-5 (continued)

CASE 3

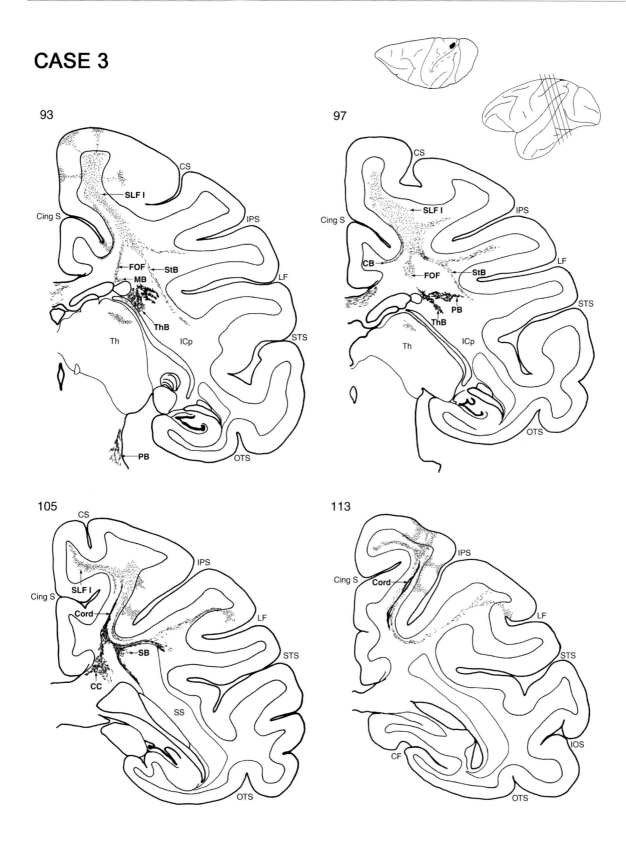

CASE 3

121

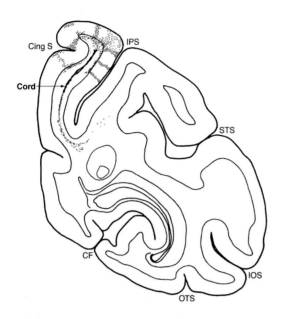

129

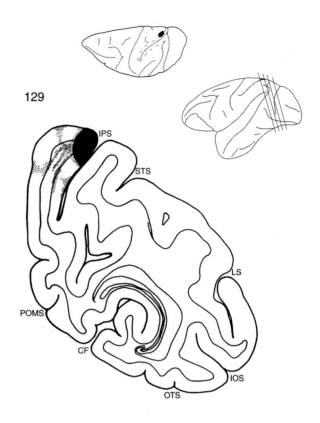

137

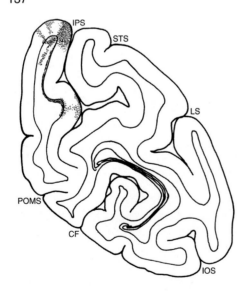

145

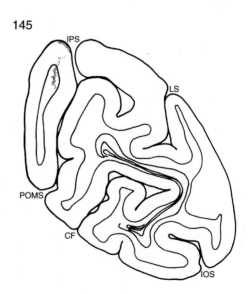

Figure 6-5 (continued)

CASE 3

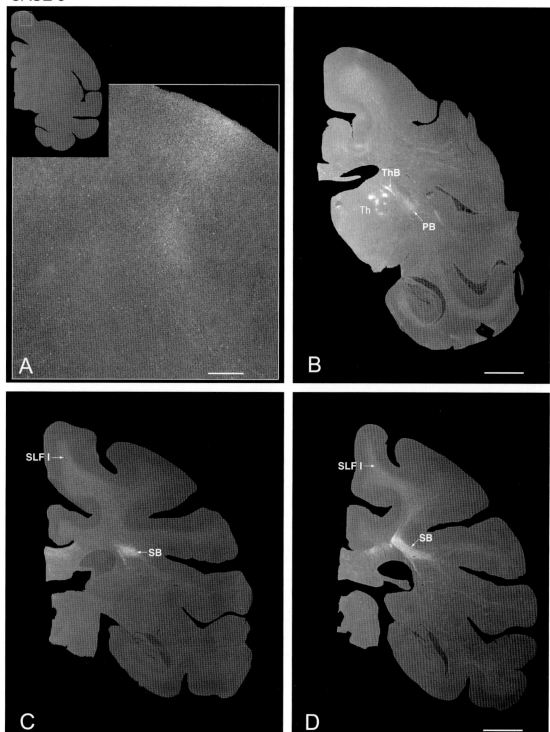

Figure 6-6

Photomicrographs of selected coronal sections of Case 3 to show the injection site in F with the injection halo in E and the resulting labeled fibers and terminations in A through F. A, High-power photomicrograph (section 73, Mag = 4×, bar = 0.5 mm), taken from the location indicated in the low-power photomicrograph in the inset to show terminations in area 6d. Photomicrographs B through F correspond to sections 85, 97, 105, 121, and 129 respectively (Mag = 0.5×, bar = 5 mm). (*Figure continued on next page*)

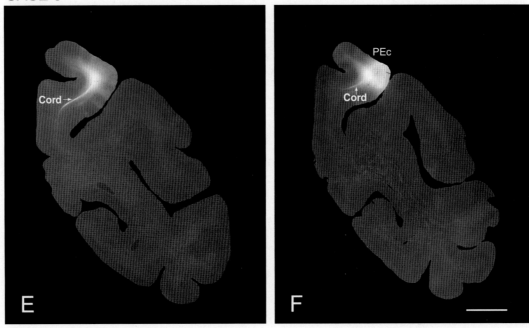

Figure 6-6 (continued)

CASE 4

Isotope was injected in the inferior parietal lobule in this case, in the caudal part of area PG and in area Opt (Scs. 121, 129, 137). See figures 6-7 and 6-8.

Fibers leave the injection site and descend medially within the white matter core of the inferior parietal lobule. In the center of the core are two parallel cords of intensely labeled fibers. Surrounding these cords and intermingling with them are the association fibers that travel both within the coronal plane of section (descending medially) and perpendicular to the coronal plane (coursing rostrally and caudally).

Association Fibers

Local Association Fibers

Local fibers travel in the white matter subjacent to the cortex and provide columnar terminations to the inferior parietal lobule in areas PG and PGop (Sc. 113). Terminations are also distributed in the depth of the intraparietal sulcus in area IPd (also termed area VIP) (Scs. 113, 121, 129, 137).

Neighborhood Association Fibers

Medially directed fibers arch around the depth of the IPS and ascend in the core of the SPL, along with the fibers of the SLF I, to provide neighborhood connections in the form of a series of columnar terminations in area PGm at the level of the injection site (Scs. 121, 129, 137).

Long Association Fibers

Caudally Directed Fibers

Association fibers traveling caudal from the injection site are situated within the preoccipital gyrus. These fibers are divided into two components. Laterally directed fibers are located in the preoccipital gyrus and terminate in the first layer in area Opt, in area V4D up to the lunate sulcus, and in area V4A in the annectant gyrus (Sc. 145). Medially directed fibers ascend in the white matter of the SPL and course caudally in the white matter of the parieto-occipital cortex. These fibers terminate in areas PGm and PO, in both a columnar manner and in the first layer (Sc. 145).

Rostrally Directed Fibers

The rostrally directed association fibers proceed medially, laterally, and ventrally. The medially directed association fibers ascend within the white matter of the SPL and terminate in area 31 below the cingulate sulcus (Scs. 105, 113). Other fibers continue forward and become incorporated into the part of the cingulum bundle (CB) situated in the white matter of the cingulate gyrus. These fibers travel rostrally and terminate first in area 23 in the cingulate gyrus and in the retrosplenial cortex in areas 30 and 29 (Scs. 93, 97, 105, 113). Further forward, the fibers terminate in area 24 in the cingulate gyrus (Scs. 57, 73, 81, 85, 89). All these terminations are columnar.

Another group of medially directed fibers destined for the ventral part of the CB courses medially from the injection site, travels within the IPL white matter, and continues medially, caudal to the splenium of the corpus callosum. These fibers then descend vertically, directed toward the retrosplenial cortex. The fibers turn laterally and lie between the calcarine cortex and the embedded caudal part of the corpus callosum. They then enter the retrosplenial portion of the cingulum bundle and continue ventrally and medially within the ventral cingulum bundle before they terminate in the presubiculum (Scs. 89, 93, 97, 105).

The lateral component of fibers emanating from the injection site travels rostrally within the IPL core and descends gradually into the white matter of the superior temporal gyrus. These fibers constitute a distinct association bundle termed the middle longitudinal fasciculus (MdLF). The fibers in this bundle course rostrally in the core of the superior temporal gyrus (STG) white matter and terminate in the upper bank of the superior temporal sulcus (STS) in area TPO in interrupted patches as the bundle moves rostrally. Terminations are also present in the depth of the STS in area PGa and in area IPa (Scs. 85, 89, 93, 97, 113).

Association fibers that course ventrally from the injection site are situated within the inferior longitudinal fasciculus (ILF) that lies between the sagittal stratum and the white matter subjacent to the STS. These fibers form a thin plate that courses rostrally. The ventral component of the bundle descends, arches over the occipitotemporal sulcus (OTS), and provides first-layer terminations to cortex medial to the OTS (area V3V) and lateral to the OTS (area V4V) (Scs. 105, 113, 121). Further rostrally, these fibers terminate in a columnar manner in area TF, lying medial to the OTS, and then in ventral temporal cortex, in area TL laterally and area TH medially (Scs. 89, 93, 97).

A major contingent of fibers leaves the injection site, enters the SLF II and runs rostrally, located in the medial part of the white matter core of the IPL. As it continues rostrally, the SLF II forms a compact bundle that runs above the Sylvian fissure and lateral to the corona radiata. Further forward these fibers course underneath the central sulcus and at the upper shoulder of the Sylvian fissure. In this position the fibers reach the frontal lobe, at which point they fan out into a thin plate that lies under the arcuate sulcus (Scs. 41–114). These fibers give rise to columnar terminations in dorsal area 6, dorsal area 8, and further rostrally in dorsal area 9 and in area 46 on both banks of the principal sulcus (Scs. 41, 49, 57, 65). Also, columnar terminations are seen in medial area 9, and in area 45 lying at the ventrolateral prefrontal convexity (Scs. 31, 41).

Commissural and Subcortical Fibers

Two parallel intensely labeled cords of fibers emanate from the injection site and descend medially in the white matter of the IPL.

The dorsal cord of fibers continues further medially and fans out as it lies above the sagittal stratum. These fibers penetrate the splenium (Scs. 105, 113) and move rostrally before passing through the midline in sector CC4 (Scs. 89, 93, 97).

The ventral part of this cord of fibers also continues medially and fans out as it enters the dorsal segment of the caudal part of sector SS-2 of the sagittal stratum (Sc. 121). These fibers turn and course rostrally in this location in SS-2 (Scs. 105, 113). Further rostrally, as they enter the retrolenticular parts of the internal capsule, ICp-5 (Sc. 97) and ICp-4 (Sc. 93), two distinct components can be discerned within these rostrally directed fibers.

A medial bundle traverses the thalamic reticular nucleus and external medullary lamina and terminates in a number of thalamic nuclei, including PM, lateral dorsal (LD), limitans (Li), and intralaminar nuclei (Scs. 89, 93, 97).

The lateral bundle of fibers coursing rostrally in the retrolenticular part of the internal capsule continues into ICp-3 (Sc. 89) and aggregates over the midpoint of the LGN. At level ICp-2 (Sc. 85), these fibers descend sharply, medial to the LGN, and enter the lateral aspect of the cerebral peduncle. These fibers course toward and terminate mostly in lateral locations in the basis pontis, in the lateral and dorsolateral pontine nuclei, and lateral parts of the peripeduncular nucleus. Some fibers leave the pontine bundle in ICp-2 before its descent into the cerebral peduncle, course above the subthalamic nucleus, and terminate in the zona incerta (Sc. 85).

Striatal Fibers

Fibers destined for the caudate nucleus travel initially with the rostrally directed association fibers lying within the IPL white matter. The striatal fibers course medially into the fronto-occipital fasciculus. They then leave the FOF, enter the MB, and then terminate throughout the rostrocaudal extent of the body and head of the caudate nucleus (Scs. 41–97). Fibers from the MB course ventrally and terminate also in the genu of the caudate nucleus (Sc. 105). As the fronto-occipital fasciculus moves rostrally, it merges with the SLF II. Some fibers within the IPL core descend into the external capsule and terminate in the ventral and middle parts of the claustrum and more rostrally in the dorsal and ventral aspects of the putamen (Scs. 49, 73, 81, 85, 89).

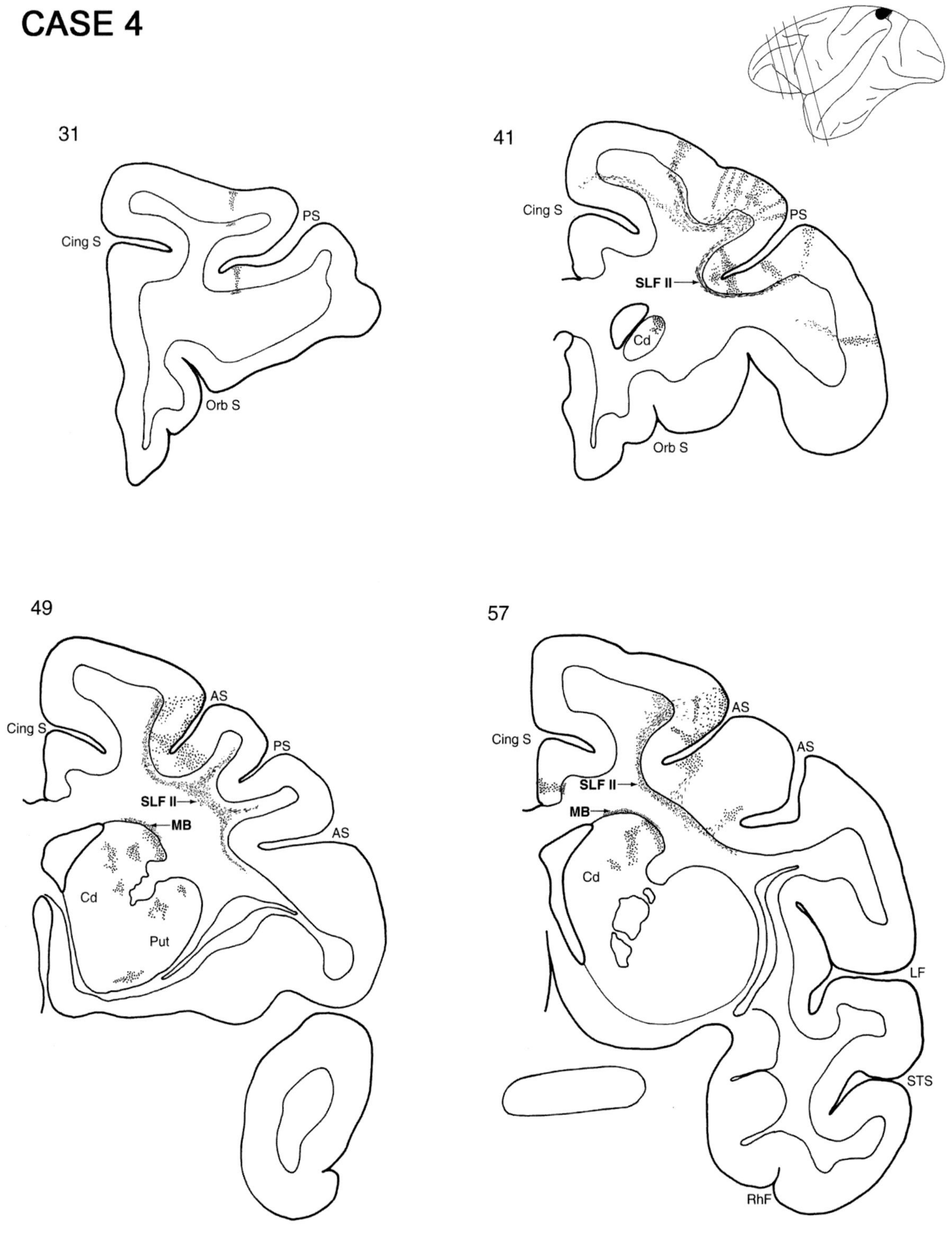

Figure 6-7

Schematic diagrams of 17 rostral–caudal coronal sections in Case 4 taken at the levels shown on the hemispheric diagram above right, to depict the isotope injection site in the inferior parietal lobule in the caudal part of area PG and in area Opt (black filled area), and the resulting trajectories of the cortical association, commissural, and subcortical fibers (dashed lines and dots) in the white matter, and the terminations in the cortex and subcortical regions (black dots).

CASE 4

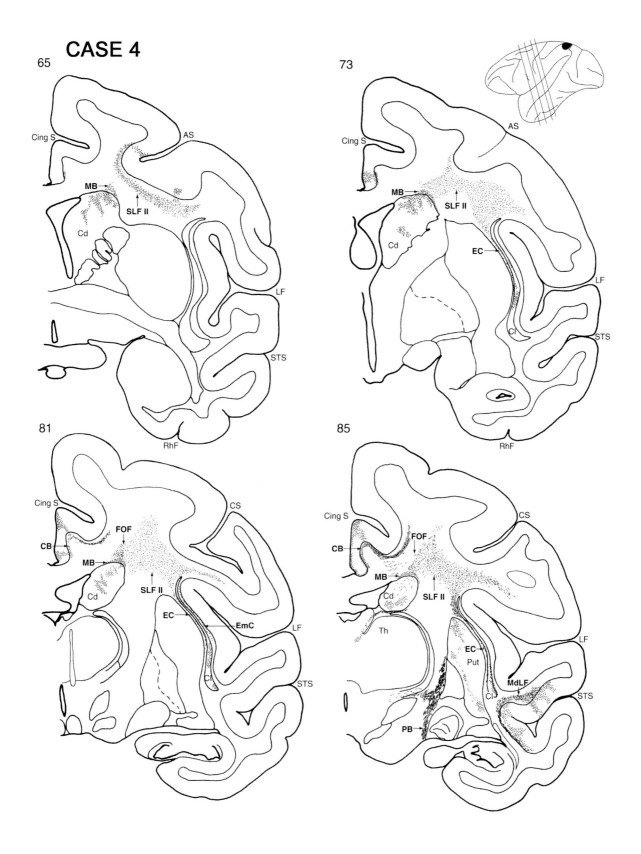

CASE 4

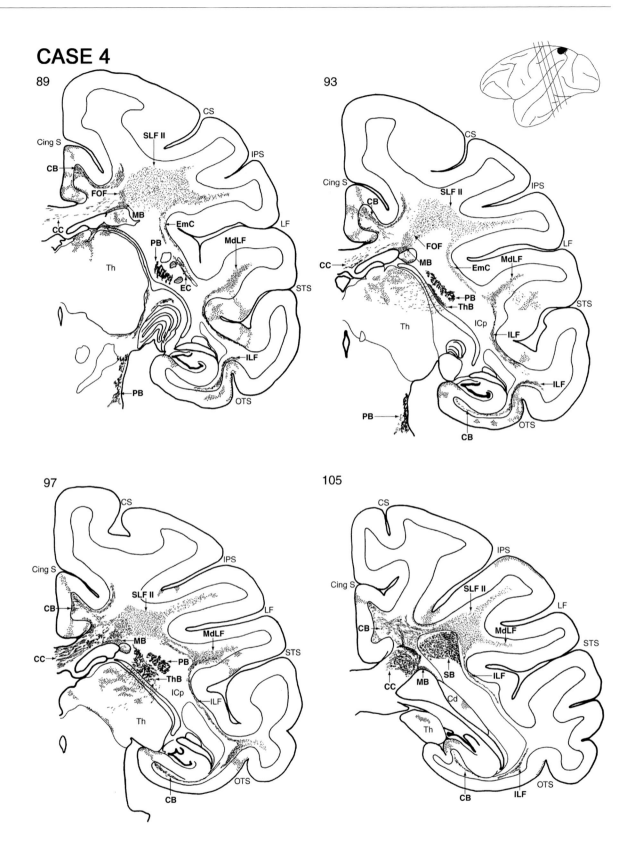

Figure 6-7 (continued)

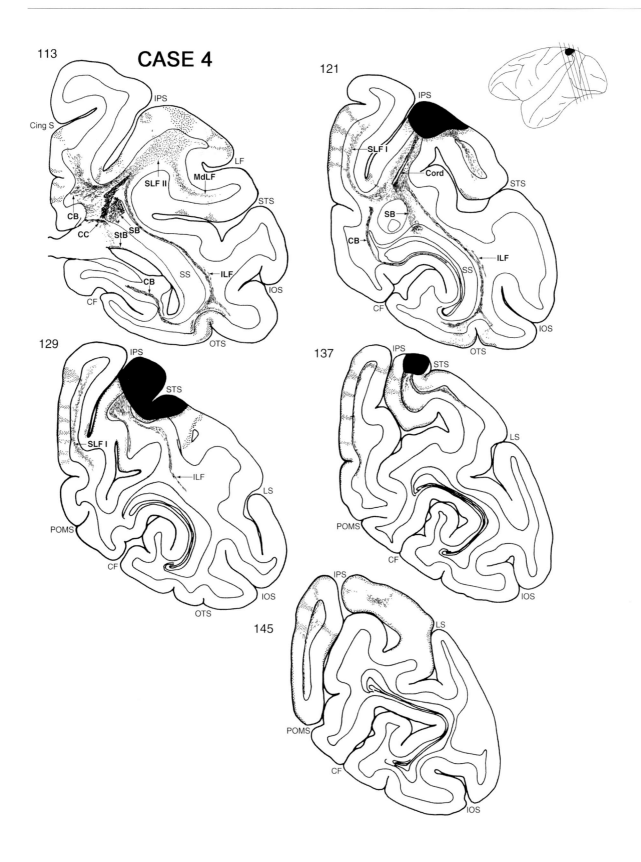

CASE 4

113

Cing S
IPS
LF
SLF II
MdLF
STS
CB
CC
StB
SB
CB
SS
ILF
CF
IOS
OTS

121

IPS
SLF I
Cord
STS
SB
CB
SS
ILF
CF
IOS
OTS

129

IPS
STS
SLF I
ILF
LS
POMS
CF
IOS
OTS

137

IPS
STS
LS
POMS
CF
IOS

145

IPS
LS
POMS
CF
IOS

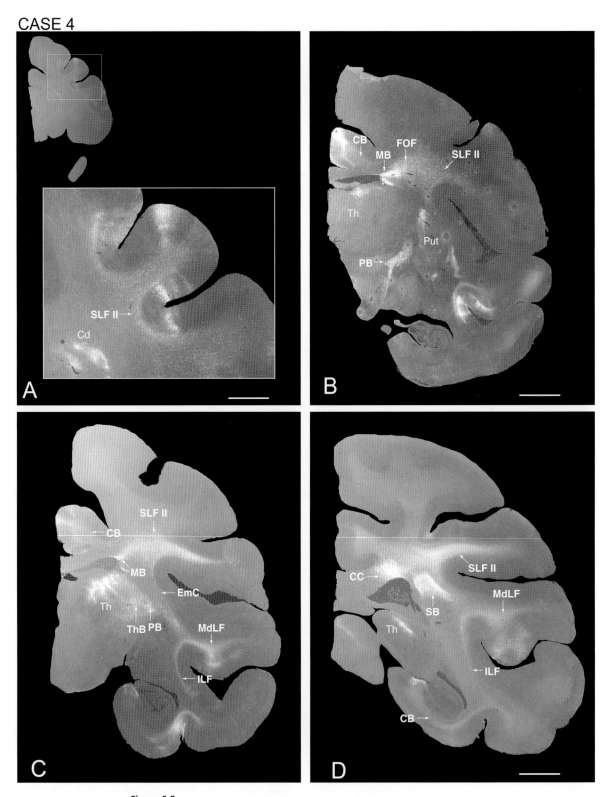

Figure 6-8

Photomicrographs of selected coronal sections of Case 4 to show the injection site in F and the resulting labeled fibers and terminations in A through F. A, High-power photomicrograph (at a level between sections 41 and 49, Mag = 1×, bar = 2.5 mm), taken from the location indicated in the low-

CASE 4

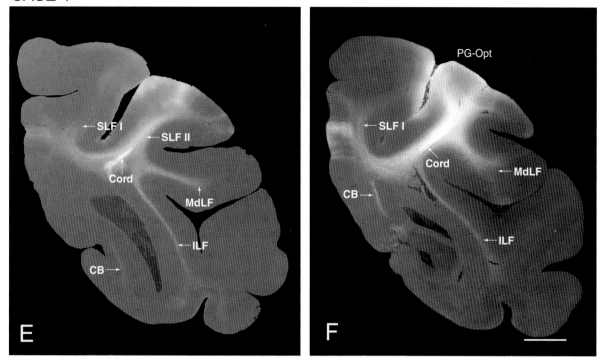

power photomicrograph in the inset to demonstrate terminations in area 8Ad, 9/46d and 9/46v, and area 6d. Photomicrographs B through F correspond to sections 85, 93, 105, 113, and 121 respectively (Mag = 0.5×, bar = 5 mm).

CASE 5

In this case, isotope injection was into the rostral inferior parietal lobule, area PF (Scs. 89, 93, 97). See figures 6-9 and 6-10.

Association Fibers

Local Association Fibers

From the injection site fibers travel within the white matter subjacent to the lower bank of the IPS and provide discrete columns of termination in areas POa and IPd (Scs. 93, 97).

Neighborhood Association Fibers

Distinct terminations are conveyed via the white matter of the superior parietal lobule to areas 1 and 3b in the lower bank of the central sulcus (Scs. 93,97). Also, columnar terminations are seen in area Ri in the depth of the Sylvian fissure, conveyed by the white matter near the injection site (Sc. 93).

Long Association Fibers

Caudally Directed Fibers

Association fibers travel caudally in the white matter in two distinct bundles.

A dorsal fiber bundle lies subjacent to the cortex of the lower bank of the IPS and terminates in a columnar manner in area POa and in area IPd (Scs. 105, 113). These fibers continue medially and then curve around the depth of the IPS to ascend in the white matter of the superior parietal lobule. They terminate in area 1 in a columnar manner and then in the first layers of areas 3b and 3a in the caudal bank and depth of the central sulcus (Sc. 105). Further caudally, these medially directed fibers terminate in a columnar manner in area 2 (Sc. 113).

The ventral fiber bundle lies subjacent to the cortex of the Sylvian fissure. It provides columnar terminations to the retroinsular vestibular cortex, area Ri (Sc. 93), situated in the depth of the Sylvian fissure, and to area PGop in the caudal part of the parietal operculum (Sc. 113).

Rostrally Directed Fibers

An association fiber bundle leaves the injection site and travels rostrally within the white matter of the parietal operculum (the SLF III). Fibers leave this bundle and terminate in the first layer in the lower bank of the central sulcus in area 3b, as well as in the first layer in areas 1 and 2 (Scs. 81, 85). The fibers also terminate in area 3a in a columnar manner (Sc. 81). A substantial contingent of fibers within the SLF III provides columnar terminations in the upper bank of the Sylvian fissure, in SII (Scs. 81, 85).

The most rostral contingent of SLF III provides columnar terminations to the ventral part of premotor area 6, the posterior bank of the ventral limb of the arcuate sulcus in area 44, and the gustatory area lying in the most rostral part of the frontal operculum (Scs. 49, 57, 65, 73).

Commissural and Subcortical Fibers

From the injection site a dense cord of fibers travels medially in the central part of the white matter of the inferior parietal lobule. In the inferior parietal lobule at a level corresponding to the caudal part of the insula, the cord of fibers divides into two main components.

One major contingent continues medially to enter the corpus callosum at sector CC4 (Sc. 93) and passes to the opposite hemisphere in the ventral and central parts of this sector (Scs. 85, 89).

The other contingent, the subcortical bundle, descends vertically from the main bundle into the posterior limb of the internal capsule, ICp-4 (Sc. 93) and travels rostrally into ICp-3 (Sc. 89).

This capsular bundle further divides into two principal parts. Within ICp-3, the more medial and dorsal part traverses the thalamic external medullary lamina and thalamic reticular nucleus and terminates in the medial, inferior, and lateral parts of the ventral posterior nucleus (VPM, VPI, VPL), and in PO and the intralaminar nuclei (CL, centromedian [CM]) (Scs. 85, 89).

The ventral and lateral part of the capsular bundle descends in ICp-3 (Sc. 89) to lie above the midpoint of the LGN. From here the fibers continue into the lateral part of the cerebral peduncle (Sc. 89), with the most rostral tip of this descending fiber bundle visible at the ventral aspect of level ICp-2 (Sc. 85) and ICp-1 (Sc. 81). These fibers terminate in the basilar pontine nuclei, concentrated most heavily in the intrapenduncular and peripeduncular nuclei, with some terminations also in the lateral, dorsal, dorsolateral, and ventral pontine nuclei. A small contingent of fibers leaves the pontine bundle in ICp-2 and travels medially above the subthalamic nucleus to terminate in the zona incerta (Sc. 85).

Striatal Fibers

The fibers destined for the striatum and claustrum travel along with the association fibers that lie at the ventral part of the white matter of the IPL, but they are distinct from the SLF III. These fibers arch over the upper shoulder of the Sylvian fissure and enter the external and extreme capsules. From here they terminate in the middle part of the claustrum, and in most rostral levels they terminate in the dorsal aspect of the claustrum (Scs. 81, 85, 89). The external capsule fibers also provide considerable terminations to the putamen, first in its middle and ventral aspects and more rostrally in its lateral and ventral sectors (Scs. 57, 65, 73, 81, 85).

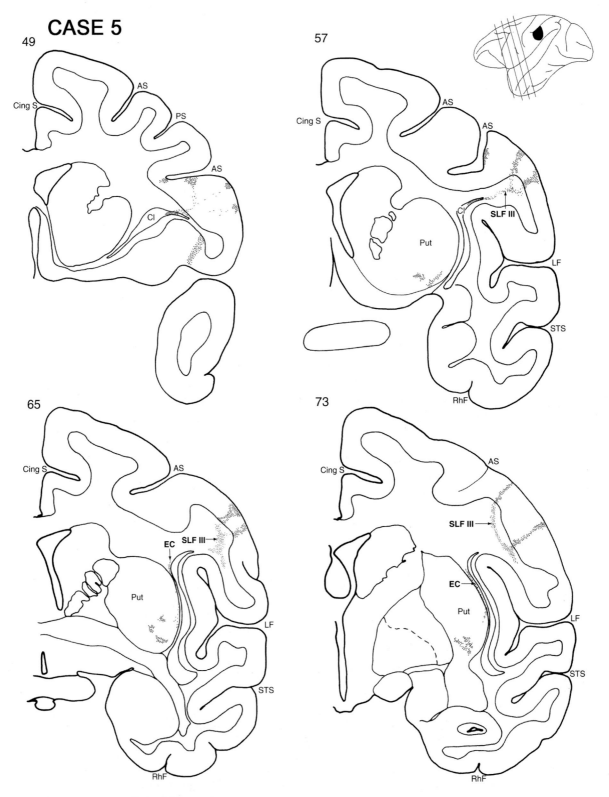

Figure 6-9

Schematic diagrams of 11 rostral–caudal coronal sections in Case 5 taken at the levels shown on the hemispheric diagram above right, to depict the isotope injection site in the rostral inferior parietal lobule, area PF (black filled area) and the resulting trajectories of the cortical association, commissural, and subcortical fibers (dashed lines and dots) in the white matter, and the terminations in the cortex and subcortical regions (black dots).

CASE 5

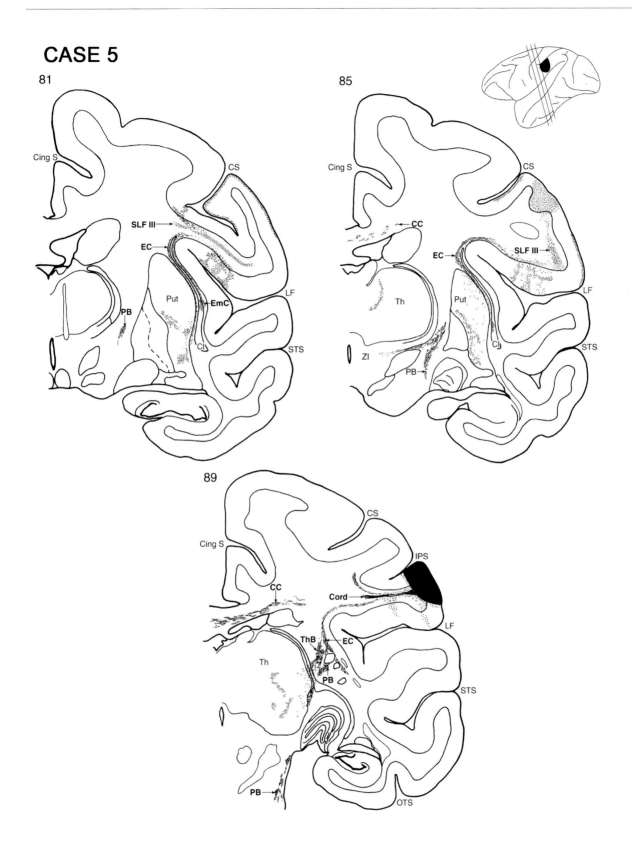

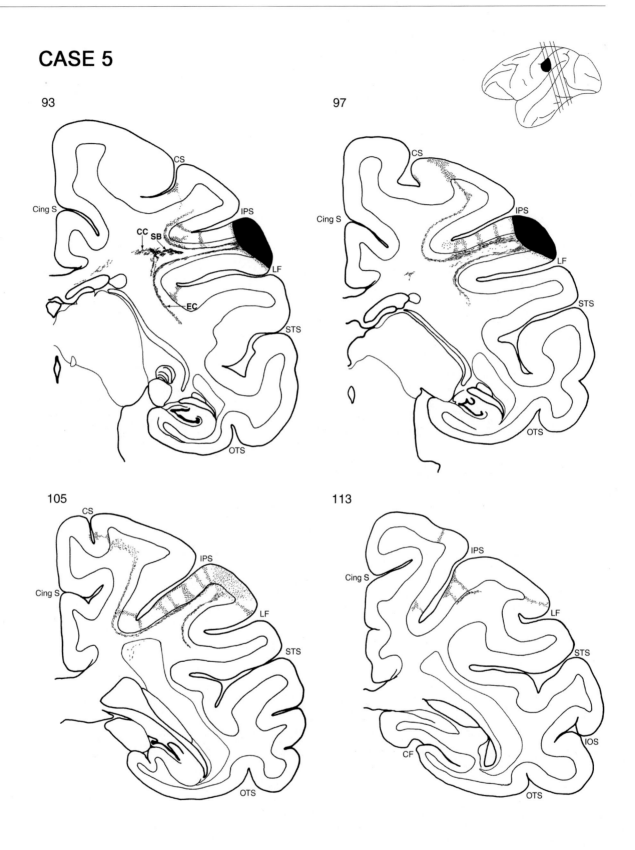

Figure 6-9 (continued)

CASE 5

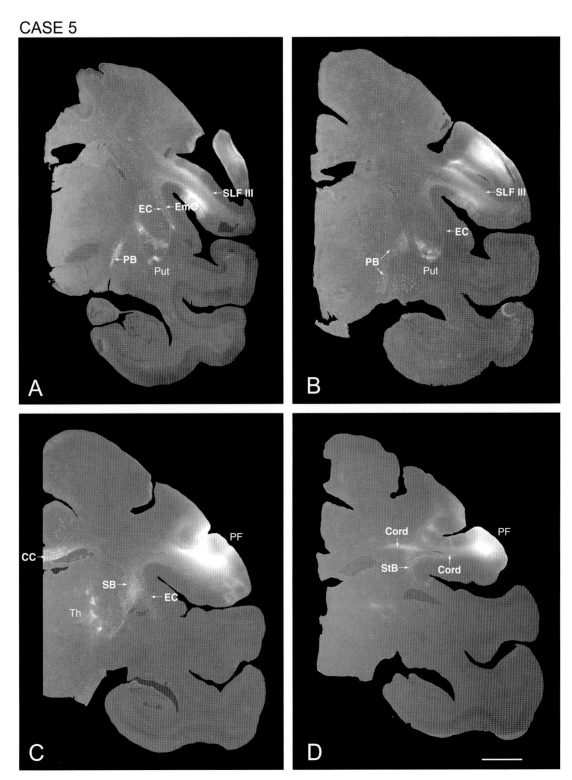

Figure 6-10

Photomicrographs of selected coronal sections of Case 5 to show the injection site in D with the injection halo in C and the resulting labeled fibers and terminations in A through D. Photomicrographs A through D correspond to sections 81, 85, 89, and 97, respectively (Mag = 0.5×, bar = 5

CASE 6

In this case, isotope was injected into the middle part of the parietal operculum (Scs. 89, 93, 97). See figures 6-11 and 6-12.

Association Fibers

Local Association Fibers

Adjacent to the injection site, terminations are noted in a columnar manner in areas PF and PFG in the inferior parietal lobule and in SII in the parietal operculum (Scs. 89, 93, 97).

Neighborhood Association Fibers

Neighborhood connections are conveyed by fibers traveling around the depth of the IPS to terminate in the first layer in areas 2 and 1 in the superior parietal lobule (Scs. 89, 93, 97).

Long Association Fibers

Caudally Directed Fibers

Fibers travel caudally from the injection site within the white matter situated immediately deep to the cortex of the intraparietal sulcus.

The fibers ventral to the intraparietal sulcus terminate in the first layer in area PGop at the parietal operculum and in area PG at the caudal inferior parietal lobule (Scs. 105, 113). As they continue caudally, these fibers give rise to terminations in the first layer in area POa at the lower bank of the intraparietal sulcus and area IPd at the depth of the intraparietal sulcus (Sc. 105).

The fibers dorsal to the intraparietal sulcus travel within the SLF I situated laterally within the white matter of the superior parietal lobule. They terminate in the first layer in area 2 and in a columnar manner in area PEa in the upper bank of the intraparietal sulcus (Scs. 105, 113, 121, 129).

Rostrally Directed Fibers

The major component of the rostrally directed long association fibers travels in the SLF III situated in the white matter of the parietal operculum and the frontal operculum. The SLF III fibers terminate in areas PF, 3b, and 2, in the first layer, and in the second somatosensory area, SII, in a columnar manner (Scs. 81, 85). More rostrally, in the frontal operculum, the SLF III fibers terminate in the ventral part of premotor area 6, in area 44 in the cortex of the lower bank of the arcuate sulcus, and in the gustatory cortex, all in a columnar manner (Scs. 49, 57, 65). As the SLF III fibers continue rostrally, they arch around the lower limb of the arcuate sulcus, course below the principal sulcus, and terminate in a columnar manner in the ventral part of area 46 in the middle part of the lower bank of the principal sulcus (Scs. 31, 41).

Some rostrally directed long association fibers leave the injection site and course medially to enter the cingulate fasciculus. These fibers terminate in the lower bank of the cingulate sulcus, in area 23c (Sc. 85).

A small contingent of fibers from the injection site moves dorsally and courses rostrally within the white matter of the superior frontal gyrus. These fibers terminate in a columnar manner in dorsal area 6 and the supplementary motor area (SMA) (Sc. 65).

A small aggregation of fibers travels medially from the injection site, descends to enter the extreme capsule, and provides terminations to the insular cortex (Sc. 81).

Commissural and Subcortical Fibers

From the injection site two dense parallel cords of fibers travel medially through the central part of the white matter of the inferior parietal lobule.

The dorsal part of the cord of fibers continues medially through the corona radiata and lies above the body of the caudate nucleus. These fibers aggregate just lateral to sector CC4 of the corpus callosum (Sc. 93) in the region of the fronto-occipital fasciculus before they stream medially across the midline in CC4 of the corpus callosum (Scs. 85, 89) and head toward the opposite hemisphere.

The ventral part of the cord of fibers descends almost perpendicularly into the internal capsule ICp-3 (Sc. 89) and ICp-2 (Sc. 85). These descending fibers consist of a medial and a lateral segment.

The medial contingent enters the thalamus in ICp-2, 3, and 4 via the lateral thalamic peduncle and terminates in the VPM, VPL, and VPI thalamic nuclei and in the medial dorsal nucleus (MD) (Scs. 85, 89, 93). The lateral contingent of fibers continues to descend and comes to lie over the dome of the midpoint of the LGN (Sc. 89). These fibers then descend medial to the LGN (Sc. 85) and enter the lateral aspect of the cerebral peduncle (Scs. 85, 89, 93) before entering and terminating in the basilar pontine nuclei, concentrated around the intrapeduncular and peripeduncular nuclei. Some fibers descending in the internal capsule level ICp-2 course medially, lie above the subthalamic nucleus, and terminate in the zona incerta (Sc. 85).

Striatal Fibers

A separate bundle of fibers leaves the injection site, heads medially, and descends to enter the external capsule that provides terminations to the middle, ventral, and lateral parts of the putamen (Scs. 57, 65, 73, 81, 89).

CASE 6

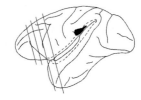

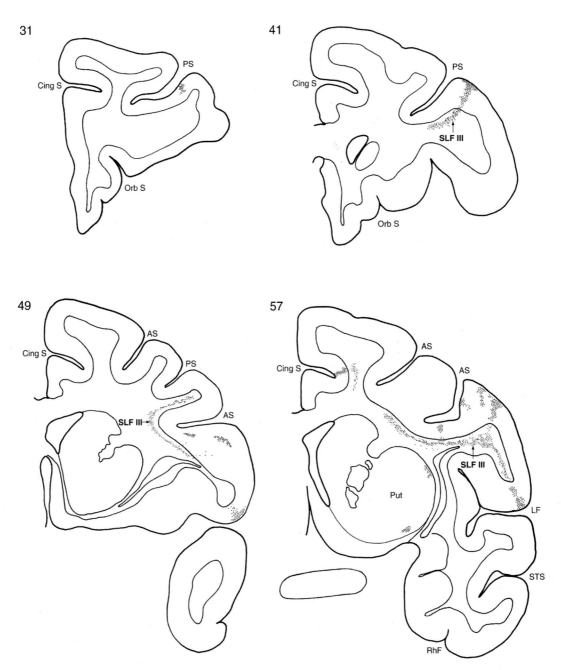

Figure 6-11

Schematic diagram of 15 rostral–caudal coronal sections in Case 6 taken at the levels shown on the hemispheric diagram above right, to depict the isotope injection site in the middle part of the parietal operculum (black filled area) and the resulting trajectories of the cortical association, commissural, and subcortical fibers (dashed lines and dots) in the white matter, and the terminations in the cortex and subcortical regions (black dots).

CASE 6

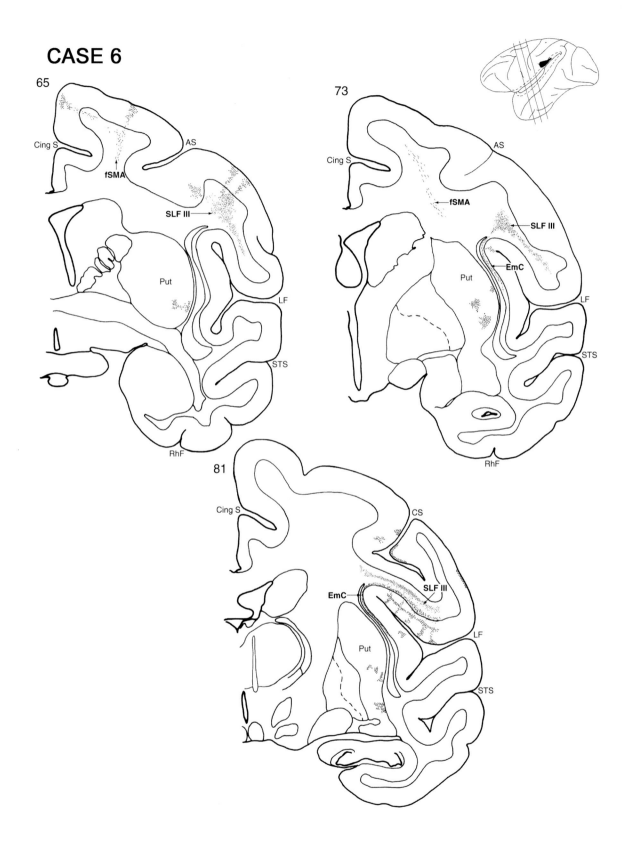

CASE 6

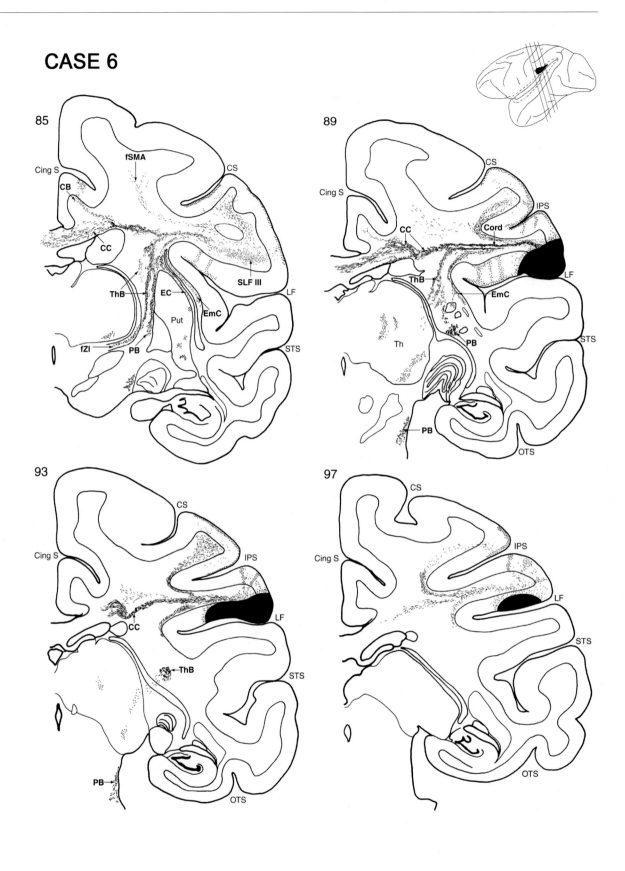

Figure 6-11 (continued)

CASE 6

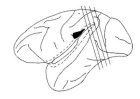

105
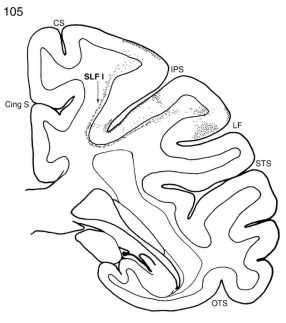

CS
Cing S
SLF I
IPS
LF
STS
OTS

113
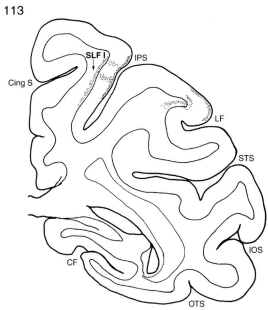

SLF I
IPS
Cing S
LF
STS
IOS
CF
OTS

121
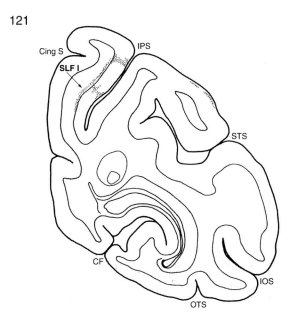

Cing S
IPS
SLF I
STS
CF
IOS
OTS

129
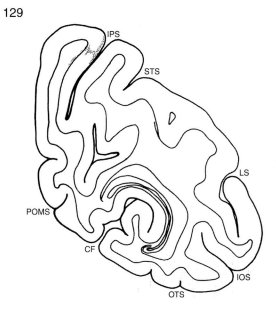

IPS
STS
LS
POMS
CF
IOS
OTS

131

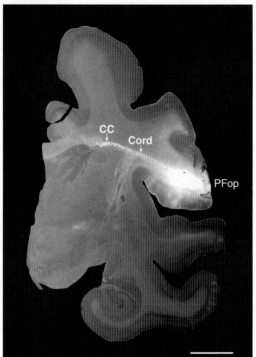

Figure 6-12
Photomicrograph of the coronal section in Case 6 at the site of the isotope injection and the resulting labeled fibers and some terminations. Photomicrograph corresponds to section 85 (Mag = 0.5×, bar = 5 mm).

Parietal Lobe Summary

Association Fibers

Long association connections of the parietal lobe are directed to the frontal lobe, the cingulate gyrus, the multimodal areas of the temporal lobe, and the parahippocampal gyrus. The parietal lobe conveys information to these cortical areas using several distinct fiber pathways: the three subdivisions of the superior longitudinal fasciculus, the middle longitudinal fasciculus, the inferior longitudinal fasciculus, the cingulum bundle, and the fronto-occipital fasciculus. The superior and medial parietal lobules convey their information predominantly via the SLF I, the FOF, and the cingulum bundle.

The caudal inferior parietal lobule sends its long association connections by the SLF II, cingulum bundle, FOF, MdLF, and ILF.

Association fibers from the rostral part of the inferior parietal lobule travel mostly within SLF III and the extreme capsule, with projections to the cingulate motor area located also within the cingulum bundle.

These fiber pathways are now summarized sequentially for each parietal region (figure 6-13).

Superior and Medial Parietal Lobule (Cases 1, 2, and 3)

1. Superior Longitudinal Fasciculus I

The superior and medial parietal lobules convey their main long association fibers through the white matter of the superior parietal lobule and the superior frontal gyrus, bounded ventrally by the depth of the cingulate sulcus. These fibers lie within a distinct fiber bundle, namely the upper segment of the superior longitudinal fasciculus (SLF I). These fibers terminate in the frontal lobe in the dorsal premotor area 6, the supplementary motor area. In the case of the medial parietal region, the terminations extend rostrally to the dorsal part of area 8. Thus, the SLF I connects the dorsal and medial parietal convexities with the dorsal premotor and supplementary motor areas in the frontal lobe. The medial parietal convexity also projects to dorsal area 8 via the SLF I.

2. Fronto-Occipital Fasciculus

Long association fibers are also conveyed from the medial and superior parietal lobule via the fronto-occipital fasciculus. The fibers from these areas become discernible as a separate bundle at the level of the caudal end of the body of the caudate nucleus. The FOF is bounded medially by the corpus callosum, laterally by the corona radiata, and ventrally by the subcallosal fasciculus of Muratoff. The parietal fibers in the FOF extend rostrally in this location up to the level of the genu of the internal capsule. At this level, the fibers course dorsally and terminate in dorsal areas 6 and 8. Many of the fibers from the FOF are also conveyed ventrally into the MB, as described below.

Like the SLF I, therefore, the FOF links superior and medial parietal cortices with the dorsal premotor area and dorsal area 8. In addition it has a second role: to provide fibers to the caudate nucleus by way of the MB.

3. Cingulum Bundle

Medial and superior parietal lobule regions commit fibers to the cingulum bundle (CB), and these extend rostrally to the level of the genu of the internal capsule. Within the CB there is a medial–lateral topography. Fibers from the medial SPL are situated medially and lie directly under the cingulate gyrus; those from the lateral part of the SPL are situated more laterally, just below the fibers of the SLF I; and the fibers from the dorsal part of the SPL occupy an intermediate position. The fibers from the dorsal and lateral SPL terminate mainly in the depth of area 24, whereas those from the medial SPL terminate in the medial portion of area 24. The CB thus links these parietal regions with the cingulate areas, and a topographic arrangement of the fibers is evident.

Caudal Inferior Parietal Lobule (Case 4)

1. Superior Longitudinal Fasciculus II

The major association fiber pathway emerging from the caudal IPL first courses through the white matter of the IPL and then crystallizes in the SLF II, the middle segment of the SLF. The SLF II is located in the white matter above the upper shoulder of the Sylvian fissure, located deep to the central sulcus, as it moves rostrally toward the frontal lobe. In the frontal lobe, the fiber bundle becomes flattened as it lies deep to the arcuate and principal sulci, and it terminates in dorsal area 6, dorsal area 8, area 9/46d, and area 46.

2. Middle Longitudinal Fasciculus

A group of fibers emerging from the caudal IPL curve around the Sylvian fissure and occupy the white matter in the central part of the superior temporal gyrus, namely the MdLF. These fibers course rostrally and terminate in interrupted patches in the multimodal areas in the upper bank and depth of the STS: areas TPO and PGa.

3. Inferior Longitudinal Fasciculus

Some fibers leave the IPL and cascade down in the ILF toward the temporal lobe. These ILF fibers, bounded laterally by the cortex in the depth of the STS and medially by the sagittal stratum, extend ventrally to the white matter surrounding the occipitotemporal sulcus (OTS), and they continue rostrally as far as the rostral end of the OTS. The ILF fibers terminate in the depth of the STS, in areas FST and IPa. Fibers situated more ventrally in the ILF terminate in the ventral temporal region, in areas TF and TL of the parahippocampal gyrus.

4. Fronto-Occipital Fasciculus

Fibers from the IPL also enter the FOF, at the level of the caudal end of the body of the caudate nucleus. These fibers travel rostrally in the FOF, and just caudal to the anterior commissure they merge laterally with the fibers of the SLF II. The FOF also gives off fibers to the MB throughout its course.

5. Cingulum Bundle

A substantial number of fibers from the IPL enter the CB at the level of the splenium of the corpus callosum and travel in both the dorsal and ventral parts of the CB. The dorsal component lies dorsally and medially within the cingulate white matter and terminates in areas 29, 30, and 23 of the caudal cingulate gyrus. Further rostrally, the fibers terminate in area 24 of the cingulate gyrus. The ventral cingulum fibers arch around the splenium of the corpus callosum. They course through the white matter of the rostral part of the calcarine sulcus and the parahippocampal gyrus, within the ventral cingulum bundle. These fibers terminate throughout the major extent of the presubiculum, and areas TH, TF and TL of the parahippocampal gyrus. The CB thus conveys information between the caudal IPL and limbic regions of the cingulate and parahippocampal gyri and the presubiculum.

Rostral Inferior Parietal Lobule (Cases 5 and 6)

1. Superior Longitudinal Fasciculus III

From the rostral part of the inferior parietal lobule and the dorsal Sylvian operculum, fibers travel rostrally through the white matter of the inferior parietal lobule within the lower segment of the superior longitudinal fasciculus, the SLF III. This fiber bundle continues rostrally in the central part of the opercular white matter until it reaches the prefrontal cortex. The fibers in the SLF III terminate first in somatic sensory areas 3, 1 and 2, as well in area SII in the cortex of the upper bank of the Sylvian fissure. In the frontal lobe, the fibers terminate in ventral area 6, area 44, and the gustatory area. Some of the fibers in the SLF III terminate also in ventral area 46, and some move medially into the white matter of the superior frontal gyrus and terminate in the supplementary motor area (area 6m) and in dorsal area 6. The SLF III thus links rostral IPL areas with the rostral and ventral premotor and prefrontal regions.

2. Extreme Capsule

Some long association fibers descend from the rostral IPL into the extreme capsule, where they move rostrally and terminate in the insular cortex.

3. Cingulum Bundle

The opercular part of the rostral IPL also sends some fibers to the dorsal part of the CB. These move medially to terminate in the cortex of the lower bank of the cingulate sulcus, in the cingulate motor area.

The SLF is thus a major white matter pathway linking the parietal and frontal lobes. The origin and termination of the fibers conveyed in the SLF, however, clearly demarcate three subdivisions in this system, each of which links distinctly different cortical areas.

The FOF carries fibers that originate in the medial, superior, and caudal inferior parietal lobules but not from the rostral part of the IPL. The FOF appears to have a dual role: it links these parietal areas with the dorsal premotor region and the dorsolateral prefrontal cortex and also conveys fibers from the parietal lobe into the striatum.

The CB conveys fibers from the medial and caudal parietal lobule, linking these areas with the caudal cingulate gyrus. CB fibers from the rostral IPL are limited and link this area with the cingulate motor region. In contrast, the CB fibers that emanate from the caudal part of the IPL are prominent, situated circumferentially in the cingulate gyrus white matter, and link the caudal IPL with both rostral and caudal cingulate cortices. In addition, the ventral part of the CB also carries fibers that link the caudal IPL with limbic cortices in the parahippocampal gyrus and the presubiculum.

The caudal IPL uses two additional fiber tracts. The MdLF carries fibers from the caudal IPL to the multimodal region of the STS, and the ILF conveys fibers to areas MT and FST, as well as to the parahippocampal gyrus.

Commissural Fibers

Most of the commissural fibers from the medial, dorsal, and inferior parts of the posterior parietal region travel through different regions of sector 4 of the corpus callosum (CC4) in a topographic manner. The fibers from the rostral part of the inferior parietal lobule and the adjacent parietal operculum travel more rostrally, whereas those from the caudal part of the inferior parietal lobule travel more caudally within CC4. The superior parietal lobule fibers course dorsally, and the medial parietal lobule fibers course caudally and more ventrally in this sector.

Subcortical Fibers

Superior Parietal Lobule

Subcortically directed fibers from the dorsal and medial parts of the superior parietal lobule descend in a compact bundle toward the sagittal stratum. The fibers continue rostrally into the posterior limb of the internal capsule, and at the level of the caudal aspect of the LGN they divide into two components. The medial aggregate of fibers traverses the upper part of the external medullary lamina to enter and terminate in the thalamus. The more lateral subcortical fiber bundle continues rostrally in the posterior limb of the internal capsule, starts to descend at the midpoint of the LGN, and enters the cerebral peduncle at the level of the rostral aspect of the LGN on its way to the pons. Fibers that leave the pontine bundle travel medially over the subthalamic nucleus and terminate in the zona incerta.

Inferior Parietal Lobule

From the caudal part of the inferior parietal lobule the cord of subcortical fibers courses ventrally and medially and enters the dorsal aspect of the sagittal stratum. These fibers then proceed rostrally into the posterior limb of the internal capsule. At the level of the pulvinar, caudal to the LGN, the subcortical bundle separates into two components. The medially situated thalamic fibers course through the upper aspect of the external medullary lamina and terminate in the thalamus. The pontine fibers continue rostrally, descending gradually until they reach the rostral aspect of the LGN, at which point they descend sharply in the capsule and enter the cerebral peduncle destined for the pons. Some fibers leave the pontine bundle, travel medially above the subthalamic nucleus, and terminate in the zona incerta.

From the rostral part of the inferior parietal lobule the cord of subcortical fibers courses medially and descends sharply into the posterior limb of the internal capsule. These fibers then divide into two segments. The medial and dorsal segment traverses the lower part of the external medullary lamina to terminate in the thalamus. The pontine fibers descend further in the posterior limb of the capsule at the level of the rostral part of the LGN before coursing into the cerebral peduncle. Some fibers leave the pontine bundle, course medially above the subthalamic nucleus, and terminate in the zona incerta.

Corticostriate Projections

Striatal fibers from association area PEc in the caudal SPL and area PGm in the medial SPL gather in the fronto-occipital bundle, descend into the MB, and course rostrally. They provide terminations to the dorsolateral sector of the head of the caudate nucleus, with lighter but consistent projections to the body of the caudate nucleus. Some of the SPL fibers traveling in the MB cross the posterior limb of the internal capsule and terminate in the intermediate and lateral parts of the putamen rostrally and in its dorsal aspect more caudally. Some SPL fibers in the external capsule lead to the claustrum and to the islands of putamen caudally.

The striatal fibers from the IPL separate into two components. One courses through the FOF that feeds the MB and progresses rostrally, providing terminations to the body and head of the caudate nucleus and the rostral part of the putamen. The other component descends and courses through the external capsule, providing terminations to the ventral part of the claustrum and the caudal part of the putamen, including the islands. Fibers from the multimodal area PG/Opt travel exclusively via the MB to terminate heavily in the dorsal, dorsolateral, and intermediate sectors of the head of the caudate nucleus, as well as to the caudate body. Some of these fibers cross the internal capsule and terminate in dorsal and ventral zones within the caudal part of the putamen, and some travel in the external capsule leading to the claustrum. The projections from the intramodality somatosensory association cortices in the rostral parts of the IPL, area PF, and the parietal operculum avoid the caudate nucleus entirely and are focused only in the putamen. The external capsule conveys these projections to the ventral region of the rostral part of the putamen and to the central and ventral parts of the middle and caudal putamen.

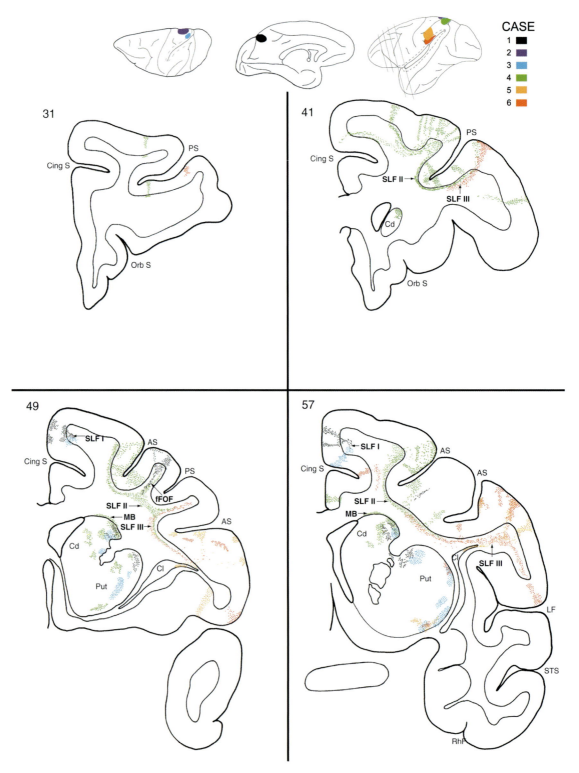

Figure 6-13

Schematic composite diagrams of rostral–caudal coronal sections of the template brain, illustrating the six parietal lobe cases (Cases 1 through 6). The injection sites, association, commissural, and sub-cortical fibers, and the termination patterns are color-coded for each case. The diagrams of the dorsal, medial, and lateral surfaces of the cerebral hemispheres (top) represent the different levels of the coronal sections and the injection sites, color-coded as follows: Case 1, black, medial parietal

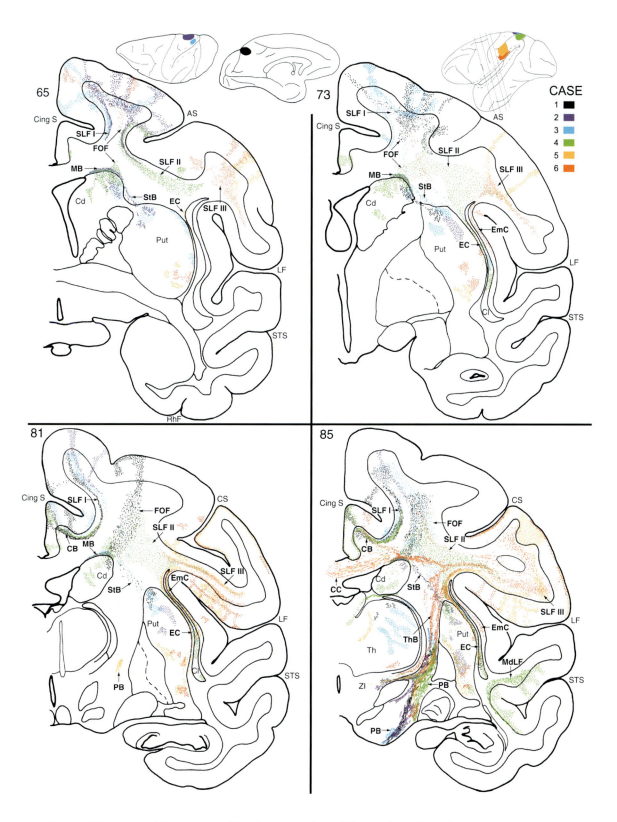

convexity area PGm, encroaching upon area PEc; Case 2, purple, medial part of area PEc at the junction of area PE; Case 3, blue, lateral part of area PEc at the junction of area PE; Case 4, green, area PG and area Opt; Case 5, orange, rostral inferior parietal lobule, area PF; Case 6, red, midregion of the parietal operculum.

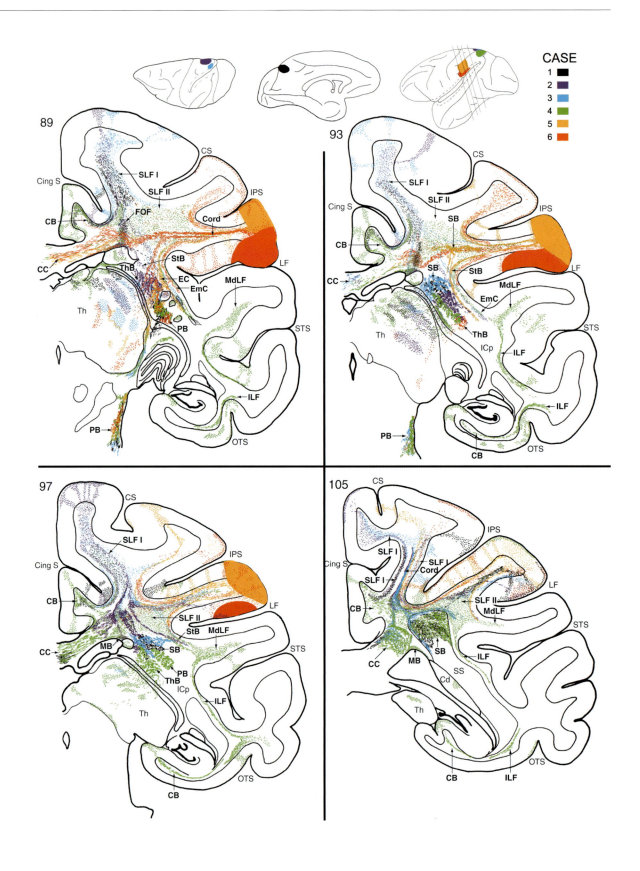

Figure 6-13 (continued)

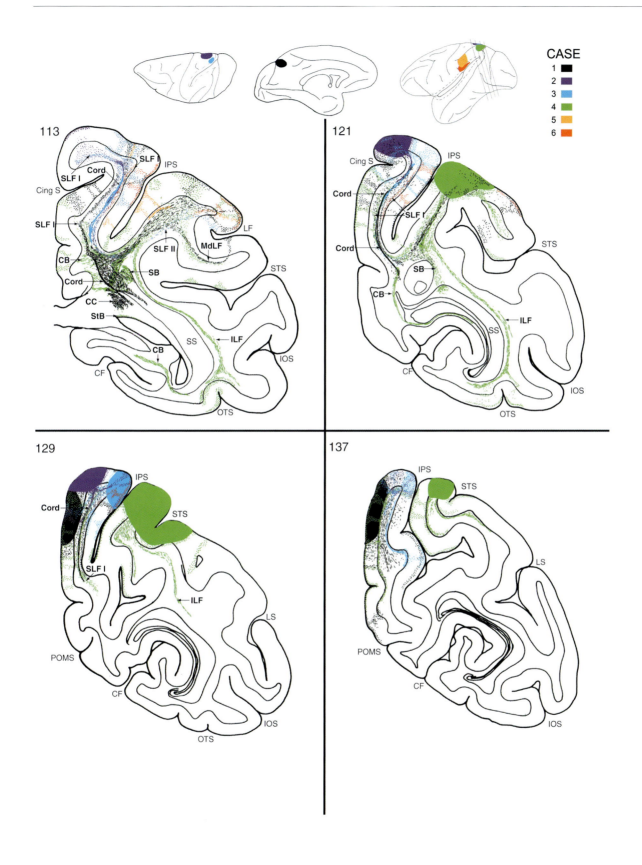

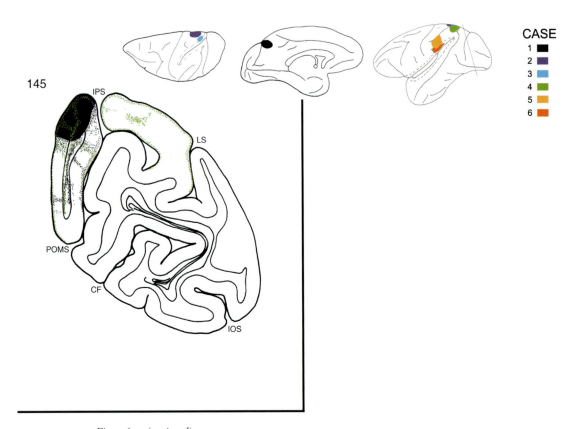

CASE
1 ■
2 ■
3 ■
4 ■
5 ■
6 ■

145

IPS

LS

POMS

CF

IOS

Figure 6-13 (continued)

Superior Temporal Region

7

In this chapter we describe the isotope injection cases in the superior temporal region of five rhesus monkeys, and we analyze the resulting association, striatal, commissural, and subcortical fiber trajectories as well as the cortical and subcortical terminations. The injections were in the caudal part of the superior temporal gyrus involving area Tpt (Case 7), the caudal part of the superior temporal gyrus in areas paAlt and Tpt (Case 8), the midportion of area TPO in the upper bank of the superior temporal sulcus, the ventral superior temporal gyrus in area TAa and the caudal part of primary auditory area KA (Case 9), the rostral part of area TS3 (Case 10), and area Pro and area TS1 encroaching on area TS2 (Case 11).

As in the previous chapter, the architectonic designations of the cortical terminations are described in the text but not identified on the coronal sections. Architectonic areas are labeled on external views of the hemisphere as in the coronal series of chapter 4. Terminations in the thalamus are shown and thalamic nuclei are referred to in the text, but the nuclei are not designated on the coronal sections. Pontine terminations are described in the text but not illustrated. Striatal terminations are illustrated and an overview of their termination patterns is presented in the text.

CASE 7

In this case the isotope injection was located in the caudal part of the superior temporal gyrus involving area Tpt. See figures 7-1 and 7-2.

Association Fibers

Local Association Fibers

The local terminations are seen mainly in the planum temporale, and in the superior temporal gyrus and cortex of the upper bank of the superior temporal sulcus. Labeled fibers travel in the white matter immediately beneath the cortex and terminate in the upper bank of the lateral (Sylvian) fissure (LF) in the first layer in area paAc (Scs. 97, 105). Fibers also terminate in area reIt (in the lower bank of the depth of the LF) and in area reIpt (in the upper bank of the depth of the LF) in a columnar manner (Scs. 105, 113). Local terminations seen caudal to the injection site are present in the caudal part of area Tpt in a columnar manner and in the caudal part of area TPO (Scs. 113,121).

Long Association Fibers

Caudally Directed Fibers

Fibers enter the ILF and travel caudally. They turn around the ventral aspect of the sagittal stratum and enter the cingulum bundle. From here, the fibers continue caudally and travel in the upper bank of the calcarine sulcus and then terminate in the retrosplenial cortex and in area 23 in a columnar manner (Scs. 113, 121, 129).

Rostrally Directed Fibers

The major rostrally directed long association fibers are conveyed by five distinct fascicles: the middle longitudinal fasciculus, SLF I, arcuate fasciculus, cingulum bundle, and ILF.

A prominent bundle of fibers leaves the injection site and runs in the middle longitudinal fasciculus (MdLF) situated in the white matter of the superior temporal gyrus. These fibers terminate in the lower bank of the Sylvian fissure in both the primary auditory area KA and in area paAc, in the first layer (Scs. 89, 93, 97). The MdLF fibers also terminate in area proK and the insular Pro in the depth of the Sylvian fissure (Scs. 81, 85, 89), as well as in area paAlt in the crown of the gyrus, and in area TAa and area TPO in the upper bank of the STS, in a columnar manner (Scs. 89, 93, 97).

Fibers directed toward the medial wall of the hemisphere travel medially in the white matter of the inferior parietal lobule (Sc. 113), traverse the SLF II, and enter the SLF I in the white matter of the superior parietal lobule. The fibers then leave the SLF I and terminate in a columnar manner in area 31 (Sc. 113), area PEci in the depth of the caudal part of the cingulate sulcus (Scs. 105), and more caudally in area PGm (Sc. 121).

A major bundle of fibers leaves the injection site and travels medially in the white matter of the superior temporal gyrus (STG), arches around the caudal end of the Sylvian fissure, and turns rostrally to form the arcuate fasciculus (AF), running along with the SLF II. The AF fibers continue rostrally deep to the white matter of the central sulcus and above the upper shoulder of the Sylvian fissure. These fibers eventually occupy a position in the white matter of the arcuate sulcus and then terminate first in area 6 and then in the dorsolateral prefrontal cortex in area 8Ad in a columnar manner (Scs. 49, 57).

A group of medially directed fibers travels along with the arcuate fasciculus, crosses the corona radiata, and enters the cingulate fasciculus before terminating in columns in the cingulate gyrus in area 23 and more rostrally in area 24 (Scs. 93, 97, 105).

Another association fiber bundle arising from the injection site descends lateral to the sagittal stratum, lying within the ILF. These fibers course around the ventral aspect of the ILF, head medially toward the parahippocampal gyrus, and become continuous with the ventral component of the cingulum bundle. From this location terminations are given off to the retrosplenial and prostriate cortices situated in the rostral end of the calcarine fissure, as mentioned above.

Commissural and Subcortical Fibers

From the injection site a dense cord of fibers moves medially within the white matter of the STG and divides into two parallel components that move toward the sagittal stratum (SS).

The sizable dorsal component enters and then traverses the dorsal aspect of the SS before it enters sector CC5 of the corpus callosum (Sc. 105). The callosal fibers then course medially to the opposite hemisphere and are evident in the midsagittal plane in callosal sectors CC5 (Sc. 105) and CC4 (Scs. 97, 93).

The ventral contingent aggregates at the lateral aspect of sector SS-2 of the sagittal stratum (Scs. 105, 113). Fibers leave this staging area, traverse the SS, where they lie at its medial aspect, and move rostrally into the retrolenticular part of the posterior limb of the internal capsule ICp-5 (Sc. 97). At the level of the thalamus a large collection of fibers traverses the reticular nucleus and terminates in the thalamus, predominantly in the PM nucleus (Sc. 97). Further rostrally in retrolenticular posterior limb ICp-4 (Sc. 93), another large contingent of thalamic fibers separates from the parent bundle and descends medially to enter and then terminate mainly in the densocellular part of the medial geniculate nucleus (Sc. 93).

As the remaining fibers continue rostrally in the posterior limb of the internal capsule into ICp-3 (Sc. 89), they come to lie above the midpoint of the lateral geniculate nucleus (LGN). At this stage they abruptly descend medial to the LGN to enter the lateral part of the cerebral peduncle. The most rostral contingent of these pontine fibers (PB) is seen below the internal capsule level ICp-2 (Sc. 85). The pontine fibers course toward the nuclei in the rostral half of the basis pontis, where they terminate in the dorsolateral and lateral nuclei and in lateral parts of the peripeduncular nucleus.

Striatal Fibers

Fibers destined for the striatum course along with those in the MdLF. They travel rostrally within the white matter of the STG, aggregate deep to the Sylvian fissure, and are incorporated mostly within the extreme capsule, although some are identified within the external capsule as well. These fibers terminate in the dysgranular insula (Sc. 81) and in the lower part of the claustrum (Scs. 73, 81). Fibers in the most dorsal part of the extreme/external capsules cross medially above the internal capsule and terminate in the body of the caudate nucleus (Scs. 81, 85).

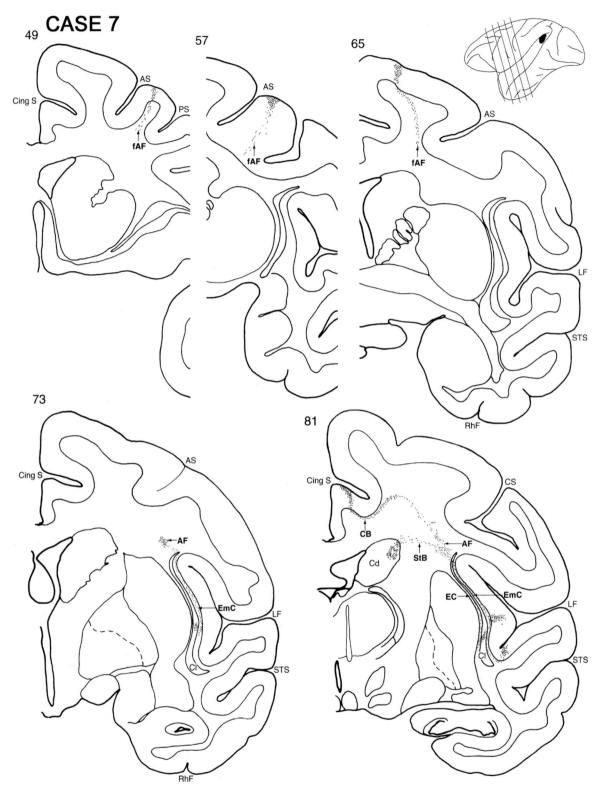

Figure 7-1

Schematic diagrams of 13 rostral–caudal coronal sections in Case 7 taken at the levels shown on the hemispheric diagram above right, showing the isotope injection site in the caudal part of the superior temporal gyrus involving area Tpt (black-filled area) and the resulting trajectories of the cortical association, commissural, and subcortical fibers (dashed lines and dots) in the white matter and the terminations in the cortex and subcortical regions (black dots). See list of abbreviations, p. 617.

CASE 7

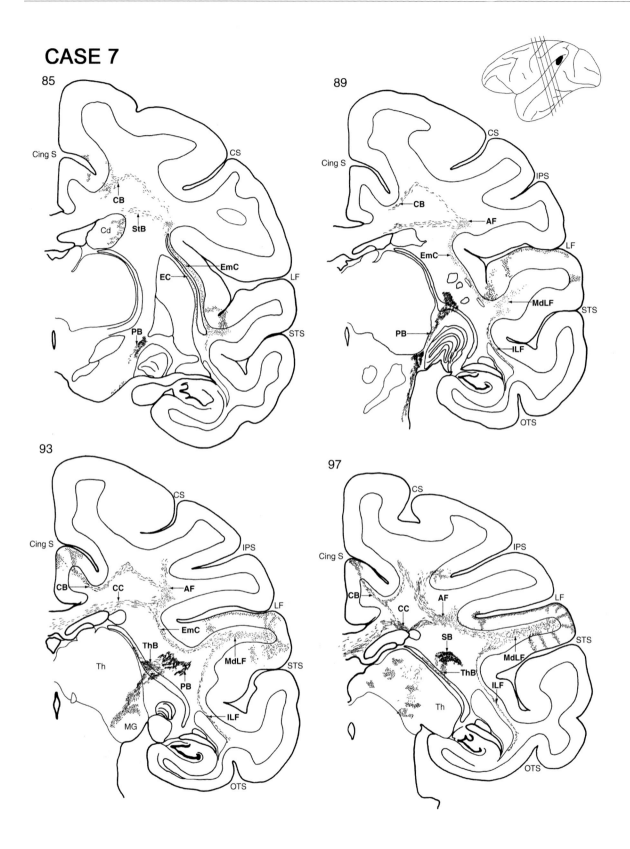

CASE 7

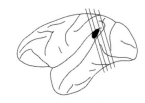

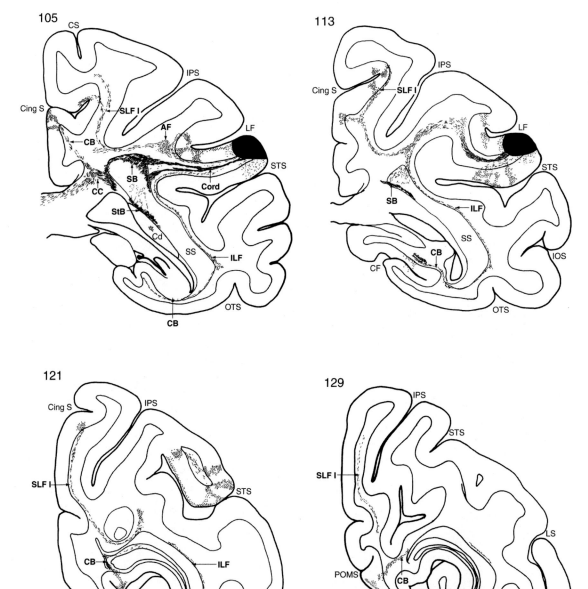

Figure 7-1 (continued)

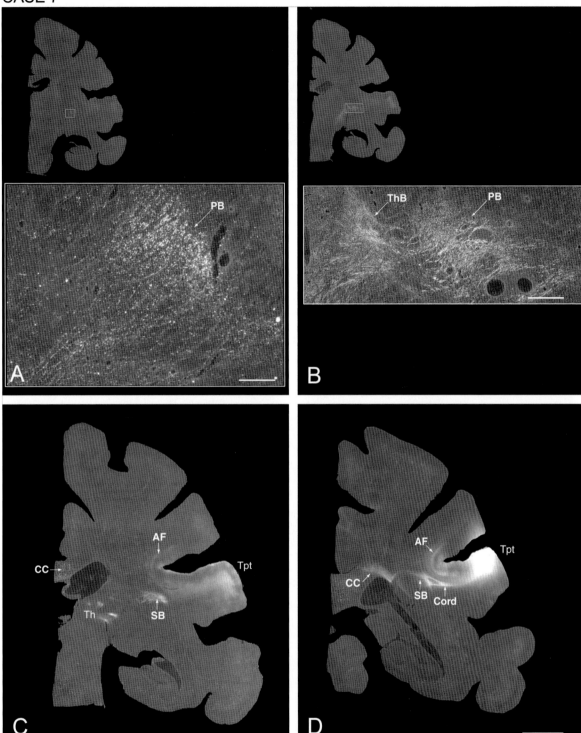

Figure 7-2

Photomicrographs of selected coronal sections of Case 7 showing the injection site in D and the resulting labeled fibers and terminations in A through D. A, High-power photomicrograph (section
89, Mag = 4×, bar = 0.5 mm) taken from the location indicated in the low-power photomicrograph
above to show pontine fibers in the subcortical fiber bundle situated within the internal capsule. B,
High-power photomicrograph (section 93, Mag = 4×, bar = 0.5 mm) taken from the location indicated in the low-power photomicrograph above to show the pontine fibers of the subcortical bundle
situated within the internal capsule laterally and the thalamic fibers traversing the reticular nucleus
coursing into the thalamus in B and C. Photomicrographs C and D correspond to sections 97 and
105, respectively (Mag = 0.5×, bar = 5 mm).

CASE 8

The isotope injection in this case was located in the caudal part of the superior temporal gyrus in areas paAlt and Tpt. See figures 7-3 and 7-4.

Association Fibers

Local Association Fibers

Local fibers leave the injection site and travel at the dorsal and ventral periphery of the white matter within the superior temporal gyrus. Near the injection site these fibers terminate dorsally in the cortex of the Sylvian fissure in area paAc mainly in the first layer, in area reIt in a columnar manner, and in area Tpt predominantly in the fourth layer (Scs. 97, 105, 113). The ventral contingent of local association fibers terminates in area TPO in a columnar manner (Sc. 105).

Long Association Fibers

Caudally Directed Fibers

Fibers leave the injection site and course medially, ascending in SLF I in the white matter of the superior parietal lobule before terminating in a columnar manner in area 31 (Scs. 105, 113) and area PEci (Sc. 121).

Rostrally Directed Fibers

From the injection site a plate of fibers runs rostrally within the white matter of the superior temporal gyrus, in the middle longitudinal fasciculus (MdLF). Fibers leave this bundle and terminate at the crown of the superior temporal gyrus mainly in the fourth layer in area paAlt and further rostrally in area TS3 (Scs. 89, 93). Terminations are also seen in the first layer in the primary auditory cortex, area KA, and area proK in a columnar manner (Scs. 85, 89).

Long association fibers are conveyed to the frontal lobe in the extreme capsule. These fibers leave the injection site and travel deep to the Sylvian fissure before coming to lie in the white matter below the lower limb of the arcuate sulcus. From this location fibers terminate in the rostral part of area 45 in a columnar manner (Sc. 41).

Another prominent fiber system arising from the injection site and lying above the cord of fibers heads medially and arches around the caudal part of the Sylvian fissure to enter the arcuate fasciculus (AF) lying within the white matter deep to the inferior parietal lobule. These AF fibers course rostrally as a compact bundle lying at the upper shoulder of the Sylvian fissure in the vicinity of the dorsal aspect of the claustrum and extreme capsule. In the frontal lobe the fibers move medially and dorsally and travel with the fibers of the SLF II. They spread out dorsally to form a flattened sheet of fibers, lying first deep to the arcuate spur and then deep to both limbs of the arcuate and the principal sulci. Fibers leave this lamella and move dorsally to terminate in dorsal area 6, dorsal area 8, area 9, and dorsal area 46 (Scs. 31, 41, 49, 57).

An intense concentration of fibers leaves the injection site and courses medially over the sagittal stratum to enter the cingulum bundle (CB). These fibers are directed medially and terminate in columns in areas 23b and 23c (Scs. 105, 113, 121). The fibers in the

CB continue caudally and terminate in the retrosplenial area, in and around the rostral end of the calcarine fissure (Sc. 121).

Commissural and Subcortical Fibers

From the injection site a dense cord of fibers moves medially within the central part of the white matter of the superior temporal gyrus. It traverses the SLF II and then lies adjacent to and penetrates the upper aspect of sector SS-2 of the sagittal stratum (Scs. 105, 113, 121).

Strands of intensely labeled fibers cross the sagittal stratum and stream dorsally within the lateral aspect of the corpus callosum, aggregating at the splenium (Sc.105), before progressing rostrally and crossing in sector CC4 of the corpus callosum to reach the opposite hemisphere (Scs. 89, 93, 97).

The fibers at the lateral aspect of sector SS-2 of the sagittal stratum move rostrally, assuming a whorled appearance. As they enter the retrolenticular part of the posterior limb of the internal capsule (ICp-5, Sc. 97), fibers leave these aggregated bundles and move medially to enter and terminate in the medial pulvinar. Fibers that enter the thalamus also move ventrally and medially as they progress rostrally and terminate in VPI, medial geniculate (densocellular [MGd] and magnocellular [MGmc]), suprageniculate (SG), and limitans nucleus (Li), as well as in the dorsomedial nucleus (MD) (Scs. 93, 97).

After the thalamic contingent of fibers has entered the thalamus, the ventral part of the whorls of fibers continues rostrally in the ICp-4 (Sc. 93) and ICp-3 (Sc. 89) until the level of the caudal aspect and midpoint of the lateral geniculate nucleus. These fibers arch over the dome of the LGN, move medial to the LGN, and descend into the cerebral peduncle (Sc. 89), from where they proceed to terminate in the basis pontis in the lateral and dorsolateral nuclei and in the lateral aspects of the peripeduncular and intrapeduncular nuclei.

Striatal Fibers

The fibers that stream medially through the sagittal stratum to enter the lateral aspect of the corpus callosum also give rise to a distinct collection of fibers lying in the subependymal zone between the lateral ventricle and the tapetum. These fibers continue rostrally, and those that are ventrally situated terminate in the genu of the caudate nucleus, whereas those that are more dorsal become continuous rostrally with the bundle of Muratoff (Sc. 105). The Muratoff bundle (MB) moves rostrally as far as the head of the caudate nucleus, all the while giving off terminations within the caudate body and head (Scs. 93, 97). The Muratoff bundle also receives inputs from the striatal bundle (StB) that courses initially along with the association fibers in the white matter core of the superior temporal gyrus before coursing medially over the internal capsule (Scs. 97, 93, 89).

Other striatal fibers lie in the lateral aspect of the sagittal stratum at the level of the genu of the caudate nucleus. These fibers continue rostrally until the level of the claustrum, at which point they turn dorsally and ascend in the ventral part of the external capsule. These fibers leave the external capsule to terminate in the ventral and dorsal parts of the putamen and in the ventral and midportions of the claustrum (Scs. 73, 81, 85).

CASE 8

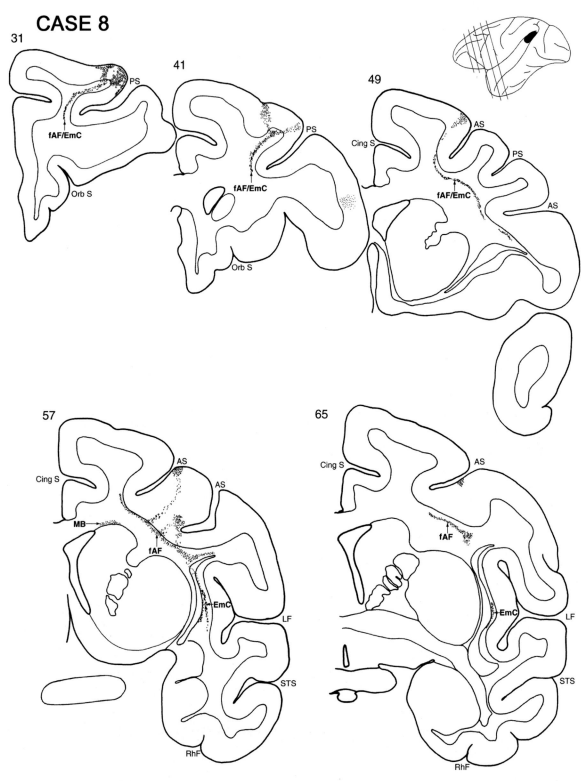

Figure 7-3

Schematic diagram of 14 rostral–caudal coronal sections in Case 8 taken at the levels shown on the hemispheric diagram above right, showing the isotope injection site in the caudal part of the superior temporal gyrus in areas paAlt and Tpt (black-filled area) and the resulting trajectories of the cortical association, commissural, and subcortical fibers (dashed lines and dots) in the white matter, and the terminations in the cortex and subcortical regions (black dots).

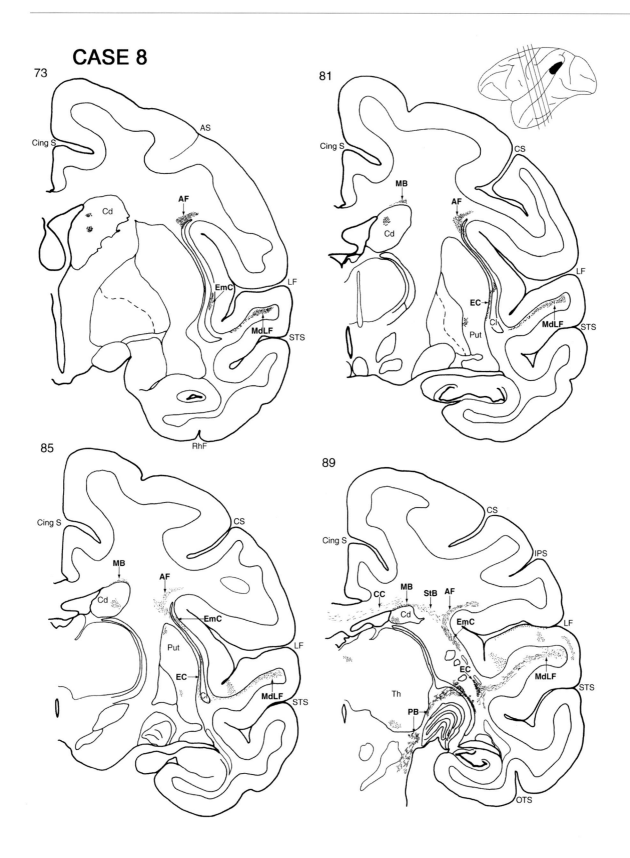

CASE 8

CASE 8

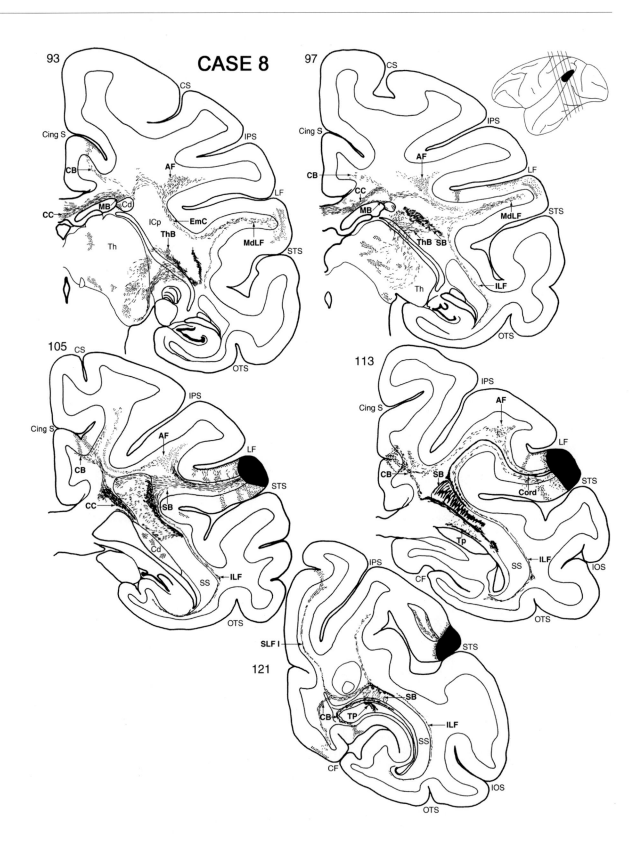

Figure 7-3 (continued)

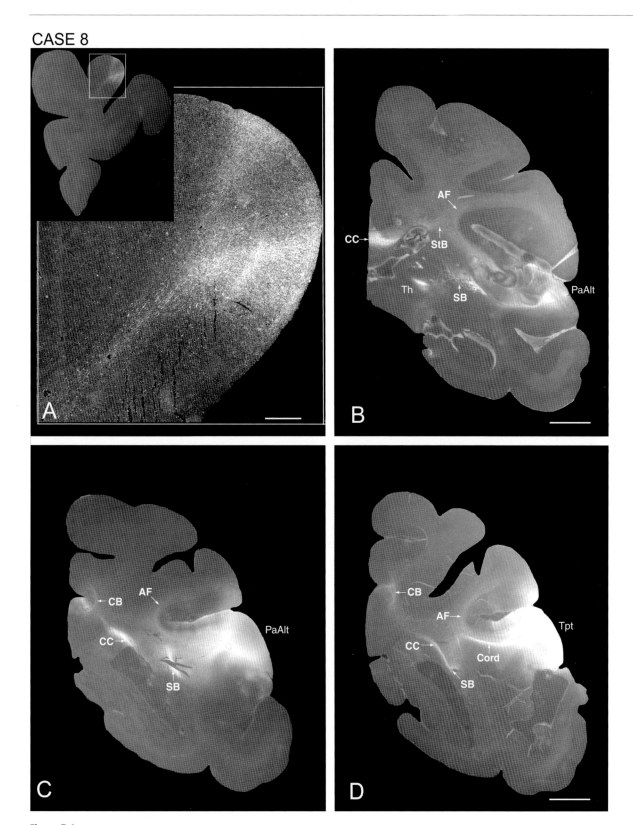

Figure 7-4

Photomicrographs of selected coronal sections of Case 8 to show the injection site in D with the injection halo in C and the resulting labeled fibers and terminations in A through D. A, High-power photomicrograph (section 31, Mag = 4×, bar = 0.5 mm) taken from the location indicated in the low-power photomicrograph in the inset to show terminations in areas 46d and 9d. Photomicrographs B through D correspond to sections 97, 105, and 113, respectively (Mag = 0.5×, bar = 5 mm).

CASE 9

The isotope injection was placed in the midportion of area TPO in the lateral part of the cortex of the upper bank of the superior temporal sulcus, the ventral part of the superior temporal gyrus, area TAa, and the caudal part of the primary auditory area KA in the supratemporal plane. See figures 7-5 and 7-6.

Association Fibers

Local Association Fibers

Labeled fibers are identified within the supratemporal plane and the upper bank of the superior temporal sulcus. The terminations in the supratemporal plane are in area paAc in the first layer and in area reIt in a columnar manner (Sc. 93). Rostrally, terminations are seen in the first layer in area KA and in area proK in a columnar manner (Sc. 85). Local terminations are also seen at the crown of the superior temporal gyrus in area paAlt and TAa (Sc. 93). The local terminations in the superior temporal sulcus are seen mainly in rostral areas TPO and PGa in a columnar manner (Scs. 89, 93).

Long Association Fibers

Caudally Directed Fibers

Association fibers travel caudally within the white matter of the superior temporal gyrus in the middle longitudinal fasciculus (MdLF). These fibers give rise to terminations in the supratemporal plane in area reIt in a columnar manner and in the first layer in area paAc (Scs. 97, 105). Terminations are also present in the superior temporal gyrus in area Tpt in the first layer (Scs. 105, 113). The MdLF fibers also terminate in the cortex of the upper bank of the superior temporal sulcus in areas Tpt, TAa, TPO, and PGa in a columnar manner and in the first layer (Scs. 97, 105, 113).

A prominent concentration of fibers leaves the injection site and descends to enter the inferior longitudinal fasciculus (ILF). These fibers course caudally and descend lateral to the sagittal stratum, giving rise to first-layer terminations in the cortex of the depth of the STS in areas FST and MST (Scs. 105, 113, 121). As the ILF travels caudally, fibers emanate from both its dorsal and ventral components.

The dorsal component bifurcates, forming laterally and medially directed contingents. Laterally directed fibers travel in the white matter of the inferior parietal lobule and terminate in area Opt in the first layer (Sc. 121). The medially directed fiber bundle passes above the sagittal stratum and divides into ascending and descending branches. The ascending component continues caudally and medially and lies within the SLF I in the white matter of the superior parietal lobule. These fibers terminate in areas PGm and PEci in a columnar manner (Sc. 121). The descending component enters the caudal part of the cingulate fasciculus, terminates in a columnar manner in area 23 (Scs. 113, 121), and then continues rostrally within the cingulate fasciculus, as described below. Further caudally some ILF fibers lie in the white matter of the occipital lobe; they terminate in area V2 in the first layer (Scs. 121, 137).

The fibers in the ventral component of the ILF curve medially and terminate in ventral area V2 and V3V, predominantly in the first layer (Sc. 121). These ILF fibers course upward around the calcarine fissure, join the fibers of the cingulum bundle, and terminate in the retrosplenial cortex in the first layer (Scs. 113, 121, 129).

Rostrally Directed Fibers

Fibers travel rostrally from the injection site in the white matter of the superior temporal gyrus, within the MdLF. These fibers terminate in areas proK and TS3 in a columnar manner, and some terminations are noted in area paAr in the first layer (Scs. 73, 81, 85). The MdLF also gives rise to terminations in the upper bank of the STS in areas PGa, TPO, and TAa in a columnar manner (Scs. 73, 81, 85).

Fibers leaving the injection site course upward into the extreme capsule and travel forward, occupying its entire extent. The extreme capsule (EmC) gives rise to columnar terminations in the granular and dysgranular insula (Scs. 81, 85). As the fibers continue forward in the extreme capsule, they first lie lateral to the claustrum, and then in the frontal lobe they are seen in the extreme capsule as it lies ventral to the claustrum. Anterior to the arcuate sulcus, the fibers provide columnar terminations to area 47/12 below the principal sulcus (Scs. 31, 41).

Another group of association fibers travels rostrally in the arcuate fasciculus (AF) that lies above the external and extreme capsules (Scs. 65, 73, 81, 85). In the frontal lobe these fibers of the arcuate fasciculus (fAF) spread out to lie beneath the arcuate sulcus and then terminate in dorsal area 8 in a columnar manner (Scs. 41, 49, 57). Further rostrally, these fibers occupy a position around the depth of the principal sulcus and provide columnar terminations in area 46 in the upper and lower banks of the principal sulcus and in area 10 above the sulcus (Scs. 20, 31).

As mentioned, some fibers that lie within the cingulate fasciculus are directed rostrally; they terminate in a columnar manner in areas 23 and 24 (Scs. 49, 73, 81).

Commissural and Subcortical Fibers

From the injection site two dense cords of fibers head medially into the white matter. The more dorsal of these cords gives rise to fibers that ascend and cross the retrolenticular capsule and head toward the caudate nucleus. The fibers arch steeply up and over the caudate body to enter sector CC4 of the corpus callosum before they traverse the midline to the opposite hemisphere (Scs. 93, 97). Some fibers also travel caudally in the periphery and center of sector SS-2 of the sagittal stratum (Scs. 113, 105) before they penetrate sector CC5 of the corpus callosum (Sc. 105).

The ventral cord of fibers that arises from the injection site gives rise to thalamic and pontine fibers.

The fibers in the thalamic bundle (ThB) lie in the retrolenticular part of the posterior limb of the internal capsule (ICp-5, Sc. 97), penetrate medially through the thalamic reticular nucleus (Sc. 93), and either travel upward in the external medullary lamina or directly penetrate the lateral thalamic peduncle. The ascending fibers terminate in the PM, CL, and MD nuclei (Scs. 93, 97). The fibers in the ventral part of the lateral thalamic peduncle enter the PL nucleus, and fibers terminate predominantly in PM, Li, and the caudal part of the MG (MGd) nucleus (Scs. 93, 97).

Fibers destined for the pons (the pontine bundle [PB]) are separate from the thalamic fiber system. They form a compact bundle lying at the ventral aspect of the posterior limb of the internal capsule in ICp-4 (Sc. 93) and ICp-3 (Sc. 89), situated above and lateral to the LGN. At the rostral aspect and midpoint of the LGN (Sc. 89), these pontine fibers move medially, descend, and assume a helmet shape lying at the most rostral and lateral aspect of the cerebral peduncle. From this point the fibers descend to the basis pontis, where they terminate throughout its rostral to caudal extent in the extreme dorsolateral, dorsolateral, and lateral pontine nuclei, with some projections also in dorsal and lateral parts of the peripeduncular nucleus.

Some fibers leave the pontine bundle above the LGN and terminate in the zona incerta (ZI, Sc. 85).

Striatal Fibers

Fibers that are destined for the head and body of the caudate nucleus and the putamen take a quite different course than fibers destined for the genu of the caudate nucleus. Those destined for the head and body of the caudate ascend in the external capsule, traverse the dorsal segment of the posterior limb of the internal capsule, enter the Muratoff bundle, and terminate in the medial aspect of the body and head of the caudate nucleus (Scs. 65, 73, 81, 85, 89). Fibers in the external capsule travel rostrally, traverse the anterior limb of the capsule, and terminate in the putamen and in the head of the caudate nucleus. Some external capsule fibers travel ventrally to terminate in the tail of the caudate (Sc. 85). The fibers destined for the genu of the caudate nucleus lie at the lateral aspect of the sagittal stratum and then move medially to the inner segment of the sagittal stratum, from which point they give rise to terminations in the genu of the caudate nucleus (Sc. 105).

Figure 7-5

Schematic diagrams of 17 rostral–caudal coronal sections in Case 9 taken at the levels shown on the hemispheric diagram above right, showing the isotope injection site in the midportion of area TPO in the lateral part of the cortex of the upper bank of the superior temporal sulcus. There is involvement also of the ventral part of the superior temporal gyrus, area TAa, and the caudal part of the primary auditory area KA in the supratemporal plane (black-filled area). The resulting trajectories of the cortical association, commissural, and subcortical fibers in the white matter are shown by dashed lines and dots, and the terminations in the cortex and subcortical regions are shown as black dots.

CASE 9

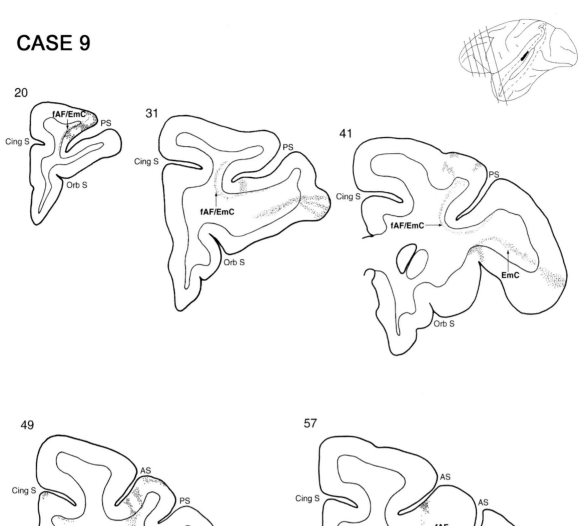

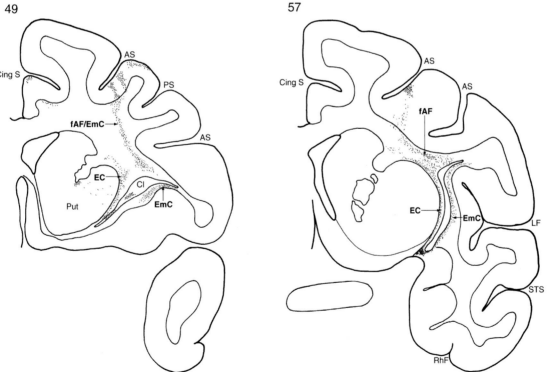

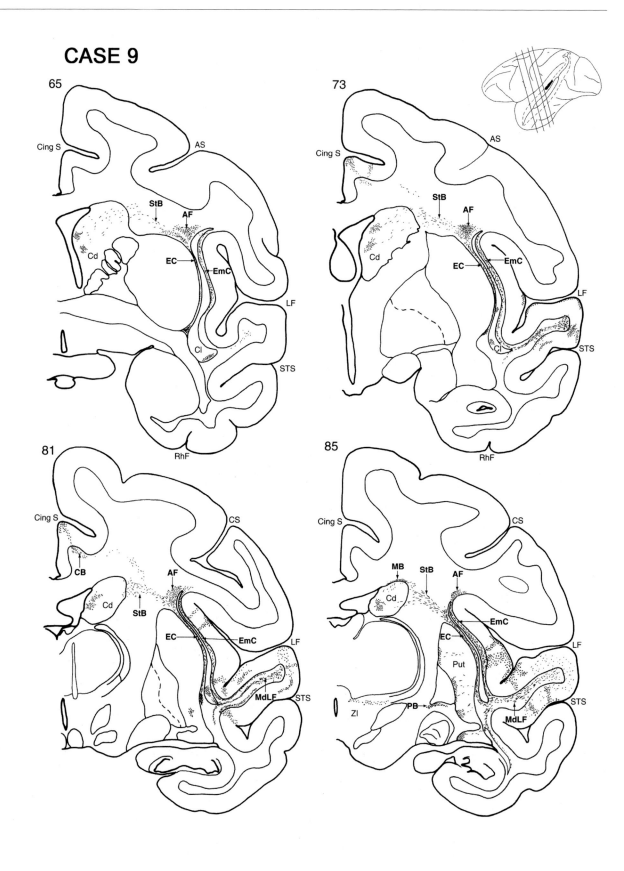

Figure 7-5 (continued)

CASE 9

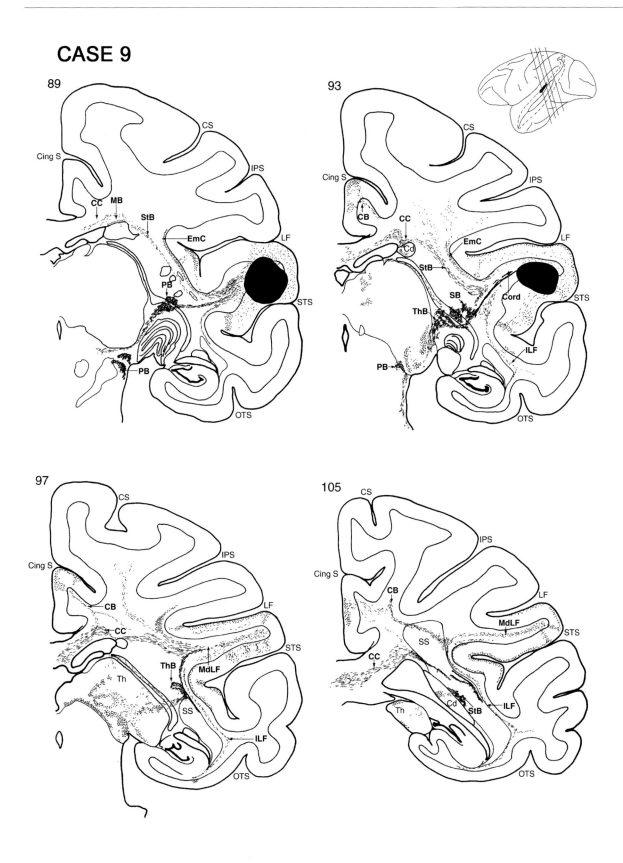

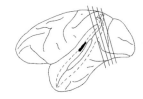

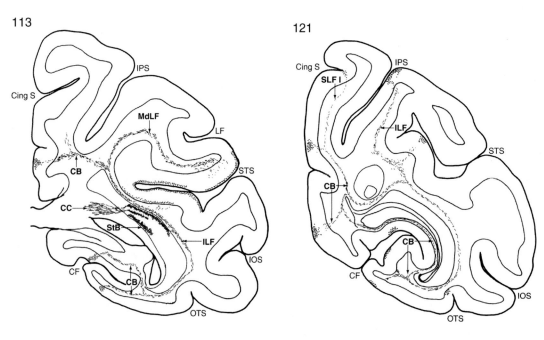

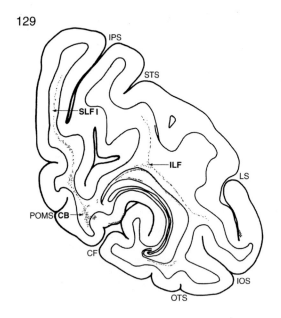

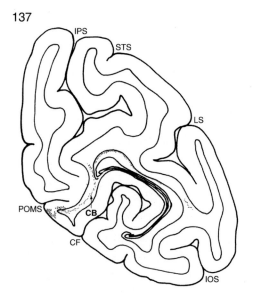

Figure 7-5 (continued)

CASE 9

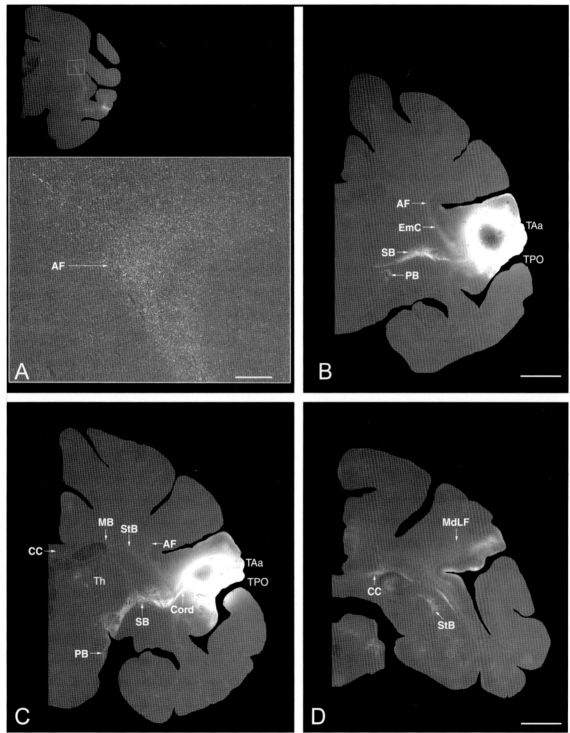

Figure 7-6

Photomicrographs of selected coronal sections of Case 9 to show the injection site in B and C and the resulting labeled fibers and terminations in A through D. A, High-power photomicrograph (section 73, Mag = 4×, bar = 0.5 mm) taken from the location indicated in the low-power photomicrograph above to show the fibers of the arcuate fasciculus. Photomicrographs B through D correspond to sections 89, 93, and 105, respectively (Mag = 0.5 ×, bar = 5 mm).

CASE 10

In this case, the isotope injection was located in the superior temporal gyrus, involving the rostral part of area TS3. See figures 7-7 and 7-8.

Association Fibers

Local Association Fibers

Adjacent to the injection site, fibers travel in the white matter immediately beneath the cortex of the superior temporal gyrus. They terminate in areas paAr, TS3, TAa, and TPO in a columnar manner (Scs. 73, 81).

Long Association Fibers

Caudally Directed Fibers

From the injection site, fibers travel caudally in the white matter of the superior temporal gyrus in the MdLF (Scs. 93, 97, 105, 113). The fibers terminate in area proK at the depth of the Sylvian fissure, area paAlt at the crown of the superior temporal gyrus, and areas TAa and TPO at the upper bank of the superior temporal sulcus in a columnar manner, and in the dysgranular insula (Scs. 85, 89). Further caudally fibers terminate in area Tpt, predominantly in the first layer (Scs. 105, 113, 121).

Other fibers lying ventral to the cord (described below) course medially through the temporal lobe white matter to join the ILF as it descends toward the ventral temporal region (Scs. 97, 105, 113). The ILF fibers course medially over the occipitotemporal sulcus and terminate in a columnar manner in the posterior parahippocampal gyrus in areas TH and TL (Scs. 85, 89, 93). The fibers that lead to the parahippocampal gyrus are also contributed to by a compact fascicle that emerges from the white matter of the superior temporal gyrus and descends in the sagittal stratum before joining the fibers of the ILF and cingulum bundle (Scs. 93, 105, 113). The fibers in the ILF that hug the lateral border of the ventral part of the sagittal stratum join medially with the fibers in the ventral portion of the cingulum bundle. These ILF and cingulate fibers together continue in a caudal direction and course dorsally and medially in the white matter deep to the calcarine cortex. They provide terminations to area prostriata and the ventral part of the retrosplenial cortex, area 30, that lies ventral to the splenium (Scs. 105, 113, 121).

Fibers lying dorsal to the cord course caudally, pass medially through the sagittal stratum, lie at its medial border, and then enter the dorsal part of the cingulate fasciculus at the level of the splenium of the corpus callosum (Scs. 105,113). These fibers terminate in the dysgranular retrosplenial cortex situated above the splenium and in areas 23 and 31 (Scs. 105, 113). Some of the cingulate fibers course around the splenium of the corpus callosum to become the ventral part of the cingulum bundle, and are joined by the fibers of the ILF. Some of the fibers in the dorsal part of the cingulate fasciculus course caudally in the white matter of the medial parietal lobe and terminate in area PGm, mostly in the first layer (Sc. 121).

Rostrally Directed Fibers

Long association fibers traveling rostrally from the injection site are located within the MdLF situated in the white matter of the superior temporal gyrus. The fibers terminate in a columnar manner in the temporal lobe within the rostral part of area TS3, and in areas TS2 and TS1 (Scs. 57, 65, 73). Fibers also terminate in the depth of the lateral fissure in area Pro and in the dorsal aspect of the temporal pole in areas TS2/Pro (Scs. 49, 57, 65, 73).

Another contingent of rostrally directed association fibers leaves the injection site and courses medially until it joins the extreme capsule (EmC). Here the fibers turn dorsally, continue upward until they cross the claustrum, and come to lie in the white matter of the prearcuate region (along with the fibers of the SLF II). Fibers leave this bundle and terminate dorsally in areas 9 and 46 (Scs. 31, 41), in area 32 at the medial wall of the hemisphere (Sc. 31), in area 45 at the ventrolateral prefrontal convexity, and in the orbital portion of area 47/12 (not shown).

Commissural and Subcortical Fibers

A dense cord of fibers emanates from the injection site and travels medially in the central part of the white matter of the superior temporal gyrus (Scs. 81, 85, 89).

From this cord of fibers, a prominent fiber bundle continues to course medially and is concentrated within the stem of the anterior commissure (Sc. 73). These fibers sweep medially, enter the anterior commissure, and course toward the opposite hemisphere (Sc. 65). Along with the association fibers that lie dorsal to the cord, a few scattered fibers are also seen in sector CC4 of the corpus callosum heading for the opposite hemisphere (Sc. 97).

An intense concentration of fibers leaves the cord and aggregates in a distinct fiber bundle below and medial to the claustrum (Scs. 85, 89). One contingent leaves this aggregation and courses caudally until the most caudal level of the LGN. At this point the fibers move medially to enter the thalamus. These thalamic bundle fibers terminate in the MG, PM, and Li nuclei (Scs. 93, 97). The other major contingent of fibers from the cord courses medially over the rostral and middle sectors of the LGN. These fibers in the pontine bundle (PB) descend medial to the LGN and enter the cerebral peduncle (Sc. 93) before terminating in the lateral part of the peripeduncular nucleus in the rostral pons.

Striatal Fibers

Some striatal fibers head medially and terminate in the ventral part of the claustrum (Sc. 65). Others travel medially and ventrally and terminate in the ventral part of the putamen and in the tail of the caudate nucleus (Scs. 73, 81, 85). One segment of fibers ascends within the extreme capsule, traverses the dorsal aspect of the claustrum to enter the external capsule, and then crosses through the internal capsule before terminating in the ventral part of the body of the caudate nucleus (Scs. 85, 89, 93).

CASE 10

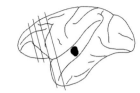

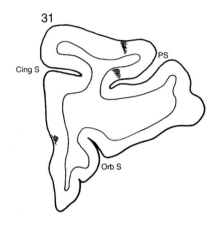

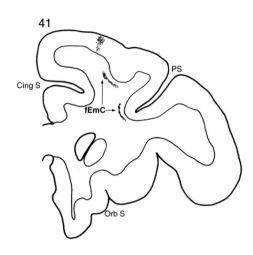

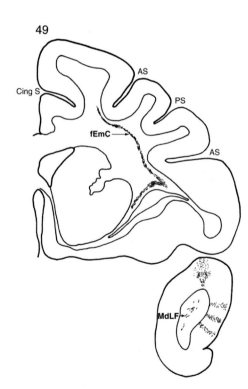

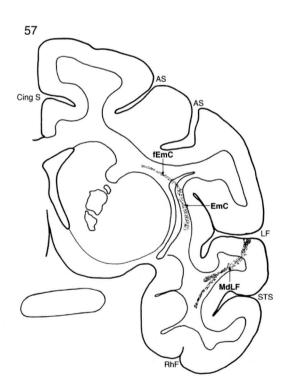

Figure 7-7

Schematic diagrams of 14 rostral–caudal coronal sections in Case 10 taken at the levels shown on the hemispheric diagram above right, showing the isotope injection site in the superior temporal gyrus involving the rostral part of area TS3 (black-filled area) and the resulting trajectories of the cortical association, commissural, and subcortical fibers (dashed lines and dots) in the white matter and the terminations in the cortex and subcortical regions (black dots).

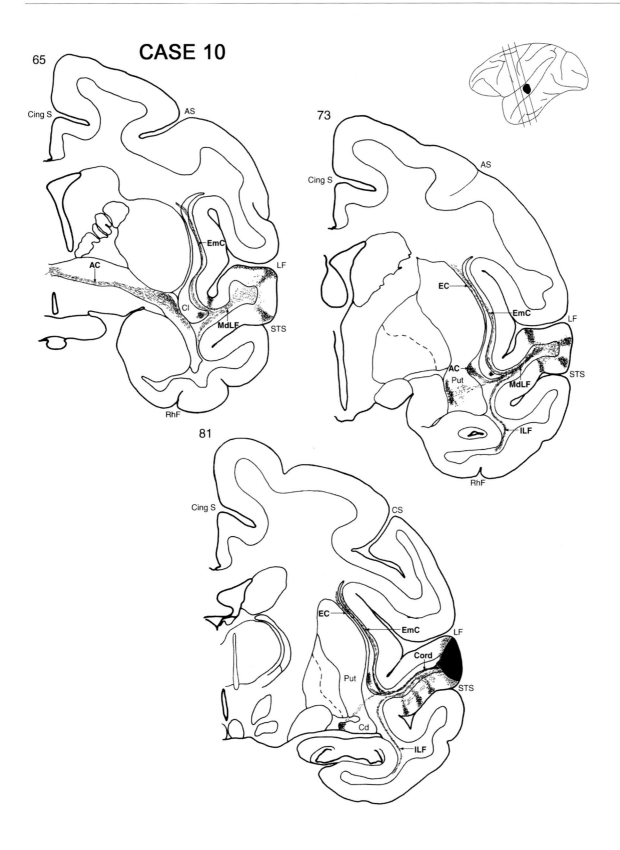

CASE 10

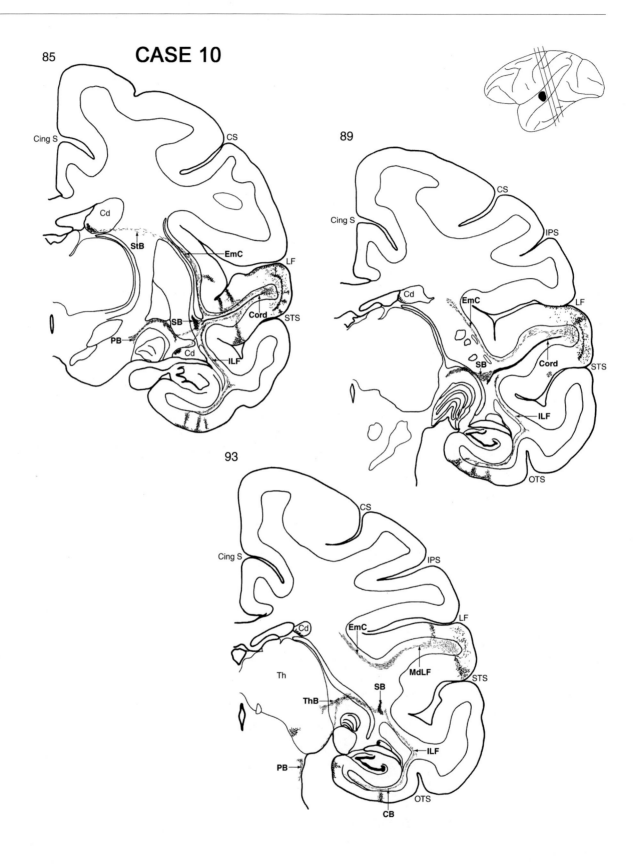

Figure 7-7 (continued)

CASE 10

97

CS
Cing S
IPS
LF
StB
STS
MdLF
Th
SS
ILF
OTS

105

CS
IPS
Cing S
LF
STS
CB
MdLF
SS
CB
ILF
CB
OTS

113

IPS
Cing S
LF
CB
STS
CB
MdLF
SS
CB
CF
ILF
IOS
OTS

121

IPS
Cing S
STS
CB
CF
IOS
OTS

169

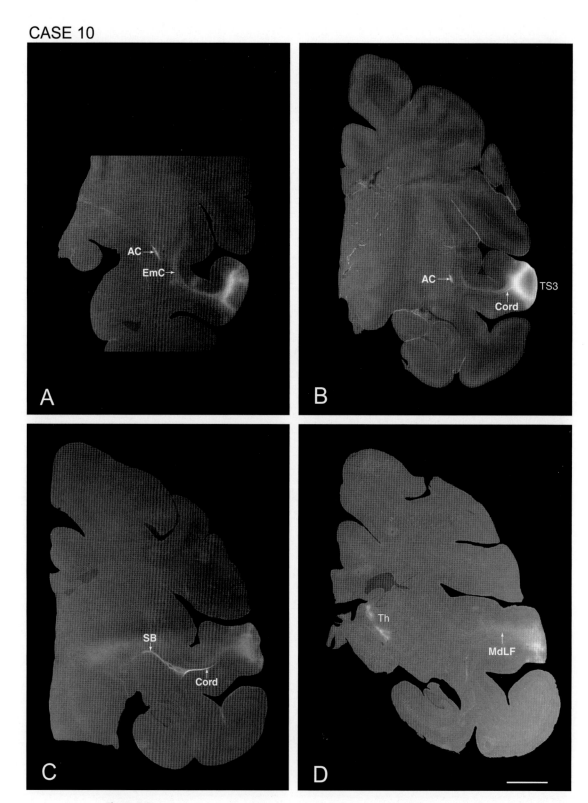

Figure 7-8
Photomicrographs of selected coronal sections of Case 10, showing the injection site in B and the resulting labeled fibers and terminations in A through D. Photomicrographs A through D correspond to sections 65, 81, 89, and 97, respectively (Mag = 0.5×, bar = 5 mm).

CASE 11

The isotope injection was placed in the rostral superior temporal gyrus in this case and involved areas Pro and TS1 and encroaching on area TS2. See figures 7-9 and 7-10.

Association Fiber Systems

Local Association Fibers

Adjacent to the injection site, terminations are seen laterally in the first layer in area TS2 and in the temporal proisocortex (Pro) and periallocortices in the medial part of the temporal pole (Scs. 49, 57). Other local fibers leave the injection site, travel beneath the cortex of the lateral fissure, and terminate in area Pro in the Sylvian fissure (Sc. 49).

Long Association Fibers

Caudally Directed Fibers

From the injection site a collection of fibers travels caudally in the middle longitudinal fasciculus (MdLF) that lies within the white matter of the superior temporal gyrus (Scs. 65, 73). These fibers give rise to terminations in the first layer in area TS2, in the lip of the upper bank of the STS in area TAa, in the cortex of the upper bank of the STS in area TPO, and in the temporal proisocortex and area paI. Some fibers from the MdLF enter the ventral part of the extreme capsule and terminate in the insular proisocortex (Sc. 81). Also, some fibers course ventrally from the injection site and terminate in the perirhinal and prorhinal cortices, area 35, and the lateral and ventrobasal nuclei of the amygdala (Scs. 57, 65).

Rostrally Directed Fibers

Fibers that travel rostrally from the injection site are situated within the uncinate fasciculus (UF) (Sc. 57). Fibers leave the injection site, travel medially, and ascend in the temporal stem toward the claustrum. Here they lie at the lateral and ventral aspect of the claustrum before passing over the limen insula and ventral to the claustrum to form a flattened plate of fibers lying above the orbital cortex (Scs. 41, 49). As fibers leave the uncinate fasciculus to terminate in the orbital cortex, they lie in the white matter immediately subjacent to the cortex and terminate in the orbital proisocortex and then more rostrally in orbital areas 12, 13, and 14 (Scs. 20, 31, 41, 49). The plate of uncinate fibers continues medially at the orbital and medial surfaces to terminate in area 25, medial area 14, and area 32 (Scs. 20, 31, 41). The fibers then move dorsally beneath the cortex of the cingulate sulcus before becoming recurved and moving caudally once more to terminate in area 24 within the depth and lower bank of the cingulate sulcus at the level of the genu of the corpus callosum (Sc. 31).

Commissural and Subcortical Fibers

A dense cord of fibers consisting of two partially separate strands leaves the injection site and descends within the white matter of the temporal stem (Scs. 57, 65).

A sizable contingent of fibers travels medially and caudally from the cord and enters the anterior commissure (AC) (Scs. 65, 73). These fibers situated in the ventral part of the AC continue to the opposite hemisphere, where they terminate.

Some of the cord fibers stream medially and then caudally from the cord and course upward at the lateral and dorsal margins of the amygdala (Sc. 65). They continue medially above the amygdala and beneath the anterior commissure, and these fibers enter the basal forebrain (f BF), where they terminate in the substantia innominata (Sc. 57).

The cord fibers continue caudally from the injection site and give rise to focal aggregations of whorls of fibers that lie in the white matter between the caudate tail and the putamen (Sc. 85). These whorls course medially and then are situated above the stria terminalis. At this point two distinct fiber components can be discerned. One travels dorsally over the dome of the LGN and collects in a helmet-shaped distribution at the medial aspect of the LGN at the entrance to the cerebral peduncle (Scs. 85, 89). Some fibers leave this helmet-shaped collection and pass medially into the zona incerta (S.85). The remaining fibers, which constitute the pontine bundle (PB), descend into the cerebral peduncle and terminate in the basilar pontine nuclei. These terminations are concentrated in the extreme dorsolateral, dorsolateral, and lateral pontine nuclei, with some in the lateral part of the peripeduncular nucleus. Other fibers lateral and ventral to the LGN continue to course caudally in this position as the thalamic fiber bundle (ThB), also termed the ventral subcortical bundle (Scs. 85, 59, 93, 97). At the level of the inferior pulvinar nucleus these fibers enter the external medullary lamina of the thalamus, course horizontally through the thalamus, and terminate in the caudal part of MGmc and then in Li, SG, and PM (Sc. 97).

Striatal Fibers

A group of fibers courses from the injection site medially and then dorsally, and some of these fibers provide terminations in the ventral aspect of the claustrum (Sc. 65). Remaining fibers enter the external capsule (EC) and provide terminations in the claustrum, while others course medially located in the most dorsal part of the anterior commissure (Sc. 65) to terminate in the ventral part of the head of the caudate nucleus and the putamen (Sc. 57, 65). Some striatal fibers traveling caudally along with the subcortical bundle terminate in the tail of the caudate nucleus and in the ventral putamen (Sc. 81).

CASE 11

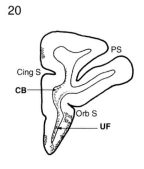

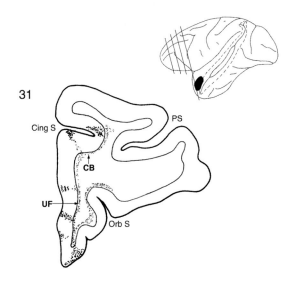

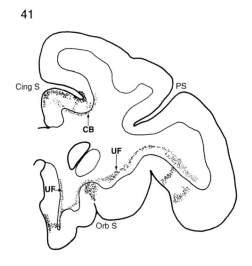

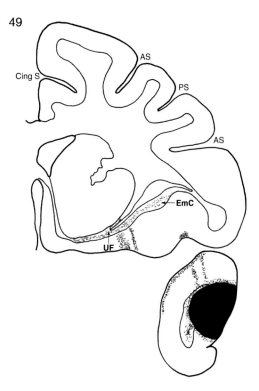

Figure 7-9

Schematic diagrams of 12 rostral–caudal coronal sections in Case 11 taken at the levels shown on the hemispheric diagram above right, showing the isotope injection site in the rostral superior temporal gyrus involving areas Pro and TS1 and encroaching on area TS2 (black-filled area) and the resulting trajectories of the cortical association, commissural, and subcortical fibers (dashed lines and dots) in the white matter and the terminations in the cortex and subcortical regions (black dots).

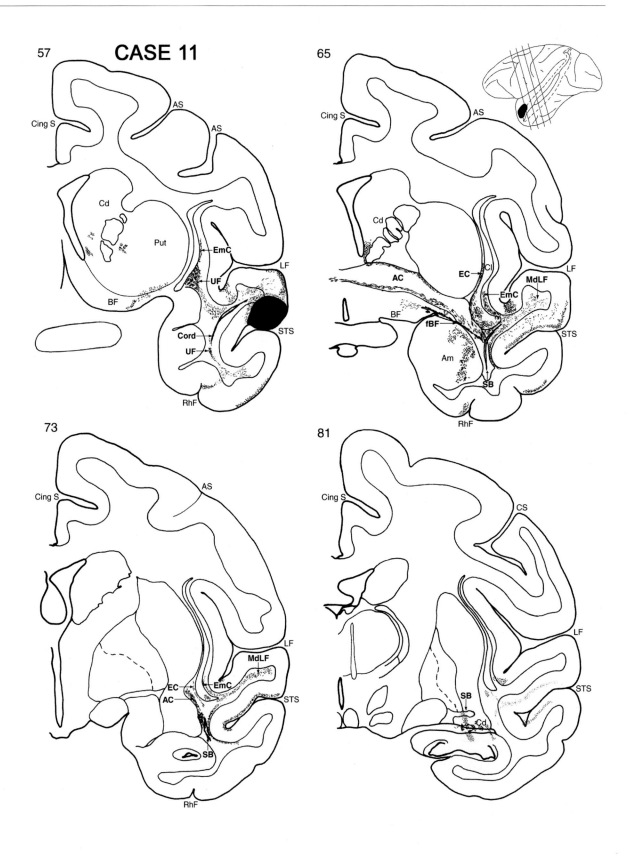

Figure 7-9 (continued)

CASE 11

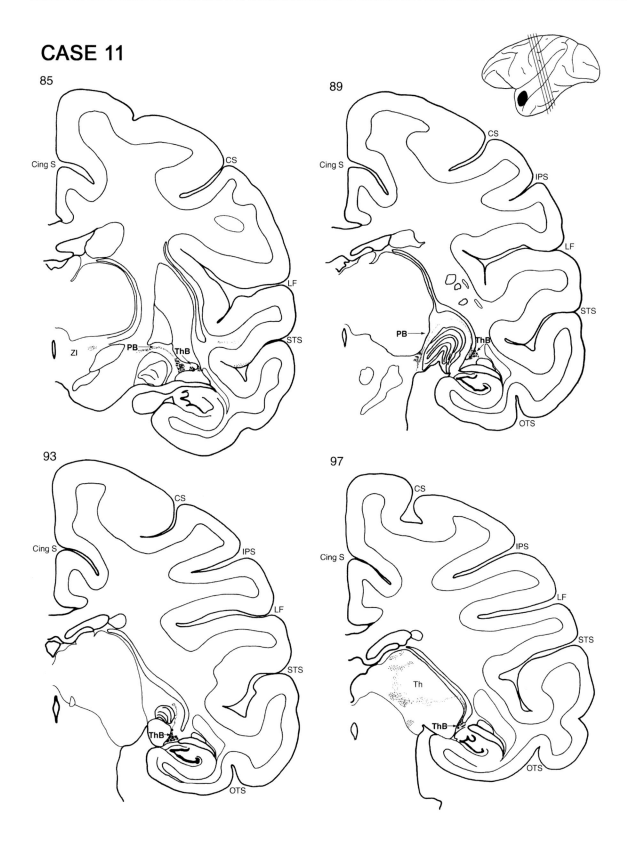

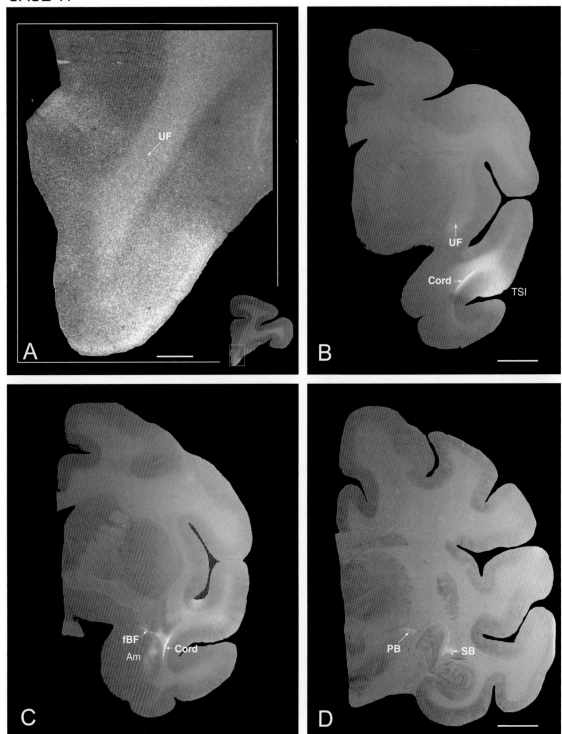

Figure 7-10

Photomicrographs of selected coronal sections of Case 11, showing the injection site in B and the resulting labeled fibers and terminations in A through D. A, High-power photomicrograph (section 31, Mag = 4×, bar = 0.5 mm) taken from the location indicated in the low-power photomicrograph below to show the uncinate fasciculus leading to terminations in area 14. Photomicrographs B through D correspond to sections 57, 65, and 75, respectively (Mag = 0.5×, bar = 5 mm).

Superior Temporal Region Summary

Association Fibers

Rostral Part of the Superior Temporal Gyrus, Area TS1 (Case 11)

This region gives rise to two major fiber bundles. The uncinate fasciculus courses rostrally, the middle longitudinal fasciculus caudally (figure 7-11).

1. Uncinate Fasciculus

The uncinate fibers emerge from the temporal polar area and provide terminations to the medial aspect of the temporal pole in the temporal proisocortex and area TS1. Onward, the fibers pass through the limen insula and course along the orbital surface of the frontal lobe. Some of these fibers terminate in area 12, as well as in the orbital proisocortex. Further rostrally, the uncinate fascicle fibers move medially and terminate in areas 12, 13, 14, and 25. At the level of the genu of the corpus callosum, the uncinate fibers course dorsally in the white matter deep to the medial wall of the hemisphere, and in front of the genu they come to lie in the white matter around the rostral part of the cingulate sulcus. From this medial part of the uncinate fasciculus, fibers terminate in area 14, rostral area 24, and area 32.

Some fibers from the rostral part of the superior temporal gyrus course medially in the temporal part of the uncinate bundle and provide terminations to the amygdala and to the perirhinal and prorhinal cortices.

2. Middle Longitudinal Fasciculus

The caudally directed fibers from the rostral temporal cortex course through the white matter of the superior temporal gyrus (the middle longitudinal fasciculus). These fibers terminate dorsally in the Sylvian fissure in areas Pro and paI. Other fibers terminate ventrally and laterally in areas TPO, TAa, and TS2.

Midsector of the Superior Temporal Gyrus, Area TS3 (Case 10)

From the midpart of the superior temporal gyrus four distinct fiber tracts are observed: the extreme capsule, the middle longitudinal fasciculus, the inferior longitudinal fasciculus, and the cingulum bundle.

1. Extreme Capsule

The fibers that leave this region and enter the extreme capsule course rostrally into the frontal lobe. They ascend dorsally along with the fibers of the SLF II and branch into a dorsal and ventral contingent. The dorsal component of fibers spreads out beneath the arcuate sulcus and terminates in dorsal area 8, dorsal area 46, and area 9. The ventral component terminates in areas 45 and 47/12.

2. Middle Longitudinal Fasciculus

The second major fiber tract courses through the middle longitudinal fasciculus in the white matter of the superior temporal gyrus. Rostrally these MdLF fibers terminate in area paAr in the lower bank of the Sylvian fissure, in areas TS2 and TAa of the superior temporal gyrus, and area TPO of the STS. The caudal contingent of the MdLF continues in the superior temporal gyrus white matter and terminates in area proK in the Sylvian fissure, areas paAlt and TAa of the superior temporal gyrus, and area TPO of the superior temporal sulcus. Further caudally, the fibers from the MdLF terminate in areas Tpt, TAa, and TPO, as well as in area PGa.

Two fiber tracts link the midpart of the superior temporal gyrus with the limbic system, running ventrally in the ILF and dorsally in the cingulum bundle.

3. Inferior Longitudinal Fasciculus

The ventrally situated fibers leave the midsector of the superior temporal gyrus and course in the ILF. These fibers terminate in areas TH and TL of the posterior parahippocampal gyrus.

4. Cingulum Bundle

The dorsally situated fibers leave the superior temporal gyrus and course medially to lie in the white matter of the cingulate gyrus. From there the fibers terminate in area 23 and area 30 of the retrosplenial cortex. These fibers course around the splenium of the corpus callosum, enter the white matter of the calcarine sulcus, and continue into the ventral part of the cingulum bundle, from where they terminate in the ventral segment of area 30 of the retrosplenial cortex.

Midportion of Area TPO in the Upper Bank of the Superior Temporal Sulcus (Case 9)

Fibers that emerge from this region travel to other cortical sites via four principal association fiber pathways: the middle longitudinal fasciculus, the extreme capsule, the arcuate fasciculus, and the cingulum bundle. In addition, the inferior longitudinal fasciculus also conveys some fibers from this region.

1. Middle Longitudinal Fasciculus

The MdLF fibers run both rostrally and caudally in the white matter of the superior temporal gyrus. Rostrally these fibers terminate in areas proK, paAr, PGa, TPO, and TAa and further rostrally in area TS3. Caudally, these MdLF fibers terminate in areas reIt and paAc of the Sylvian fissure, areas Tpt and TAa of the superior temporal gyrus, and areas TPO and PGa of the STS.

2. Extreme Capsule

Fibers traveling in the extreme capsule course rostrally and terminate first in the granular and dysgranular insula. In the frontal lobe, these fibers terminate in area 45 and area 47/12.

3. Arcuate Fasciculus

Fibers course rostrally in the AF situated in the white matter above the Sylvian fissure until they reach the prefrontal cortex. Here the fibers surround the arcuate sulcus and terminate in dorsal area 8. Further rostrally, these fibers surround the principal sulcus and terminate in dorsal area 46.

4. Cingulum Bundle

Another group of fibers that stems from area TPO moves medially and becomes part of the cingulum bundle lying in the white matter of the cingulate gyrus. One contingent of fibers runs rostrally and terminates in area 24. The other contingent runs caudally and terminates in area 23. Some of these cingulum bundle fibers move dorsally in the superior parietal lobule and terminate in areas 31, PEci (SSA) and PGm. Other cingulum fibers course ventrally in the white matter of the calcarine sulcus and join the ILF fibers, as described below. These fibers terminate in areas V2 and V3V.

5. Inferior Longitudinal Fasciculus

Ventrally directed fibers arising from area TPO course in the ILF lateral to the sagittal stratum. These fibers continue caudally, and at the level of the end of the Sylvian fissure they divide into dorsal and ventral components. The dorsal contingent of the ILF fibers ascends in the white matter of the inferior parietal lobule and terminates in areas Opt and MST. The ventral contingent of the fibers joins with the cingulum bundle, as described above.

Caudal Superior Temporal Gyrus (Cases 7 and 8)

Six long association fiber bundles emanate from the caudal part of the superior temporal gyrus (STG). These are principally the arcuate fasciculus and cingulum bundle, in addition to the SLF I, middle longitudinal fasciculus, extreme capsule, and inferior longitudinal fasciculus.

1. Arcuate Fasciculus

The arcuate fasciculus fibers arch upward, deep to the caudal part of the Sylvian fissure. These fibers run forward, located above the upper shoulder of the Sylvian fissure, where they are situated ventral to the main bulk of fibers of the SLF II. After coursing through the parietal and precentral white matter in this location, the AF fibers reach the white matter deep to the arcuate sulcus and terminate in area 8Ad above the principal sulcus and in dorsal area 6.

2. Cingulum Bundle

Medially directed fibers from the caudal STG course toward the cingulum bundle. These fibers course through two separate fascicles. The dorsal fascicles course along with the SLF I before heading medially beneath the cingulate sulcus to enter the cingulate white matter. The ventral fibers travel along with those destined for the callosum; at the level of the caudal part of the body of the caudate nucleus, they become incorporated into the cingulum bundle (CB). From there the fibers run in the CB in both rostral and caudal directions. Rostrally the fibers terminate in the caudal part of area 24, and area 23. The caudally directed CB fibers arch around the splenium of the corpus callosum in the ventral part of the CB situated in the white matter deep to the calcarine sulcus. These fibers terminate in the caudal part of area 23 and in the retrosplenial cortex in the calcarine sulcus. The ventral CB fibers receive a contribution also from the inferior longitudinal fasciculus that originates from the caudal STG.

3. Superior Longitudinal Fasciculus I

The caudal part of the STG gives rise to fibers that course medially in the white matter deep to the intraparietal sulcus and then turn dorsally around the depth of the intraparietal sulcus to become incorporated in the SLF I. These fibers then proceed caudally in the white matter of the superior parietal lobule and terminate medially in areas 31 and PEci and laterally in the cortex in the depth of the intraparietal sulcus, in area IPd.

4. Middle Longitudinal Fasciculus

Another group of fibers runs rostrally in the MdLF in the white matter of the superior temporal gyrus. In their course, the MdLF fibers provide terminations to areas reIt, reIpt, paAc, and proK and the caudal part of area KA in the Sylvian fissure. Terminations are also distributed in the cortex of the superior temporal gyrus, in areas Tpt, TAa, and paAlt, and in the upper bank of the superior temporal sulcus, in area TPO.

5. Extreme Capsule

A small contingent of fibers from the caudal STG courses rostrally in the ventral part of the extreme capsule and terminates in the ventral part of the insula.

6. Inferior Longitudinal Fasciculus

Fibers from the caudal STG descend in the vertical limb of the ILF, course medially toward the parahippocampal gyrus, where they become continuous with the ventral component of the cingulum bundle, and terminate in the retrosplenial and prostriate cortices.

Commissural Fibers

Commissural fibers from the caudal part of the superior temporal gyrus and the adjacent part of the superior temporal sulcus course across the midline through the rostral part of the most caudal fifth of the corpus callosum (CC5), rostral to the splenium, in a topographic manner. Commissural fibers from the middle part of the superior temporal gyrus course through sector CC5, as well as the anterior commissure. In contrast, fibers from the rostral part of the superior temporal gyrus course through the anterior commissure only. Within the anterior commissure, the superior temporal region fibers tend to be situated ventrally.

Subcortical Fibers

Rostral Part of the Superior Temporal Region

The subcortical fibers from the rostral part of the superior temporal region gather in the central core of the white matter. These fibers then travel caudally as a compact bundle, course ventrally, and enter the white matter above the caudate tail as they proceed further caudally. At the level of the rostral part of the lateral geniculate nucleus, this subcortical bundle differentiates into two parts. The pontine system arches over the midportion of the LGN and enters the cerebral peduncle. The thalamic contingent of subcortical fibers continues caudally, and at the level of the caudal end of the LGN the fibers move dorsally and enter the ventral part of the external medullary lamina. From there the fibers terminate in the thalamus.

Middle Part of the Superior Temporal Gyrus

From the middle part of the superior temporal gyrus the dense cord of fibers continues caudally in the central core of the white matter of the gyrus. At the level of the midpoint of the LGN, the fibers separate, with the pontine fiber system arching over the LGN and descending into the cerebral peduncle. The thalamic fiber contingent lies in the ventral part of the external medullary lamina and penetrates the thalamus at the level of the caudal end of the LGN.

Caudal Part of the Superior Temporal Gyrus

The subcortical fibers from the caudal part of the superior temporal gyrus head medially in the cord and enter the dorsal part of the sagittal stratum. From here the fibers travel rostrally in the lateral aspect of the sagittal stratum, enter the posterior limb of the internal capsule, and separate into two components. The medially situated thalamic fibers enter the thalamus through the midportion of the external medullary lamina, at the level of the pulvinar and caudal to the LGN. The pontine fiber bundle continues rostrally until the midpoint of the LGN, arches over the LGN, and descends into the cerebral peduncle.

Corticostriate Projections

Fibers from the rostral superior temporal region (temporal proisocortex and rostral part of area TS1) lead to terminations in the ventral aspect of the head of the caudate nucleus, including its most ventral component in the nucleus accumbens. These fibers reach their destination in a unique fashion, traveling medially beneath the striatum along the dorsal aspect of the anterior commissure. Some fibers from the rostral temporal region terminate in the ventral part of the claustrum, and those that travel in the external capsule terminate in the ventral putamen and the tail of the caudate nucleus.

The striatal system arising from the midpart of the superior temporal gyrus (area paAlt) and adjacent midportion of the superior temporal sulcus (area TPO) has a dorsal and a ventral contingent. The dorsal part ascends in the extreme and then external capsules, crosses the posterior limb of the internal capsule, and terminates in the ventral part of the body of the caudate nucleus. The ventral striatal system travels initially in the external capsule and terminates in discrete patches in the medial part of the ventral aspect of the putamen and in the rostral part of the tail of the caudate nucleus.

The caudal part of the superior temporal gyrus (area Tpt) gives rise to a contingent of striatal fibers that moves medially and dorsally, enters the Muratoff bundle, and terminates in the caudate body as it moves rostrally. These terminations are situated lateral to those arising from the mid-STG. Other striatal fibers ascend in the extreme and then external capsules, terminating in the midpart of the claustrum and in the medial aspect of the caudal part of the putamen. A third contingent moves ventrally, passes medially through the sagittal stratum, and enters the genu of the caudate nucleus, where it terminates.

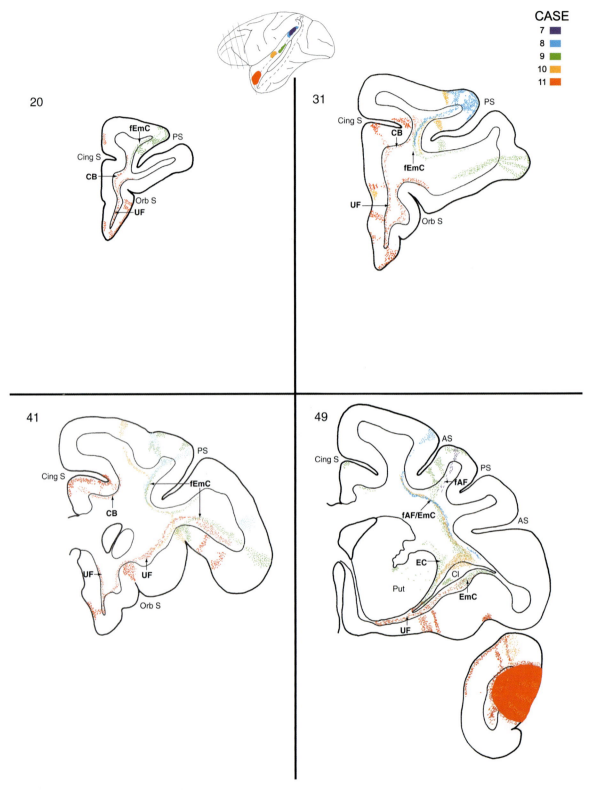

Figure 7-11

Schematic composite diagrams of rostral–caudal coronal sections of the template brain, illustrating the five superior temporal region cases (Cases 7 through 11). The injection sites and the association, commissural, and subcortical fibers, as well as the termination patterns, are color-coded for each case. The schematic diagram of the lateral surface of the cerebral hemisphere (at top) represents the different levels of the coronal sections and the injection sites. Color-coding is as follows: Case 7—purple,

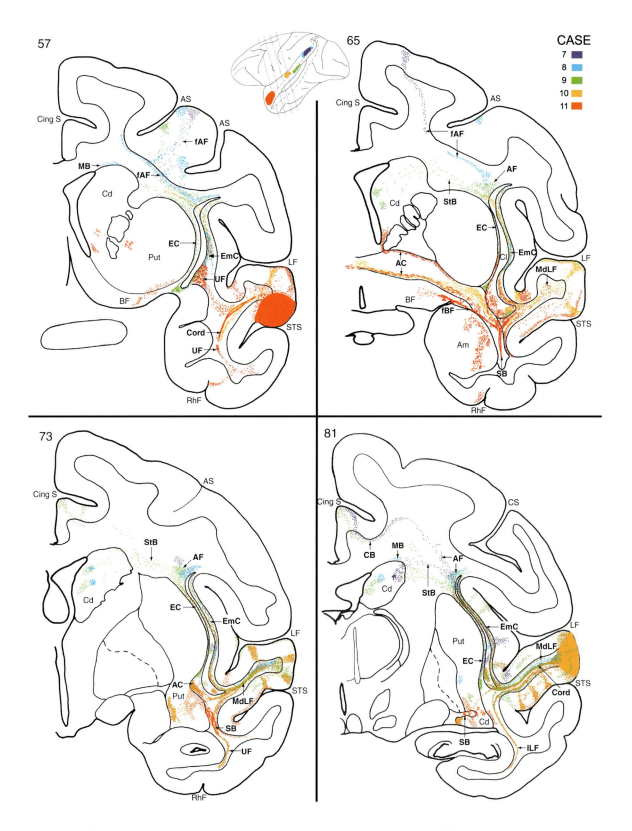

caudal part of the superior temporal gyrus involving area Tpt; Case 8—blue, caudal part of the superior temporal gyrus in areas paAlt and Tpt; Case 9—green, midportion of area TPO, ventral superior temporal gyrus area TAa, and caudal part of primary auditory area KA; Case 10—orange, rostral part of area TS3 in the superior temporal gyrus; Case 11—red, rostral part of superior temporal gyrus in areas Pro and TS1, encroaching on area TS2.

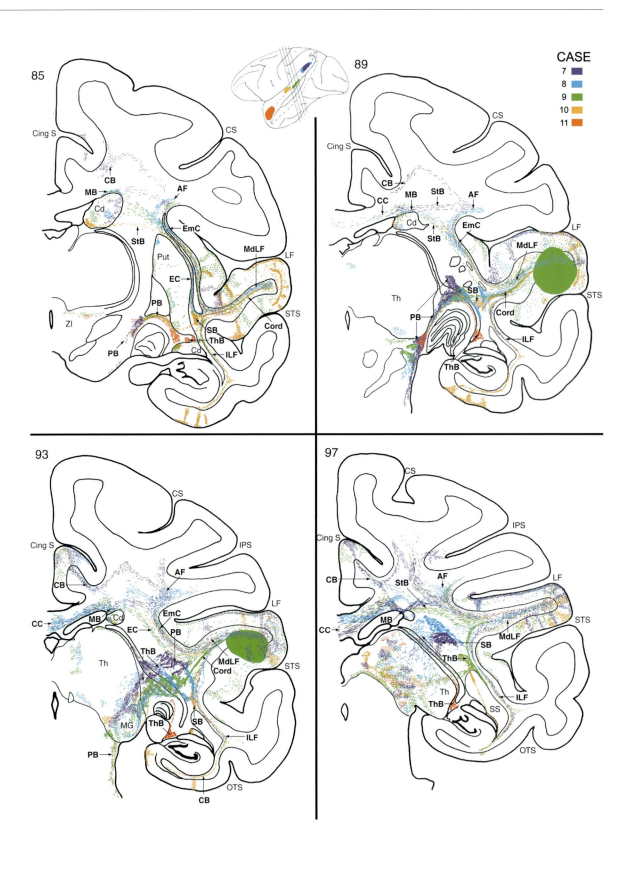

Figure 7-11 (continued)

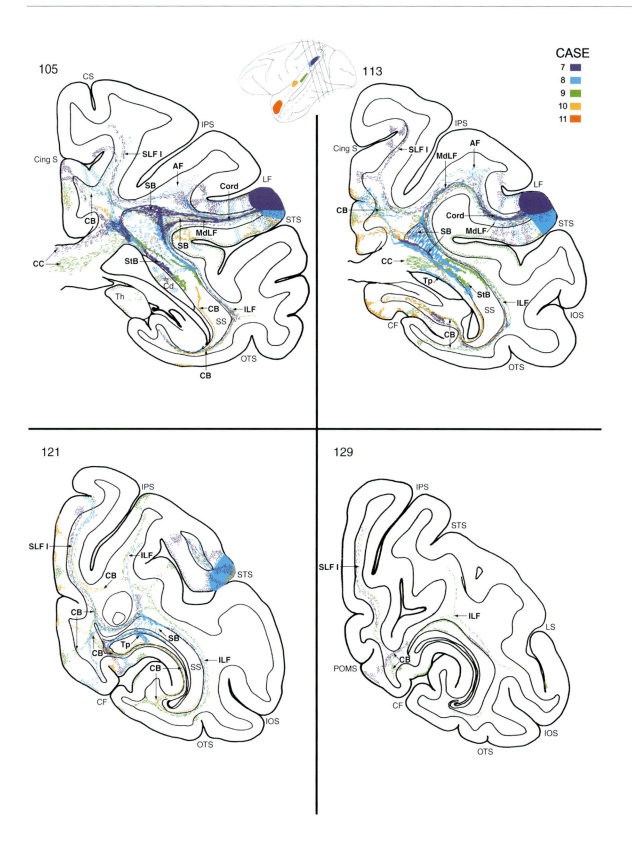

185

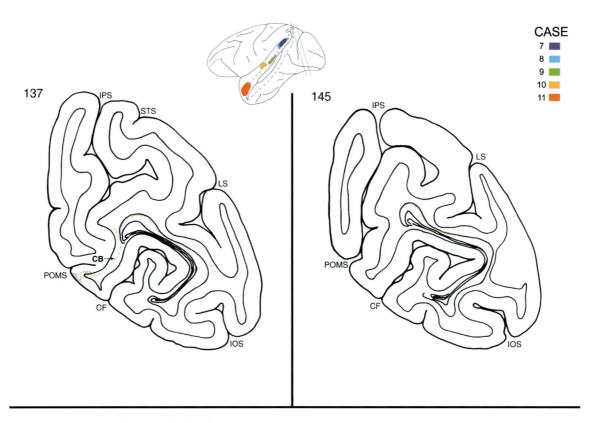

Figure 7-11 (continued)

Inferior Temporal Region

8

In this chapter we describe the isotope injection cases in the inferior temporal region of five rhesus monkeys and analyze the resulting association, striatal, commissural, and subcortical fiber trajectories, as well as the cortical and subcortical terminations. The injections were in the ventral part of the temporal lobe in areas TE2 and TE3 (Case 12), the ventral temporal region, area TF (Case 13), cortex in the rostral part of the superior temporal sulcus involving area IPa, and encroaching on the lateral border of the hippocampus (Case 14), the medial part of the inferior temporal gyrus in areas TE1 and TE2 (Case 15), and the rostral temporal lobe in the midportion of area TE2 (Case 16).

As in the previous chapters, the architectonic designations of the cortical terminations are described in the text but not identified on the coronal sections. Architectonic areas are labeled on external views of the hemisphere as well as in the coronal series of chapter 4. Terminations in the thalamus are shown and thalamic nuclei are referred to in the text, but the nuclei are not designated on the coronal sections. Pontine terminations are described in the text but not illustrated. Striatal terminations are illustrated and an overview of their termination patterns is presented in the text.

CASE 12

Isotope injections were made in this case in the midportion of the inferotemporal region in areas TE2 and TE3. See figures 8-1 and 8-2.

Association Fibers

Local Association Fibers

Local terminations are seen in cortices adjacent to the injection site, in areas TE3, TEO, and MT, in the first layer (Scs. 93, 97, 105).

Long Association Fibers

Caudally Directed Fibers

Fibers leave the injection site and travel caudally in the inferior longitudinal fasciculus (ILF). Most of the fibers are concentrated in the ventral part of the ILF, occupying the white matter between the inferior occipital sulcus (IOS) and the occipitotemporal sulcus (OTS), as well as between the IOS and the superior temporal sulcus (STS). These fibers progress in a longitudinal and caudal direction, and they terminate in ventral area V4 around the IOS, in area TEO, and in area MT, principally in the first layer (Scs. 113,

121, 129). Other fibers leave the injection site and ascend to enter the dorsal segment of the ILF within the white matter deep to the STS. As these fibers travel caudally they terminate in the fourth layer in area POa in the cortex of the lower bank of the intraparietal sulcus (Scs. 105, 113) and in the first layer of area V4D above the lunate sulcus (Sc. 137), as well as in areas V3D and V2 in the depth in the lower bank of the lunate sulcus (Scs. 137, 145).

Rostrally Directed Fibers

Rostrally directed association fibers leave the injection site and travel in the ILF contained within the white matter of the rostral part of the inferotemporal region. The fibers terminate in areas MT and FST within the cortex of the STS (Scs. 85, 89) and in areas TE1, TE2, and TE3 ventrally in the inferotemporal region (Scs. 73, 81, 85, 89). The terminations in these areas are principally located around the fourth layer in a columnar manner. The ILF also carries fibers dorsally to terminate in the middle part of area POa in the fourth layer (Scs. 105, 113). A few fibers terminate in the ventral aspect of area 8Av (Sc. 49), although the exact course of the fibers destined for this cortical area are not reliably discerned.

Commissural and Subcortical Fibers

From the injection site a dense cord of labeled fibers heads medially and enters the external segment of the sagittal stratum (SS). Some of these fibers traverse both the external and internal segments of the ventral part of sector SS-2 of the SS (Scs. 105, 113), enter the tapetum medially, and turn sharply upward. They ascend in the tapetum, penetrate the splenium of the corpus callosum (CC5), and progress to the opposite hemisphere (Sc. 113). Other commissural fibers (anterior commissure, AC) course rostrally in the subcortical bundle, enter the anterior commissure, and then cross to the opposite hemisphere (Scs. 65, 73).

The major component of the cord of labeled fibers that emanates from the injection site traverses the external segment of the sagittal stratum and concentrates in the internal segment of SS-2 (Scs. 113, 105). This dense bundle of fibers moves further rostrally in the internal segment of the sagittal stratum into sector SS-1. At the lateral border of the thalamus at the level of the pulvinar, most of these fibers leave the SS-1, gather at the lower part of the retrolenticular portion of the internal capsule (ICp-5, Sc. 97), and enter the thalamus via the lateral and ventral thalamic peduncles. These fibers terminate predominantly in the PI and PL nuclei and to a lesser extent in LP (Sc. 97).

Striatal Fibers

One contingent of striatal fibers (StB) aggregates ventral to the tail of the caudate nucleus before terminating in the genu and tail and in the ventral aspect of the putamen (Scs. 81, 85, 89, 105). Other fibers in the striatal bundle (StB) travel along with the ILF, traverse the retrolenticular aspect of the internal capsule, and terminate in the body of the caudate nucleus, the caudal part of the putamen, and the ventral aspect of the claustrum (Scs. 73, 81, 85, 89).

CASE 12

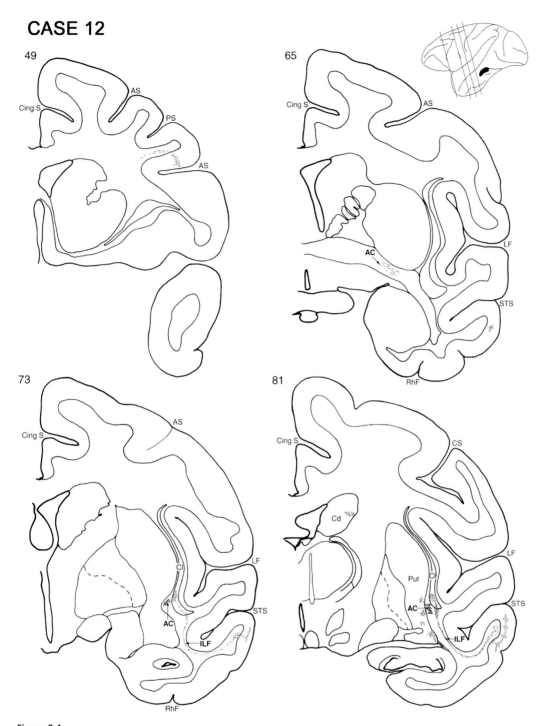

Figure 8-1

Schematic diagrams of 16 rostral–caudal coronal sections in Case 12 taken at the levels shown on the hemispheric diagram above right, showing the isotope injection site in the ventral part of the temporal lobe, in areas TE2 and TE3 (black-filled area), and the resulting trajectories of the cortical association, commissural, and subcortical fibers (dashed lines and dots) in the white matter and the terminations in the cortex and subcortical regions (black dots). See list of abbreviations, p. 617.

CASE 12

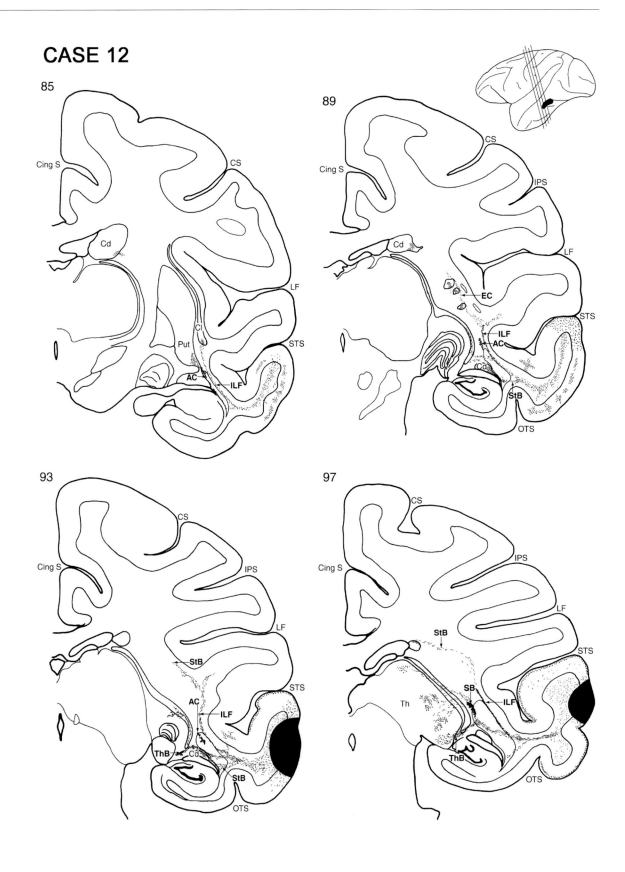

Figure 8-1 (continued)

CASE 12

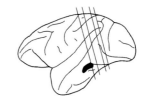

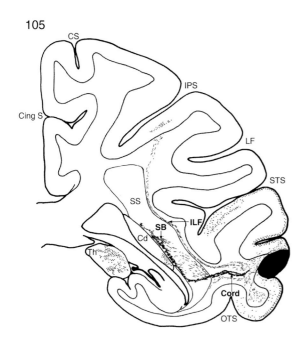

105

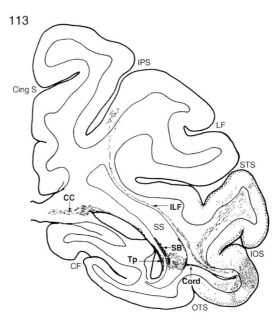

113

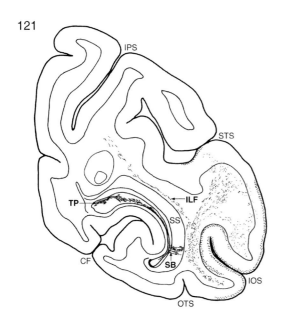

121

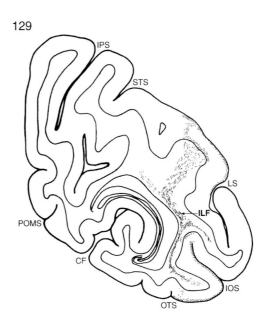

129

CASE 12

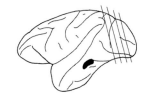

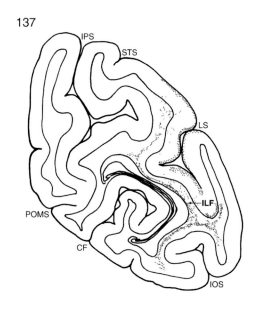

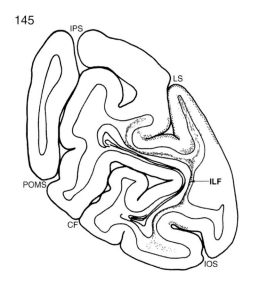

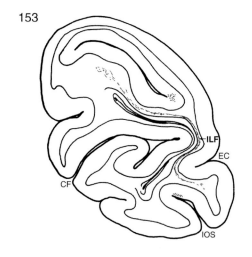

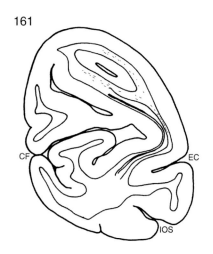

Figure 8-1 (continued)

CASE 12

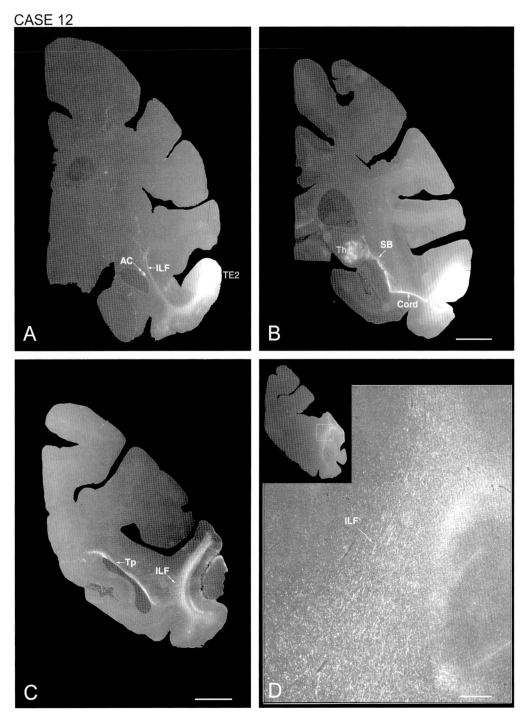

Figure 8-2

Photomicrographs of selected coronal sections of Case 12 showing the injection site in A and B and the resulting labeled fibers and terminations in A through D. Photomicrographs A through C correspond to sections 89, 97/105, and 113, respectively (Mag = 0.5×, bar = 5 mm). D, High-power photomicrograph (section 129, Mag = 4×, bar = 0.5 mm) taken from the location indicated in the low-power photomicrograph above, showing labeled fibers in the inferior longitudinal fasciculus and terminations in the ventral part of area V4.

CASE 13

In this case the isotope injection was in the ventral temporal region, area TF. See figures 8-3 and 8-4.

Association Fibers

Local Association Fibers

Adjacent to the injection site, local terminations are seen in the parahippocampal gyrus in areas TH and TL and the parasubiculum in a columnar manner (Scs. 93, 97).

Long Association Fibers

Caudally Directed Fibers

From the injection site fibers travel caudally in several subcomponents of the ILF. Fibers in the ventral aspect of the ILF are contiguous with those in the ventral part of the cingulum bundle medially. These ILF fibers terminate in a columnar manner in the ventral temporal cortex around the occipitotemporal sulcus, first in transitional areas TFO and TLO of the parahippocampal gyrus, and more caudally in areas V3V and TEO. Also, first-layer terminations are seen in area V4V (Scs. 105, 113, 121).

The fibers that travel in the ascending component of the ILF enter the white matter within the inferior parietal lobule and terminate in the inferior parietal lobule in area PG (Sc. 113). Further caudally, they terminate in the upper bank of the superior temporal sulcus in area MST (Sc. 121), in the most caudal part of the inferior parietal lobule in area Opt, and in the cortex of the lower bank of the intraparietal sulcus in area POa in a columnar manner (Scs. 121, 129, 137). The fiber system in the ILF and inferior parietal lobule continues caudally and terminates in the occipital lobe in the first layer of area V4D (Scs. 137, 145).

A bundle of fibers leaves the ascending part of the ILF and turns sharply medially, coursing above the annectant gyrus, and heads medially towards area PGm at the medial parietal convexity, where it terminates in a columnar manner (Scs. 129, 137).

A contingent of fibers in the medial aspect of the ventral cingulum bundle lying within the ventral temporal white matter courses upward in the white matter of the rostral part of the calcarine sulcus and then heads medially toward the cingulate gyrus, where it terminates in area 23 (Scs. 105, 113).

Rostrally Directed Fibers

From the injection site an intense bundle of labeled fibers enters the ILF and ascends in the ILF lateral to the sagittal stratum. These form a plate of fibers that moves rostrally until it reaches the rostral aspect of the hippocampus.

At the fundus of the occipitotemporal sulcus, a ventral-lateral group of fibers leaves the main bundle and moves laterally within the white matter of the inferotemporal cortex. These fibers terminate in the ventral temporal region in areas TE3, TE2, and TE1 as they move rostrally (Scs. 81, 85, 89). This same bundle gives off fibers that move dorsally within the white matter of the inferior temporal gyrus and terminate in the lower bank of the superior temporal sulcus in areas IPa, TEa, and TEm. These terminations are all columnar (Scs. 81, 85).

The ascending component of the fibers in the ILF courses toward the white matter of the superior temporal gyrus and moves laterally within the gyrus as the middle longitudinal fasciculus (MdLF). These fibers terminate in the upper bank of the STS in areas TPO and PGa (Scs. 57, 65, 73, 81, 85, 89).

From the injection site fibers travel medially in the ventral part of the cingulum bundle lying in the white matter of the parahippocampal gyrus. These fibers terminate in areas TF, TL, and TH (Scs. 81, 85, 89). They also terminate in the parasubiculum and presubiculum and further rostrally in the perirhinal and lateral entorhinal cortices (Scs. 65, 73, 81). The terminations are all columnar.

Some of the fibers from the injection site that course along with the ILF leave this bundle at the point where the MdLF originates. These fibers ascend medially and dorsally through the corona radiata before becoming incorporated into the cingulum bundle (CB). The CB fibers then run rostrally and terminate in the cingulate gyrus in the caudal part of area 23 and in area 24 in a columnar manner (Scs. 49, 81, 89).

Another group of fibers travels rostrally in the uncinate fasciculus (UF), situated deep to the superior temporal sulcus, until it reaches the rostral aspect of the hippocampus. These fibers ascend in the white matter at a level anterior to the most rostral component of the sagittal stratum and aggregate lateral to the ventral part of the claustrum. The UF fibers move rostrally, first lateral to and then ventral to the claustrum. As they continue in the rostral direction they move medially and obliquely and flatten out so that they come to lie in a plate-like manner in the white matter immediately deep to the orbital cortex. As they move forward these fibers terminate in columns in the orbitofrontal cortex in areas 12, 13, 11, and 10 (Scs. 20, 31, 41).

Some fibers leading to the basal forebrain region emerge from the cord of subcortical fibers and travel along with the fibers that ascend toward the staging area for the anterior commissure. They then pass medially beneath the anterior commissure toward the nucleus basalis and the substantia innominata, where they terminate (Sc. 57).

A group of fibers enters the extreme capsule from the dorsal aspect of the ILF as it moves laterally into the white matter of the superior temporal gyrus. These extreme capsule fibers continue rostrally in the frontal lobe, where they ascend and join with the SLF II fibers lying deep to the principal sulcus, and they terminate in columns in area 46 and area 9 of the prefrontal cortex (Sc. 41).

Commissural and Subcortical Fibers

Fibers travel caudally from the injection site, situated ventral to the sagittal stratum, and are incorporated into the alveus of the hippocampus (Sc. 97). They travel dorsally and medially in the fornix (Scs. 105, 113). They move rostrally and cross to the opposite hemisphere in the dorsal hippocampal commissure situated beneath sector CC4 of the corpus callosum (Scs. 89, 93, 97).

The dense cord of fibers that leaves the injection site ascends medial to the sagittal stratum, just lateral to the inferior horn of the lateral ventricle. Fibers destined for the anterior commissure leave the cord and ascend medial to the sagittal stratum until they reach a staging area lateral to the ventral part of the putamen. Fibers move rostrally within this bundle until they reach the anterior commissure (AC), at which point they stream medially in a dense concentration toward the opposite hemisphere (Scs. 65, 73, 81).

A major contingent of cord fibers continues rostrally, courses over the tail of the caudate nucleus and the stria terminalis, and occupies a position medial to and above the stria terminalis just lateral to the pulvinar inferior and the LGN (Sc. 93). We have termed this aggregate of thalamic bundle fibers the "ventral subcortical bundle." From this position, two main contingents of fibers terminate in the thalamus. One sizable bundle of fibers continues to run caudally and then heads medially to enter the pulvinar inferior, where the fibers terminate (Scs. 93, 97). A second contingent of fibers leaves the ventral subcortical bundle and ascends in the thalamic external medullary lamina, from which fibers move medially into the thalamus and terminate in the anteroventral (AV), CL, LD, and PM nuclei (Scs. 85, 89, 93, 97). A small bundle of fibers can also be seen traversing the pulvinar to enter the limitans nucleus (Sc. 97). A few fibers terminate in the basal part of the amygdala (Sc. 65).

Striatal Fibers

Fibers leading to the tail of the caudate nucleus leave the injection site, ascend in the subependymal white matter and course medially toward the tail of the caudate nucleus, where they terminate (Scs. 73, 81, 85). Fibers destined for the head and body of the caudate nucleus ascend along with the ILF, from which they become distinct at the ventral aspect of the claustrum (Scs. 65, 73, 81, 85). These fibers cradle the ventral aspect of the claustrum, and the medially situated fibers in the external capsule provide terminations to the ventral claustrum. Other fibers in the external capsule, and some fibers from the extreme capsule, ascend in a plate-like manner and traverse the internal capsule before crystallizing in the bundle of Muratoff. In this location, the fibers move rostrally before they descend into the body and head of the caudate nucleus, where they terminate (Scs. 41, 49, 57, 65, 73, 81, 85).

CASE 13

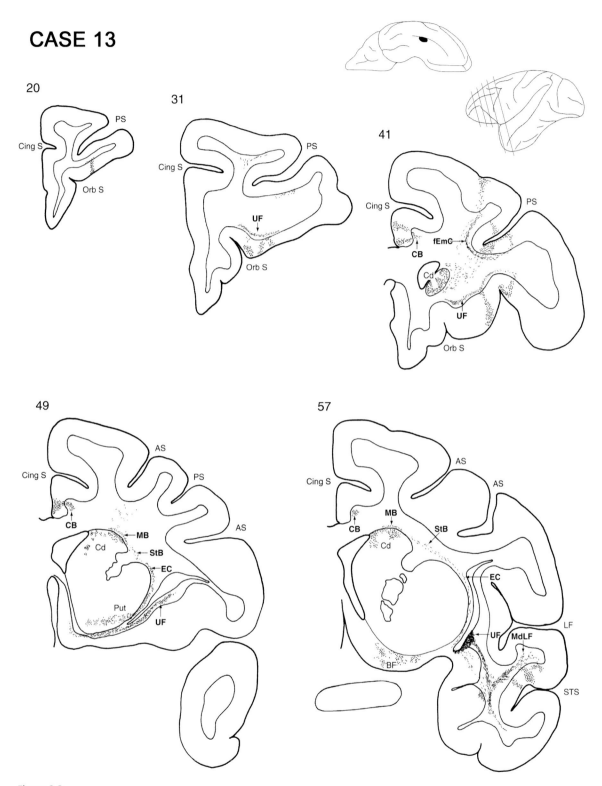

Figure 8-3

Schematic diagrams of 19 rostral–caudal coronal sections in Case 13 taken at the levels shown on the hemispheric diagram above right, showing the isotope injection site in the ventral temporal region, area TF (black-filled area), and the resulting trajectories of the cortical association, commissural, and subcortical fibers (dashed lines and dots) in the white matter and the terminations in the cortex and subcortical regions (black dots).

CASE 13

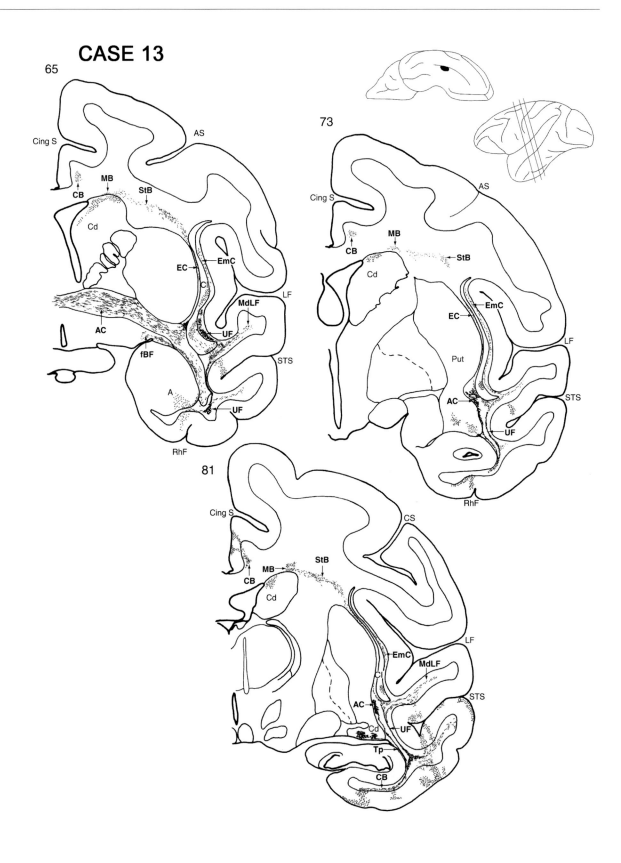

Figure 8-3 (continued)

CASE 13

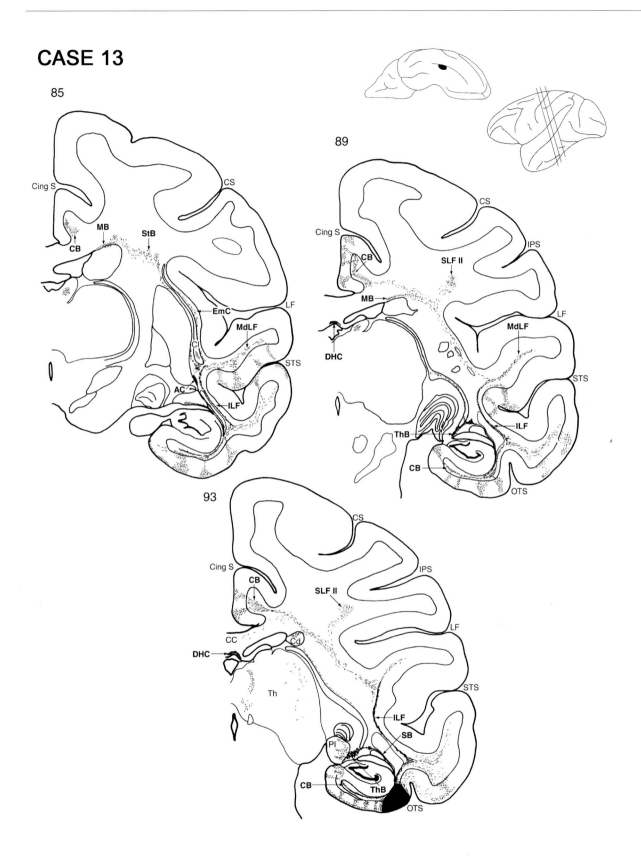

CASE 13

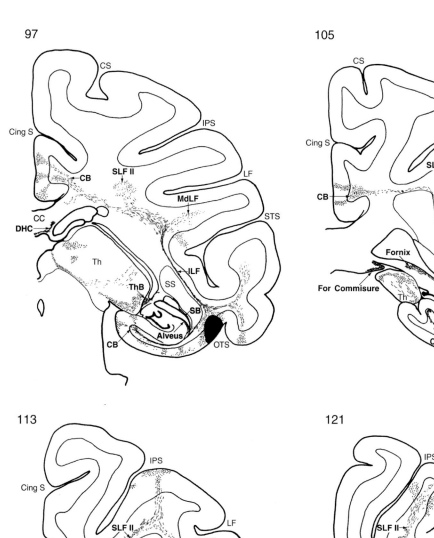
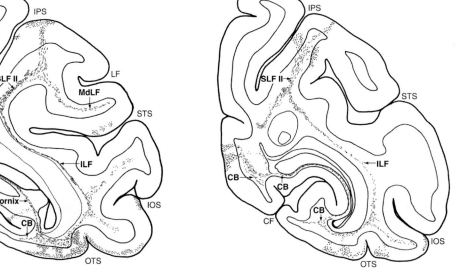

Figure 8-3 (continued)

CASE 13

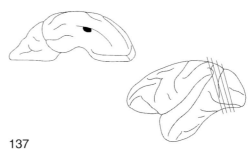

129

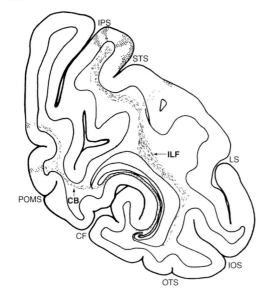

137

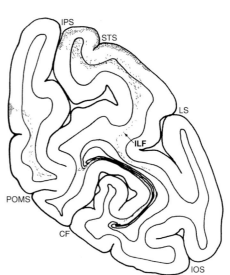

145

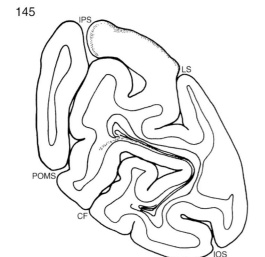

153

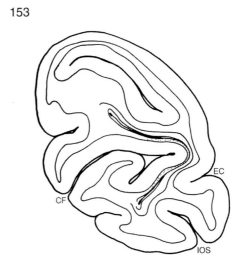

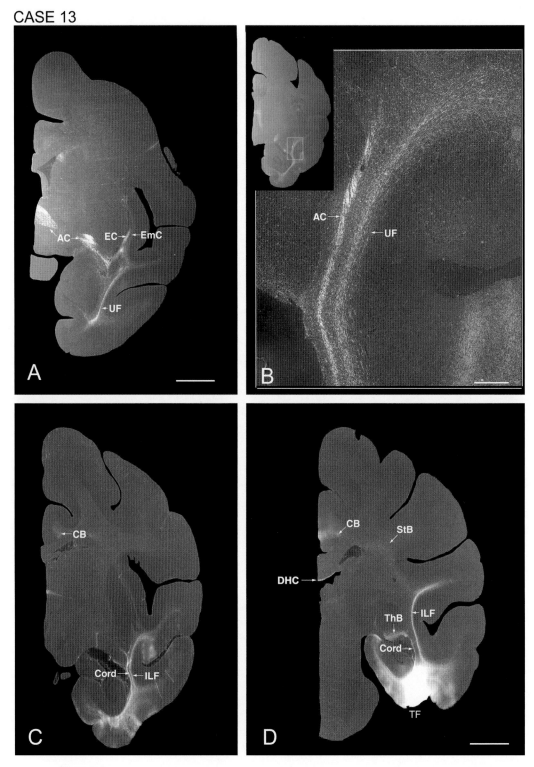

CASE 13

Figure 8-4
Photomicrographs of selected coronal sections of Case 13 showing the injection site in D and the resulting labeled fibers and terminations in A through F. B, High-power photomicrograph taken from the location indicated in the low-power photomicrograph above, showing the uncinate fasciculus and fibers coursing to run in the anterior commissure (section 81, Mag = 4×, bar = 0.5 mm). Photomicrographs A, C, D, E, and F correspond to sections 65, 85, 93, 105, and 113, respectively (Mag = 0.5×, bar = 5 mm).

CASE 13

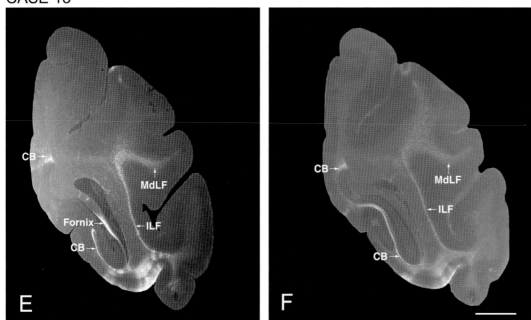

CASE 14

Isotope was injected in this case in the depth of the rostral superior temporal sulcus involving area IPa, as well as the adjacent part of the underlying white matter. See figures 8-5 and 8-6.

Association Fibers

Local Association Fibers

Local terminations adjacent to the injection site are seen in areas TEa and TEm in the cortex of the lower bank of the superior temporal sulcus (Scs. 65, 73).

Long Association Fibers

Caudally Directed Fibers

From the injection site fibers progress caudally within the ventral and dorsal components of the ILF. Fibers within the ventral component of the ILF travel in both the medial and the lateral aspects of the ventral temporal region. Fibers in the medial aspect terminate in the first layer in area TL rostrally and area TF caudally (Scs. 81, 85, 89). Fibers in the lateral aspect progress caudally and terminate in the first layer of area TE2 and TE3 (Scs. 81, 85, 89, 93, 97, 105). Fibers in the dorsal component of the ILF ascend and proceed caudally. They provide terminations in the cortex lying within the depth of the STS, in the rostral part of area FST in the superficial and deep layers, and in the lower bank of the STS in the rostral part of area MT, predominantly in the first layer (Scs. 89, 93, 97, 105). Some fibers are also noted in areas TPO and PGa in the cortex of the upper bank of the STS (Sc. 85).

Some fibers that continue to ascend in the ILF course along with the SLF III in the white matter of the inferior parietal lobule. These fibers terminate in the first layer in the cortex of the rostral part of the lower bank of the intraparietal sulcus, both in the vestibular area at the tip of the sulcus and more caudally in area POa (corresponding to area LIP) (Scs. 85, 89, 93, 97, 105).

Rostrally Directed Fibers

The fibers that leave the injection site and travel rostrally comprise three main groups. One is found in the inferotemporal region, a second progresses dorsally, and a third heads medially.

The fibers that aggregate deep to the injection site in the inferotemporal region terminate in the perirhinal cortex in area 35 (Scs. 57, 65, 73).

Fibers that head dorsally lie in the extreme capsule, then turn laterally and descend into the white matter of the frontal operculum within the SLF III before they terminate in the rostral aspect of SII, in the first layer (Sc. 81). Fibers also leave the extreme capsule within the depth of the lateral fissure. These fibers terminate in the dysgranular insula in the first layer and more rostrally in the agranular insula in a columnar manner (Scs. 57, 65, 73). The extreme capsule fibers continue further rostrally into the frontal lobe and terminate in columns in the lateral parts of area 47/12 and area 10 (Scs. 20, 41, 49).

The uncinate fasciculus (UF) is the other major component of the rostrally directed association fibers that leave the injection site. The UF fibers travel rostrally in the white matter of the temporal pole and terminate in columns in area TL (Scs. 49, 57). Uncinate fibers lying within the temporal stem occupy a position lateral to the amygdala before entering and terminating within the lateral and central nuclei of the amygdala (Sc. 57).

The majority of the UF fibers ascend in the temporal stem and come to lie ventral to the claustrum before passing medially to lie ventral to the anterior commissure. Throughout its course the UF lies ventrally adjacent to the fibers of the extreme capsule. Continuing in a medial and ventral direction (lateral and ventral to the putamen), the UF fibers terminate in forebrain areas, including the olfactory tubercle, nucleus basalis of Meynert, and the diagonal band of Broca (Scs. 49, 57, 65). As the UF fibers lie ventral and lateral to the putamen, they terminate in the orbital proisocortex (Sc. 49). The UF fibers then continue rostrally and medially to form a plate-like fiber bundle hugging the white matter deep to the orbital cortex. From the medial aspect of this plate-like bundle, fibers emerge to terminate in a columnar fashion in areas 13 and 14 of the orbital cortex (Scs. 31, 41).

Commissural and Subcortical Fibers

From the injection site a dense cord of fibers ascends in the temporal stem and heads medially to enter the lateral aspect of the anterior commissure (AC). The AC fibers progress rostrally and medially before they cross to enter the opposite hemisphere (Sc. 65).

The cord also gives rise to a dense fiber bundle that progresses in a caudal direction and heads medially before occupying two distinct positions related to the lateral geniculate nucleus, one dorsal to the LGN and one ventral and lateral to the LGN (Sc. 85).

The dorsally situated fibers arch over the dome of the most rostral aspect of the LGN before they descend medially, lying in an oblique striated fashion, and then move medially to terminate in the hypothalamus (Sc. 85). Further caudally, the fibers at the dome of the LGN ascend medially to enter the thalamus and terminate in the rostral part of the thalamus in the CL, SG, and PO nuclei (Scs. 85, 89, 93).

The ventral subcortical fiber bundle lying ventral and lateral to the LGN continues caudally, situated between the LGN and the stria terminalis. At the level of the pulvinar, fibers leave this bundle, proceed medially, and give rise to terminations in the PM and limitans nuclei (Sc. 97).

Striatal Fibers

A sizable number of fibers leave the temporal stem, enter the lower part of the external capsule, and ascend. These fibers continue rostrally and enter the striatum, resulting in prominent terminations in distinct patches in the rostral part of the putamen, as well as in the head of the caudate nucleus (Scs. 49, 57). Finally, some fibers leave the cord and ascend toward and terminate in the ventral aspect of the claustrum (Scs. 57, 65, 73, 81).

CASE 14

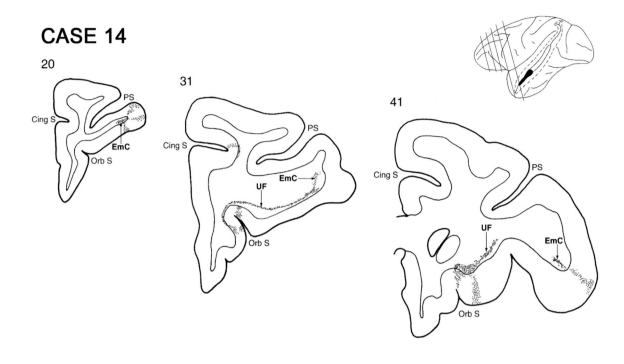

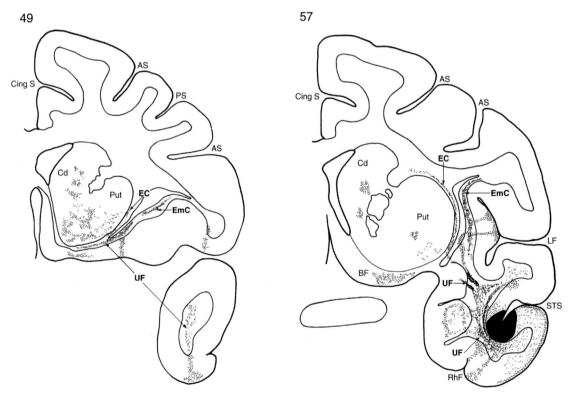

Figure 8-5

Schematic diagram of 13 rostral–caudal coronal sections in Case 14 taken at the levels shown on the hemispheric diagram above right, showing the isotope injection site in the depth of the rostral superior temporal sulcus involving area IPa, as well as the adjacent part of the underlying white matter (black-filled area). The resulting trajectories of the cortical association, commissural, and subcortical fibers in the white matter are shown (dashed lines and dots), as well as the terminations in the cortex and subcortical regions (black dots).

CASE 14

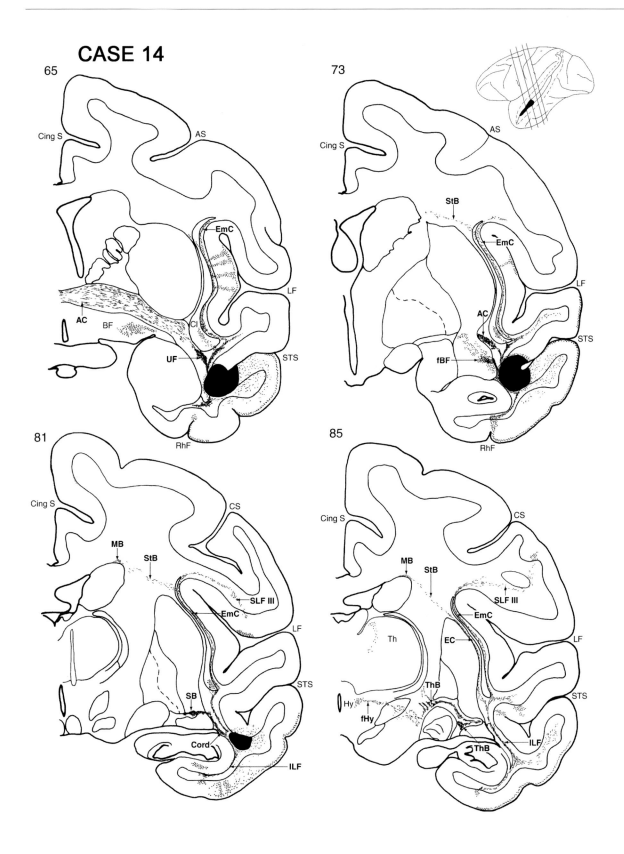

65

Cing S

AS

EmC

LF

AC

BF

CI

UF

STS

73

Cing S

AS

StB

EmC

LF

AC

STS

fBF

RhF

81

Cing S

CS

MB

StB

SLF III

EmC

LF

STS

SB

Cord

ILF

85

Cing S

CS

MB

StB

SLF III

EmC

EC

LF

Th

ThB

STS

Hy

fHy

ILF

ThB

CASE 14

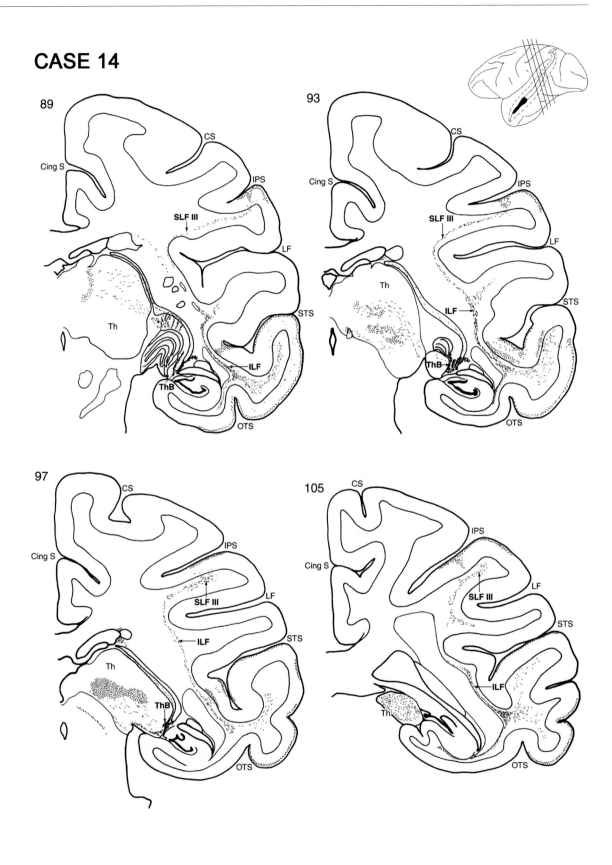

Figure 8-5 (continued)

CASE 14

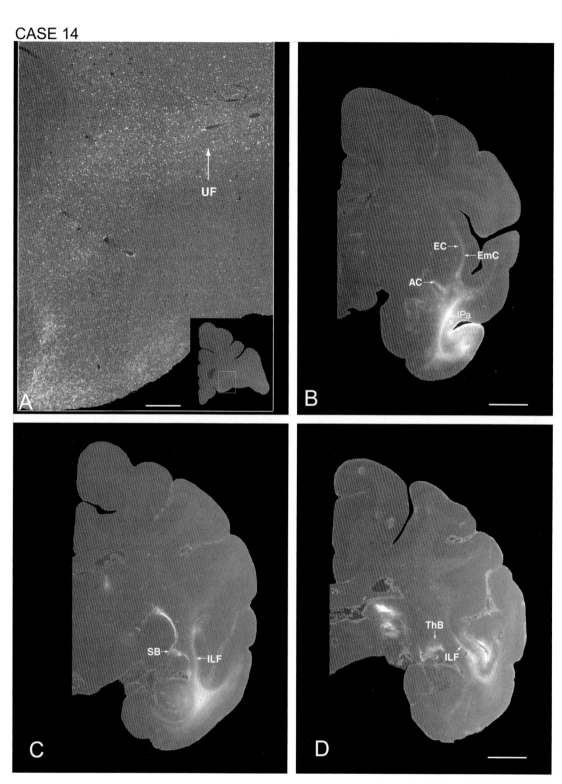

Figure 8-6

Photomicrographs of selected coronal sections of Case 14 to show the injection site in B and the resulting labeled fibers and terminations in A through D. A, High-power photomicrograph (section 41, Mag = 4×, bar = 0.5 mm) taken from the location indicated in the low-power photomicrograph below, showing the uncinate fasciculus and terminations in the orbital cortex, area 13. Photomicrographs B through D correspond to sections 57, 85, and 93, respectively (Mag = 0.5×, bar = 5 mm).

CASE 15

Isotope was injected in the medial part of the inferior temporal gyrus in areas TE1 and TE2 in this case. See figures 8-7 and 8-8.

Association Fibers

Local Association Fibers

Local association fibers leave the injection site and terminate in the cortex at the depth of the superior temporal sulcus (STS) in area IPa, in the cortex of the lower bank of the STS in area TEa, and in area TEm in the inferotemporal area (Sc. 73).

Long Association Fibers

Caudally Directed Fibers

There are three main association fiber bundles that emanate from the injection site and travel in a caudal direction. One group of fibers ascends in the ILF and terminates in the depth of the rostral part of the STS in areas PGa and FST and the caudal part of area TEa (Scs. 81, 85, 89). A second component, continuous with the ventral aspect of the ILF, runs caudally in the periphery of the white matter of the inferotemporal gyrus and terminates in the first layer of areas TE2, TE3, and V4V (Scs. 97, 105, 113, 121). The third contingent of fibers courses medially from the injection site lying within the ventral aspect of the cingulum bundle and terminates in a columnar manner in the medial aspect of the ventral temporal region in areas TH and TF and in the first layer of area TL (Sc. 97).

Rostrally Directed Fibers

Fibers leave the injection site and ascend in the temporal lobe white matter. Some fibers continue dorsally around the lateral aspect of the claustrum into the extreme capsule (EmC) and terminate in columns in the lower part of the insular proisocortex (Sc. 73).

A contingent of fibers travels rostrally from the injection site within the white matter of the ventral temporal lobe. These fibers terminate in the ventral temporal cortex in areas TE1, TL, and in the perirhinal cortex in area 35 (Scs. 49, 57, 65). Just caudal to the level of the anterior commissure a contingent of fibers leaves the ascending bundle and moves medially to enter the basal forebrain area. These fibers travel rostrally and medially before terminating in the substantia innominata and the medial forebrain (Scs. 57, 65).

The majority of the long association fibers that travel rostrally from the injection site within the ventral part of the temporal lobe white matter course through the uncinate fasciculus. These fibers continue forward to the level of the anterior commissure, situated just medial to the thin plate of neurons that correspond to the extension of the ventral part of the claustrum. At the level of the anterior commissure the fibers ascend within the temporal stem and move medially to lie at the ventral and medial aspect of the claustrum. From this point, as the UF fibers move rostrally and medially they come to lie in a flattened plate-like manner ventral to the claustrum and putamen. The fibers move rostrally in this location and terminate in the ventral prefrontal convexity in area 47/12, in the orbital cortex in area 13, and more rostrally in area 11 (Scs. 20, 31, 41, 49).

Commissural and Subcortical Fibers

A dense cord of fibers leaves the injection site and ascends in the white matter wedged between the ILF and the tapetum. A large contingent of fibers within the cord leaves the main bundle and enters the anterior commissure before traveling to the opposite hemisphere (Sc. 65). Fibers in the cord destined for the thalamus (ThB) course lateral to the tail of the caudate nucleus. The bulk of the fiber bundle continues medially, situated between the tail of the caudate ventrally and the putamen dorsally, and in this location consists of dense whorls of caudally directed fibers. As they move caudally, these fibers shift medially over the stria terminalis and are concentrated in the ventral subcortical bundle lateral and ventral to the LGN (Sc. 89). Next they arch over the dome of the LGN and extend medial to the LGN to enter the PI nucleus of the thalamus (Sc. 93). From this point the fibers distribute their terminations within the inferior and medial pulvinar (PI and PM) and the limitans nucleus (Scs. 97, 105).

Striatal Fibers

Fibers destined for the striatum emanate from the site of the injection, course along with the thalamic fibers, and terminate in both the tail of the caudate nucleus and the ventral part of the putamen (Sc. 73). Rostrally directed striatal fibers travel via the external capsule and terminate in the rostral part of the putamen and the head of the caudate nucleus (Scs. 41, 49, 57, 65). Terminations in the ventral aspect of the claustrum are derived from fibers that ascend in the extreme capsule. Caudally directed fibers course adjacent to the ependyma of the inferior horn of the lateral ventricle (these may represent the ventral equivalent of the Muratoff bundle), and they terminate in the ventral part of the putamen and in the tail of the caudate nucleus (Sc. 73).

A small bundle of fibers travels with the cord and lies at the lateral border of the amygdala before terminating within the amygdala in the lateral and basoventral nuclei (Sc. 65).

CASE 15

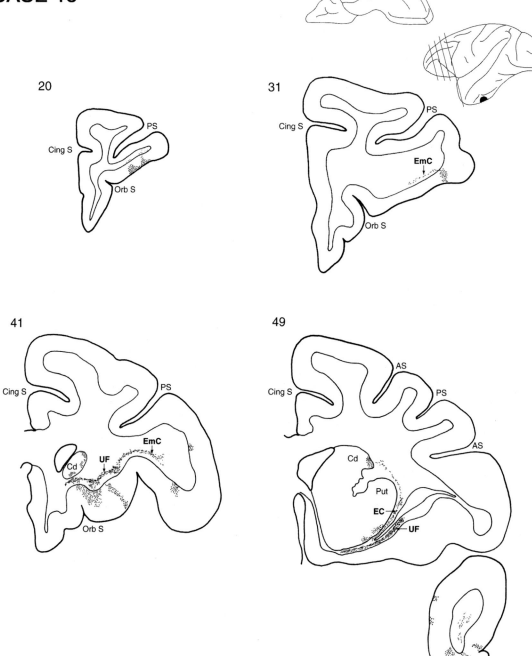

Figure 8-7

Schematic diagram of 15 rostral–caudal coronal sections in Case 15 taken at the levels shown on the hemispheric diagram above right, showing the isotope injection site in the medial part of the inferior temporal gyrus in areas TE1 and TE2 (black-filled area) and the resulting trajectories of the cortical association, commissural, and subcortical fibers (dashed lines and dots) in the white matter and the terminations in the cortex and subcortical regions (black dots).

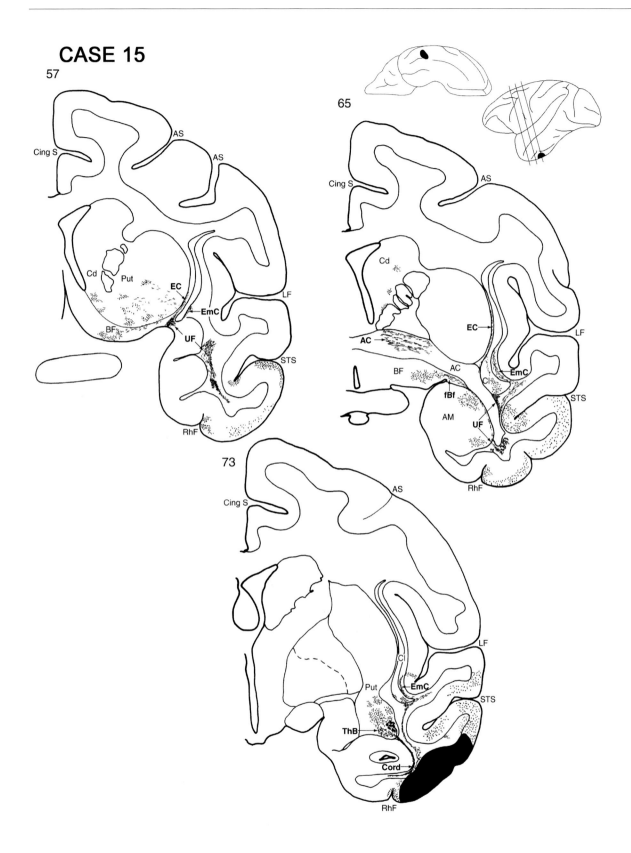

CASE 15

CASE 15

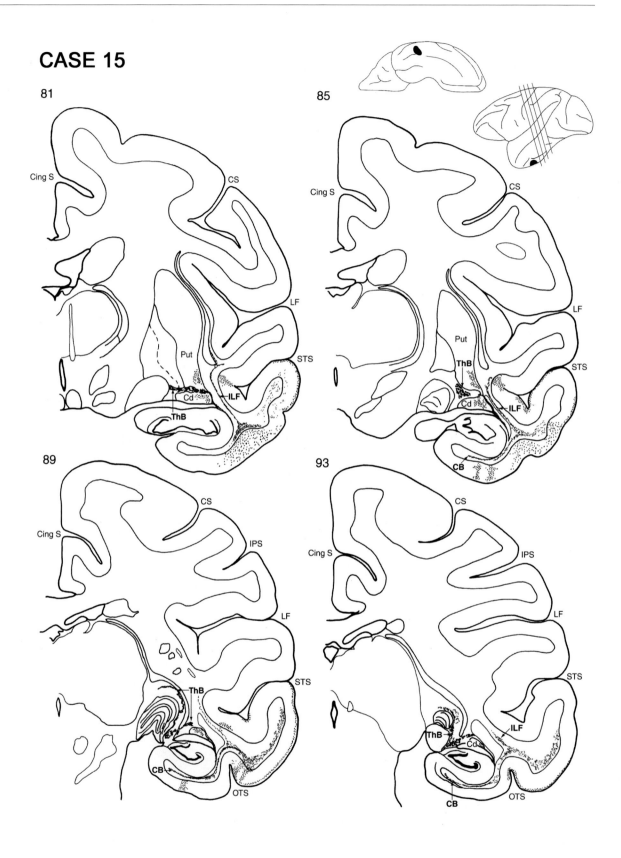

Figure 8-7 (continued)

CASE 15

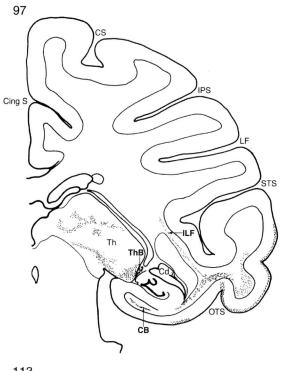

97

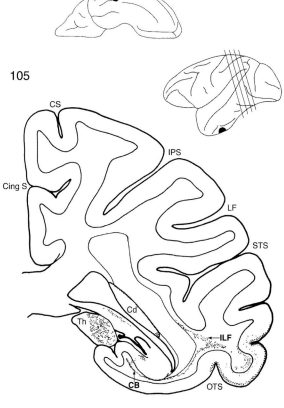

105

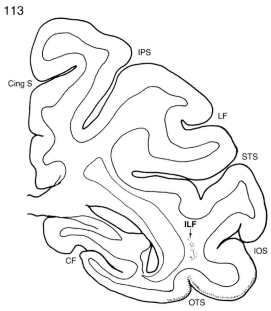

113

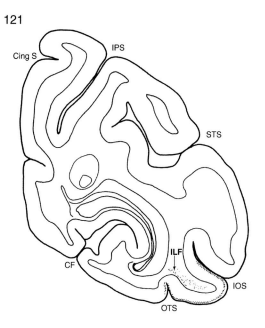

121

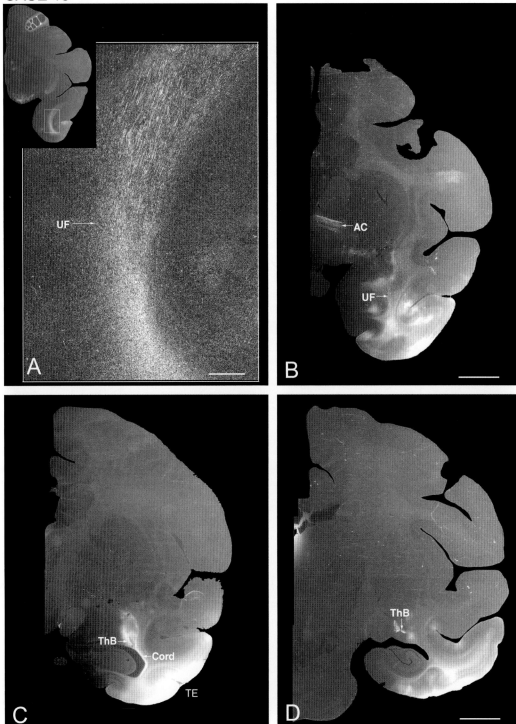

Figure 8-8
Photomicrographs of selected coronal sections of Case 15 to show the injection site in C with spread
into B and D, and the resulting labeled fibers and terminations in A through D. A, High-power photomicrograph (section 57, Mag = 4×, bar = 0.5 mm) taken from the location indicated in the low-
power photomicrograph above, showing the uncinate fasciculus. Photomicrographs B through D
correspond to sections 65, 73, and 85, respectively (Mag = 0.5×, bar = 5 mm).

CASE 16

In this case isotope was injected in the rostral temporal lobe in the midportion of area TE2. See figures 8-9 and 8-10.

Association Fibers

Local Association Fibers

Fibers leave the injection site and terminate in adjacent cortex in area TE2.

Long Association Fibers

Caudally Directed Fibers

Fibers leave the injection site and travel caudally in the ventral sector of the ILF lying within the central portion of the white matter of the inferotemporal area. These fibers terminate in the ventral bank of the superior temporal sulcus (STS) in area TEa in a columnar manner; further caudally, terminations are in area FST, also in a columnar manner (Scs. 81, 85, 89). The other contingent of the caudal terminations are in areas TE2 and TE3. In area TE2, terminations are columnar as well as in the first layer, whereas in TE3 they are mainly in the first layer (Scs. 81, 85, 89, 93).

Rostrally Directed Fibers

Rostral to the injection site, the association fibers travel within the rostral component of the ILF situated in the white matter of the inferotemporal region. These fibers terminate in a columnar manner in areas TE1, TL, and TEa, as well as in area 35 (Scs. 49, 57, 65). Some fibers leave the injection site and ascend in the uncinate fasciculus, move rostrally, and terminate in the amygdala (Scs. 57, 65).

Commissural and Subcortical Fibers

Fibers leave the injection site and aggregate within a dense cord situated within the white matter immediately adjacent to the lateral aspect of the uncus of the hippocampus. A large contingent of fibers arising from the cord travels rostrally, enters the anterior commissure, and is directed toward the opposite hemisphere (Sc. 65). The thalamic contingent of fibers travels medially over the tail of the caudate nucleus, moves caudally, and occupies a position in the ventral subcortical bundle wedged between the ventral aspect of the lateral geniculate nucleus and the stria terminalis (ThB, S.73). This bundle then travels further caudally until it reaches the pulvinar inferior (PI), at which point the fibers move medially and terminate within the PI (Sc. 97).

Striatal Fibers

Fibers destined for the striatum ascend along with the cord and terminate in the ventral aspect of the putamen and in the tail of the caudate nucleus (Scs. 73, 81). Some of the fibers in the striatal bundle ascend from the injection site along with the uncinate fasciculus and terminate in the claustrum (Sc. 65).

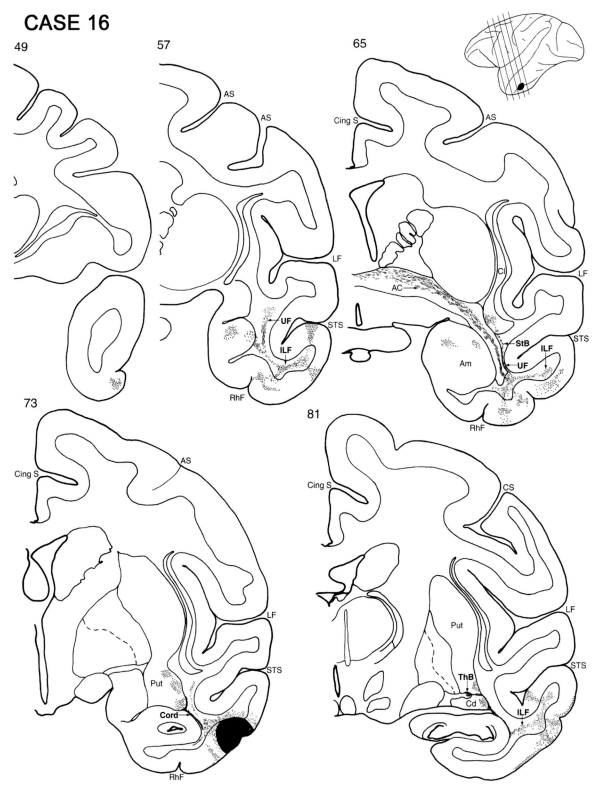

CASE 16

Figure 8-9
Schematic diagram of nine rostral–caudal coronal sections in Case 16 taken at the levels shown on the hemispheric diagram above right, showing the isotope injection site in the rostral inferotemporal regions in the midportion of area TE2 (black-filled area) and the resulting trajectories of the cortical association, commissural, and subcortical fibers (dashed lines and dots) in the white matter and the terminations in the cortex and subcortical regions (black dots).

CASE 16

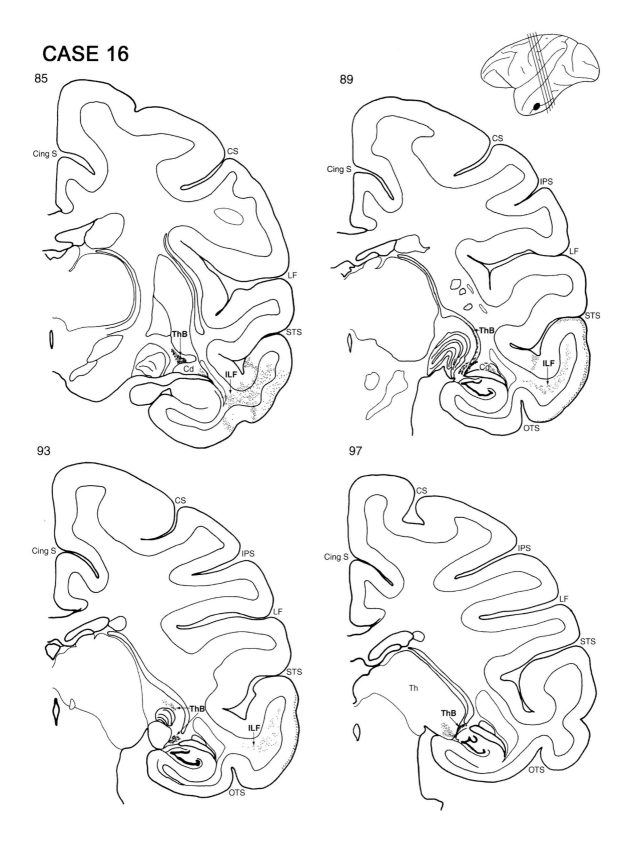

CASE 16

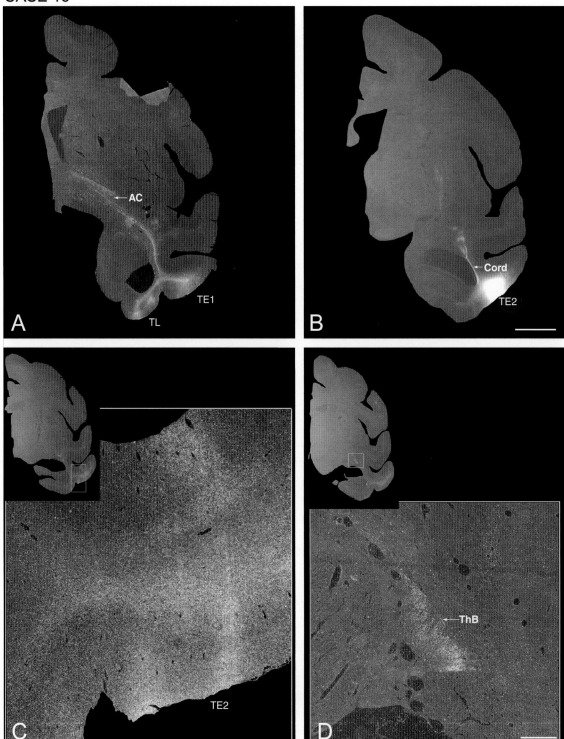

Figure 8-10

Photomicrographs of selected coronal sections of Case 16 to show the injection site in B and the resulting labeled fibers and terminations in A through D. Photomicrographs A through D correspond to sections 65, 73, 81, and 85, respectively. C and D are high-power photomicrographs (Mag = 4×, bar = 0.5 mm) showing terminations in inferior temporal area TE2 (C) and subcortical fibers in the thalamic peduncle (D) (A and B, Mag = 0.5×, bar = 5 mm).

Inferior Temporal Region Summary

Association Fibers

Ventral Temporal Region (Lateral Parahippocampal Gyrus) (Area TF, Case 13)

The long association fibers leave this region in five distinct fiber bundles: the inferior longitudinal fasciculus (ILF), uncinate fasciculus, extreme capsule, cingulum bundle, and middle longitudinal fasciculus (see figure 8–11).

1. Inferior Longitudinal Fasciculus

The ILF courses in both rostral and caudal directions. Rostrally directed ILF fibers travel in the white matter of the inferotemporal cortex and terminate in areas TE2, TE1, TEa, TEm, and IPa. Caudally directed ILF fibers course through the white matter of the inferotemporal cortex, as well as in the white matter between the sagittal stratum and the superior temporal sulcus. Those in the inferotemporal area terminate in area TE3. The major segment of the ILF that courses lateral to the sagittal stratum ascends dorsally into the white matter of the inferior parietal lobule. From there the fibers terminate in areas PG and Opt, POa, and MST and further caudally in areas V4D and DP.

2. Uncinate Fasciculus

The uncinate fasciculus ascends from the parahippocampal gyrus in the white matter of the depth of the superior temporal sulcus and enters the temporal stem. One group of fibers runs medially around the amygdala and provides terminations to it. These fibers continue into the orbital cortex and terminate in the basal forebrain area in the caudal part of the orbital cortex. The bulk of the fibers in the uncinate fasciculus course dorsally in the white matter deep to the superior temporal sulcus and ascend further before congregating ventral and lateral to the base of the claustrum. They then move medially through the limen insulae and course in the ventral part of the white matter of the orbital surface in a plate-like manner. These fibers terminate in areas 12, 13, 11, and 25.

3. Extreme Capsule

The fibers in the extreme capsule course rostrally, and in the frontal lobe they move dorsally and aggregate around the principal sulcus. From there the fibers terminate in areas 9 and 46.

4. Cingulum Bundle

Another group of fibers ascends in the ILF before spreading out rostrally and caudally to enter the cingulum bundle. The rostrally directed cingulate fibers are situated first around the ventral and medial aspects of the cingulate white matter, and further rostrally they are in the core of the cingulum bundle. These fibers terminate in much of the extent of area 24. The caudally directed cingulate fibers terminate in area 23 before coursing around the splenium of the corpus callosum and run in the white matter deep to the calcarine sulcus to become incorporated into the ventral part of the cingulum bundle. From there, as the fibers move rostrally they terminate in areas V3V, V4V, TF, TL, TH, area prostriata, and the presubiculum.

5. Middle Longitudinal Fasciculus

A contingent of fibers ascends from the parahippocampal gyrus and becomes incorporated in the middle longitudinal fasciculus in the white matter of the superior temporal gyrus. These fibers terminate in the midpart of the superior temporal sulcus in areas TPO and PGa.

Rostral Inferotemporal Region (Cases 15 and 16)

The association fibers from the rostral part of the inferotemporal region are conveyed by the inferior longitudinal fasciculus, the uncinate fasciculus, fibers to the basal forebrain, the extreme capsule, and the middle longitudinal fasciculus.

1. Inferior Longitudinal Fasciculus

The fibers that emanate from the rostral inferotemporal area and course through the ILF terminate in areas IPa, TEa, and TEm, as well as in area TE1. The ILF fibers that are caudally directed run mainly through the white matter of the inferotemporal region. These fibers terminate laterally in areas TE2, TE3, TEO, and V4V. Some of the ILF fibers run medially and terminate in the perirhinal cortex, area TL, and area TF.

2. Uncinate Fasciculus

The fibers in the uncinate fasciculus move rostrally in the white matter of the temporal stem and ascend until they lie ventral and lateral to the claustrum. They then cross the limen insulae and course in the white matter on the floor of the orbital cortex. These uncinate fibers terminate in areas 12, 13, and 11.

3. Fibers to the Basal Forebrain

The fibers to the basal forebrain also ascend in the white matter of the temporal stem, situated at the medial border of the amygdala. Some of these fibers terminate in the amygdala and others continue into the frontal lobe, passing through the limen insulae. From there the fibers terminate in the basal forebrain region.

4. Extreme Capsule

Caudal to the uncinate fasciculus, a fiber bundle leaves the inferotemporal region and runs in the white matter of the depth of the superior temporal sulcus. Some of the fibers from this system ascend into the extreme capsule and terminate in the lower part of the insula (IPro).

5. Middle Longitudinal Fasciculus

Association fibers derived from the cortex of the superior temporal sulcus enter the middle longitudinal fasciculus lying in the white matter of the superior temporal gyrus. These fibers terminate in areas TAa, TPO, and PGa of the superior temporal sulcus.

Caudal Inferotemporal Area (Case 12)

The ILF is the principal bundle by which the caudal inferior temporal region sends association fibers to other cortical areas. The ILF moves rostrally and caudally from the caudal-inferotemporal region. Rostrally the ILF fibers lie within the white matter of the inferior temporal gyrus. These fibers terminate in areas FST, TEm, TE2, and TE1. Caudally, the ILF fibers run in two main streams. One group of ILF fibers ascends dorsally in the white matter lateral to the sagittal stratum. These fibers enter the white matter of the inferior parietal lobule and terminate in area POa. Further caudally, the ILF fibers terminate in area V4D. The ILF fibers in the inferotemporal white matter terminate in areas MT, TE3, TEO, V4V, V3D, V2, and V1.

Commissural Fibers

Most of the interhemispheric fibers arising from the inferotemporal region and parahippocampal gyrus course through the anterior commissure with some degree of topographic overlapping. They course via the dorsal and caudal sectors of the anterior commissure in the midsagittal plane. The caudal part of the inferotemporal region has some fibers traversing the corpus callosum through sector CC5 in the splenium. The posterior parahippocampal gyrus also has interhemispheric fibers traveling in the dorsal hippocampal commissure.

Subcortical Fibers

Parahippocampal Gyrus

The cord of subcortical fibers that emerges from the parahippocampal region ascends medial to the sagittal stratum and lateral to the inferior horn of the lateral ventricle and the tail of the caudate nucleus. The fibers enter the ventral subcortical bundle (VSB); some terminate in the pulvinar inferior nucleus while others ascend in the thalamic external medullary lamina before terminating in the thalamus.

Rostral Inferotemporal Region

The cord of fibers from this region gives rise to fibers that course caudally in the white matter between the putamen and the tail of the caudate nucleus. These fibers occupy the VSB. At a level corresponding to the caudal end of the LGN, the fiber system moves dorsally and medially and enters the thalamus through the ventral part of the external medullary lamina.

Caudal Part of the Inferotemporal Region

The thalamic fibers that leave the cord fibers enter the ventral portion of the sagittal stratum and course rostrally within the VSB. The fibers enter the thalamus via the ventral and lateral parts of the external medullary lamina.

Corticostriate Projections

Fibers from the rostral inferotemporal region and the rostral part of the superior temporal sulcus are conveyed through the external capsule and then the Muratoff bundle to the midportion of the head of the caudate nucleus and the ventral striatum. A sizable contingent of fibers from the rostral STS ascends in the white matter of the temporal stem and terminates in the ventral putamen, the tail of the caudate nucleus, and ventral regions of the claustrum.

Striatal fibers from the caudal part of the inferotemporal region move dorsally to reach the genu of the caudate nucleus, where they terminate. Further rostrally, this bundle of striatal fibers courses along with the ventral subcortical bundle above the tail of the caudate nucleus and terminates in the tail of the caudate nucleus and the ventral portion of the putamen. Other striatal fibers course dorsally along with the ILF and terminate in the ventral part of the claustrum before entering the external capsule and terminating in the islands of the putamen and the body of the caudate nucleus.

The external capsule conveys striatal fibers from the parahippocampal gyrus (area TF) in the ventral temporal region. These fibers cross the internal capsule, enter the Muratoff bundle, and terminate in the dorsal part of the head and body of the caudate nucleus, as well as in the nucleus accumbens. Projections from this region are also directed to the caudate tail, the ventral part of the putamen, and the claustrum, as the fibers course directly dorsally from the ventral temporal cortex into these nuclei.

Figure 8-11

Schematic composite diagrams of rostral–caudal coronal sections of the template brain, illustrating the five inferior temporal region cases (Cases 12 through 16). The injection sites and association, commissural, and subcortical fibers, as well as the termination patterns, are color-coded for each case. The schematic diagrams of the basal and lateral surfaces of the cerebral hemispheres (at top) represent the different levels of the coronal sections and the injection sites. Color-coding is as follows: Case 12—purple, caudal part of the inferior temporal region areas TE2 and TE3; Case 13—red, ventral temporal region area TF; Case 14—orange, cortex in the depth of the rostral superior temporal sulcus involving area IPa; Case 15—green, medial part of the inferior temporal gyrus areas TE1 and TE2; Case 16—blue, rostral part of the inferior temporal lobe in the midportion of area TE2.

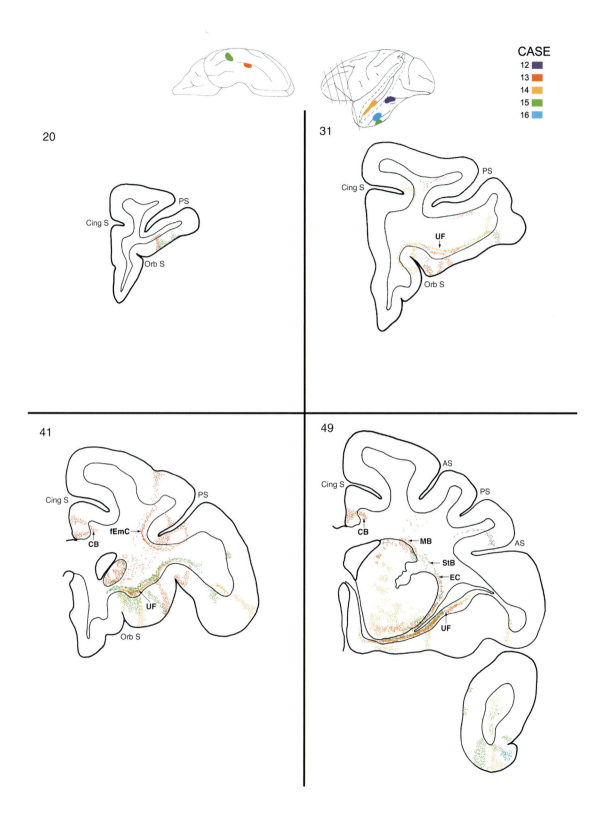

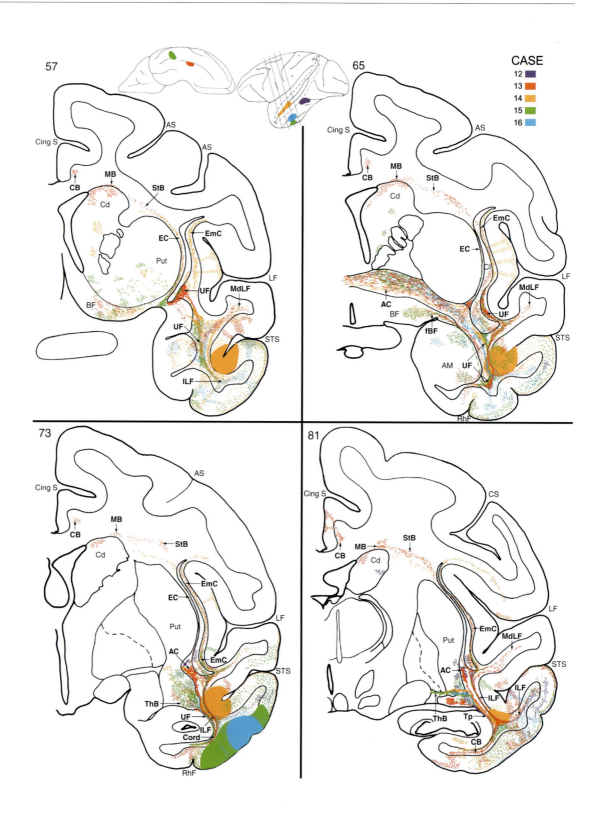

Figure 8-11 (continued)

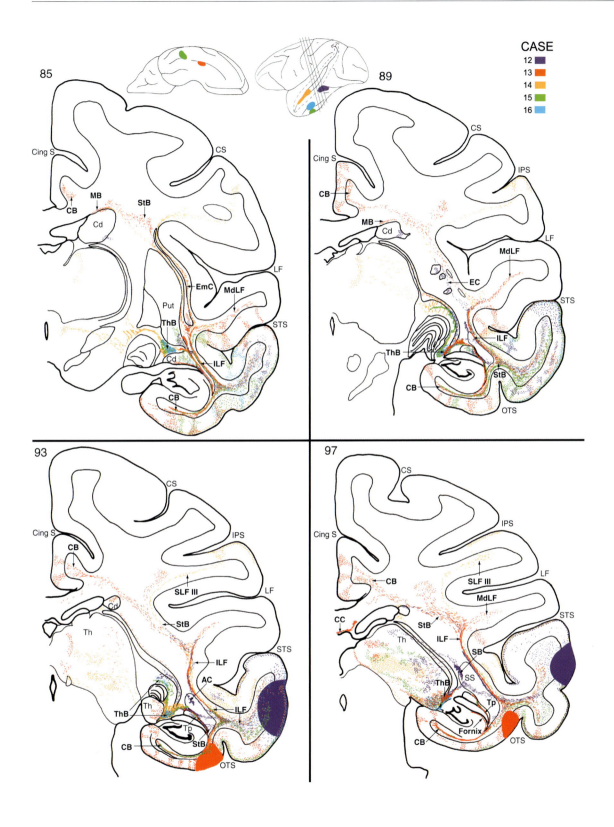

CASE
12
13
14
15
16

85

Cing S
CB
MB
StB
CS
Cd
EmC
MdLF
Put
ThB
Cd
ILF
CB
LF
STS

89

Cing S
CB
MB
Cd
EC
MdLF
ThB
ILF
StB
CB
OTS
CS
IPS
LF
STS

93

Cing S
CB
Cd
Th
SLF III
StB
ILF
AC
ThB
Th
Tp
ILF
CB
StB
OTS
CS
IPS
LF
STS

97

Cing S
CB
CC
Th
SLF III
MdLF
StB
ILF
SB
ThB
SS
Tp
Fornix
CB
OTS
CS
IPS
LF
STS

227

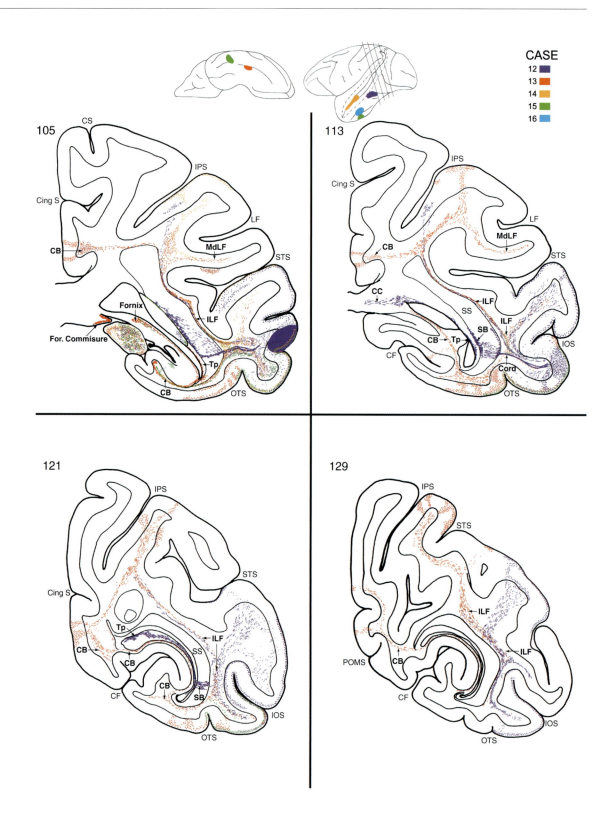

Figure 8-11 (continued)

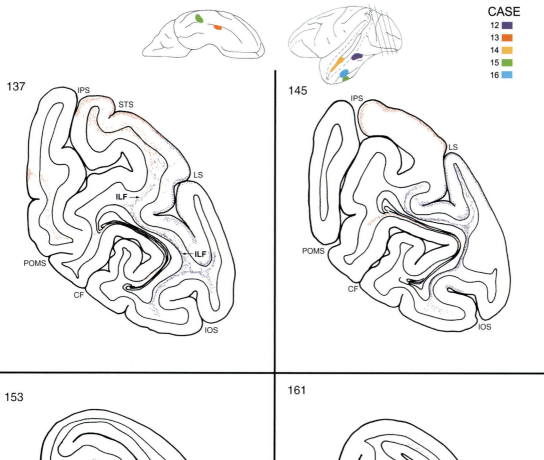

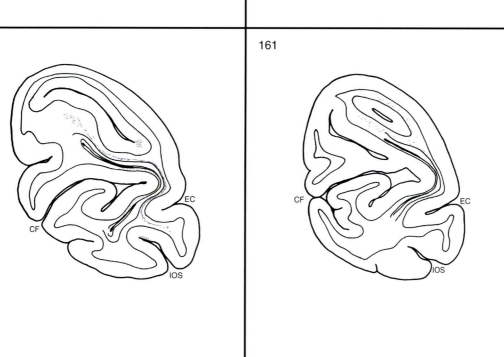

Occipital Lobe

9

In this chapter we describe the isotope injection cases in the occipital lobe of five rhesus monkeys and analyze the resulting association, striatal, commissural, and subcortical fiber trajectories, as well as the cortical and subcortical terminations. The injections were in the medial preoccipital gyrus involving the medial part of area 19 (area PO) and area PGm (Case 17), the dorsal preoccipital gyrus in area DP and the upper part of area V4D (Case 18), the dorsal part of area V4 and the adjacent area V4T (Case 19), the ventral preoccipital gyrus above inferior occipital sulcus in area V4 (Case 20), and in ventral area V4, with some encroachment in ventral area V3 (Case 21).

As in the previous chapters, the architectonic designations of the cortical terminations are described in the text but not identified on the coronal sections. Architectonic areas are labeled on external views of the hemisphere as well as in the coronal series of chapter 4. Terminations in thalamus are shown and thalamic nuclei are referred to in the text, but the nuclei are not designated on the coronal sections. Pontine terminations are described in the text but not illustrated. Striatal terminations are illustrated and an overview of their termination patterns is presented in the text.

CASE 17

In this case, the isotope injection was placed in the medial part of the preoccipital gyrus, involving medial area 19 (area PO) and area PGm (Scs. 137, 145). See figures 9-1 and 9-2.

Association Fibers

Local and Neighborhood Association Fibers

Local association fibers travel immediately beneath the cortex. Medially directed fibers remain in the medial preoccipital gyrus and terminate in a columnar manner in area 19 (medial V4) and area PGm (Scs. 137, 145). These fibers are directed caudally and travel within the dorsal part of the white matter and terminate predominantly in the first layer of dorsal areas 17 and 18 (Scs. 157, 161). Rostrally the fibers travel in the white matter of the preoccipital gyrus and terminate in a columnar manner in area 31 and PGm (Scs. 121, 129).

Laterally directed local association fibers hug the undersurface of the annectant gyrus as they move rostrally in a ventral then lateral and then dorsal direction. These fibers terminate in the first layer of area 18 (V3A) and area 19 (S.137). Dorsally they terminate in area V4 in a columnar manner (Sc. 137). As these fibers move rostrally from the injection site they travel immediately under the cortex of the medial surface of the intraparietal sulcus and give rise to terminations in the upper bank of the intraparietal sulcus in area PEa (PIP) and in the depth of the intraparietal sulcus in area IPd (Scs. 121, 129). These fibers then turn around the fundus of the intraparietal sulcus, continue within the center of the white matter of the inferior parietal lobule, and terminate in a columnar manner in areas PG and Opt (Scs. 121, 129).

Long Association Fibers

Rostrally Directed Fibers

Long association fibers leave the injection site and course rostrally in the white matter of the superior parietal lobule. At the level of the splenium of the corpus callosum these fibers separate into three subcomponents that run in the superior longitudinal fasciculus (SLF) I, the fronto-occipital fasciculus (FOF), and the cingulum bundle (CB).

As the fibers within the SLF I move rostrally, they are situated in a curvilinear fashion around the cingulate sulcus, first in the parietal lobe and then in the frontal lobe. These fibers terminate in the supplementary motor area and in the prefrontal cortex in area 9 in a columnar manner (Scs. 41, 49).

The fibers that enter the FOF course rostrally, remaining above the caudate nucleus, and between the fibers of the corpus callosum and corona radiata. In the frontal lobe these fibers move dorsally and provide terminations to dorsal area 6, area 8Ad, and dorsal areas 46 and 9 (Scs. 41, 49, 57, 65).

The fibers that enter the CB travel rostrally, lying beneath the lower bank of the cingulate sulcus. These CB fibers terminate in a columnar manner in the cortex in the depth of the cingulate sulcus, in area 24 (Sc. 81).

Commissural and Subcortical Fibers

A dense cord of fibers emerges from the injection site and descends within the center of the medial preoccipital gyrus, bounded on each side by the medial and lateral local association fibers. As it travels rostrally, fibers from the cord aggregate in an intense bundle of obliquely oriented fibers lying within the superior and medial aspects of sector SS-2 of the sagittal stratum (Sc. 113). A small contingent of fibers is also present more ventrally at the medial aspect of the internal segment of the sagittal stratum.

A group of fibers separates from the cord and enters the splenium in sector CC5 of the corpus callosum (Sc. 113). They course rostrally and medially and traverse the midsagittal plane in the dorsal part of sector CC5 (Sc. 105) to enter the opposite hemisphere.

The labeled fibers that remain in the sagittal stratum descend obliquely and ventrally as they move forward in SS-2 and enter the retrolenticular part of the internal capsule (ICp-5, Sc. 97). At this point the fibers divide into medial (ThB) and lateral (PB) components (Sc. 97).

The medial component enters the thalamus through the external medullary lamina to terminate in the LP and medial pulvinar nuclei, with some terminations also in the CL nucleus (Scs. 97, 93, 89).

The lateral component continues to descend in the posterior limb of the internal capsule (ICp-5, Sc. 97, and ICp-4, Sc. 93) and courses medially over the midpoint of the LGN in ICP-3 (Sc. 89). It then descends into the lateral aspect of the cerebral peduncle (Sc. 85) and courses to the basilar pontine nuclei. The fibers terminate throughout the rostral to caudal extent of the pons in the lateral, dorsolateral, and extreme dorsolateral and lateral parts of the peripeduncular nuclei, with some projections also in the ventral and NRTP nuclei. Before entering into the peduncle, some fibers leave the descending bundle to reach the zona incerta (Sc. 85).

Striatal Fibers

Some fibers leave the FOF (see above) and enter the compact Muratoff bundle situated above the body of the caudate nucleus. These fibers course rostrally to terminate in the dorsal and lateral aspects of the body and head of the caudate nucleus (Scs. 57, 65, 73, 81, 85, 89, 93).

Other fibers derived from both the Muratoff bundle and the FOF descend and cross over the internal capsule. Some of these terminate in the putamen, and others continue in the external capsule to terminate in the claustrum (Scs. 73, 81, 85, 89).

CASE 17

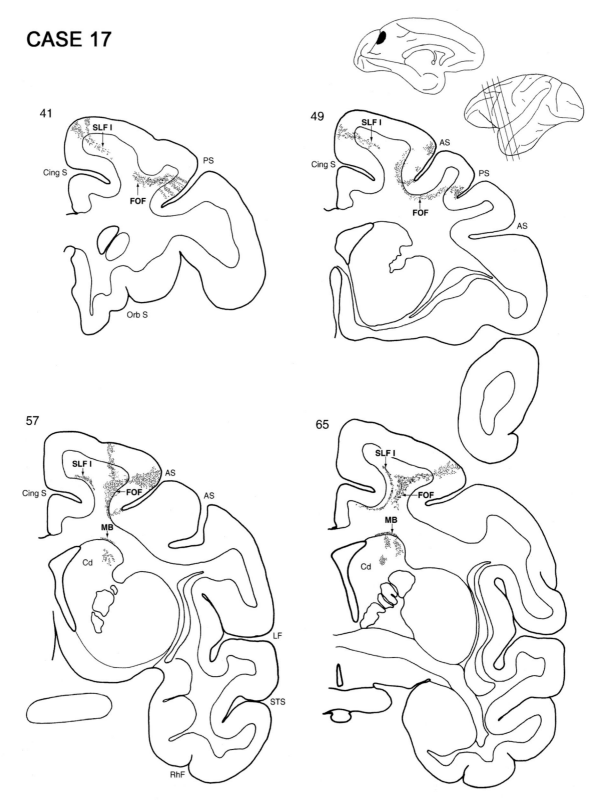

Figure 9-1

Schematic diagrams of 18 rostral–caudal coronal sections in Case 17 taken at the levels shown on the hemispheric diagrams above right, showing the isotope injection site in the medial part of the preoccipital gyrus, involving medial area 19 (area PO) and area PGm (injection site shown in the black-filled area). The figure illustrates the resulting trajectories of the cortical association, commissural, and subcortical fibers (dashed lines and dots) in the white matter and the terminations in the cortex and subcortical regions (black dots). See list of abbreviations, p. 617.

CASE 17

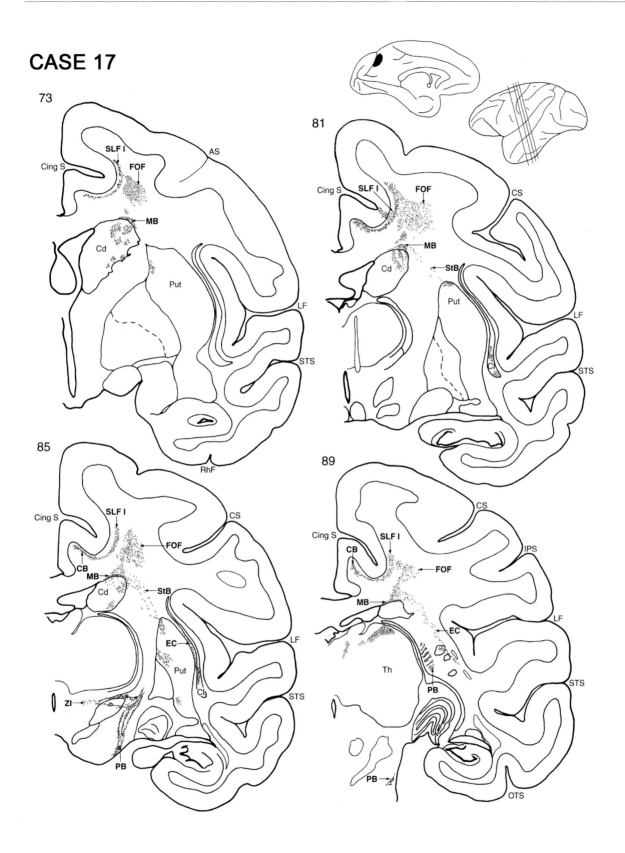

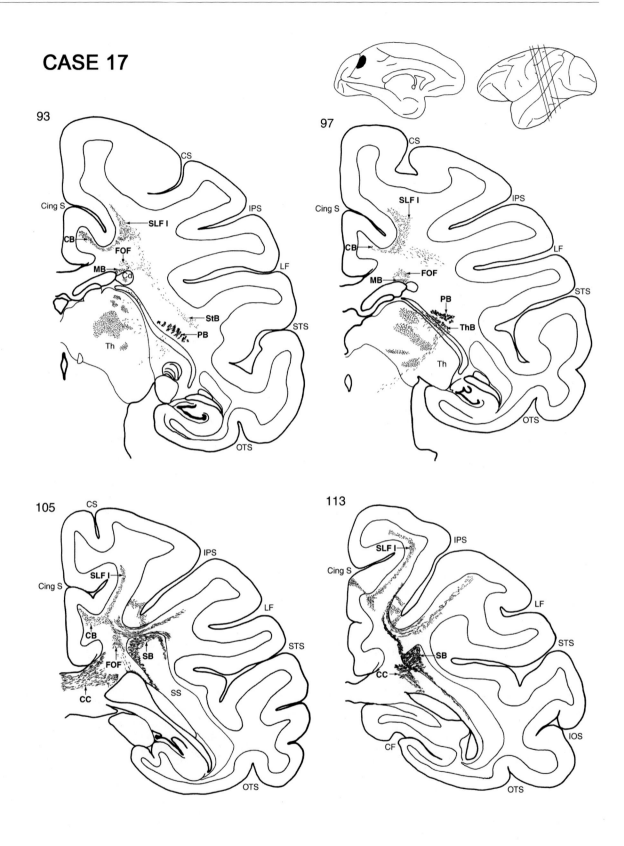

CASE 17

Figure 9-1 (continued)

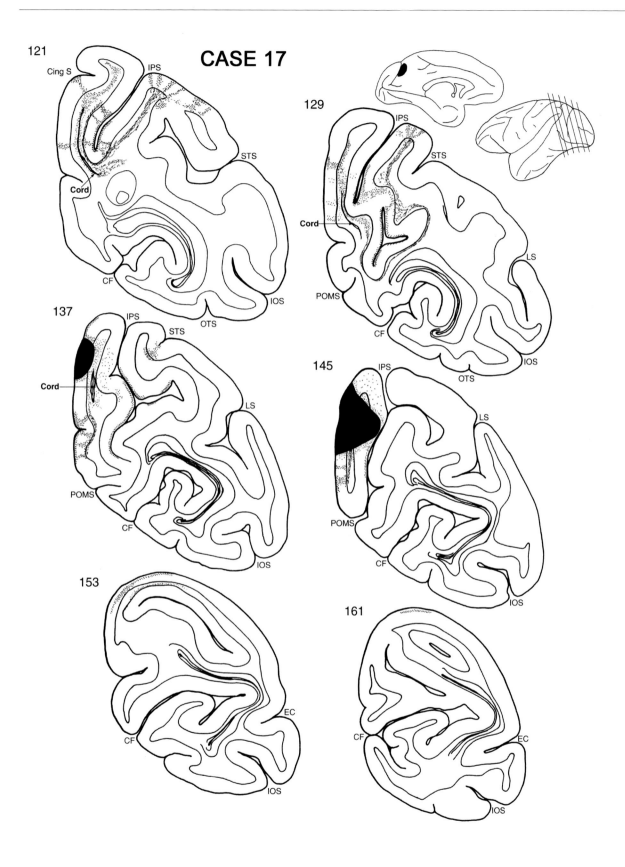

CASE 17

121

Cing S   IPS

Cord

CF

STS

IOS

129

IPS

STS

Cord

POMS

CF

LS

OTS

IOS

137

IPS   STS

Cord

POMS

CF

LS

IOS

145

IPS

LS

POMS

CF

IOS

153

CF

EC

IOS

161

CF

EC

IOS

237

CASE 17

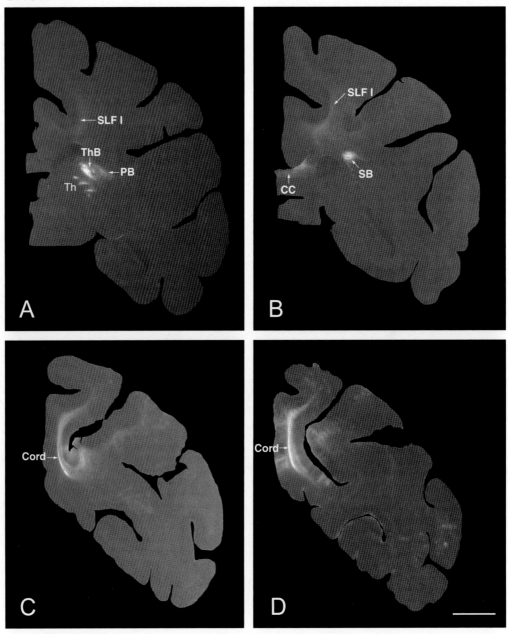

Figure 9-2

Photomicrographs of selected coronal sections of Case 17 to show the labeled fibers and terminations in A through D. The injection site is caudal to these images. Photomicrographs A through D correspond to sections 97, 105, 121, and 129, respectively (Mag = 0.5×, bar = 5 mm).

Striatal Fibers

Some fibers that leave the subcortical bundle in the sagittal stratum course upward and are incorporated into the Muratoff bundle that lies above the body of the caudate nucleus (Sc. 97). As these fibers move rostrally they are joined also by fibers from the FOF and the SLF II. Fibers leave the Muratoff bundle and terminate throughout the body and in the head of the caudate nucleus (Scs. 41, 49, 57, 65, 73, 81, 85, 89, 93, 97).

A group of fibers in the striatal fiber bundle (StB) descends obliquely from the SLF II and courses ventrally to lie within the ventral part of the external capsule. From there, fibers terminate in the caudal part of the putamen and in the ventral portion of the claustrum (Scs. 73, 81, 85, 89).

CASE 18

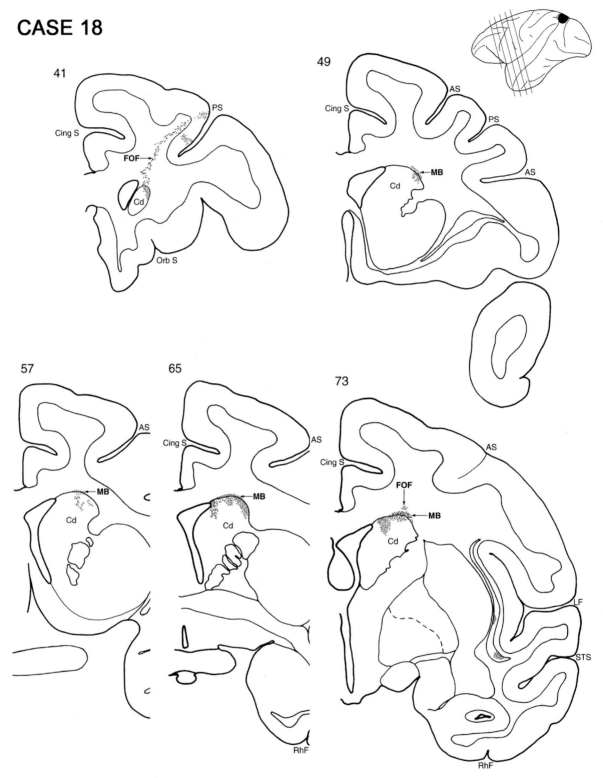

Figure 9-3

Schematic diagrams of 19 rostral–caudal coronal sections in Case 18 taken at the levels shown on the hemispheric diagram above right, showing the isotope injection site in the dorsal part of the preoc-cipital gyrus, corresponding to area DP, and the upper part of area V4D (black-filled area) and the resulting trajectories of the cortical association, commissural, and subcortical fibers (dashed lines and dots) in the white matter and the terminations in the cortex and subcortical regions (black dots).

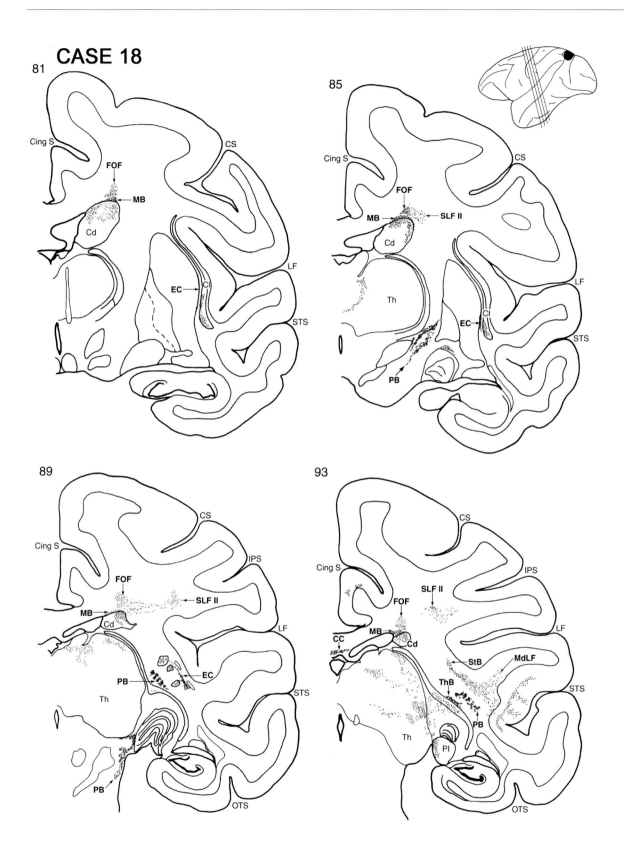

CASE 18

81

Cing S
CS
FOF
MB
Cd
EC
Cl
LF
STS

85

Cing S
CS
FOF
MB
SLF II
Cd
Th
EC
Cl
LF
STS
PB

89

Cing S
CS
IPS
FOF
SLF II
MB
Cd
LF
PB
EC
STS
Th
PB
OTS

93

Cing S
CS
IPS
SLF II
FOF
LF
CC
MB
Cd
StB
MdLF
ThB
STS
PB
Th
Pl
OTS

243

CASE 18

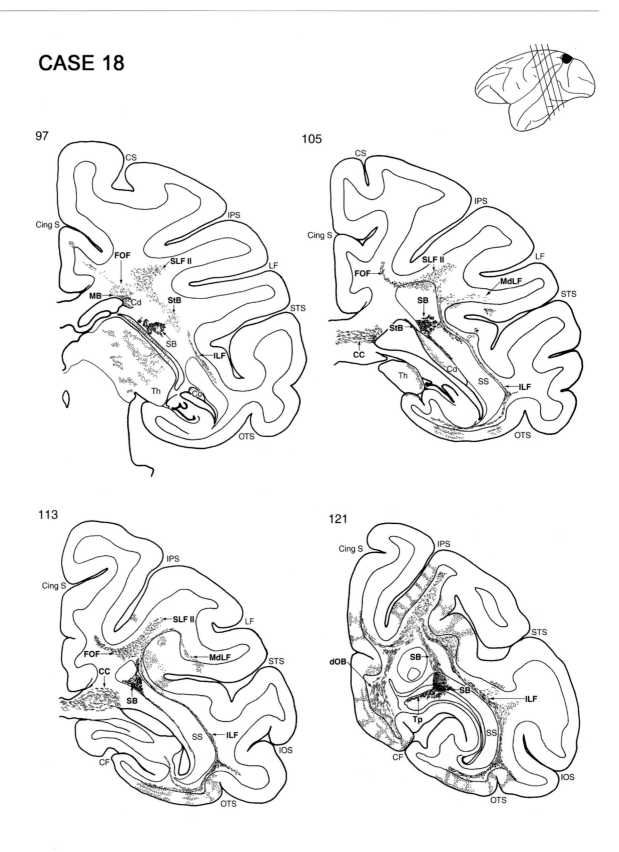

Figure 9-3 (continued)

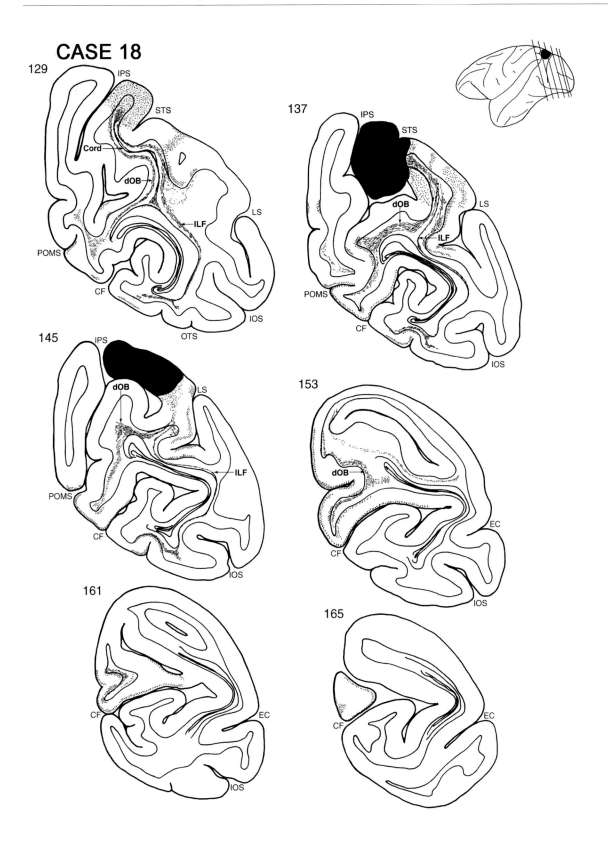

CASE 18

CASE 18

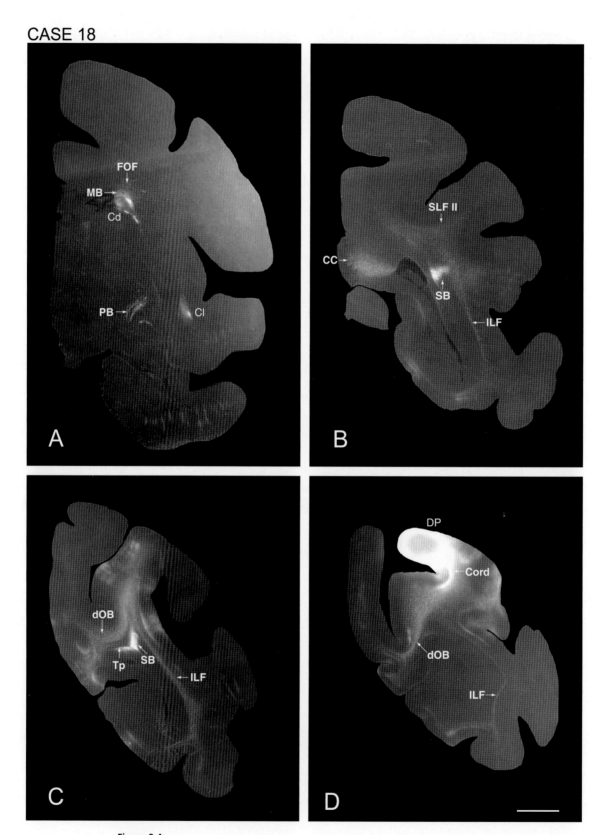

Figure 9-4
Photomicrographs of selected coronal sections of Case 18 to show the injection site in D and the resulting labeled fibers and terminations in A through D. Photomicrographs A through D correspond to sections 85, 105, 121, and 137, respectively (Mag = 0.5×, bar = 5 mm).

CASE 19

In this case the isotope injection was in dorsal area V4 and adjacent area V4T (Scs. 129, 137). See figures 9-5 and 9-6.

Association Fibers

Local Association Fibers

Fibers leave the injection site and travel in the preoccipital gyrus. They terminate dorsally in area V4D and ventrally in V3 in the cortex of the upper bank of the lunate sulcus, in columns and in the first layer (Sc. 137).

Long Association Fibers

Caudally Directed Fibers

These fibers travel from the injection site within two major components. A dorsomedial component (the dorsal occipital bundle [dOB]) courses medially in the white matter of the annectant gyrus, and a ventral component occupies the inferior longitudinal fasciculus.

The dorsomedial component, dOB, courses dorsally under the annectant gyrus, hugging the lateral and superior border of the sagittal stratum. It provides terminations first to area V3A in the annectant gyrus and then further caudally in the occipital lobe to areas V2 and V1 (Scs. 145, 153, 161, 165). As these fibers continue further caudally they descend in the white matter of the medial aspect of the annectant gyrus and distribute terminations in area V3 at the medial aspect of the annectant gyrus, as well as in the dorsal aspects of areas V1 and V2 (Scs. 153, 161, 165). These terminations are in the first and sixth layers in areas V3A and V2 and in the first and fourth layers in the caudal part of area V1.

The ventrally directed fibers enter the inferior longitudinal fasciculus (ILF), descend ventrally, curve around the lateral aspect of the sagittal stratum, and then course medially. From there the fibers terminate in the ventral occipital gyrus in areas V3V and V3 in the first and sixth layers (Scs. 137, 145, 153).

Rostrally Directed Fibers

Ventrally directed fibers leave the injection site and enter the ILF situated deep to the superior temporal sulcus (STS) and lateral to the sagittal stratum. Some fibers leave the ILF at this stage and terminate in the caudal segment of areas FST, V4T, and MT (Scs. 105, 113, 121). The remaining ILF fibers descend to the region of the occipitotemporal sulcus (OTS), where they divide into a medial and a lateral component. The medial component terminates in the rostral and lateral part of area V4V that lies medial to the OTS (Scs. 105, 113, 121). The lateral component terminates in the ventral part of TE3 that lies lateral to the OTS (Scs. 105, 113, 121). In all these areas (FST, MT, TE3, and rostral V4), terminations are seen in a columnar manner, but they are predominantly in layer 4.

Dorsally directed fibers from the ILF course upward and medially toward the lower bank of the intraparietal sulcus, where they terminate in the caudal portion of area POa (LIP) in a columnar manner (Scs. 113, 121).

Some of the fibers turn medially around the dorsal aspect of the sagittal stratum and enter the fronto-occipital fasciculus (FOF) lying above the Muratoff bundle. The labeled fibers in the FOF course rostrally to the level of the anterior commissure, at which point they turn laterally, and these fibers of the FOF (fFOF) course along with those of the SLF II before terminating in the ventral part of area 8 (Scs. 49, 57).

Commissural and Subcortical Fibers

A dense cord of fibers leaves the injection site and courses ventrally and medially towards the upper-middle part of the sagittal stratum (Sc. 129). Fibers enter the rostral part of sagittal stratum sector SS-3 (Sc. 129), travel medially through the external segment of the sagittal stratum (SSe), and coalesce as a dense bundle in the internal segment of the sagittal stratum (SSi) throughout sector SS-2 (Scs. 105, 113, 121, 129). Some fibers continue further medially into the adjacent tapetum (Sc. 121) and then course medially to enter the splenium in sector CC5 of the corpus callosum at its midsection (in the dorsal-ventral dimension) before they enter the opposite hemisphere (Scs. 105, 113).

The subcortical fiber bundle (SB) in the internal segment of the sagittal stratum contains fibers destined for the thalamus, brainstem, and striatum. The bulk of the fibers in the internal segment of the sagittal stratum throughout SS-2 (Scs. 105, 113, 121) course rostrally until they enter the retrolenticular part of the posterior limb of the internal capsule (ICp-5, Sc. 97) and traverse the external medullary lamina of the thalamus. Some of these fibers course medially and terminate in the thalamus, most heavily in the inferior and lateral pulvinar nuclei (Scs. 97, 93). Few fibers traverse the thalamus to terminate in the superior colliculus.

Other fibers traveling rostrally in the sagittal stratum enter ICp-5 (Sc. 97) and continue rostrally as the pontine bundle (PB) in the posterior limb of the internal capsule until they reach level ICp-3 (Sc. 89). At this level and just rostral to it, corresponding also to the rostral and midpoint of the lateral geniculate nucleus (Sc. 85), the PB fibers course medially over the LGN and descend in the lateral aspect of the cerebral peduncle to the dorsal and lateral parts of the rostral pons before they terminate in the lateral, dorsolateral, and lateral parts of the peripeduncular pontine nuclei.

Striatal Fibers

Some of the fibers from the FOF gather above the genu of the caudate nucleus. They travel rostrally within the Muratoff bundle and provide terminations in the body and head of the caudate nucleus (Scs. 65, 73, 81, 85, 89, 93, 97). Some of the fibers situated at the internal segment of the sagittal stratum provide terminations to the immediately adjacent genu of the caudate nucleus as well (Sc. 105).

Some of the fibers within the lateral sector of the sagittal stratum continue rostrally as a striatal bundle (StB, Sc. 93) and enter the external capsule. From here, fibers terminate in the caudal part of the putamen and in the tail of the caudate nucleus (Scs. 89, 93). Further rostrally, these external capsule fibers terminate in the ventral portion of the claustrum (Scs. 73, 81, 85). Some fibers traverse dorsally through the posterior limb of the internal capsule and enter the Muratoff bundle.

CASE 19

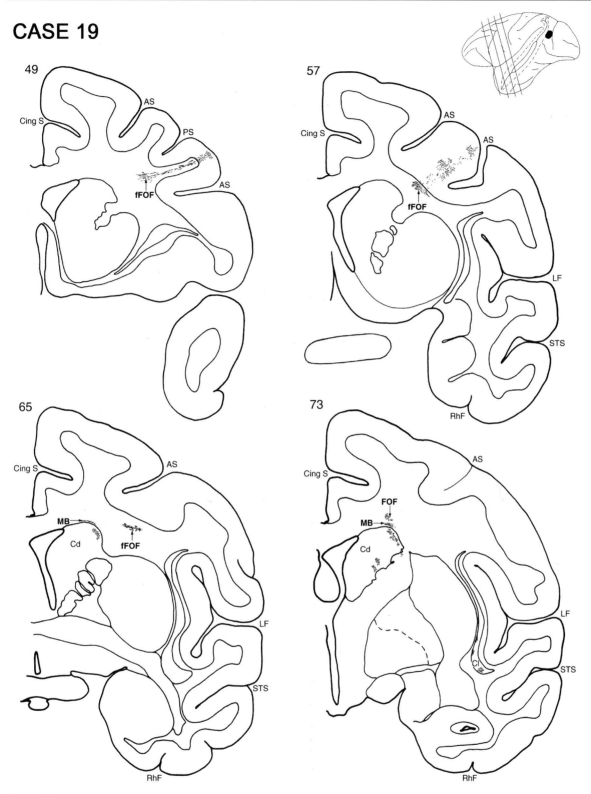

Figure 9-5

Schematic diagrams of 18 rostral–caudal coronal sections in Case 19 taken at the levels shown on the hemispheric diagram above right, showing the isotope injection site in dorsal area V4 and adjacent area V4T (black-filled area) and the resulting trajectories of the cortical association, commissural, and subcortical fibers (dashed lines and dots) in the white matter and the terminations in the cortex and subcortical regions (black dots).

CASE 19

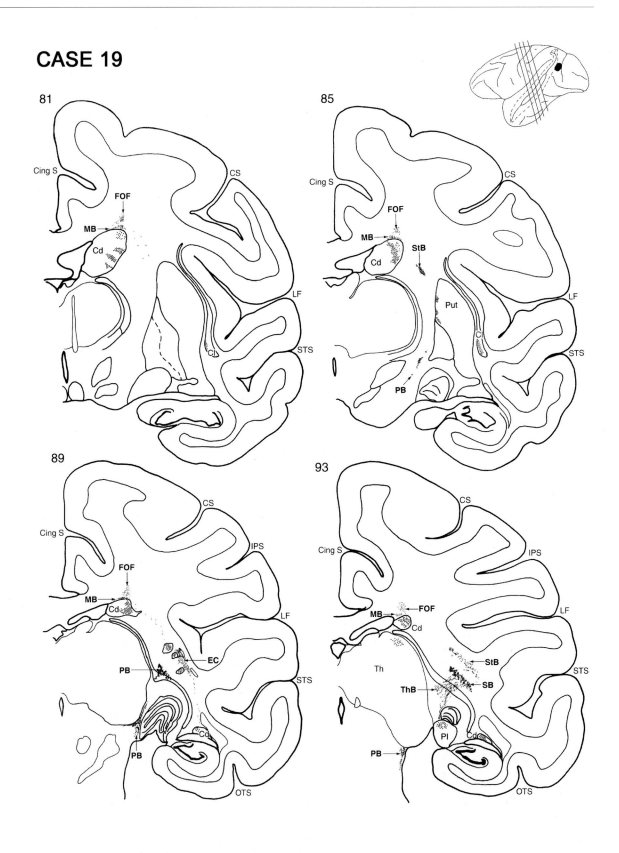

Figure 9-5 (continued)

CASE 19

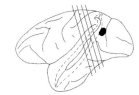

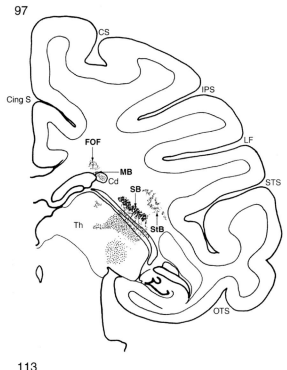

97

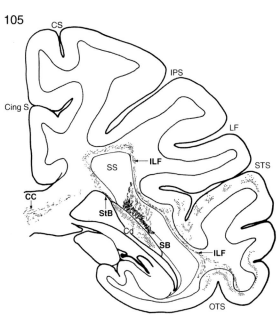

105

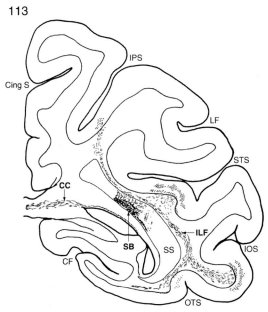

113

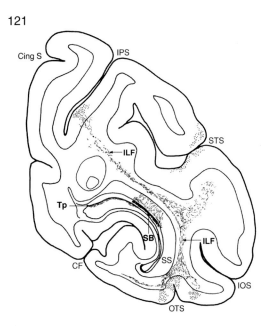

121

CASE 19

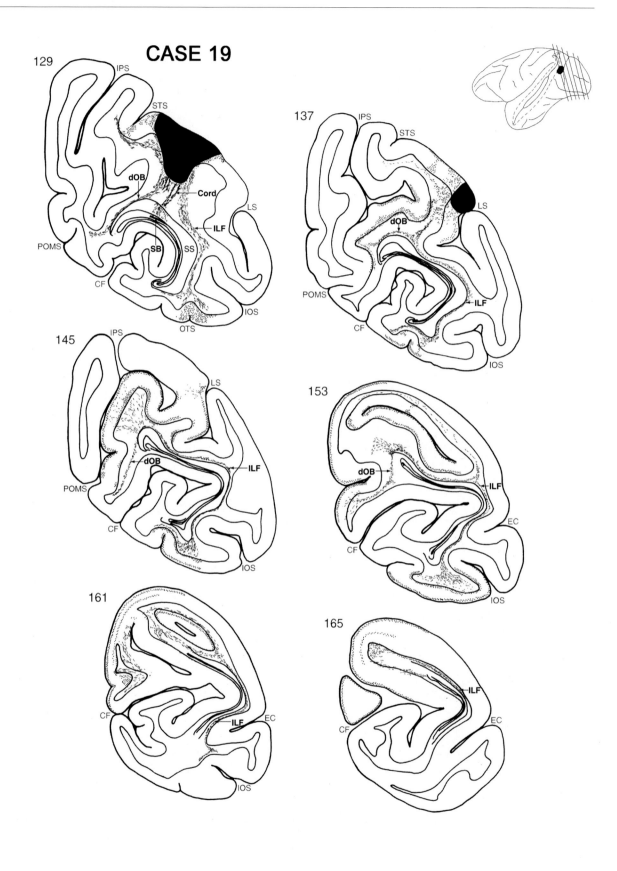

Figure 9-5 (continued)

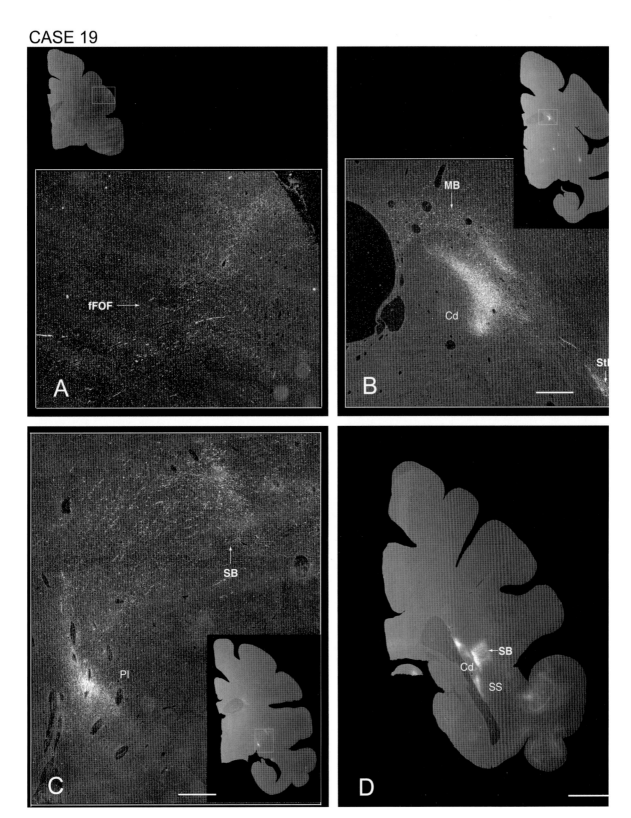

Figure 9-6

Photomicrographs of selected coronal sections of Case 19 to show the injection site in F with the resulting labeled fibers and terminations in A through F, corresponding to sections 49, 85, 93, 105, 121, and 129, respectively. A, B, and C are high-power photomicrographs (Mag = 4×, bar = 0.5 mm) taken from the areas shown in the insets in the low-power photomicrographs, showing fibers from the fronto-occipital fasciculus terminating in area 8Av (A), fibers of the Muratoff bundle and terminations in the head of the caudate nucleus (B), and the subcortical bundle with fibers entering and terminating in the pulvinar inferior nucleus (C). (Photomicrographs D through F, Mag = 0.5×, bar = 5 mm.)

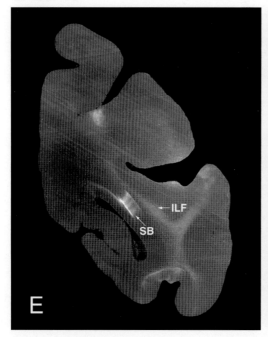
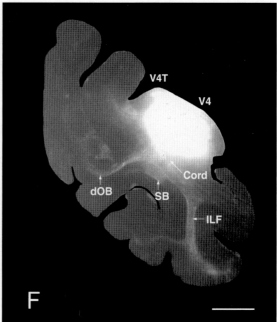

Figure 9-6 (continued)

CASE 20

Isotope was injected in this case in the ventral part of the preoccipital gyrus above the inferior occipital sulcus, in area V4 (Scs. 113, 121, 129). See figures 9-7 and 9-8.

Association Fibers

Local Association Fibers

Local fibers adjacent to the injection site terminate in area V4D above the injection (Sc. 129).

Long Association Fibers

Caudally Directed Fibers

From the injection site, caudally directed fibers enter the white matter and occupy a position between the sagittal stratum and the local fibers, lying within the caudal limb of the inferior longitudinal fasciculus (ILF). These ILF fibers continue into the caudal part of the occipital lobe. They terminate locally in the first layer in areas V4, V3, and V2 in the lunate sulcus (Scs. 137, 145). Dorsally directed ILF fibers are concentrated in the white matter deep to the annectant gyrus. They terminate in the first layer in area V3A in the annectant gyrus, as well as in the dorsal part of area V1 (Scs. 137, 145, 153, 161, 165).

Ventrally directed ILF fibers extend to the white matter around the inferior occipital sulcus. These fibers terminate in the first layer in the cortex of the inferior occipital sulcus (IOS) in area V3 (Scs. 137, 145).

Rostrally Directed Fibers

These fibers are conveyed mainly by the ILF. The dorsal segment of the ILF leads to regions adjacent to the injection site, including area V3A in the annectant gyrus, areas POa and IPd in the intraparietal sulcus, and area MST at the caudal aspect of the STS (Scs. 105, 113, 121, 129). The ventral segment of the ILF directs fibers to area V3 in the IOS. All these terminations are columnar.

Rostrally directed long association fibers are conveyed via the rostral segment of the ILF, remaining predominantly in the white matter of the inferotemporal region. These fibers terminate in a columnar manner in areas PGa, MST, and MT in the depths of the superior temporal sulcus and in areas TE3 and TEO, mainly in the fourth layer (Scs. 93, 105).

Commissural and Subcortical Fibers

Fibers emanate from the injection site in the form of a broad cord in the center of the white matter of the inferotemporal area (Scs. 121, 129). The fibers aggregate at the lateral aspect of the external segment of the sagittal stratum at the junction of sectors SS-2 and SS-3 (Scs. 121, 129). From there fibers course medially in a radial direction leading to two intense fiber bundles. One group of fibers (the subcortical bundle [SB]) lies in the medial aspect of the internal segment of sector SS-2 of the sagittal stratum (Scs.

105, 113, 121). The other, further medially situated, lies within the tapetum (Scs. 113, 121, 129).

The tapetal fibers enter the splenium of the corpus callosum (Sc. 113) and then course rostrally and medially to enter the opposite hemisphere in the dorsal part of CC5 (Sc. 105).

The fibers lying within the internal segment of the sagittal stratum (SSi) continue rostrally as the main subcortically directed bundle (SB) that gives rise to a number of target-specific fiber systems.

At the level of the retrolenticular part of the internal capsule (ICp-5, Sc. 97), the thalamic fibers leave the subcortical bundle, course medially, and reach the thalamus via the external medullary lamina. These fibers terminate in the lateral and inferior pulvinar nuclei (Sc. 97).

The pontine fibers (PB) in the SSi continue to course rostrally in the posterior limb of the internal capsule in ICp-5 (Sc. 97) and ICp-4 (Sc. 93). When these fibers come to lie above and lateral to the midpoint of the lateral geniculate nucleus (LGN) at level ICp-3 (Sc. 89), they course medially over the LGN and enter the lateral aspect of the cerebral peduncle on their way to terminate in the lateral and dorsolateral pontine nuclei and the lateral and dorsolateral parts of the peripeduncular nucleus.

Striatal Fibers

Fibers destined for the striatum travel in the sagittal stratum and terminate first in the genu of the caudate nucleus (Sc. 105). Further rostrally, a dorsal contingent of these striatal fibers enters the Muratoff bundle and terminates in the body and caudal part of the head of the caudate nucleus (Scs. 81, 85, 89, 93, 97). The ventral segment of striatal fibers courses rostrally and terminates in the tail of the caudate nucleus and the caudal part of the putamen (Scs. 89, 93, 97). Further rostrally, these ventral striatal fibers occupy a position in the ventral part of the external capsule before terminating in the claustrum (Scs. 81, 85).

CASE 20

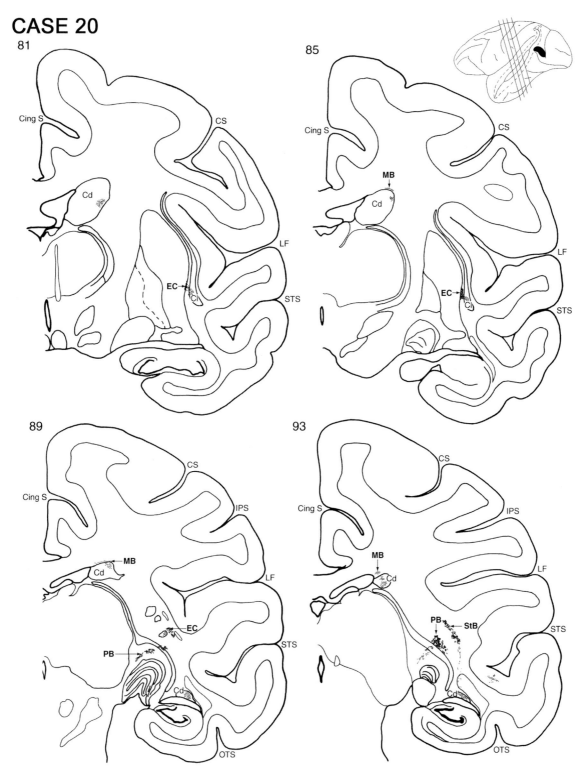

Figure 9-7

Schematic diagrams of 14 rostral–caudal coronal sections in Case 20 taken at the levels shown on the hemispheric diagram above right, showing the isotope injection site in the ventral part of the preoccipital gyrus above the inferior occipital sulcus, in area V4 (black-filled area), the resulting trajectories of the cortical association, commissural, and subcortical fibers (dashed lines and dots) in the white matter, and the terminations in the cortex and subcortical regions (black dots).

CASE 20

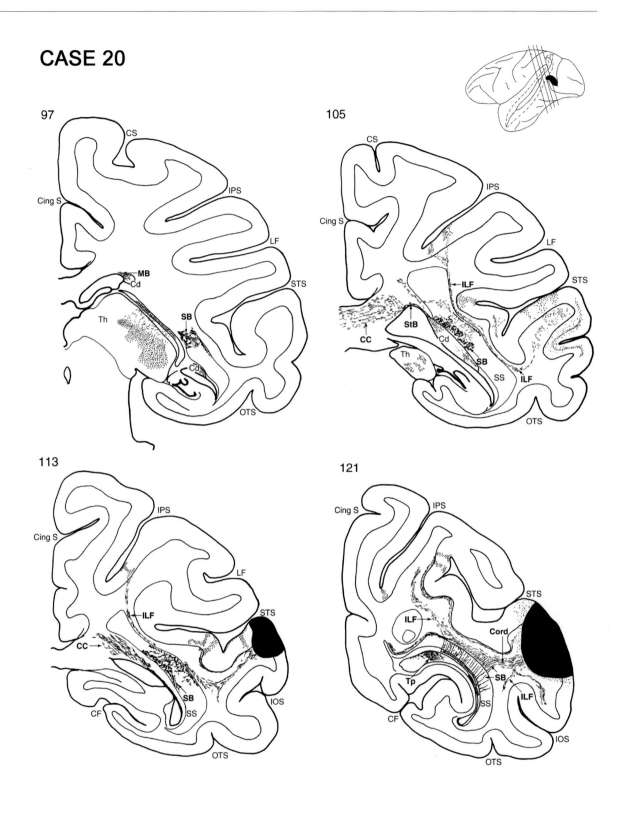

Figure 9-7 (continued)

CASE 20

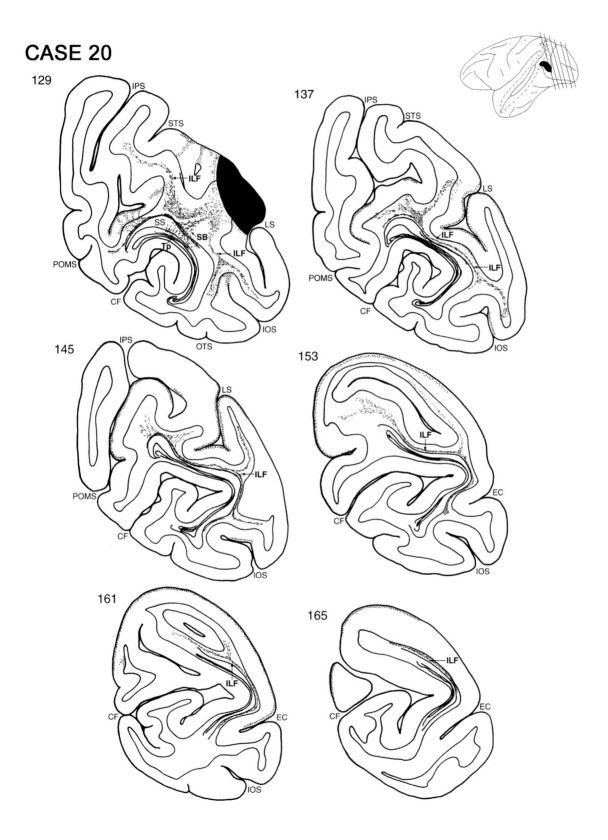

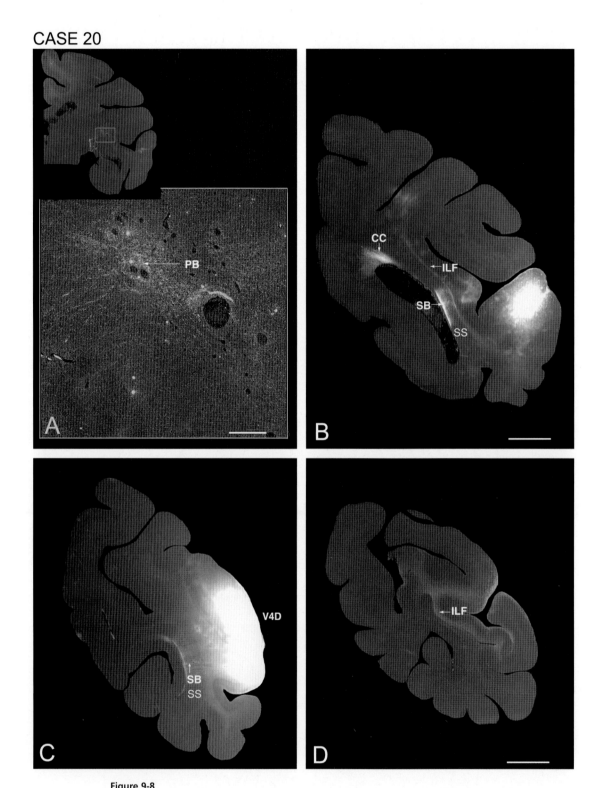

Figure 9-8

Photomicrographs of selected coronal sections of Case 20 to show the injection site in C with the injection halo in B and the resulting labeled fibers and terminations in A through D. A, High-power photomicrograph (section 93, Mag = 4×, bar = 0.5 mm) taken from the location indicated in the low-power photomicrograph above, showing the pontine bundle. B through D correspond to sections 113, 121, and 137, respectively (Mag = 0.5×, bar = 5 mm).

CASE 21

In this case the isotope injection was in the ventral part of area V4, with some encroachment in ventral area V3 (Scs. 121, 129, 137, 145). See figures 9-9 and 9-10.

Association Fibers

Local Association Fibers

Near the injection site, fibers terminate in areas V3 and V4D (Scs. 129, 137, 145).

Long Association Fibers

Caudally Directed Fibers

Fibers leave the injection site and travel caudally in two distinct fiber bundles. Medially situated fibers lie within the white matter deep to the occipitotemporal sulcus (OTS) and terminate in the first layer in the ventral and ventromedial parts of area V2 (Scs. 153, 161, 165). Dorsally directed fibers ascend in the inferior longitudinal fasciculus (ILF) lateral to the sagittal stratum and deep to the inferior occipital sulcus (IOS) and then further dorsally curve medially and lie dorsal to the sagittal stratum. These fibers terminate in areas V3 in the lunate sulcus, area V4A, and area V4 in the buried caudal part of the annectant gyrus, predominantly in the first layer (Sc. 161).

Rostrally Directed Fibers

These association fibers travel rostrally within the ventral part of the ILF. Some fibers course laterally and rostrally within the dorsal part of the white matter of the inferotemporal region and terminate principally in the fourth layer in areas V4D, MT, and FST (Scs. 89, 93, 97, 105, 113). Other ILF fibers continue rostrally in the white matter of the ventral part of the inferotemporal region and terminate predominantly in the fourth layer of areas TE3 and TE2 ventrally, as well as around the OTS, where they terminate in area TF (Scs. 73, 81, 85, 89, 93, 97, 105, 113).

Commissural and Subcortical Fibers

A dense cord of fibers leaves the injection site and courses toward the ventral aspect of the sagittal stratum in the rostral part of sector SS-3 (Sc. 129). Fibers traverse the ventral part of this sector of the sagittal stratum and aggregate within its internal segment (SSi). From this position, a distinct group of fibers separates, ascends in the tapetum (Scs. 113, 121), and enters the splenium of the corpus callosum (Scs. 105, 113). These fibers traverse through the midsagittal plane in the ventral part of sector CC5 (Sc. 105).

The major concentration of fibers lying within the SSi travels rostrally in the ventral aspect of sectors SS-2 and SS-1 of the sagittal stratum. At the level of the pulvinar inferior (the caudal part of sector SS-1) these fibers course medially, enter the thalamus, and terminate heavily in the thalamus, principally in PI (Sc. 97).

Striatal Fibers

The striatal fibers are conveyed by two fiber contingents. Ventrally situated fibers penetrate the sagittal stratum before terminating in the genu and tail of the caudate nucleus and the caudal and ventral parts of the putamen (Scs. 81, 85, 89, 93, 97, 105). Some fibers terminate in the claustrum (Sc. 73). A dorsal group of striatal fibers runs with the ILF and becomes continuous rostrally with the external capsule, and then the fibers curve medially, crossing the posterior limb of the internal capsule. These fibers terminate in the body and caudal part of the head of the caudate nucleus or enter the Muratoff bundle before terminating in the caudate nucleus (Scs. 85, 89, 93, 97).

CASE 21

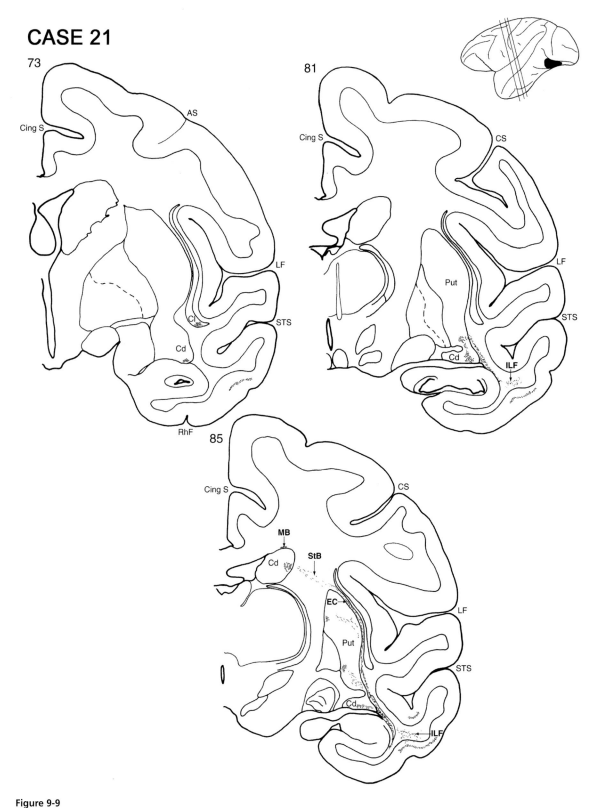

Figure 9-9

Schematic diagram of 15 rostral–caudal coronal sections in Case 21 taken at the levels shown on the hemispheric diagram above right, showing the isotope injection site in ventral area V4, with some encroachment in ventral area V3 (black-filled area), the resulting trajectories of the cortical association, commissural, and subcortical fibers (dashed lines and dots) in the white matter, and the terminations in the cortex and subcortical regions (black dots).

CASE 21

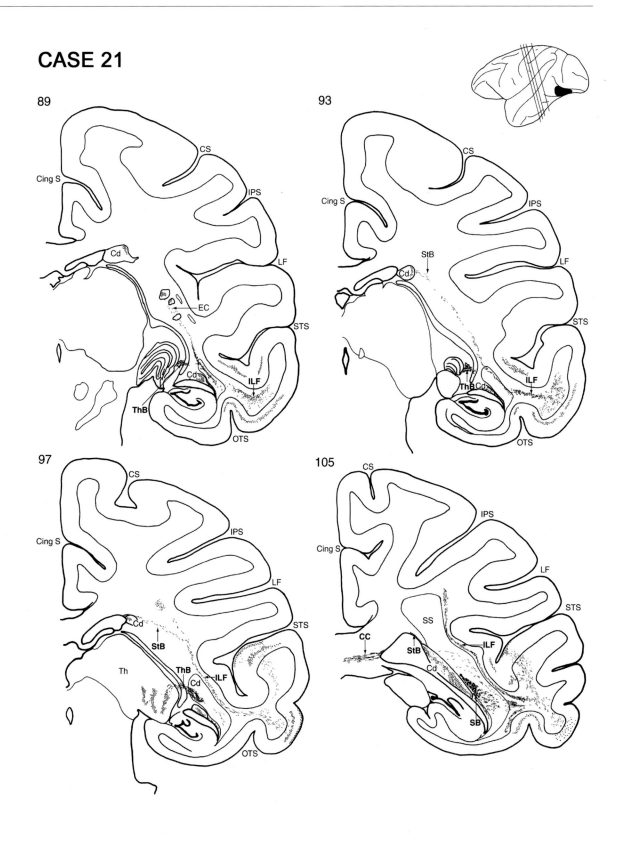

Figure 9-9 (continued)

CASE 21

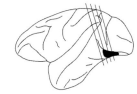

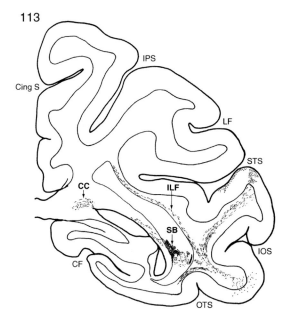

113

Cing S

IPS

LF

STS

CC

ILF

SB

CF

IOS

OTS

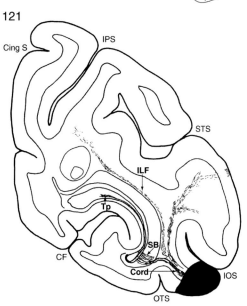

121

Cing S

IPS

STS

ILF

Tp

SB

CF

Cord

IOS

OTS

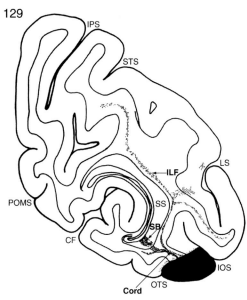

129

IPS

STS

ILF

LS

POMS

SS

SB

CF

IOS

Cord

OTS

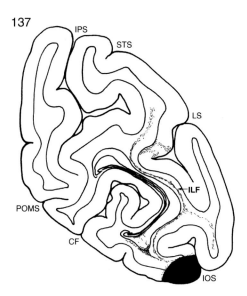

137

IPS

STS

LS

ILF

POMS

CF

IOS

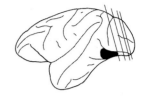

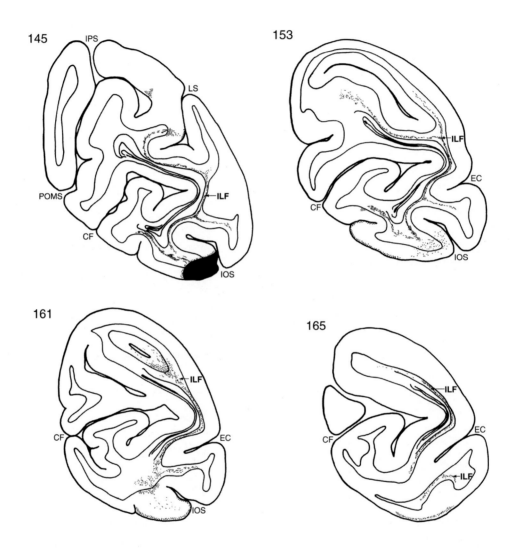

Figure 9-9 (continued)

CASE 21

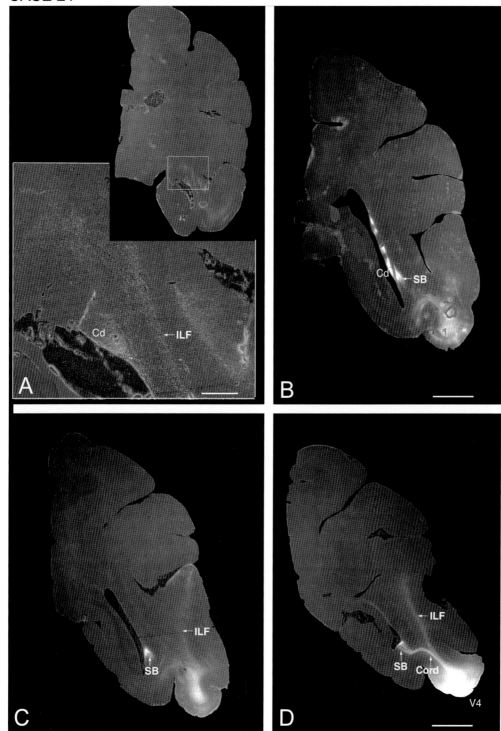

Figure 9-10

Photomicrographs of selected coronal sections of Case 21 to show the injection site in D and the resulting labeled fibers and terminations in A through D. A, High-power photomicrograph (section 93, Mag = 4×, bar = 0.5 mm) taken from the location indicated in the low-power photomicrograph above, showing fibers in the inferior longitudinal fasciculus. B through D correspond to sections 105, 113, and 121, respectively (Mag = 0.5×, bar = 5 mm).

Occipital Lobe Summary

Association Fibers

Medial Occipital Region (Area PO, Case 17)

Rostrally directed fibers limited to the parietal lobe course through the white matter of the superior parietal lobule, curve around the depth of the intraparietal sulcus, and reach the white matter of the inferior parietal lobule (see figure 9-11). These fibers terminate in area PEa in the upper bank of the intraparietal sulcus and in area POa in the lower bank. These fibers terminate also in areas PG and Opt, and some terminations are directed to the annectant region, area V3A.

A minor contingent of fibers from the medial occipital region courses caudally through the dorsal white matter of the occipital lobe and terminates in areas PO, V2, and V1.

The long association fibers that emanate from the medial occipital region course principally within SLF I and the FOF. A small contingent of fibers also travels in the dorsal part of the cingulate fasciculus.

1. Superior Longitudinal Fasciculus I

The SLF I fibers course rostrally in the white matter of the superior parietal lobule, situated around the cingulate sulcus. As they move rostrally, the fibers terminate in area PGm and area 31 in the medial parietal cortex. The SLF I fibers in this location continue into the frontal lobe, lying within the white matter of the superior frontal gyrus. In the frontal lobe the SLF I fibers move dorsally and terminate in medial area 6 (the supplementary motor) and area 9.

2. Cingulum Bundle

The fibers in the cingulum bundle also course rostrally deep to the cingulate sulcus and terminate in a limited manner in the depth of the cingulate sulcus, in the caudal part of area 24d.

3. Fronto-Occipital Fasciculus

At the level of the caudal end of the body of the caudate nucleus, a distinct group of fibers separates laterally from the fiber bundle in the SLF I. These fibers situated in the FOF occupy a position between the corpus callosum and corona radiata. As they course rostrally in the frontal lobe, the FOF fibers move dorsally from this location to lie deep to the upper limb of the arcuate sulcus before terminating in dorsal area 6, area 8Ad, and dorsal area 46.

Dorsal Preoccipital Gyrus Area DP (Case 18)

The major association fiber bundles emerging from the dorsal occipital area are the inferior longitudinal fasciculus (ILF), the dorsal occipital bundle (dOB), and the FOF. Some fibers also run in the middle longitudinal fasciculus (MdLF), SLF I, SLF II, and the cingulate fasciculus.

1. Inferior Longitudinal Fasciculus

Fibers emerging from the dorsal preoccipital gyrus course ventrally and run in the ILF situated between the superior temporal sulcus and the sagittal stratum. As they descend into the ILF, they provide terminations to areas MST and FST. Further, the ILF fibers proceed in both a caudal and a rostral direction.

Caudally directed ILF fibers terminate in areas V4D and V3. Rostrally, the fibers curve medially around the lateral convexity of the sagittal stratum, course medially, and terminate in areas V3V and V4V. A contingent of fibers runs along with the ILF, enters the white matter of the superior temporal gyrus, and runs forward in the MdLF to terminate in the caudal part of areas TPO and PGa.

2. Dorsal Occipital Bundle

A separate fiber bundle, the dorsal occipital bundle (dOB), descends in the white matter of the preoccipital gyrus and the inferior parietal lobule, running parallel and medial to the fibers descending into the ILF. At the level of the upper segment of the sagittal stratum, these fibers course medially into the white matter of the annectant gyrus and the dorsal bank of the calcarine fissure. From there they terminate in the dorsal segments of area V1 in the calcarine fissure, the dorsal part of areas V2 and V3, and a part of ventral area PO. These fibers course rostrally in the white matter of the medial occipital and parietal cortices and terminate in areas V2, V3, and V4. A small contingent of fibers moves medially and dorsally as a part of the SLF I and terminates in area PGm.

3. Fronto-Occipital Fasciculus

The FOF fibers are situated above and medial to the sagittal stratum, move rostrally, and come to lie dorsal to the caudate nucleus. Some fibers from the FOF course medially and terminate in area 23. The remaining fibers continue rostrally in the FOF into the frontal lobe and terminate in dorsal area 46.

Lateral Preoccipital Gyrus (Cases 19 and 20)

The association fibers emerging from the lateral preoccipital gyrus travel in the inferior longitudinal fasciculus, the dorsal occipital bundle, and the FOF.

1. Inferior Longitudinal Fasciculus

The fibers that course medially from the lateral preoccipital gyrus enter the ILF lying lateral to the sagittal stratum, and proceed in caudal and rostral directions.

The fibers traveling caudally terminate first in the lateral parts of areas V3 and V2. Further caudally, the ILF fibers course in two directions, ventrally and dorsally. The ventral fibers terminate primarily in area V3V, whereas the dorsal fibers terminate in the dorsal, medial, and lateral parts of areas V2 and V1.

The ILF also conveys associative fibers rostrally in the parietal and temporal lobes. These rostrally directed fibers lying between the sagittal stratum and the white matter of the superior temporal sulcus terminate dorsally in areas POa and IPd of the intraparietal sulcus, as well as in areas MST, FST, and MT in the caudal part of the STS. More ventrally, the ILF fibers terminate in areas TEO and TE3, as well as in area TF.

2. Fronto-Occipital Fasciculus

The fibers that travel rostrally in the FOF leave the lateral preoccipital gyrus, course along with the dorsal segment of the ILF fibers, and move medially into the FOF at the level of the caudal end of the body of the caudate nucleus. These fibers travel within the FOF until they reach the prefrontal cortex. At the level of the anterior commissure, the FOF fibers move laterally and enter the white matter of the arcuate sulcus in a location corresponding to the position of the SLF II before terminating in the ventral part of area 8 (area 8Av).

3. Dorsal Occipital Bundle

Fibers traveling caudally from the lateral preoccipital gyrus enter the dorsal occipital bundle (dOB) and course through the white matter between the sagittal stratum and the annectant gyrus. These fibers then terminate mainly in area V3A of the annectant gyrus.

Inferior Occipital Gyrus (Ventral Parts of Areas V3 and V4, Case 21)

The bulk of the long association fibers from the ventral occipital lobe are contained within the ILF and run both caudally and rostrally. Caudally the ILF fibers course in the white matter between the lunate sulcus and the sagittal stratum. These fibers terminate in the occipital lobe in the caudal part of area V3A and in areas V4D, V3, and ventral V2. Rostrally directed ILF fibers course between the sagittal stratum and the white matter of the superior temporal gyrus. These fibers travel for a considerable distance rostrally within the white matter of the inferotemporal cortex. They terminate within areas V4, MT, FST, TF, TE3, and TE2 and the caudal part of area TE1.

Commissural Fibers

The commissural fibers from the various regions of the preoccipital gyrus course through the most caudal sector of the corpus callosum, sector CC5. Those from the medial preoccipital gyrus course dorsally and rostrally in this sector, whereas those from the dorsolateral preoccipital region course caudal to the fibers from the medial region. From the ventral preoccipital gyrus, fibers course through the ventral part of CC5.

Subcortical Fibers

Medial and Dorsal Aspects of the Preoccipital Gyrus

The subcortical fibers descend in a cord traveling in the white matter of the superior and inferior parietal lobules. Fibers then enter the dorsal portion of the sagittal stratum, the fibers from the medial preoccipital gyrus located more superiorly. These fibers travel rostrally and enter the posterior limb of the internal capsule; at the level of the pulvinar caudal to the lateral geniculate nucleus, they separate into thalamic and pontine fiber bundles. The thalamic fibers cross the lateral and ventral parts of the external medullary lamina and enter the thalamus. The pontine fibers continue further rostrally, and at the level of the rostral aspect of the LGN they continue into the peduncle as they descend caudally into the pons.

Lateral Preoccipital Gyrus

The subcortical fibers course medially into the midsector of the sagittal stratum, move medially within the stratum, and divide into two segments. The thalamic fibers cross the lateral medullary lamina and enter the pulvinar. The pontine fibers continue rostrally in the posterior limb of the internal capsule until the midpoint of the LGN, at which stage they arch over the LGN to enter the cerebral peduncle on their way to the basis pontis.

Ventral Preoccipital Region

The subcortical fibers course through the ventral part of the sagittal stratum. They aggregate at the medial portion of the sagittal stratum and enter the ventral part of the external medullary lamina before terminating in the thalamus.

Corticostriate Projections

The parastriate cortices in the occipital lobe project predominantly to the body and the tail of the caudate nucleus, with less consistent input to the caudal part of the head of the caudate nucleus and caudal sectors of the putamen.

The striatal fibers from area PO at the medial convexity and area DP in the preoccipital gyrus are situated lateral and dorsal to the sagittal stratum. A dorsal contingent of fibers courses first through the FOF and then the Muratoff bundle and leads to the dorsal and dorsolateral parts of the head and body of the caudate nucleus. The ventral component of striatal fibers courses rostrally in the external capsule and terminates in the medial part of the caudal putamen and in the ventral part of the claustrum. Some ventral striatal fibers from the dorsal preoccipital region also terminate in the genu and the tail of the caudate nucleus.

The striatal fibers from the lateral preoccipital gyrus traverse the sagittal stratum to reach their terminations in the genu of the caudate nucleus. Some fibers course dorsally and gather in the Muratoff bundle and proceed rostrally as they terminate in the body and head of the caudate nucleus. Ventrally situated striatal fibers descend and terminate in the islands of the putamen and in the tail of the caudate nucleus. Some of these fibers also terminate in the ventral part of the claustrum.

Fibers destined for the striatum from the ventral preoccipital region traverse the sagittal stratum and terminate in the genu of the caudate nucleus. Other fibers run in the ILF and move dorsally and rostrally, course through the extreme capsule, enter the Muratoff bundle, and terminate medially in the body of the caudate nucleus. Fibers in the ILF that course ventrally terminate in the tail of the caudate nucleus, the caudal part of the putamen, and the claustrum. Ventral area V4 uses the external capsule to convey fibers that terminate in the caudate tail and the ventral and medial putamen, as well as the islands of putamen, and fibers cross into the Muratoff bundle before providing light terminations more ventrally in the lateral part of the body of the caudate nucleus.

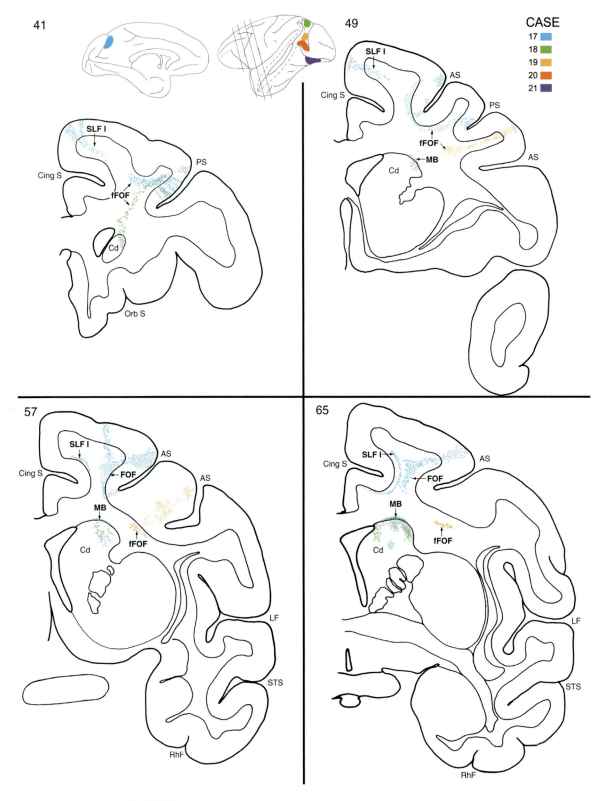

Figure 9-11

Schematic composite diagrams of the rostral–caudal coronal sections of the template brain, illustrating the five occipital lobe cases (Cases 17–21). The injection sites and the association, commissural, and subcortical fibers, as well as the termination patterns, are color-coded for each case. The schematic diagrams of the medial and lateral surfaces of the cerebral hemispheres (at top) represent the different

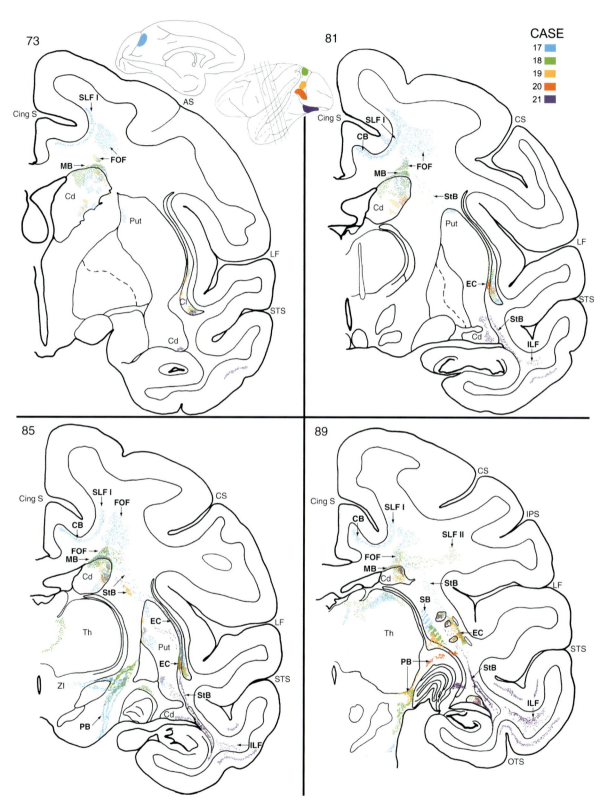

levels of the coronal sections and the injection sites. Color-coding is as follows: Case 17—blue, medial preoccipital gyrus, medial area 19 (area PO) and area PGm; Case 18—green, dorsal preoccipital gyrus, area DP, and upper part of area V4D; Case 19—orange, preoccipital gyrus in dorsal area V4 and adjacent area V4T; Case 20—red, ventral preoccipital gyrus above the inferior occipital sulcus, in area V4; Case 21—purple, area TEO and ventral area V4, with encroachment in ventral area V3.

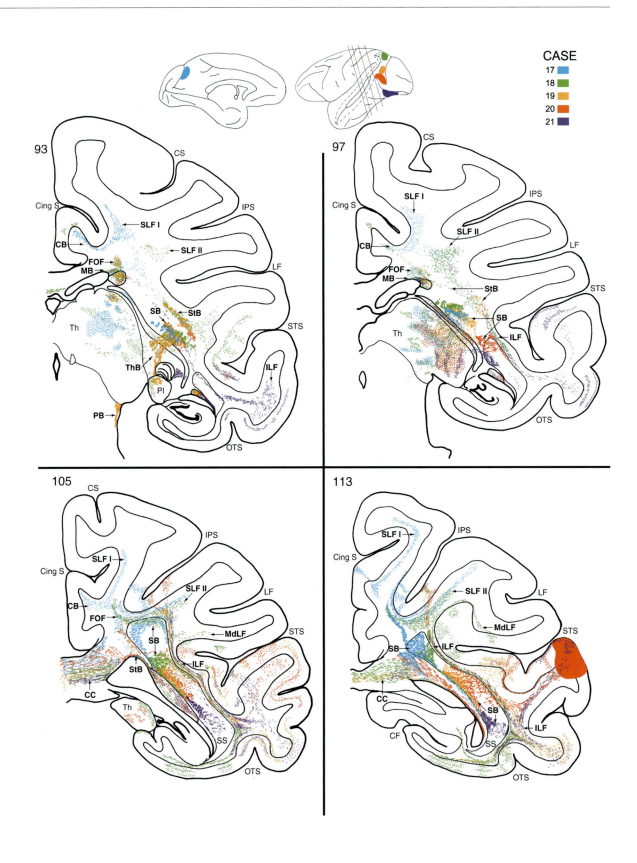

Figure 9-11 (continued)

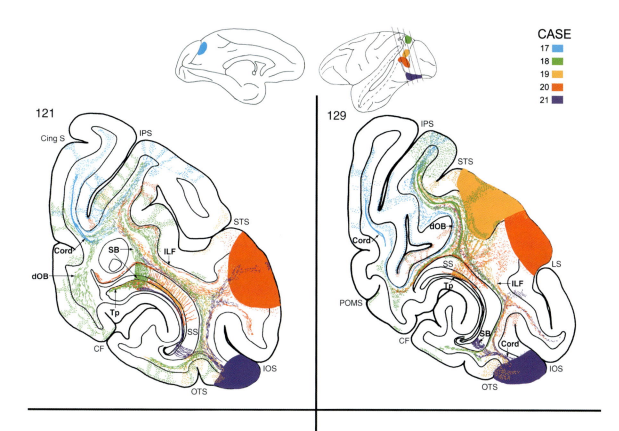

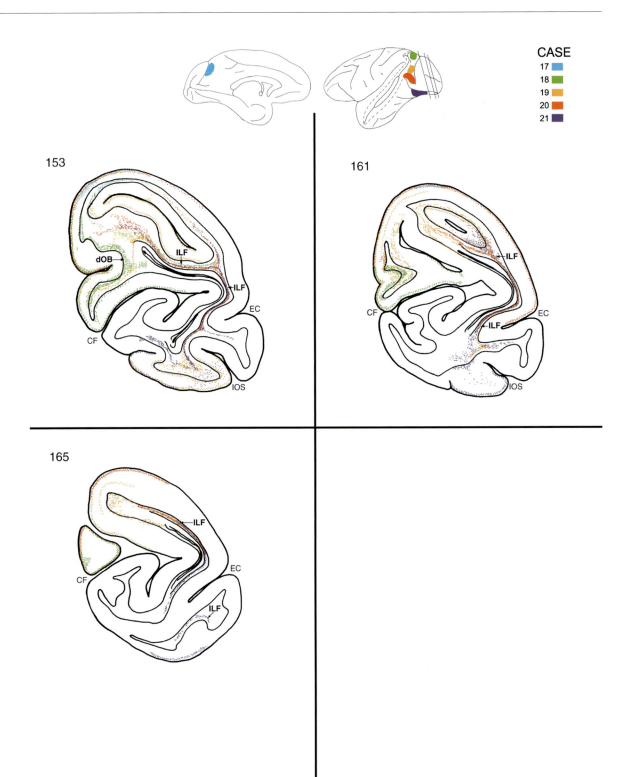

Figure 9-11 (continued)

Cingulate Cortex

10

In this chapter we describe the isotope injection cases in the cingulate gyrus of two rhesus monkeys and analyze the resulting association, striatal, commissural, and subcortical fiber trajectories, as well as the cortical and subcortical terminations. The injections were in the retrosplenial cortex in area 30 and in area 23 (Case 22) and in the rostral cingulate gyrus in area 24 (Case 23).

As in the previous chapters, the architectonic designations of the cortical terminations are described in the text but not identified on the coronal sections. Architectonic areas are labeled on external views of the hemisphere as well as in the coronal series of chapter 4. Terminations in the thalamus are shown and thalamic nuclei are referred to in the text, but the nuclei are not designated on the coronal sections. Pontine terminations are described in the text but not illustrated. Striatal terminations are illustrated and an overview of their termination patterns is presented in the text.

CASE 22

The isotope injection in this case was in the retrosplenial cortex in area 30 and in area 23 (Scs. 105, 113). See figures 10-1 and 10-2.

Association Fibers

Local Association Fibers

From the injection site, fibers traveling within the ventral component of the cingulum bundle terminate locally in the cingulate gyrus in area 23 and in the retrosplenial cortex in area 29/30 (Scs. 105, 113, 117). Fibers that ascend from the injection site traverse the cingulate fasciculus and terminate in areas 23b and 23c (Sc. 105). Fibers that ascend further to join the superior longitudinal fasciculus I (SLF I) terminate in the medial parietal cortex in area 31 (Sc. 113). All these local terminations are columnar.

Long Association Fibers

Caudally Directed Fibers

Fibers that pass caudally from the injection site form two main bundles, one medial and one lateral. The medial fiber bundle has an ascending component (SLF I) that travels in the white matter of the superior parietal lobule and terminates in area PGm, mostly in the superficial layers (Scs. 121, 129). The descending component of this bundle terminates in the rostral portion of area PO and in area V2 above the calcarine fissure (Scs.

121, 129). The lateral bundle that runs in the inferior parietal lobule leads to terminations in area TPO, area MST (not shown), and area Opt in the most caudal part of the inferior parietal lobule (Scs. 121, 129).

Rostrally Directed Fibers

One group of fibers leaves the injection site and courses almost horizontally in the lateral direction. These fibers pass through the white matter underlying the depth of the intraparietal sulcus, skirt the superior border of the sagittal stratum, traverse the SLF II, and enter the white matter of the superior temporal gyrus to lie in the middle longitudinal fasciculus (MdLF). The MdLF fibers progress rostrally and terminate in the upper bank of the superior temporal sulcus in area TPO, and in area Tpt, in a columnar manner (Scs. 93, 97, 105).

Fibers that leave the injection site and course rostrally in the cingulum bundle (CB) form two distinct components, one dorsal and one ventral. The dorsal component of the cingulum bundle lies in the white matter deep to the cingulate gyrus and the cingulate sulcus. Fibers lying within this bundle course medially and terminate in a columnar manner in the cingulate gyrus in area 23 (23a, 23b, and 23c) and in area 24 (Scs. 81, 85, 89, 93, 97). A sizable contingent of fibers leaves the dorsal part of the CB and runs laterally, traversing the lateral aspect of the corpus callosum, to enter both the Muratoff bundle (described further below) and the fronto-occipital fasciculus (FOF). Fibers then travel rostrally toward the frontal lobe within the dorsal part of the CB and the FOF. Within the dorsal prefrontal white matter, fibers ascend from the FOF and become intermingled with fibers that course laterally from the CB. These FOF and CB fibers terminate in a columnar manner in area 9, and the midportion of area 46 both at the gyrus and in the depth of the upper bank of the principal sulcus (Scs. 20, 31, 41). Some fibers leave the CB and travel medially to terminate in a columnar manner in area 24 in prefrontal cortex (Sc. 41). Beyond the genu of the corpus callosum, the CB becomes a flattened plate of fibers that extends medially and ventrally toward the orbital surface. These fibers terminate in area 32, and also in the medial portions of area 11 and in area 14 in the orbital surface, in a columnar manner (Scs. 20, 31).

Fibers that enter the ventral component of the cingulum bundle leave the injection site and descend in the white matter lying between the splenium of the corpus callosum laterally and the retrosplenial cortex medially (Sc. 117). These fibers continue their ventral course, lying first deep to the calcarine fissure and then lying within the white matter of the parahippocampal gyrus. They provide columnar terminations to the ventral temporal region in areas TL and TH and more rostrally in area TF, as well as areas TL, TH, area prostriata, and the presubiculum (Scs. 85, 89, 93, 97, 105, 113, 121).

Commissural and Subcortical Fibers

A dense cord of fibers distinct from the association fibers leaves the injection site and moves laterally into the white matter (Sc. 117). One aggregate of fibers from the cord moves laterally and descends sharply into the white matter caudal and lateral to the splenium of the corpus callosum (Sc. 117). From this staging area fibers stream rostrally and medially to enter CC5 in the splenium (Sc. 113) before coursing medially toward the opposite hemisphere through the full dorsoventral extent of the corpus callosum in CC5 (Scs. 113, 105) and CC4 (Scs. 97, 93).

A second major concentration of fibers emerges from the cord and lies within the white matter above and medial to the SS-2 sector of the sagittal stratum. As this compact fiber bundle descends, it enters the sagittal stratum in midsector SS-2 (Sc. 113); it occupies a dorsal position as it moves rostrally into SS-1 (Sc. 105). This subcortical bundle (SB) then enters the retrolenticular capsule (ICp-5, Sc. 97), at which point it divides into two components. The thalamic fibers (ThB) lie dorsally and the pontine fibers (PB) are more ventrally situated.

The thalamic fibers move medially to lie at the superior and lateral aspect of the thalamus within retrolenticular capsule levels ICp-4 and ICp-5 (Scs. 93, 97). Fibers then emanate from this bundle, traverse the reticular nucleus of the thalamus, and enter the thalamus to terminate in clusters in the pulvinar nucleus (PO, PL, and PM) and the LP nucleus, and a small contingent continues medially to terminate in the limitans nucleus (Scs. 93, 97, 105). A substantial number of fibers at the superior and lateral aspect of thalamus enter the superior thalamic peduncle and result in intense terminations in LD, AD, AV, and AM nuclei, as well as in intralaminar nuclei (CL) and in midline nuclei including reuniens (Scs. 81, 85, 89, 97). Some of the fibers that enter the thalamus from its lateral aspect pass through the thalamus and terminate in the midbrain (Sc. 97).

The pontine fibers lying within the sagittal stratum (SS-2) continue rostrally within the retrolenticular capsule (ICp-5 and ICp-4, Scs. 97, 93) and come to lie above the midpoint of the LGN in the ICp-3 (Sc. 89). From there, fibers descend sharply into the lateral aspect of the cerebral peduncle and terminate in clusters in the lateral and ventral aspects of the basilar pontine nuclei (Sc. 89). A small contingent of fibers leaves the pontine bundle above the LGN and descends medially between the thalamic reticular nucleus and the subthalamic nucleus to terminate in the zona incerta and hypothalamus (Scs. 81, 85).

Striatal Fibers

Over a considerable rostrocaudal extent, a prominent stream of fibers leaves the dorsal part of the cingulum bundle, descends through the corpus callosum, and joins the subcallosal fasciculus of Muratoff. The Muratoff bundle also receives fibers from the superiorly adjacent FOF. The Muratoff bundle courses rostrally at the dorsal aspect of the body and the head of the caudate nucleus, and fibers enter and terminate in distinct clusters in the dorsomedial aspect of the body and head of the caudate nucleus (Scs. 41, 49, 57, 65, 73, 81, 85, 89, 93, 97). Further rostrally, fibers descend through the head of the caudate nucleus and terminate in the ventral portion of the putamen and in the nucleus accumbens septi (Sc. 49). Some fibers also appear to leave the Muratoff bundle and move laterally into the external capsule before terminating in the ventral part of the claustrum (Scs. 73, 85).

CASE 22

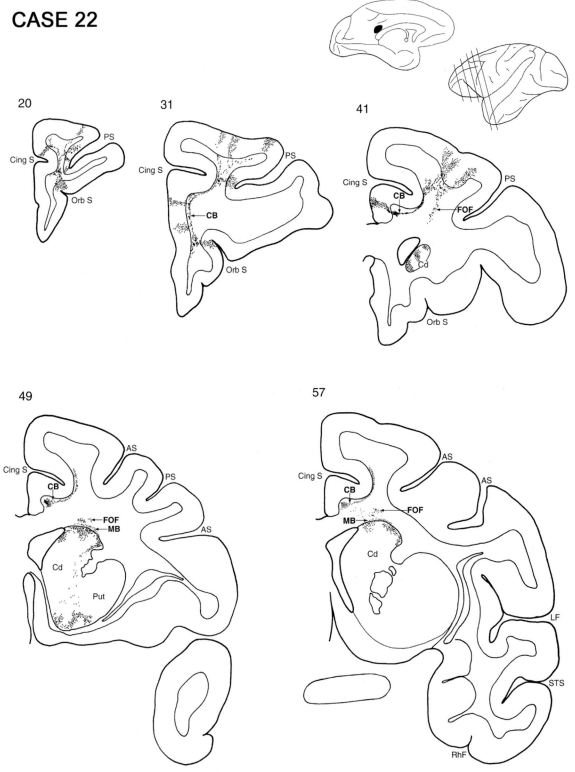

Figure 10-1

Schematic diagrams of 17 rostral–caudal coronal sections in Case 22 taken at the levels shown on the hemispheric diagrams above right, showing the isotope injection site in the retrosplenial cortex in area 30 and in area 23 (black-filled area), the resulting trajectories of the cortical association, commissural, and subcortical fibers (dashed lines and dots) in the white matter, and the terminations in the

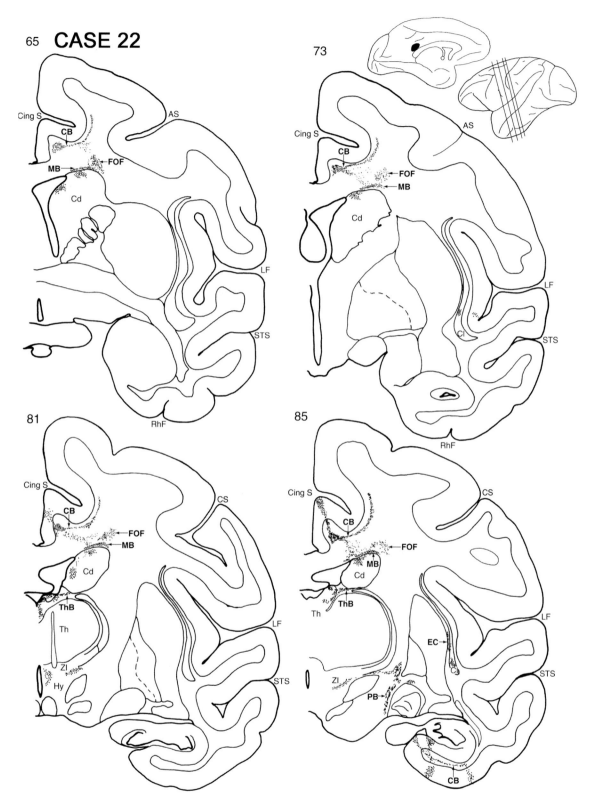

cortex and subcortical regions (black dots). An additional section, 117, interposed between template sections 113 and 121, was added to show a pattern of fibers emanating from the injection site that was unique to this case. See list of abbreviations, page 617.

CASE 22

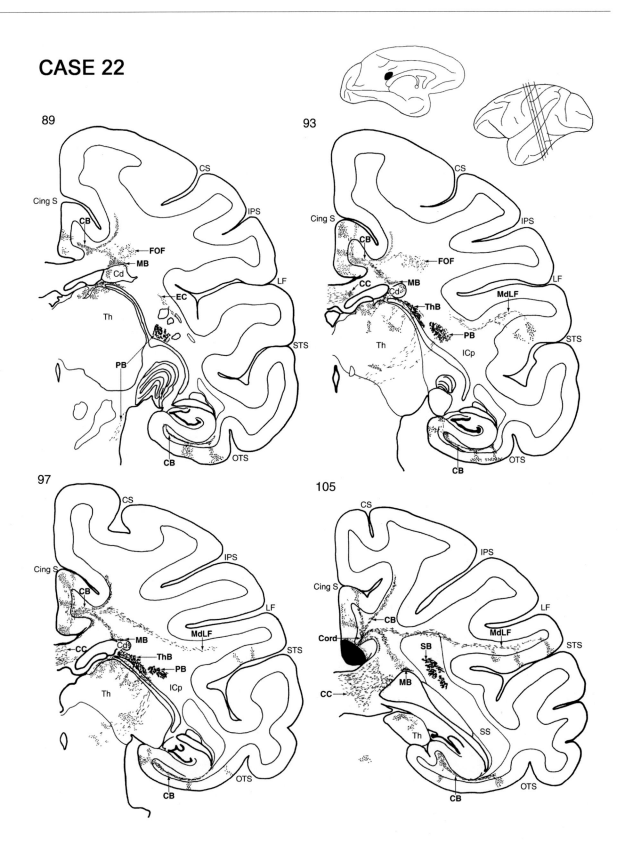

Figure 10-1 (continued)

CASE 22

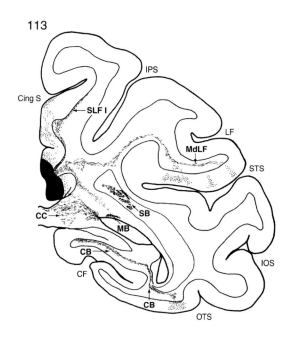

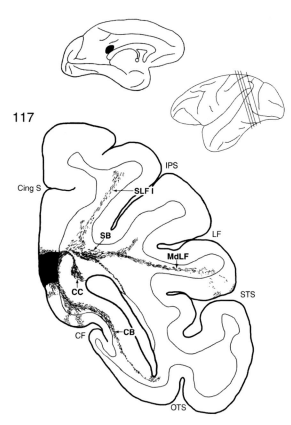

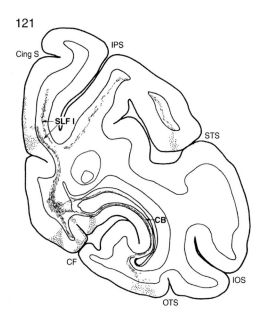

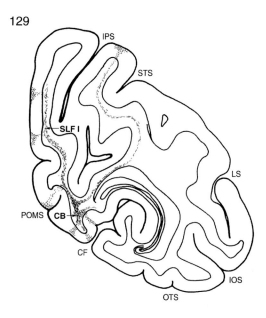

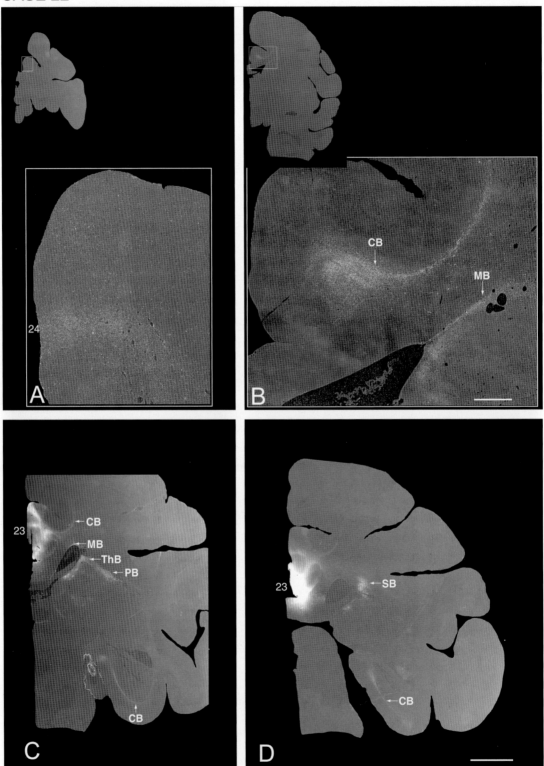

Figure 10-2

Photomicrographs of selected coronal sections of Case 22 showing the injection site in D and the resulting labeled fibers and terminations in A through D. A and B are high-power photomicrographs (sections 41 and 73, respectively) taken from the location indicated in the low-power photomicro-graphs above (Mag = 4×, bar = 0.5 mm), showing the cingulum bundle fibers terminating in area 24 (A) and fibers in the cingulum bundle and the Muratoff bundle (B). C and D correspond to sections 93 and 105, respectively (Mag = 0.5×, bar = 5 mm).

CASE 23

Isotope was injected in this case in the rostral cingulate gyrus in area 24 (Scs. 31, 41, 49). See figures 10-3 and 10-4.

Association Fibers

Local Association Fibers

Fibers adjacent to the injection site terminate in the first layer in the medial prefrontal cortex (area 32) and in area 24 in the cingulate gyrus. Some fibers descending to area 32 also travel within the substance of the cortex (Scs. 31, 41, 49).

Neighborhood Association Fibers

Near the injection site, terminations are distributed in the first layer of the dorsal pre- frontal cortex (area 9) and the ventral prefrontal cortex (area 13) (Scs. 41, 49). There are some terminations in area 47/12 on the orbitofrontal surface.

Long Association Fibers

Rostrally Directed Fibers

Fibers travel rostrally from the injection site in the white matter of the medial prefrontal cortex and terminate in the depth of the cingulate sulcus in area 32, as well as in the first layer in area 14 (Sc. 20). Few fibers traveling in the white matter of the orbital frontal cortex terminate in area 11 (Sc. 20).

Caudally Directed Fibers

The long association fibers traveling caudally from area 24 are served by three fiber bundles: the cingulum bundle, the uncinate fasciculus, and the extreme capsule.

   The cingulum bundle fibers leave the injection site and travel caudally. These fibers terminate in a columnar manner in area 24 and mainly in the first layer in the rostral part of area 23 (Scs. 57, 65, 73, 81).

   An intense bundle of fibers descends from the injection site, rostral to the genu of the corpus callosum, and enters the ventral part of the cingulum bundle. These fibers continue into the white matter of the medial prefrontal cortex and provide termina- tions to the medial wall of the orbital cortex in area 25 (Sc. 49). The fibers then turn laterally to enter the uncinate fasciculus at the undersurface of the orbital cortex. Some of these fibers terminate in the medial forebrain area, namely the vertical limb of the diagonal band of Broca and the nucleus basalis of Meynert (Sc. 57). Further caudally, these fibers arch around the limen insulae and occupy a position under the claustrum and extreme capsule (Sc. 57) and at the level of the anterior commissure (Sc. 65). From there some of the fibers are directed to the amygdala, where they terminate mainly in the lateral basal nucleus (Scs. 65, 73). The remaining fibers enter the temporal pole and terminate in the temporal polar proisocortex (Sc. 49) and in the first layer of the perirhinal cortex in the medial bank of the rhinal fissure (Sc. 65).

   Fibers destined for the extreme capsule leave the injection site and travel initially along with the fibers coursing through the anterior limb of the internal capsule (ICa).

Lateral to the ICa, the fibers separate into two bundles; one enters the ICa and the other enters the extreme capsule. Some fibers from the extreme capsule terminate in the rostral insular cortex (Sc. 73). Others enter the white matter of the superior temporal gyrus in the MdLF and terminate in area TPO in the cortex of the upper bank of the superior temporal sulcus, mainly in the first layer (Scs. 81, 85, 89).

Commissural and Subcortical Fibers

From the injection site a dense cord of fibers travels laterally and immediately divides into two segments.

The medial and ventral group of fibers descends into the lateral aspect of the CC1 sector of the corpus callosum in its genu and rostrum (Scs. 41, 49). At these levels, the fibers course medially and cross the midline to the opposite hemisphere, with some fibers also traveling through the dorsal part of rostral CC2 (Sc. 57).

The lateral group of fibers (the subcortical bundle [SB]) crystallizes laterally in the white matter, at the level of the anterior pole of the caudate nucleus, in the most rostral part of the anterior limb of the internal capsule, in ICa-1 (Sc. 41). The fibers travel in the anterior limb of the internal capsule and descend gradually as they travel caudally throughout the entire length of the ICa. At the genu of the internal capsule, these fibers segregate into two distinct components. One of these enters the reticular nucleus of thalamus and gives rise to terminations to the VA nucleus and further caudally to AD, AV, and MDpc, as well as midline thalamic nuclei (Sc. 81). Some fibers in the reticular nucleus continue ventrally to terminate medially in the zona incerta (Sc. 81).

The other component of fibers in the internal capsule continues to descend within the rostral part of the posterior limb (ICp-1, Sc. 81), enters the cerebral peduncle (PB), and terminates in medially situated pontine nuclei.

Striatal Fibers

A substantial number of fibers emerges from the injection site, situated between the fibers to the callosum and the subcortical bundle. These fibers move ventrally and surround the head of the caudate nucleus. As they move caudally, the fibers that remain at the dorsal aspect of the caudate nucleus become part of the Muratoff bundle. These fibers penetrate the head and body of the caudate nucleus, where they terminate in distinct patches in its dorsal and medial parts (Scs. 41, 49, 57, 65, 73, 81). Other fibers aggregate laterally and then ventrally to become part of the external capsule. These fibers surround the putamen and the nucleus accumbens and provide terminations to the middle and ventral putamen and to the nucleus accumbens and claustrum (Scs. 49, 57, 65, 73).

CASE 23

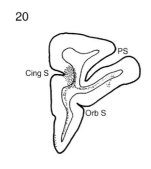

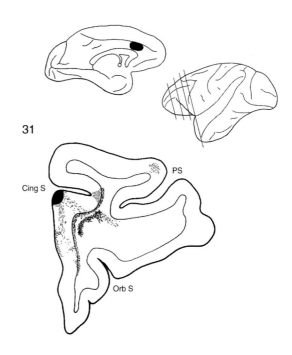

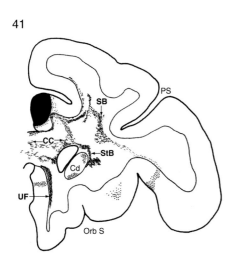

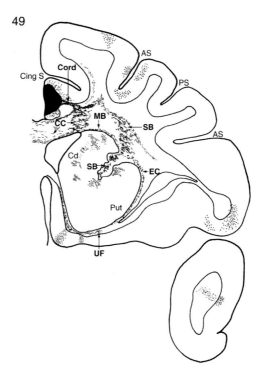

Figure 10-3

Schematic diagrams of eleven rostral–caudal coronal sections in Case 23 taken at the levels shown on the hemispheric diagrams above right, showing the isotope injection site in the rostral cingulate gyrus in area 24 (black-filled area), the resulting trajectories of the cortical association, commissural, and subcortical fibers (dashed lines and dots) in the white matter, and the terminations in the cortex and subcortical regions (black dots).

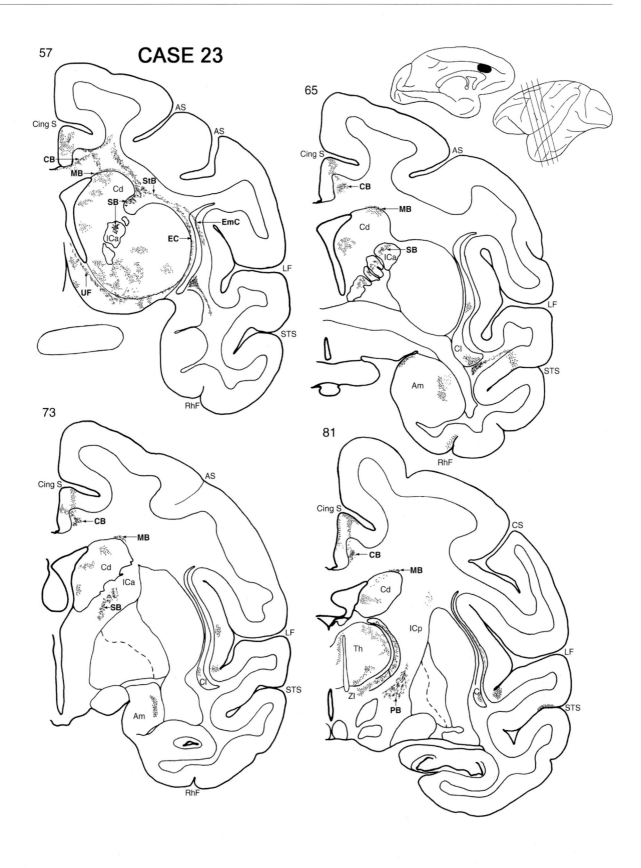

Figure 10-3 (continued)

CASE 23

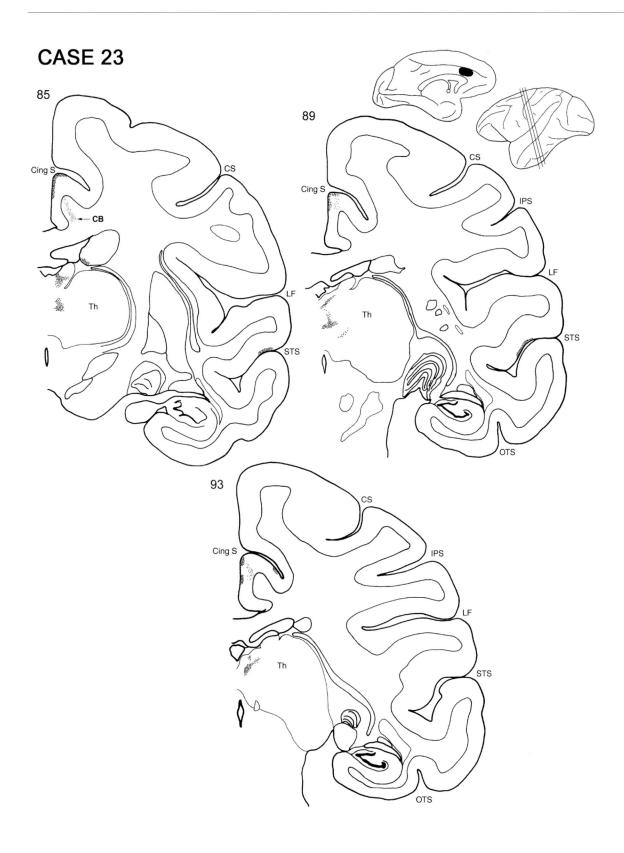

CASE 23

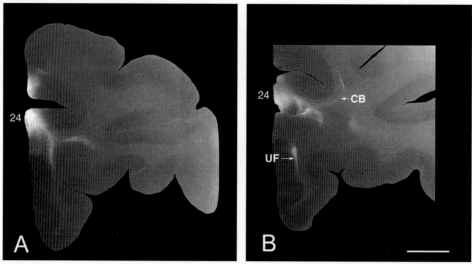

Figure 10-4
Photomicrographs of selected coronal sections of Case 23 to show the injection site in A and B and the resulting labeled fibers and terminations in both sections. A and B correspond to sections 31 and 41, respectively (Mag = 0.5×, bar = 5 mm).

Cingulate Cortex Summary

Association Fibers

Caudal Part of the Cingulate Gyrus (Areas 23 and 30; Case 22)

Four major long association fibers emerge from the caudal part of the cingulate gyrus (figure 10-5). Fibers travel rostrally and caudally in the cingulum bundle (CB); some are situated dorsally within the superior longitudinal fasciculus I (SLF I); a lateral fiber system is contained within the middle longitudinal fasciculus (MdLF); and fibers directed to the frontal lobe are in the fronto-occipital fasciculus (FOF).

Rostrally directed cingulate fibers travel in the ventral and medial parts of the cingulum bundle and terminate in the cingulate gyrus first in area 23 and further rostrally in area 24. The CB fibers also provide terminations to areas 9 and 46. Anterior to the genu of the corpus callosum, the fibers in the CB arch around the white matter of the ventromedial prefrontal cortex and terminate in areas 32 and 11.

The caudal segment of the CB arches around the splenium of the corpus callosum and enters the white matter lying deep to the calcarine fissure. The fibers provide terminations to the retrosplenial cortex and the cingulate gyrus before continuing in the ventral part of the cingulum bundle to terminate in areas TF, TL, and TH, as well as in the parasubiculum and presubiculum.

The SLF I fibers course caudally in the white matter of the superior parietal lobule and terminate in areas 31, PGm, and PO. Some fibers at this level course laterally under the annectant gyrus and then dorsally in the white matter of the inferior parietal lobule. These fibers terminate in area Opt in the caudal inferior parietal lobule.

From the caudal part of the cingulate gyrus, white matter fibers course laterally and occupy the middle longitudinal fasciculus situated in the white matter of the superior temporal gyrus. These fibers terminate in the upper bank of the superior temporal sulcus (STS) in area TPO and area TAa, and in area Tpt.

Another group of fibers emerges from the caudal cingulate gyrus and courses laterally and ventrally. These fibers enter the FOF that lies between the corpus callosum and the corona radiata at the level of the caudal end of the body of the caudate nucleus. In the prefrontal cortex the FOF fibers terminate along with those from the CB in areas 9 and 46.

Rostral Part of the Cingulate Gyrus (Area 24; Case 23)

The long association fibers emanating from the rostral part of the cingulate gyrus area 24 include the cingulum bundle, uncinate fasciculus (UF), and extreme capsule (EmC).

The cingulum bundle fibers course caudally and terminate mainly in area 24 and in the rostral part of area 23. Rostrally directed cingulate fibers course around the cingulate sulcus and move ventrally and laterally. The ventral fibers terminate medially in areas 32 and 14. The lateral contingent of fibers courses in the white matter toward the region of the principal sulcus and terminates ventrally in the orbital cortex area 11 and dorsally in the cortex above the principal sulcus in area 46d, as well as in areas 8Ad and 6d. Area 4 projections have also been noted by Baleydier and Mauguiere (1980).

Some fibers course ventrally from the rostral cingulate cortex, situated between the caudal medial prefrontal cortex and the caudate nucleus. These fibers move laterally in the white matter of the caudal part of the orbital surface of the frontal lobe to become part of the uncinate fasciculus. On its course, the UF fibers terminate in area 25, as well as in basal forebrain areas. Further laterally, the uncinate fibers course around the limen insulae and enter the rostral part of the temporal lobe. These fibers terminate in the amygdala, as well as in the perirhinal cortex.

A third group of fibers from the rostral cingulate area courses laterally and enters the extreme capsule to provide terminations in the dysgranular insula and the insular Pro.

Commissural Fibers

The interhemispheric fibers from the rostral cingulate area 24 course ventrally to enter CC1 in the rostrum and genu of the corpus callosum, and they cross the midline at these levels, as well as slightly more caudally in the rostral part of CC2. The commissural fibers from caudal cingulate area 23 traverse the midsagittal plane through a broad area of sectors CC4 and CC5.

Subcortical Fibers

Caudal Cingulate Gyrus

The cord of subcortical fibers that emanates from the caudal cingulate gyrus travels medially into the dorsal aspect of the sagittal stratum. These fibers course rostrally into the posterior limb of the internal capsule and segregate into two components at the level of the pulvinar. The dorsal and medial segment (thalamic bundle [ThB]) traverses the dorsal part of the external medullary lamina to enter and terminate in the thalamus. The pontine bundle (PB) continues to travel rostrally as it descends gradually in the posterior limb of the internal capsule, and at the level of the rostral part of the LGN it descends sharply into the cerebral peduncle on its way to the basis pontis. At this level it gives off fibers that travel medially to terminate in the zona incerta and the hypothalamus.

Rostral Cingulate Gyrus

The subcortical fibers from the rostral cingulate gyrus course laterally and then curve ventrally into the anterior limb of the internal capsule at the level of the anterior aspect of the caudate-putamen. These fibers course caudally, descending gradually in the capsule, until just rostral to the genu. At this level thalamic fibers continue caudally into thalamus, while the pontine fibers continue to descend on their way via the cerebral peduncle to the basis pontis. The fibers in the thalamic reticular nucleus continue medially and ventrally to terminate in the zona incerta.

Corticostriate Projections

Both the rostral cingulate gyrus, area 24, and the caudal cingulate region, including area 23 and the retrosplenial cortex area 30, project to the head of the caudate nucleus. Rostral regions project to dorsal and intermediate sectors; caudal regions project only dorsally. These projections are conveyed mainly by the Muratoff bundle. Both the rostral and caudal cingulate areas have strong projections to the nucleus accumbens.

Striatal fibers from the rostral cingulate gyrus, area 24, move laterally and surround the head of the caudate nucleus. As these fibers move caudally, they occupy a position above and below the anterior limb of the internal capsule. The dorsal fibers course in the Muratoff bundle and terminate in the head of the caudate nucleus. The ventral fibers curve around the lateral border of the putamen, course within the external capsule, and turn ventrally and medially to terminate within the ventral striatum, in the rostral part of the putamen, and in the ventral part of the claustrum.

The striatal fibers from the caudal cingulate gyrus area 23 and the retrosplenial cortex gather in the Muratoff bundle at the level of the atrium of the lateral ventricle and move rostrally into the prefrontal region. These fibers terminate throughout the rostral-caudal extent of the body and head of the caudate nucleus, as well as in the rostral part of the putamen. Nucleus accumbens projections from area 23 and the retrosplenial cortex are carried by fibers that descend from the Muratoff bundle through the head of the caudate nucleus before reaching the ventral striatum. Some of the striatal fibers course through the external capsule and terminate ventrally in the caudal part of the claustrum.

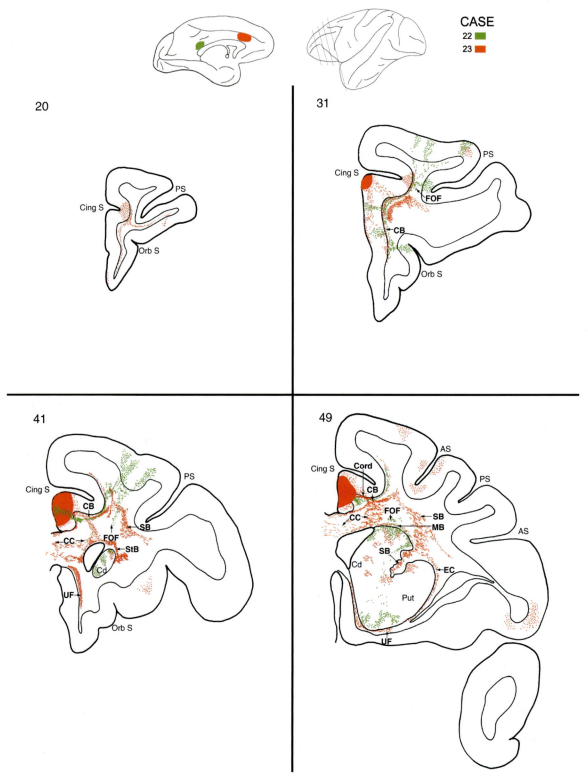

Figure 10-5

Schematic composite diagrams of the rostral–caudal coronal sections of the template brain, illustrating the two cingulate cases (Cases 22 and 23). The injection sites and the association, commissural, and subcortical fibers, as well as the termination patterns, are color-coded for each case. The schematic

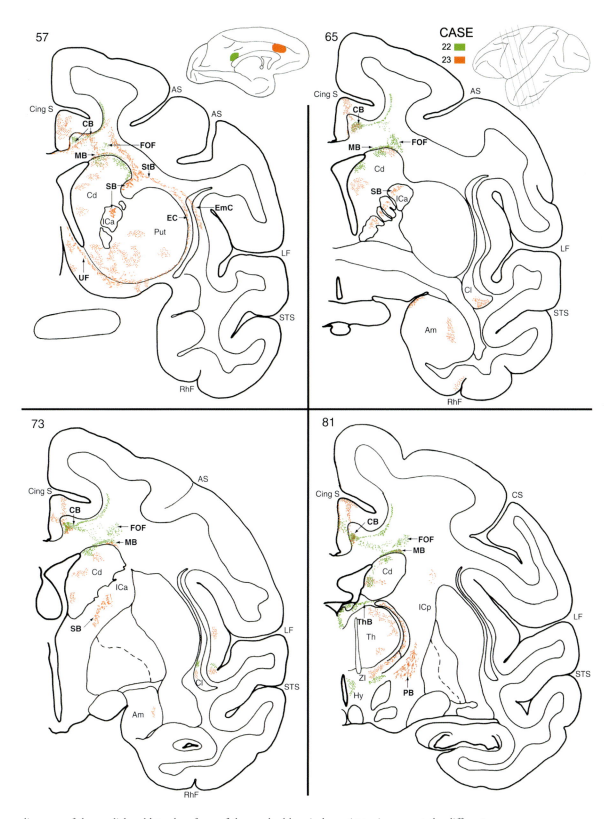

diagrams of the medial and lateral surfaces of the cerebral hemispheres (at top) represent the different levels of the coronal sections and the injection sites. Color-coding is as follows: Case 22—green, caudal cingulate area 23 and retrosplenial cortex area 30; Case 23—red, rostral cingulate gyrus area 24.

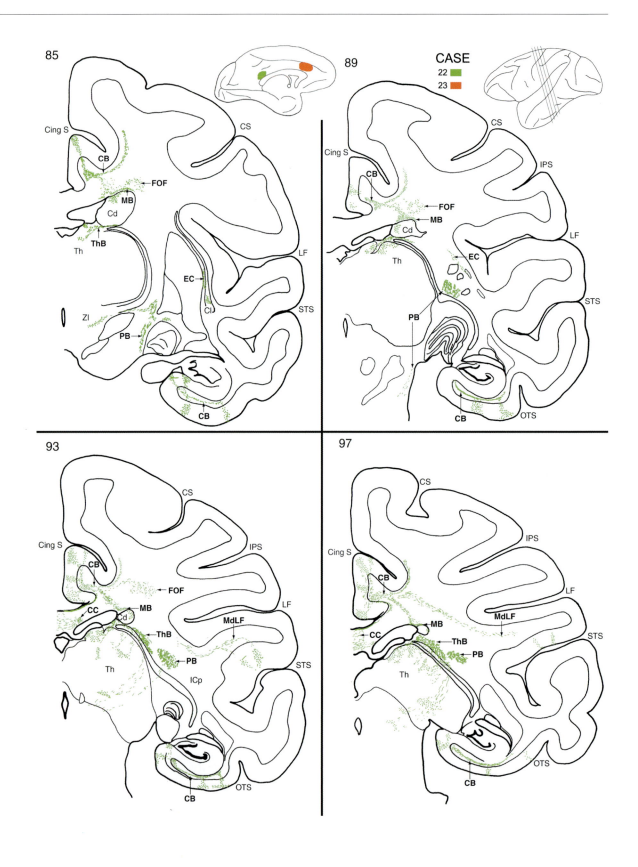

Figure 10-5 (continued)

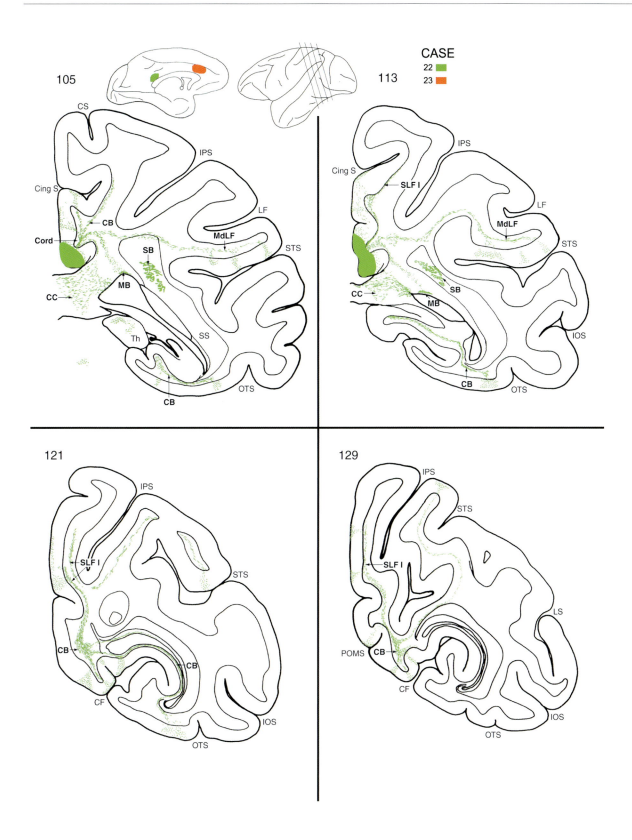

Motor Cortex

In this chapter we describe the isotope injections placed in the motor cortex of six rhesus monkeys and analyze the resulting association, striatal, commissural, and subcortical fiber trajectories, as well as the cortical and subcortical terminations. The injections were in the frontal operculum in the precentral aspects of areas 1 and 2 (Case 24), ventral area 4 in the face representation (Case 25), area 4 behind the arcuate spur in the hand representation (Case 26), the dorsal precentral gyrus in the trunk representation region of area 4 (Case 27), the dorsal part of area 4 in the foot representation (Case 28), and the medial part of the superior frontal gyrus, rostral area MII, involving the face representation (Case 29).

As in the previous chapters, the architectonic designations of the cortical terminations are described in the text but not identified on the coronal sections. Architectonic areas are labeled on external views of the hemisphere as well as in the coronal series of chapter 4. Terminations in thalamus are shown and thalamic nuclei are referred to in the text, but the nuclei are not designated on the coronal sections. Pontine terminations are described in the text but not illustrated. Striatal terminations are illustrated and an overview of their termination patterns is presented in the text.

CASE 24

In this case isotope injections were placed in the frontal operculum in the precentral aspects of areas 1 and 2 (Scs. 65, 73). See figures 11-1 and 11-2.

Association Fibers

Local Association Fibers

Fibers leave the injection site and travel in the opercular white matter immediately beneath the cortex of the upper bank of the Sylvian fissure. These fibers provide diffuse terminations in the cortex of the frontal operculum, in area ProM, the second somatosensory area (SII), and precentral area 3b (Scs. 65, 73).

Long Association Fibers

Caudally Directed Fibers

Fibers leave the injection site and travel in the white matter of the parietal operculum and are situated within the superior longitudinal fasciculus III (SLF III). These fibers terminate in SII principally in the first layer and in postcentral areas 3b and 2 in a columnar manner (Scs. 81, 85, 89).

Rostrally Directed Fibers

Fibers coursing rostrally from the injection site also travel via SLF III in the white matter subjacent to the upper bank of the Sylvian fissure. These fibers form an arch that includes an opercular section laterally, a segment lying above the shoulder of the upper bank of the Sylvian fissure, and a medial component that enters the extreme capsule (EmC).

The fibers in the lateral component of the SLF III provide diffuse terminations in all layers of the precentral portion of area 3 and first-layer terminations in ventral area 6 (Scs. 49, 57).

At the upper shoulder of the Sylvian fissure the fibers terminate in the deep layers of the rostral SII type cortex in the upper bank of the Sylvian fissure and in a columnar manner in the gustatory area of the frontal operculum (Scs. 49, 57).

The fibers in the extreme capsule terminate in the rostral, agranular insular cortex in a columnar manner, principally in the fourth layer (Sc. 57).

Commissural and Subcortical Fibers

From the injection site a dense cord of fibers travels upward and medially (Sc. 73). One prominent contingent continues medially through the corona radiata into the corpus callosum at the level of the injection site in CC3 and then courses toward the opposite hemisphere (Scs. 65, 73).

The other major contingent of fibers descends sharply from the parent bundle to enter the caudal part of the anterior limb of the internal capsule (ICa-6, Sc. 73). As they move caudally into the posterior limb, these capsular fibers separate into medial and lateral components.

The medial component in ICp-1 (the thalamic bundle [ThB], Sc. 81) enters the reticular nucleus of the thalamus and provides terminations in the reticular nucleus, as well as in the VPM, VPMpc, and CL nuclei (Scs. 85, 89).

The fibers lying more laterally within ICp-1 descend into the cerebral peduncle (pontine bundle [PB]), travel toward the basis pontis, and terminate in the medial part of the rostral third of the pontine nuclei (Sc. 81).

Striatal Fibers

The fibers destined for the striatum leave the injection site and travel with the SLF III fibers. They cross through the extreme capsule, descend in the external capsule, and terminate in the medial aspect of the midportion of the putamen (Scs. 65, 73, 81).

CASE 24

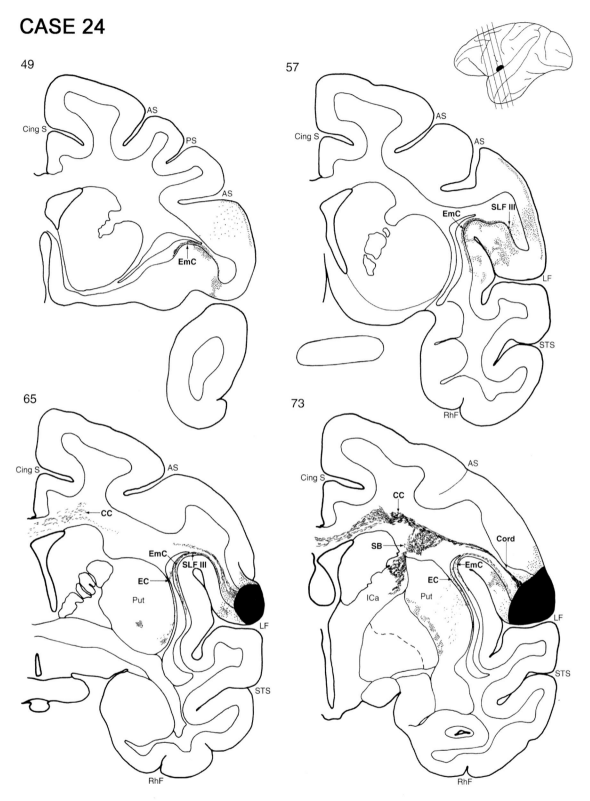

Figure 11-1

Schematic diagrams of seven rostral–caudal coronal sections in Case 24 taken at the levels shown on the hemispheric diagram above right, showing the isotope injection site in the frontal operculum in the precentral aspects of areas 1 and 2 (black-filled area), the resulting trajectories of the cortical association, commissural, and subcortical fibers (dashed lines and dots) in the white matter, and the terminations in the cortex and subcortical regions (black dots). See list of abbreviations, page 617.

CASE 24

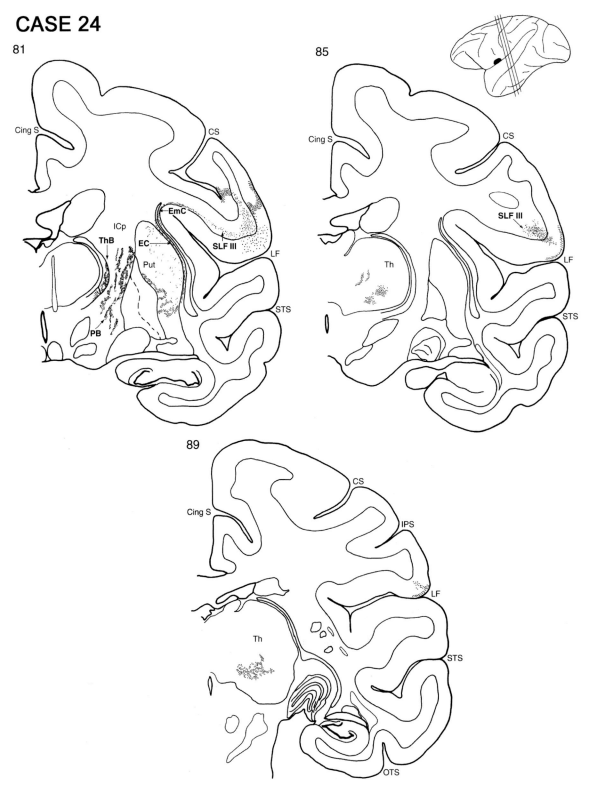

Figure 11-1 (continued)

CASE 24

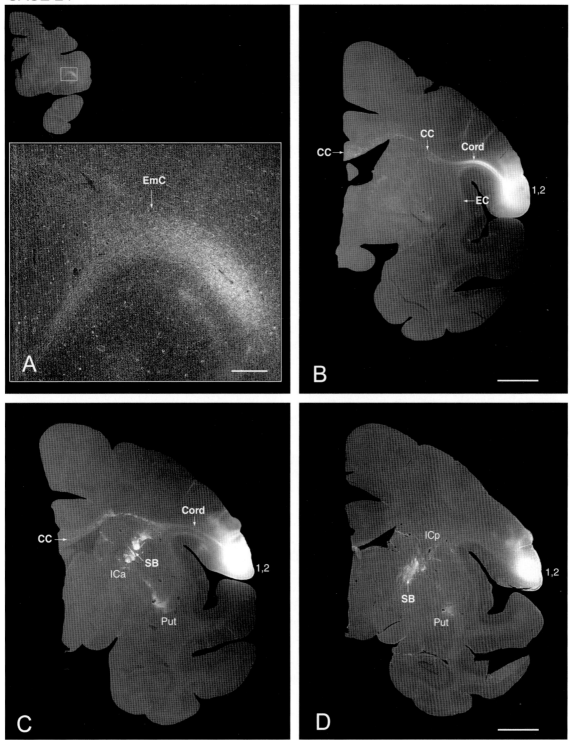

Figure 11-2

Photomicrographs of selected coronal sections of Case 24 showing the injection site in B and C with the injection halo in D and the resulting labeled fibers and terminations in A through D. A, High-power photomicrograph (section 49, Mag = 4×, bar = 0.5 mm) taken from the location indicated in the low-power photomicrograph above, showing fibers in the extreme capsule. B through D correspond to sections 65, 73, and 81, respectively (Mag = 0.5×, bar = 5 mm).

CASE 25

Isotope was injected in the ventral part of area 4 in the precentral gyrus corresponding to the face motor representation in this case (Scs. 65, 69). See figures 11-3 and 11-4.

Association Fibers

Local Association Fibers

Adjacent to the injection site, fibers travel ventrally to terminate in the precentral portion of areas 3, 1, 2, and SII (Scs. 65, 69).

Long Association Fibers

Caudally Directed Fibers

Caudally directed association fibers leave the injection site and travel in the white matter of the dorsal Sylvian operculum in the superior longitudinal fasciculus III (SLF III). These fibers provide terminations to the face area of SII lying at the outer edge of the Sylvian operculum and to postcentral areas 3a and 3b (Scs. 73, 78). These terminations are predominantly in the first layer. Further caudally, terminations in areas 1 and 2 are also noted in the deeper layers (Scs. 81, 85).

Rostrally Directed Fibers

Fibers leave the injection site and travel rostrally in the frontal opercular white matter in SLF III. These fibers terminate in ventral area 6 in a columnar manner with an emphasis on the first layer (Sc. 57). Some fibers in SLF III continue to course rostrally in the frontal lobe. Fibers situated ventrally in SLF III terminate in area ProM (Sc. 49). Other rostrally directed fibers course dorsally toward the white matter of the superior frontal gyrus and terminate in the supplementary motor area corresponding to the face representation (Sc. 49).

Commissural and Subcortical Fibers

From the injection site two paired cords of fibers, one above the other, move medially and dorsally into the white matter of the ventral part of the precentral gyrus. One group of fibers moves dorsally and medially to enter the corpus callosum at the junction of CC2 and CC3 (Scs. 65, 69) and passes to the opposite hemisphere at these levels and slightly caudally (Sc. 73).

A spray of fibers descends from the lower cord of fibers to enter the midcaudal aspect of the anterior limb of the internal capsule, ICa-5 (Sc. 69). These fibers, which constitute the subcortical bundle (SB), descend gradually as they move caudally into the genu of the internal capsule and the rostral part of the posterior limb of the internal capsule (ICp), occupying its central and lateral aspects. At the genu of the capsule the subcortical bundle separates into two distinct components.

The more dorsal component within ICp-1 (Sc. 81) lies within the lateral thalamic peduncle and provides terminations to the reticular nucleus as it traverses it to enter the thalamus. Thalamic terminations are then present in the VA nucleus, as well as in nucleus X, VLm, CM, and Pcn (Scs. 81, 85, 89).

The ventral component of fibers in the subcortical bundle occupies the breadth of the rostral part of the posterior limb (ICp-1 and the ventral part of ICp-2) as it descends toward the cerebral peduncle. Some fibers leave the subcortical bundle to enter and terminate in the zona incerta (Scs. 81, 85, 89). Most of the fibers in the capsule (the pontine bundle [PB]) arch medially around the globus pallidus as they cascade into the medial and intermediate parts of the cerebral peduncle. Terminations predominantly in the caudal half of the pons are situated in the paramedian and dorsomedial nuclei and the medial parts of the peripeduncular and intrapeduncular nuclei, with some in the dorsal, ventral, and NRTP nuclei. Other fibers contained within the corticofugal fiber bundles in the pons continue to descend to the spinal cord.

Striatal Fibers

From the injection site two distinct fiber bundles descend in the external and extreme capsules. The extreme capsule (EmC) provides terminations to the central part of the claustrum (Scs. 69, 73, 78). The fibers in the external capsule (EC) terminate in patches in the ventral and medial portions of the putamen (Scs. 65, 69, 73, 78, 81, 85, 89).

CASE 25

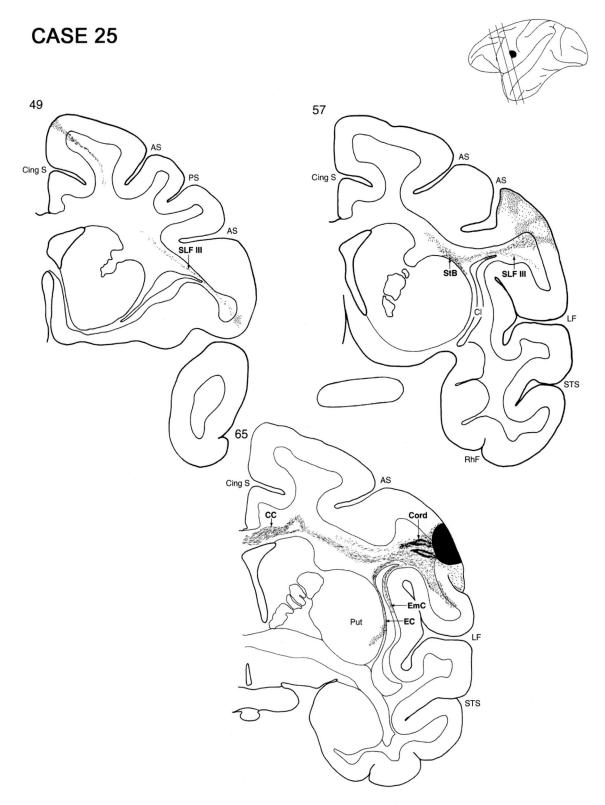

Figure 11-3

Schematic diagrams of nine rostral–caudal coronal sections in Case 25 taken at the levels shown on the hemispheric diagram above right, showing the isotope injection site in the ventral part of area 4 in the precentral gyrus corresponding to the face motor representation (black-filled area). The result-

CASE 25

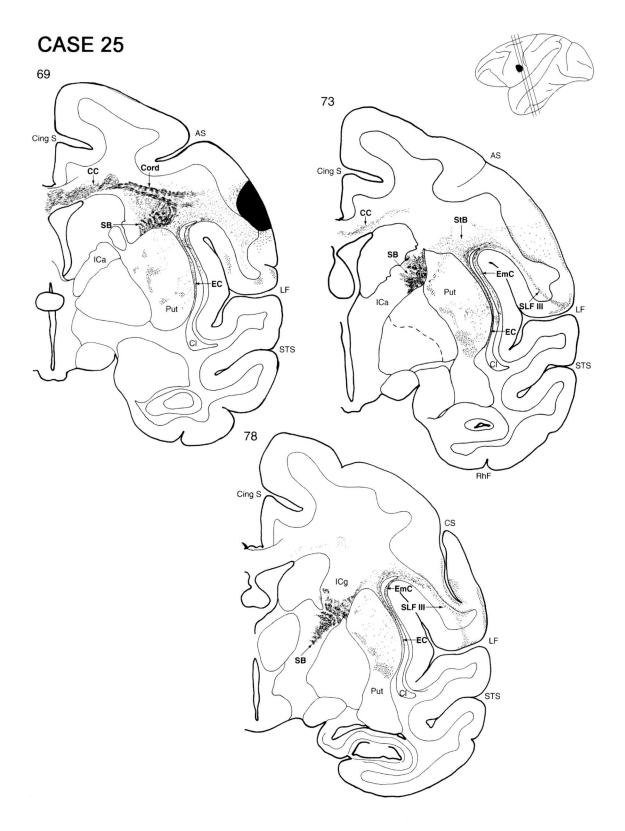

ing trajectories of the cortical association, commissural, and subcortical fibers (dashed lines and dots) in the white matter are shown, as well as the terminations in the cortex and subcortical regions (black dots).

CASE 25

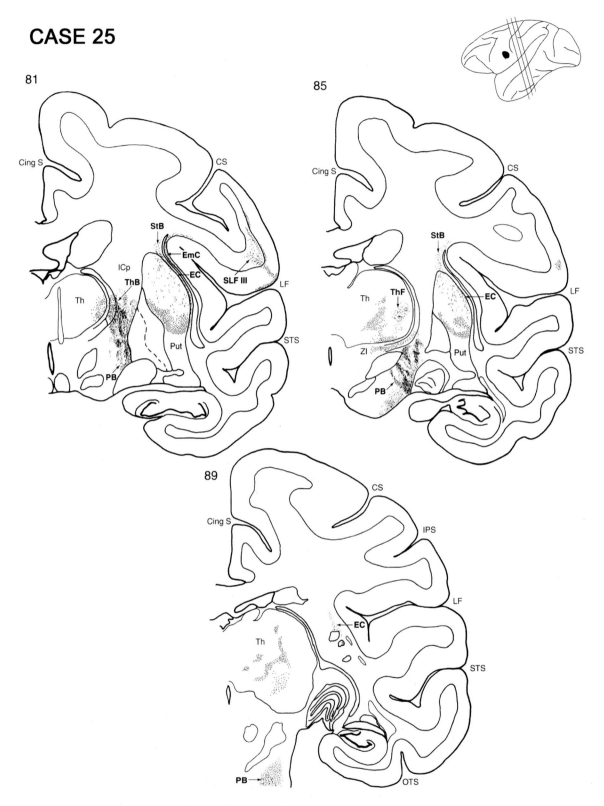

Figure 11-3 (continued)

CASE 25

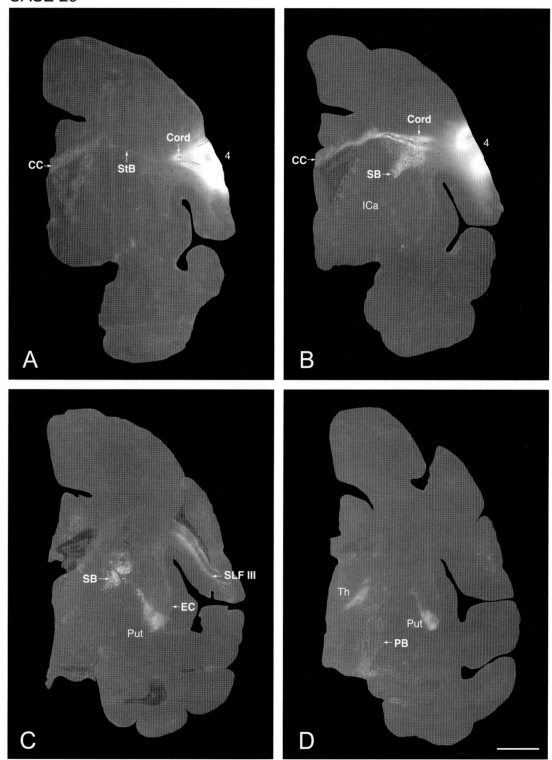

Figure 11-4

Photomicrographs of selected coronal sections of Case 25 to show the injection site in A and B and the resulting labeled fibers and terminations in A through D. A through D correspond to sections 45, 69, 78, and 85, respectively (Mag = 0.5×, bar = 5 mm).

CASE 26

In this case the isotope injection was in area 4 in the precentral gyrus in the hand motor representation (Scs. 78, 81). The location of the hand motor area was confirmed by physiological stimulation. See figures 11-5 and 11-6.

Association Fibers

Local Association Fibers

Surrounding the injection site, diffuse terminations are seen in area 4 (Scs. 78, 81).

Long Association Fibers

Caudally Directed Fibers

Fibers located immediately beneath the cortex travel caudally and curve around the depth of the central sulcus into the white matter of the postcentral gyrus. Some of these fibers terminate in areas 1 and 2 above the intraparietal sulcus in a columnar manner, with a first-layer preference (Scs. 89, 93, 97). Some terminations are also noted in area 3a (Scs. 89, 93). These fibers then continue caudally in the white matter of the superior parietal lobule and provide predominantly first-layer terminations in area 2 of the superior parietal lobule and intraparietal sulcus and in the first layer in area PE (Scs. 105, 113). A few fibers leave the white matter of the superior parietal lobule, enter the white matter of the inferior parietal lobule, and terminate at the outer lip of the Sylvian fissure, in area SII (Sc. 97).

Rostrally Directed Fibers

Fibers travel rostrally from the injection site and are situated in the white matter beneath the spur of the arcuate sulcus, within the area corresponding to the superior longitudinal fasciculus II (SLF II). Fibers leave this bundle and terminate in dorsal area 6 and ventral to the arcuate spur in area 6/4C (Scs. 65, 69, 73). These terminations are columnar, with a first-layer preference.

One group of fibers ascends medially from the SLF II and is directed toward SLF I, from which position they provide terminations in the supplementary motor area (area MII), as well as in the depth of the cingulate sulcus (Scs. 65, 69).

Commissural and Subcortical Fibers

From the injection site a dense and broad cord of fibers courses medially in the white matter (Scs. 78, 81). One contingent of fibers continues medially and rostrally from the cord, enters the corpus callosum in sector CC3 (Sc. 78), and passes to the opposite hemisphere in this sector (Scs. 78, 73, 69).

A massive contingent of fibers takes a sharp vertical descent from the cord and enters the posterior limb of the internal capsule at the genu and just caudal to it in ICp-1 (Scs. 78, 81). Within this subcortical bundle (SB) in the ICp, two principal components can be discerned.

A dorsal group of fibers (thalamic bundle [ThB]) moves medially and crystallizes in the lateral thalamic peduncle lateral to the thalamic reticular nucleus (Scs. 81, 85). These fibers enter the thalamus and terminate first in the reticular nucleus and then in the VL, VPL, CM, and CL nuclei (Scs. 81, 85, 89). A small contingent of the dorsal fibers within the ICp descends ventrally into the external medullary lamina and terminates in the zona incerta (ZI), subthalamic nucleus (STN), red nucleus (RN), and interstitial nucleus of Cajal (Scs. 81, 85, 89).

The ventral group of fibers (pontine bundle [PB]) in the ICp cascades vertically down within capsular level ICp-1 (Sc. 81). The fibers enter the central portion of the cerebral peduncle (Scs. 85, 89) before descending into the brainstem, where they terminate in the rostral more than the caudal pons. The terminations lie within a semicircular lamella closed medially and open laterally, concentrated in the peripeduncular, intrapeduncular, paramedian, dorsomedial, medial, and NRTP nuclei, with some terminations in the ventral, lateral, and dorsolateral nuclei as well. A sizable contingent of fibers continues to descend in the corticofugal fiber bundles into the medullary pyramid destined for the spinal cord.

Striatal Fibers

Fibers destined for the striatum are distinct from both the association fibers and the internal capsule fibers. The striatal fibers (striatal bundle [StB]) descend from the injection site and lie above the upper shoulder of the Sylvian fissure and progress rostrally as well as caudally for a short distance. The rostrally directed fibers travel mainly via the external capsule (EC) and terminate in distinct patches in the dorsal and central putamen (Scs. 65, 69, 73, 78, 81, 85, 89). Fibers in the external capsule, and some also in the extreme capsule (EmC), terminate in the dorsal part of the claustrum (Scs. 65, 69, 73).

CASE 26

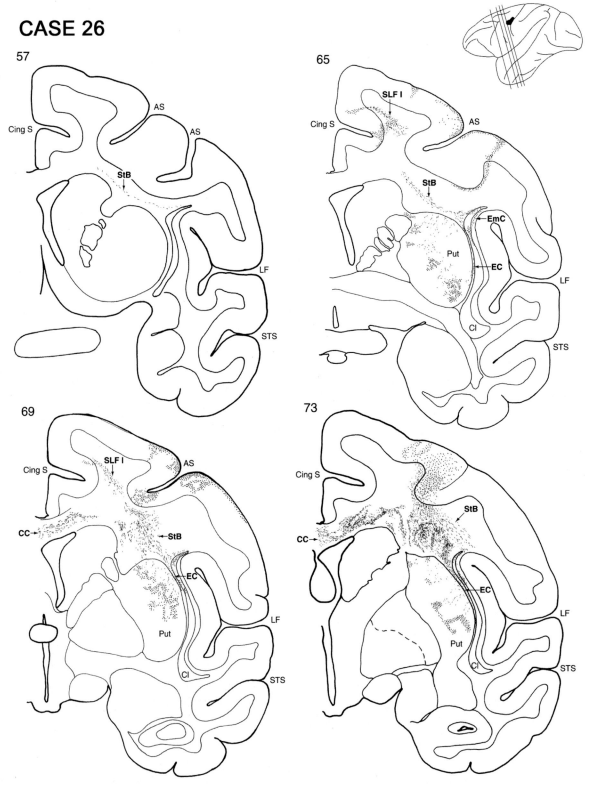

Figure 11-5

Schematic diagrams of 12 rostral-caudal coronal sections in Case 26 taken at the levels shown on the hemispheric diagram above right, showing the isotope injection site in area 4 in the precentral gyrus behind the arcuate spur, in the hand motor representation (black-filled area). The resulting trajectories of the cortical association, commissural, and subcortical fibers (dashed lines and dots) in the white matter are shown, as well as the terminations in the cortex and subcortical regions (black

CASE 26

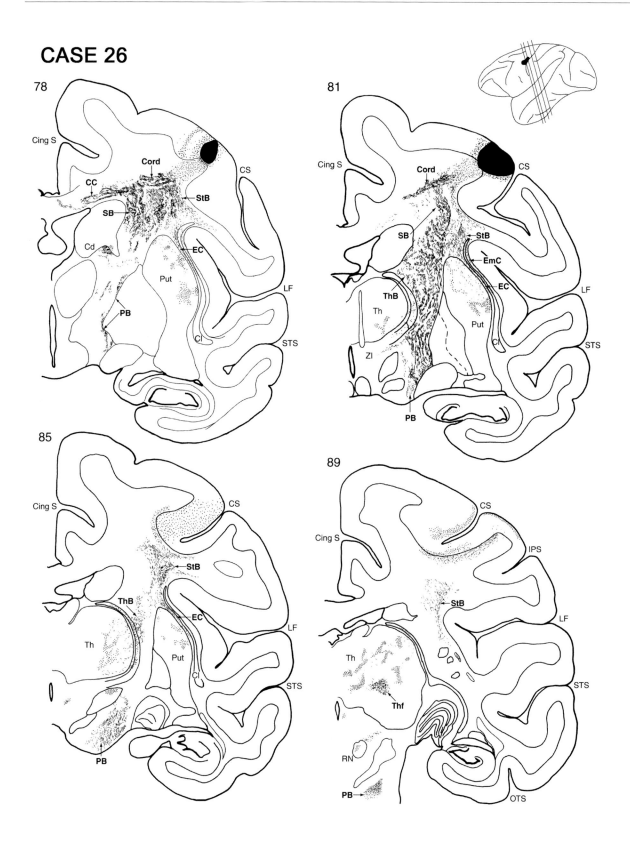

CASE 26

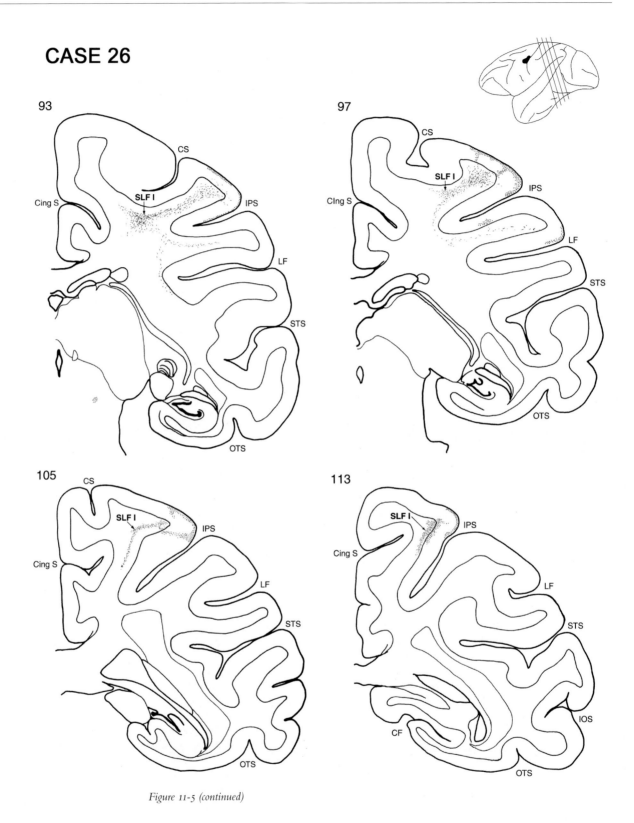

Figure 11-5 *(continued)*

CASE 26

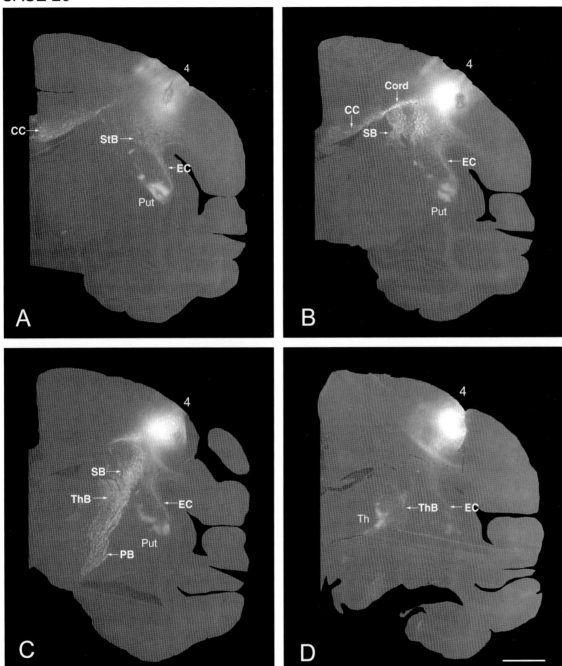

Figure 11-6

Photomicrographs of selected coronal sections of Case 26 showing the injection site in B and C with the injection halo in A and D and the resulting labeled fibers and terminations in A through D. A through D correspond to sections 73, 78, 81, and 85, respectively (Mag = 0.5×, bar = 5 mm).

CASE 27

Isotope was injected in this case in the dorsal part of the precentral gyrus involving area 4 corresponding to the motor trunk representation (Scs. 78, 81, 85, 89). See figures 11-7 and 11-8.

Association Fibers

Local Association Fibers

Adjacent to the injection site fibers travel in the white matter immediately beneath the cortex of the superior frontal gyrus. They terminate dorsally in area 6 and ventrally in area 4 in a columnar manner (Scs. 78, 81, 85, 89). At the level of the injection site, terminations are seen in the supplementary motor area (SMA) and the cingulate motor area (CMA) (Scs. 78, 81, 85, 89).

Long Association Fibers

Caudally Directed Fibers

A medially directed group of long association fibers leaves the injection site and courses dorsally and then medially in the white matter of the superior frontal gyrus to come to lie within the superior longitudinal fasciculus I (SLF I). These SLF I fibers travel caudally and provide terminations in the SMA (area MII) and CMA in the upper bank of the cingulate sulcus (Sc. 93).

From the injection site two distinct ventrally directed association fiber bundles are also observed. One occupies the white matter deep to the central sulcus and the superior parietal lobule and provides terminations to the deep layers of areas 3a and 3b, to the first layer in area 2 (Scs. 93,97), and in columns in areas PEa and PE (Scs. 105, 113). The other group of fibers descends through the SLF II and lies in the white matter deep to the Sylvian fissure. From this location terminations are noted in the deep layers of the cortex lying in the depth of the Sylvian fissure, corresponding to the trunk representation of area SII (Sc. 93).

Rostrally Directed Fibers

Fibers leave the injection site, traveling immediately beneath the cortex of the superior frontal gyrus, and terminate in a columnar manner below the superior precentral dimple in area 6 (Scs. 57, 65, 69, 73). Fibers within the SLF I (see above) progress rostrally from the injection site and terminate in columns in the SMA and CMA (Scs. 57, 65, 69, 73).

Commissural and Subcortical Fibers

From the injection site a thick cord of fibers descends obliquely into the white matter (Scs. 78, 81).

One group of fibers continues medially from the cord, enters the corpus callosum in sector CC3 (Sc. 78), and crosses to the opposite hemisphere in this sector at this level and adjacent to it (Scs. 73, 78, 81). From the main body of the cord of fibers, a massive contingent of subcortically directed fibers (SB) rains down into the corona radiata; although some fibers enter the genu (Sc. 78), most of the fibers enter the rostral part of the posterior limb of the internal capsule (ICp-1, Sc. 81). The bulk of these fibers aggregates at the lateral border of the thalamus in ICp-1 and ICp-2 before entering through the reticular nucleus as the fibers continue caudally within the substance of the thalamus (ThB). These fibers give rise to terminations in the reticular nucleus and in the VL, VPL, CM, and CL nuclei (Scs. 81, 85, 89, 93).

The other contingent of the subcortical bundle within ICp-1 and ICp-2 (the pontine bundle [PB]) continues to descend, arching medial to the globus pallidus, and enters the cerebral peduncle at the level of the rostral aspect of the lateral geniculate nucleus. Some fibers leave this bundle and move medially beneath the thalamus to terminate in the subthalamic nucleus (STN), zona incerta (ZI), and red nucleus (RN) (Scs. 85, 89).

The remaining ICp fibers that descend into the lateral to intermediate part of the cerebral peduncle (Scs. 85, 89) provide terminations particularly to the caudal parts of the pons, focused most heavily in the peripeduncular and intrapeduncular nuclei, with involvement of the paramedian, dorsal, dorsolateral, lateral, and ventral nuclei, as well as the NRTP. A prominent contingent of fibers continues caudally through the medullary pyramid into the spinal cord.

Striatal Fibers

Fibers destined for the striatum leave the injection site lateral to and distinct from the cord fibers (StB) and lie in the white matter lateral to the ICp and deep to the upper shoulder of the Sylvian fissure. From this location the fibers enter the external and extreme capsules and provide terminations to the dorsal and lateral portions of the putamen, as well as the upper part of the claustrum (Scs. 57, 65, 69, 73, 78, 81, 85, 89). A small contingent of fibers leaves the striatal bundle to enter the Muratoff bundle (MB); there these fibers travel rostrally and give rise to light terminations in the head of the caudate nucleus (Sc. 65).

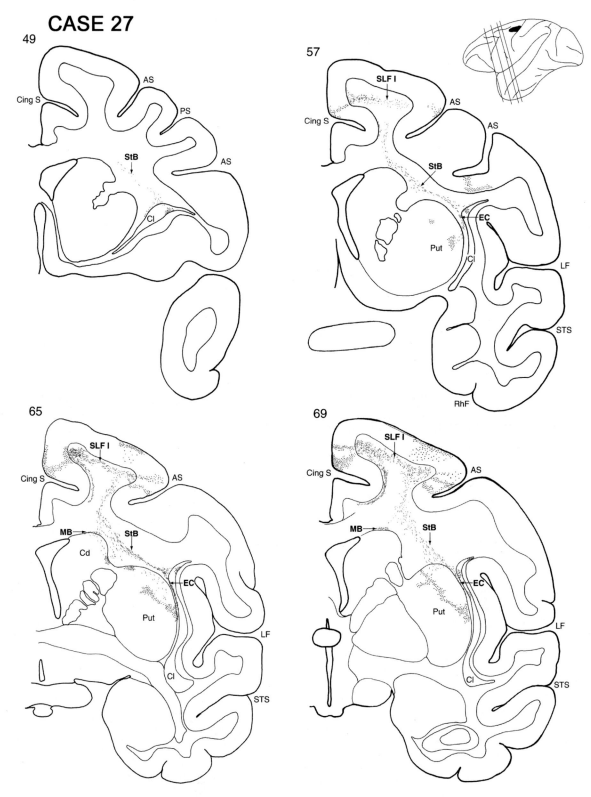

CASE 27

Figure 11-7

Schematic diagrams of 13 rostral-caudal coronal sections in Case 27 taken at the levels shown on the hemispheric diagram above right showing the isotope injection site in the dorsal part of the precentral gyrus involving area 4 corresponding to the motor trunk representation (black-filled area), the resulting trajectories of the cortical association, commissural, and subcortical fibers (dashed lines and dots) in the white matter, and the terminations in the cortex and subcortical regions (black dots).

CASE 27

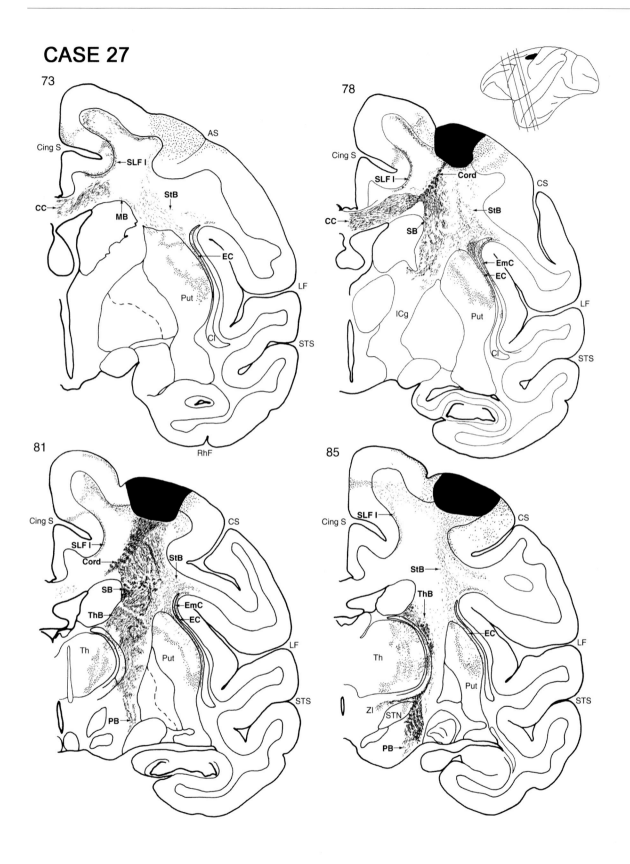

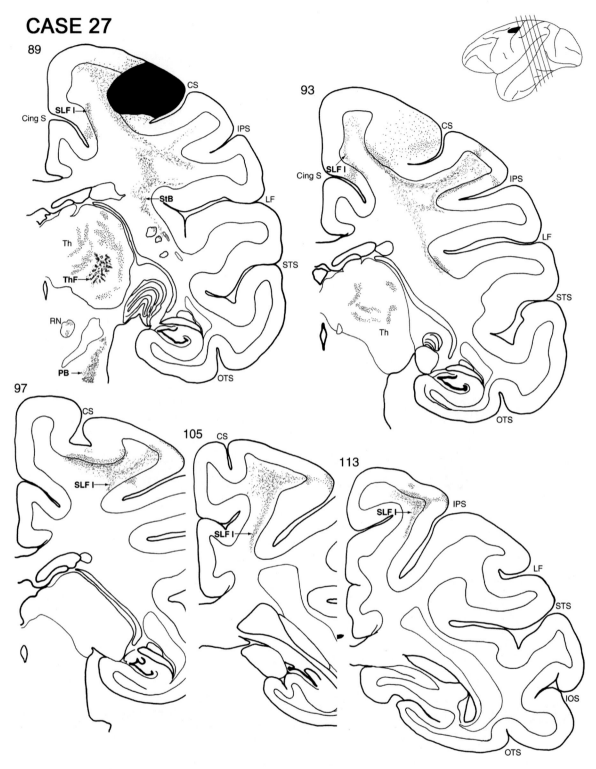

CASE 27

Figure 11-7 (continued)

CASE 27

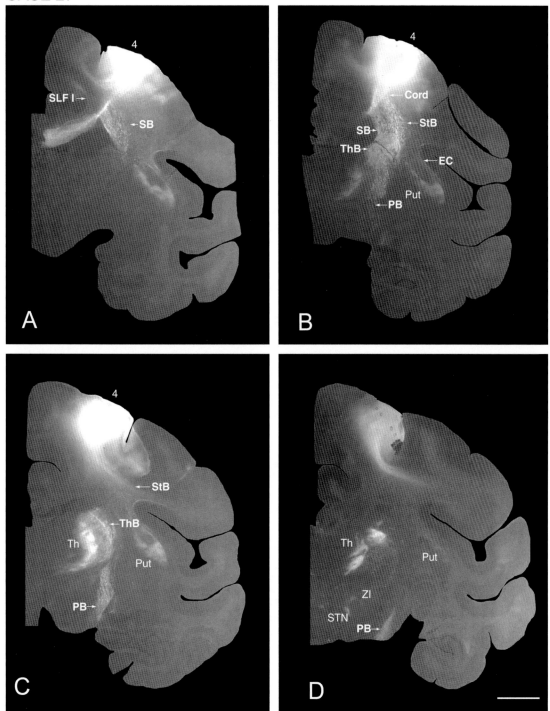

Figure 11-8

Photomicrographs of selected coronal sections of Case 27 showing the injection site in A through C with the injection halo in D and the resulting labeled fibers and terminations in A through D. A through D correspond to sections 78, 81, 85, and 89, respectively (Mag = 0.5×, bar = 5 mm).

CASE 28

In this case isotope was injected in the dorsal part of area 4 in the precentral gyrus corresponding to the foot motor representation (Scs. 89, 93, 97). The location of the foot motor representation was confirmed by physiological stimulation. See figures 11-9 and 11-10.

Association Fibers

Local Association Fibers

Diffuse terminations adjacent to the injection site are seen in area 4. Immediately caudal to the injection site, fibers terminate in medial area 3.

Long Association Fibers

Caudally Directed Fibers

From the injection site association fibers enter the superior longitudinal fasciculus I (SLF I) and proceed caudally in the white matter of the superior parietal lobule. These fibers terminate in the first layer of area 1, and further caudally they terminate in a columnar manner with a first-layer preference in the supplementary sensory area (Murray and Coulter, 1981) in the caudomedial part of the superior parietal lobule and in the upper bank of the cingulate sulcus (Scs. 105, 113, 121). A small contingent of fibers descends from the SLF I and moves laterally and ventrally heading toward the cortex in the depth of the upper bank of the Sylvian fissure. Here the fibers terminate in the deep layers in the area corresponding to the leg representation of SII (Sc. 105).

Rostrally Directed Fibers

Rostral to the injection site fibers travel in the white matter of the precentral gyrus and terminate in the rostral and dorsal part of area 4 in a columnar manner (Scs. 78, 81, 85). A small contingent of fibers near the injection site gathers at the upper bank and depth of the cingulate sulcus. These fibers terminate in the cortex at the depth of the cingulate sulcus in a region corresponding to the leg representation of the cingulate motor area, M3 (Sc. 81). The association fibers in the white matter of the superior frontal gyrus continue rostrally and terminate in the dorsal premotor area 6 in a columnar manner (Scs. 65, 69, 73). Further rostrally these fibers gather in the SLF I and result in two discrete loci of columnar terminations in the upper bank of the cingulate sulcus, corresponding to area MII (Sc. 57).

Commissural and Subcortical Fibers

From the injection site a dense paired cord of labeled fibers descends into the white matter of the precentral gyrus (Scs. 85, 59, 93, 97).

The fibers in the medial segment of the cord descend and course rostrally as they curve deep to the cingulate sulcus white matter. At a level just rostral to the lateral geniculate nucleus (LGN), the fibers leave the cord and move medially to enter sector CC3 of the corpus callosum (Sc. 81) and head toward the opposite hemisphere (Scs. 78, 81).

The fibers in the lateral segment of the cord continue to descend in the corona radiata and enter the posterior limb of the internal capsule at level ICp-2 (Sc. 85). At this level the subcortical fibers (SB) are distinguishable as two broad bundles.

One of these fiber bundles (ThB) moves medially at the superior aspect of ICp-2 and is discernible as an aggregate of fibers that is incorporated into the rostral and caudal parts of the lateral thalamic peduncle. The rostral fibers traverse the reticular nucleus while also providing terminations to it (Scs. 81, 85). They then penetrate into the thalamus and provide terminations to the VL nucleus (Sc. 85). The more caudal fibers that enter the thalamus terminate in the VPL nucleus, as well as in the CL and CM nuclei (Scs. 89, 93).

The other fibers in the subcortical bundle (pontine bundle [PB]) continue to descend in the central and medial parts of the rostral posterior limb ICp-2 and ICp-1 (Scs. 85, 81). As the fibers descend in the capsule they form an anteriorly convex arch just medial to the globus pallidus (Sc. 78). The bulk of these fibers enters the cerebral peduncle and lies within the midlateral part of the peduncle as they continue into the brainstem (Scs. 78, 81, 85, 89). These fibers provide terminations mostly to the caudal half of the pons, situated within a curved lamella closed laterally and open medially, in the intrapeduncular, peripeduncular, dorsal, lateral, and NRTP pontine nuclei. A number of fibers continue within the corticofugal pontine fiber tracts to the spinal cord.

A small contingent of fibers peels medially off the capsular fibers before they descend into the peduncle, to head toward and terminate in the zona incerta (ZI) and subthalamic nucleus (STN) (Sc. 81).

Striatal Fibers

The striatal bundle (StB) constitutes a distinct fiber system that descends from the injection site. It lies lateral to the fibers in the cord and passes through the white matter of the precentral gyrus before entering the corona radiata. These striatal fibers enter the dorsal aspect of the external capsule and terminate in the dorsal segment of the claustrum, as well as in patches within the dorsal and lateral sectors of the putamen throughout most of its rostrocaudal extent (Scs. 49, 57, 65, 69, 73, 78, 81, 85, 89).

A small contingent of fibers leaves the striatal bundle to enter the Muratoff bundle (MB). These fibers course rostrally before terminating in the body and head of the caudate nucleus. Some fibers from the MB traverse the dorsal aspect of the ICp to terminate in the putamen (Scs. 65, 69, 73, 78).

CASE 28

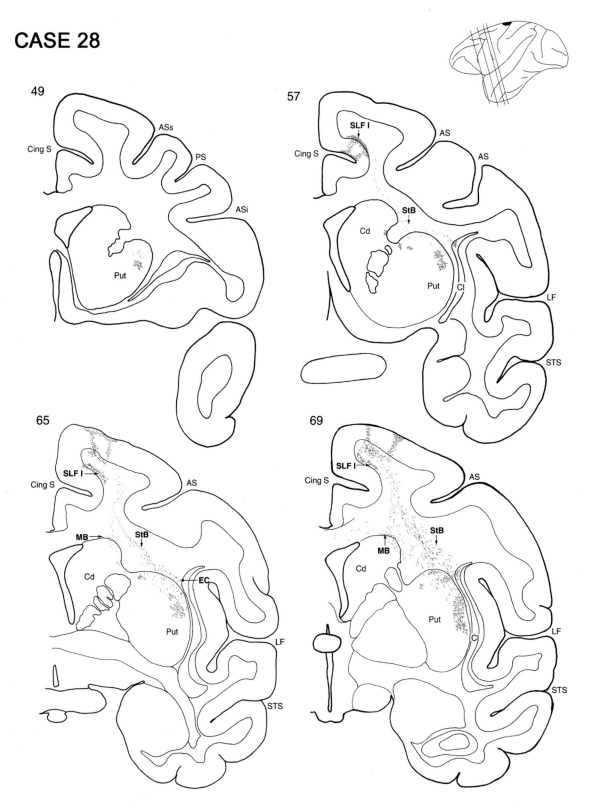

Figure 11-9

Schematic diagrams of 14 rostral-caudal coronal sections in Case 28 taken at the levels shown on the hemispheric diagram above right, showing the isotope injection site in the dorsal part of area 4 in the precentral gyrus corresponding to the motor representation of the foot. The injection site is illus-

CASE 28

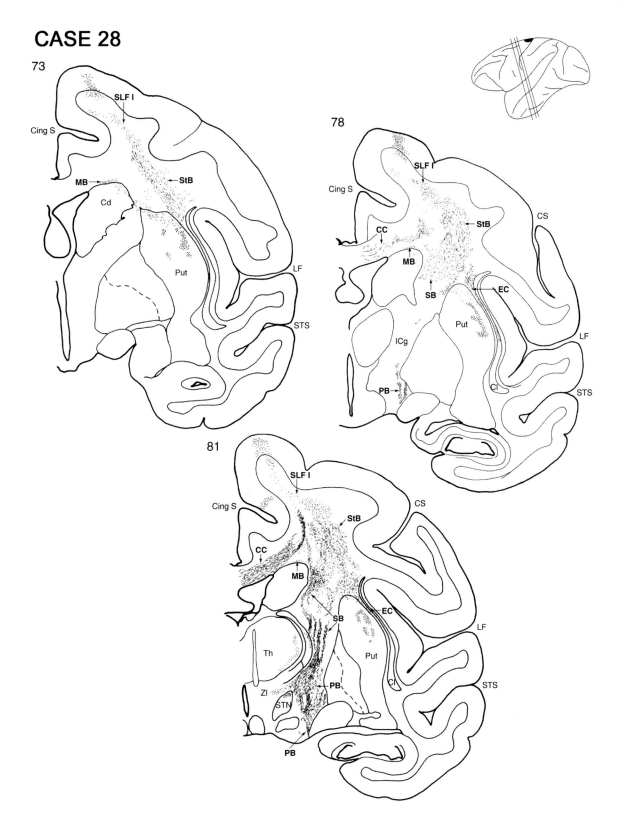

trated (black-filled area), along with the resulting trajectories of the cortical association, commissural, and subcortical fibers (dashed lines and dots) in the white matter and the terminations in the cortex and subcortical regions (black dots).

CASE 28

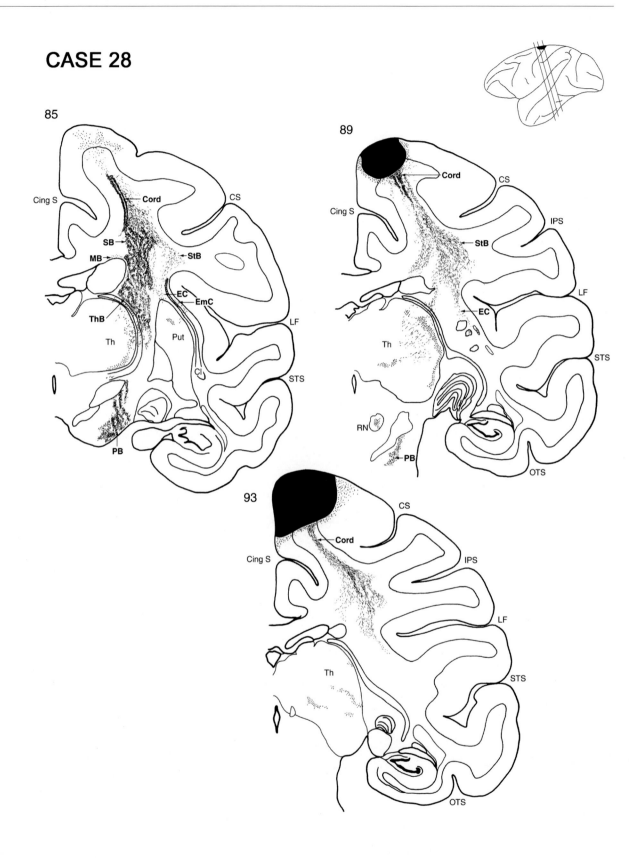

Figure 11-9 (continued)

CASE 28

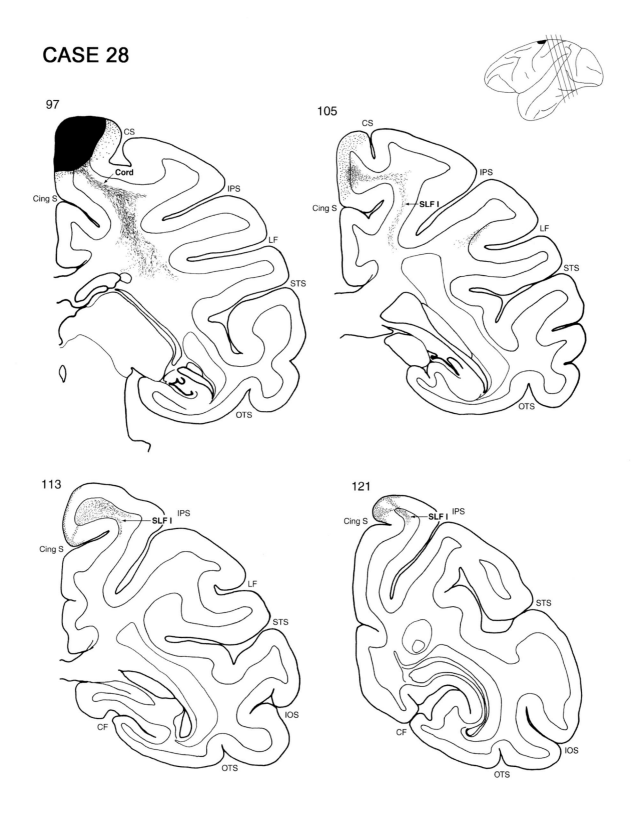

CASE 28

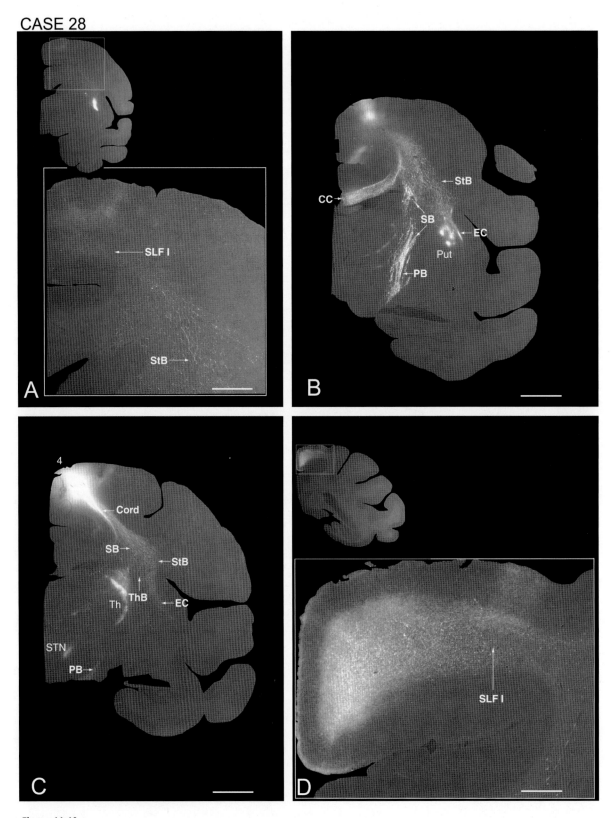

Figure 11-10

Photomicrographs of selected coronal sections of Case 28 to show the injection site in C and the resulting labeled fibers and terminations in A through D. A and D (sections 69 and 113, respectively, Mag = 1×, bar = 2.5 mm) are taken from the locations indicated in the low-power photomicrographs above to show fibers destined for the striatum (StB), fibers from the SLF I terminating in area 6d (A), and fibers in the SLF I (D). B and C correspond to sections 81 and 89, respectively (Mag = 0.5×, bar = 5 mm).

CASE 29

Isotope was injected in this case in the medial part of the superior frontal gyrus in the rostral part of area MII, corresponding to the face representation of the supplementary motor area (Sc. 41). See figures 11-11 and 11-12.

Association Fibers

Local Association Fibers

Adjacent to the injection site, terminations are seen in area 24 in the cingulate gyrus, predominantly in the first layer (Sc. 41).

Long Association Fibers

Caudally Directed Fibers

Caudal to the injection site, fibers travel via the white matter of the superior frontal gyrus in the superior longitudinal fasciculus I (SLF I) and in the cingulum bundle (CB).

The fibers in SLF I terminate in the supplementary motor area and in area 6 in the dorsal superior frontal gyrus. These terminations are columnar, with a first-layer predominance (Scs. 49, 57, 65, 69, 73). The SLF I continues caudally for a considerable distance until the splenium of the corpus callosum. At this level fibers terminate in area 31 in the first layer (Scs. 105, 113).

The fibers in the cingulum bundle terminate in area 24, the rostral part of area 23, and area 31, mainly in the first layer (Scs. 49, 57, 65, 69, 73, 78, 81, 85, 89, 93, 97). Some of these fibers terminate in a columnar manner with a first-layer preference in the motor regions of the cingulate gyrus designated M3 and M4 (Morecraft and Van Hoesen, 1998).

Some association fibers course ventrally in the white matter through the SLF II. These fibers terminate predominantly in the first layer in ventral area 6 and in area 44 in the cortex of the lower bank of the inferior limb of the arcuate sulcus (Sc. 49).

Rostrally Directed Fibers

Association fibers course rostrally from the injection site within the SLF I. They terminate in the medial part of area 9 and in the cortex of the lower bank of the cingulate sulcus in area 24c in a columnar manner (Sc. 31).

Commissural and Subcortical Fibers

From the injection site a dense cord of labeled fibers descends and arches around the cingulate sulcus (Scs. 41, 49). At the ventral aspect of the cord the fibers divide into two distinct bundles (Sc. 41).

The medial fiber bundle continues to descend medially to penetrate the corpus callosum in sector CC1 (Sc. 49) and course to the opposite hemisphere at this level.

The lateral group of fibers arches ventrally and laterally and enters the anterior limb of the internal capsule at level ICa-2 (Sc. 49). These fibers in the subcortical bundle

(SB) lie within the medial and central aspects of the ICa and descend gradually until they reach level ICa-6. Here the fibers segregate into two distinct components (Sc. 73).

The medially situated thalamic fiber bundle (ThB) continues caudally and enters the thalamus via the superior part of the lateral thalamic peduncle. The fibers penetrate the reticular nucleus, providing terminations to the nucleus as they pass through. Terminations within the thalamus are then noted in the VA and AV nuclei and further caudally in the VLm and VLc nuclei, nucleus X, and Csl. Fibers continue further caudally within the thalamus and terminate additionally in the MD nucleus and in the intralaminar nuclei, CM, Pf, and CL (Scs. 81, 85, 89, 93).

The capsular fibers that lie more laterally (the pontine bundle [PB]) continue to descend at the level of the genu of the internal capsule (Sc. 78), from which point they enter the medial part of the midportion of the cerebral peduncle and continue in a medial position within the corticofugal fiber bundles of the pons (Scs. 78, 81, 85). Terminations are present in the median, paramedian, and dorsomedial pontine nuclei, as well as in medial parts of the peripeduncular and ventral nuclei and in the NRTP. Some fibers in the corticofugal bundles are seen to descend caudal to the pons.

A number of fibers that leave the internal capsule move medially and head toward the subthalamic nucleus (STN) and zona incerta (ZI), to which they provide terminations (Scs. 81, 85). Some of these fibers also terminate in the red nucleus (RN) (Sc. 89).

Striatal Fibers

A group of fibers that leads to the striatum emerges from the central core of the white matter behind the injection site and gathers first in the fronto-occipital fasciculus (FOF) before descending into the Muratoff bundle (MB). These fibers terminate in the dorsal and lateral aspects of the head and body of the caudate nucleus (Scs. 41, 49, 57, 65, 69, 73, 78, 81, 85, 89, 93).

Another group of striatal fibers, situated lateral to the FOF, runs ventrally, crosses the internal capsule and enters the external capsule. These fibers terminate predominantly in the dorsal and medial aspects of the putamen and in the midsector of the claustrum throughout much of its rostrocaudal extent (Scs. 49, 57, 65, 69, 73, 78, 81, 85, 89).

CASE 29

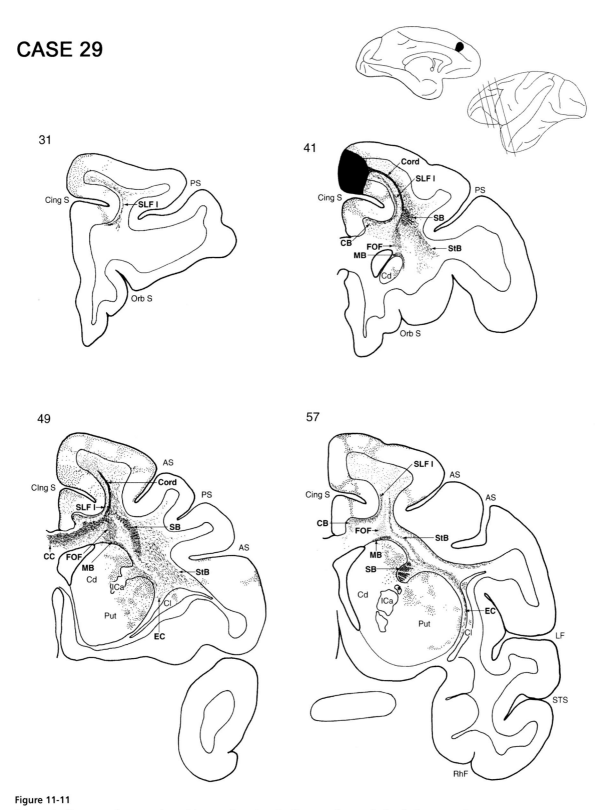

Figure 11-11

Schematic diagrams of 15 rostral-caudal coronal sections in Case 29 taken at the levels shown on the hemispheric diagrams above right, showing the isotope injection site in the medial part of the superior frontal gyrus corresponding to the face representation of the supplementary motor area (black-filled area). The resulting trajectories of the cortical association, commissural, and subcortical fibers (dashed lines and dots) are depicted, along with the terminations in the cortex and subcortical regions (black dots).

CASE 29

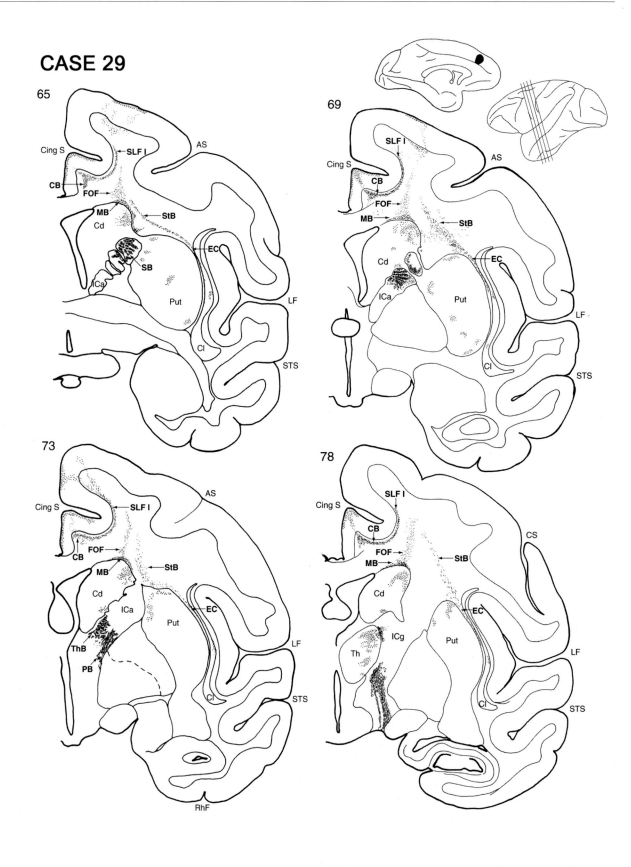

Figure 11-11 (continued)

CASE 29

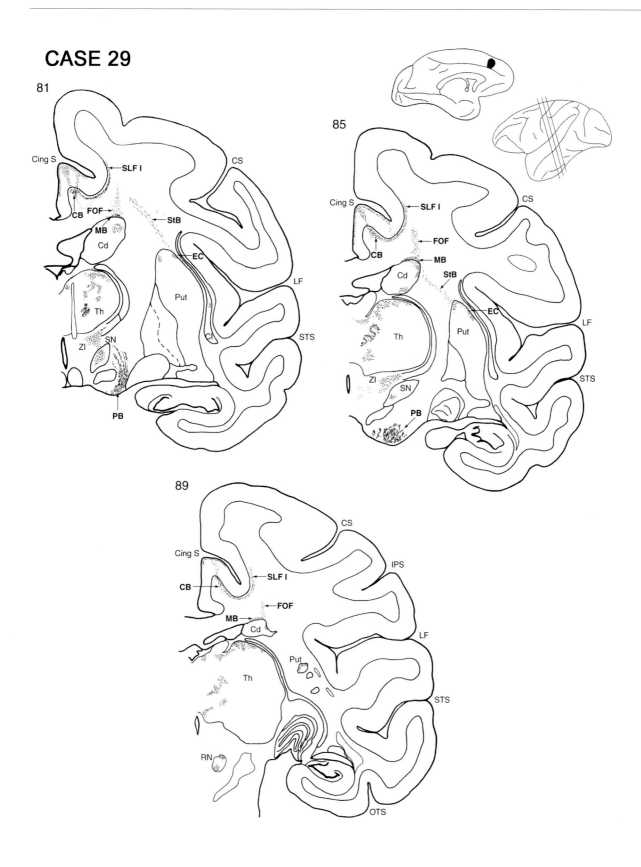

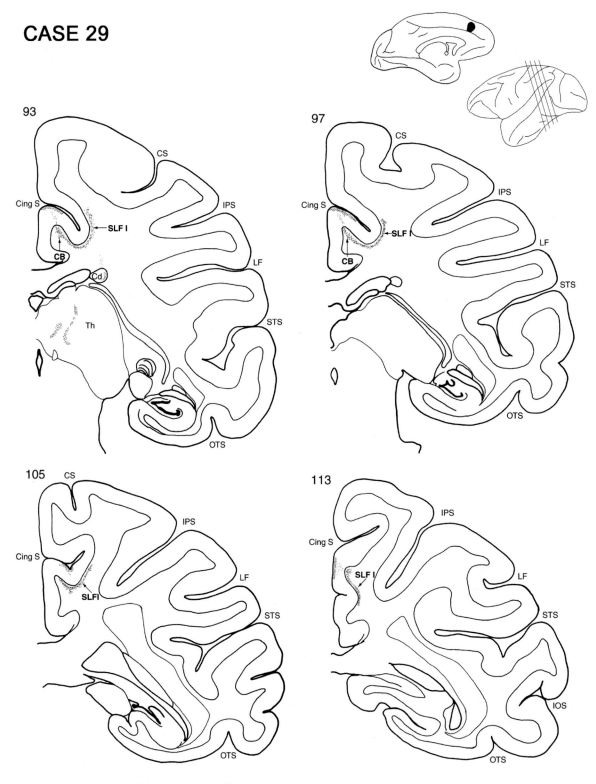

Figure 11-11 (continued)

CASE 29

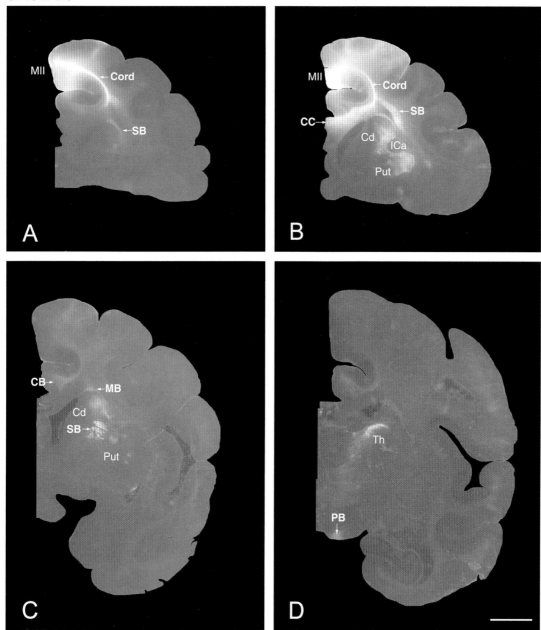

Figure 11-12

Photomicrographs of selected coronal sections of Case 29 to show the injection site in A and B and the resulting labeled fibers and terminations in A through D. Photomicrographs A through D correspond to sections 41, 49, 65, and 85, respectively (Mag = 0.5×, bar = 5 mm).

Motor Cortex Summary

Association Fibers

Frontal Operculum (Case 24)

The frontal opercular cortex that contains the precentral components of areas 1 and 2 conveys its long association fibers mainly via the SLF III and the extreme capsule (figure 11-13).

The SLF III fibers terminate in the gustatory area, SII, precentral portion of area 3, and ventral area 6, as well as in the postcentral portion of areas 3b and 2.

The frontal opercular fibers that travel in the upper part of the extreme capsule terminate in the rostral part of the insula.

Lower Part of the Precentral Gyrus (Motor Face Area; Case 25)

Association fibers emanating from the lower part of the precentral gyrus course in the white matter immediately beneath the cortex of the precentral and premotor region and in the SLF III lying in the frontal operculum. The fibers lying immediately beneath the cortex terminate in ventral area 6, whereas those within the SLF III terminate in area ProM.

A few fibers leave the lower part of the precentral gyrus and course dorsally and medially in the white matter of the superior frontal gyrus before terminating in medial area 6, in the supplementary motor area.

Caudally directed fibers travel mainly via the SLF III in the white matter of the frontal and parietal operculum and terminate in the precentral portion of area SII and areas 1, 2, and 3. Further caudally, the SLF III fibers terminate in the postcentral portion of area SII, as well as in areas 3, 1, and 2.

Midsector of the Precentral Gyrus (Motor Hand Area; Case 26)

Rostral to the midsector of the precentral gyrus, fibers travel in the white matter beneath the central sulcus and provide terminations to the dorsal and ventral parts of the area around the arcuate spur and to area 4C below the spur. Further rostrally, these fibers occupy the SLF I in the white matter of the superior frontal gyrus, and they terminate in the depth and upper bank of the cingulate sulcus involving the cingulate motor area and the supplementary motor area.

Caudally directed fibers course in the white matter beneath the central sulcus and then in the white matter of the superior parietal lobule. These fibers terminate in areas 3a, 1, and 2, area PEa, and area PE. Some fibers descend from the white matter of the superior parietal lobule, course around the depth of the intraparietal sulcus, and occupy the white matter of the inferior parietal lobule. From here the fibers terminate in area POa in the lower bank of the intraparietal sulcus and in the upper bank of the Sylvian fissure, area SII.

Dorsomedial Portion of the Precentral Gyrus (Motor Foot Area; Case 28)

The rostrally directed association fibers course via the SLF I in the white matter of the superior frontal gyrus. They terminate in the cingulate motor area in the upper bank of the cingulate sulcus, in dorsal area 6, and in the supplementary motor area.

The caudally directed association fibers course through the white matter of the precentral and postcentral gyri, as well in SLF I. These fibers terminate in medial areas 3, 1, and 2 and areas PE and PEci. A few fibers from the SLF I course around the depth of the intraparietal sulcus and reach the caudal part of the Sylvian fissure, where they terminate in SII.

Rostral and Dorsal Precentral Gyrus (Motor Trunk Area; Case 27)

Association fibers emerge from the rostral and dorsal parts of the precentral gyrus and travel rostrally within the SLF I subjacent to the cingulate sulcus and the cortex of the superior frontal gyrus. These fibers terminate in the supplementary motor area, dorsal area 6, and the cingulate motor area lying in the depth and upper bank of the cingulate sulcus.

Caudally directed fibers course mainly in SLF I in the white matter of the precentral, postcentral, and superior parietal lobules. These fibers terminate in the dorsal part of area 3a, area 2 above the intraparietal sulcus, and area PEa in the depth of the intraparietal sulcus. Further caudally these fibers also terminate in area PE. Some fibers leave these fascicles, course ventrally, and terminate in the depth of the Sylvian fissure, in area SII.

Medial Prefrontal Area (Rostral Part of the Supplementary Motor Area; Case 29)

The long association bundles emanating from the supplementary motor area course in the SLF I and the cingulum bundle.

The fibers in the SLF I proceed rostrally in the medial aspect of the white matter of the superior frontal gyrus and terminate in medial area 9. The caudally directed SLF I fibers lead to dorsal area 6 and the caudal parts of the supplementary motor area.

The cingulum bundle lies within the white matter of the lower bank and depth of the cingulate sulcus. From there, the fibers terminate rostrally in areas 24b and 24c and caudally in areas 23c and 31.

Commissural Fibers

Fibers arising in the precentral motor cortex course to the opposite hemisphere through sector CC3 of the corpus callosum in a topographic manner. Those from the opercular cortex are most rostral and involve part of the CC2 sector as well. These are followed caudally in a sequential manner by fibers from the face representation, then those from the hand, trunk, and foot. There is some overlap between face and hand fibers. Those from the trunk area overlap rostrally with fibers from the hand and caudally with fibers from the foot. The callosal fibers from the leg representation are distinct from those derived from the hand and face areas.

In contrast to the fibers that travel mostly in CC3 from the precentral motor cortex, those arising from the supplementary motor cortex are restricted within callosal sector CC1.

Subcortical Fibers

Precentral Operculum (Case 24)

The subcortically directed fibers that emanate from the precentral operculum ascend medially in the cord and descend sharply from the cord of fibers to enter the anterior limb of the internal capsule. The fibers in the ICa segregate into two components. The medial component enters the reticular nucleus of thalamus and provides terminations in the reticular nucleus, as well as in the VPM, VPMpc, and CL nuclei. The fibers that lie more laterally in the ICa continue to descend, and at the level of the rostral part of the posterior limb of the internal capsule they descend into the cerebral peduncle before terminating in the nuclei of the basis pontis.

Lower Part of the Precentral Gyrus (Motor Face Area; Case 25)

The subcortical fibers from the lower portion of the precentral gyrus (corresponding to the face representation of the motor cortex) form a cord in the white matter of the frontal operculum that courses dorsally and medially. As the cord passes over the anterior limb of the internal capsule (ICa), a prominent contingent of fibers descends obliquely into the capsule. These ICa fibers move caudally until the genu of the internal capsule. At this level, fibers situated medially within the capsule penetrate the lower part of the external medullary lamina and terminate in the VA nucleus, as well as in the VLm and Pcn nuclei, and nucleus X. At the level of the genu of the internal capsule, fibers continue to descend toward the cerebral peduncle. Some head medially and terminate in the zona incerta, but the majority descend to terminate in the basilar pontine nuclei and lower brainstem.

Midportion of the Precentral Gyrus (Motor Hand Area; Case 26)

The subcortical fibers first course medially and then descend straight down in the rostral part of the posterior limb of the internal capsule, reaching from the corona radiata to the cerebral peduncle at the same level. One segment of these fibers crosses the lateral part of the external medullary lamina, enters the thalamus, and progresses caudally within the thalamus while giving rise to terminations in the reticular nucleus as well as in the VL, VPL, CL and CM nuclei. The most ventral fibers in the ICp descend further into the midpart of the cerebral peduncle, destined for the pons and spinal cord. Some of the capsular fibers course ventral to the thalamus and terminate in the zona incerta, red nucleus, and interstitial nucleus of Cajal.

Dorsal and Dorsomedial Precentral Gyrus (Motor Foot Area; Case 28)

The subcortically directed fibers from the dorsal portions of the precentral gyrus descend ventrally in the cord of fibers situated in the central part of the white matter of the precentral gyrus. A prominent contingent of fibers leaves the cord and descends through the corona radiata into the posterior limb of the internal capsule (ICp). One segment of this subcortical bundle in the ICp enters the midportion of the external medullary lamina and terminates in the lateral parts of thalamus in the VL nucleus, and more caudally in the VPL, as well as in the CM and CL nuclei. The fibers that remain in the capsule continue ventrally, medial to the globus pallidus. Some of these fibers course medially and terminate in the zona incerta and red nucleus, whereas most of the fibers enter the cerebral peduncle and descend to terminate in the basilar pontine nuclei and provide terminations in the spinal cord.

Medial Prefrontal Area (Rostral Part of the Supplementary Motor Area; Case 29)

From the medial superior frontal gyrus that corresponds to the supplementary motor area, subcortically directed fibers course in the form of a cord into the white matter of the superior frontal gyrus. The bulk of the fibers leaves the cord and descends obliquely laterally to enter the anterior limb of the internal capsule (ICa). The capsular fibers course obliquely caudally, and at the level of the genu the fibers enter the thalamus. They terminate in the VA and AV nuclei rostrally, and then continue caudally within the thalamus to terminate in the VLm and VLc nuclei, as well as in nucleus X and Csl, and further caudally in MD and the intralaminar nuclei (CM, Pf, CL). At the level of the genu of the internal capsule, the remaining fibers descend into the cerebral peduncle. Some of these fibers enter the subthalamic nucleus, zona incerta, and red nucleus, where they terminate. The remaining fibers in the peduncle descend into the pons and terminate in the basilar pontine nuclei.

Corticostriate Projections

The precentral motor cortex (MI) projections to the striatum are conveyed almost exclusively by the external capsule to the dorsal two thirds of the middle and caudal parts of the putamen. The ventral precentral gyrus (opercular cortex and face representation) projects to the ventral and medial regions of the dorsal half of the putamen; dorsal precentral regions (leg and foot areas) project to the dorsal and lateral putamen; and projections from the upper limb representation are situated between these two termination fields.

Opercular fibers travel first with those in the SLF III and cross through the extreme capsule before descending into the external capsule to terminate in the medial part of the midportion of the putamen. Fibers from the face region course over the upper shoulder of the rostral Sylvian fissure, enter the external capsule, proceed caudally, and terminate in the ventral and medial parts of the putamen, as well as in dorsal aspects of the claustrum. Hand motor fibers course through the external capsule to dorsal parts of the putamen and claustrum. Fibers from the dorsal and dorsomedial precentral gyrus (foot and trunk representations) move ventrally, progress rostrally within the dorsal aspect of the external capsule, and terminate in the lateral and dorsal aspects of the putamen throughout its rostral-to-caudal extent, with some terminations in the dorsal part of the claustrum. Some of these foot/trunk fibers gather in the Muratoff bundle and terminate in the dorsal portion of the head of the caudate nucleus, while others leave the Muratoff bundle, cross the internal capsule, and enter the external capsule before terminating in the putamen.

The striatal projections and fiber bundles of the face representation of the supplementary motor area (SMA) are distinctly different than those of MI. One contingent of fibers courses medial to the thalamic fibers, passes through the fronto-occipital bundle, gathers in the Muratoff bundle, and terminates in the dorsolateral part of the head of the caudate nucleus, with projections also to the dorsal and lateral regions of the caudate body. A second contingent of SMA fibers courses via the external capsule to the dorsal and lateral aspects of the rostral putamen, with lesser input to the dorsal aspect of the putamen more caudally, and some fibers terminate in midregions of the claustrum.

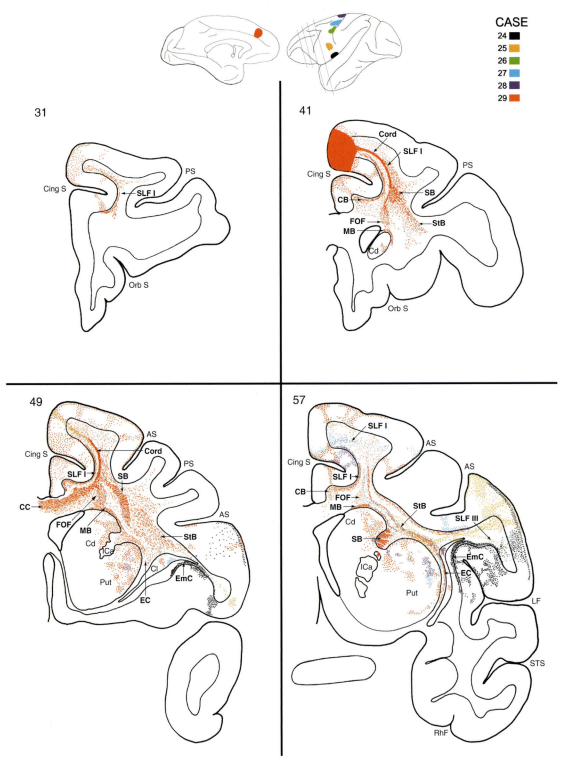

Figure 11-13

Schematic composite diagrams of the rostral-caudal coronal sections of the template brain, illustrating the six precentral motor cases (Cases 24–29). The injection sites and the association, commissural, and subcortical fibers, as well as the termination patterns, are color-coded for each case. The schematic diagrams of the medial and lateral surfaces of the cerebral hemispheres (at top) represent the different levels of the coronal sections and the injection sites. Color-coding is as follows:

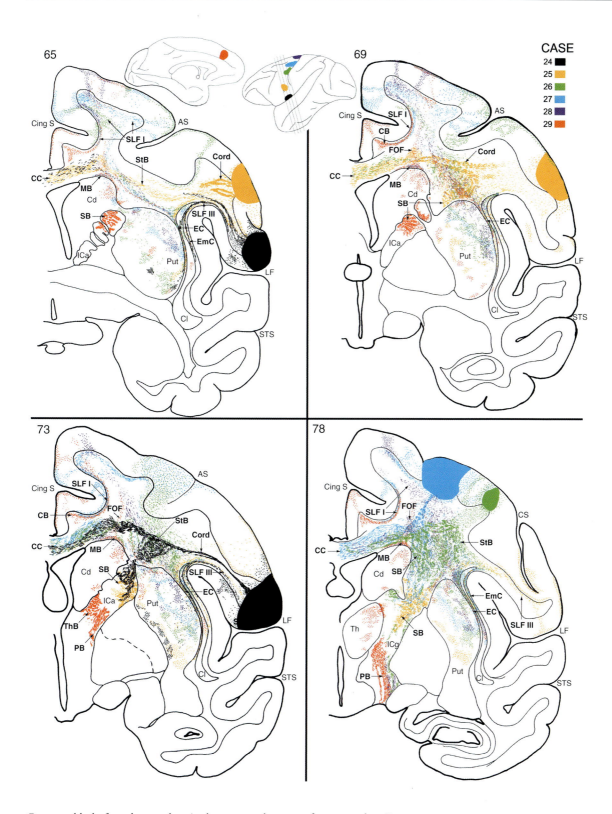

Case 24—black, frontal operculum in the precentral aspects of areas 1 and 2; Case 25—orange, ventral area 4, face motor representation; Case 26—green, area 4 behind the arcuate spur, hand motor representation; Case 27—blue, dorsal precentral gyrus area 4, trunk motor representation; Case 28—purple, dorsal area 4, foot motor representation; Case 29—red, medial part of the superior frontal gyrus, rostral area MII, supplementary motor face representation.

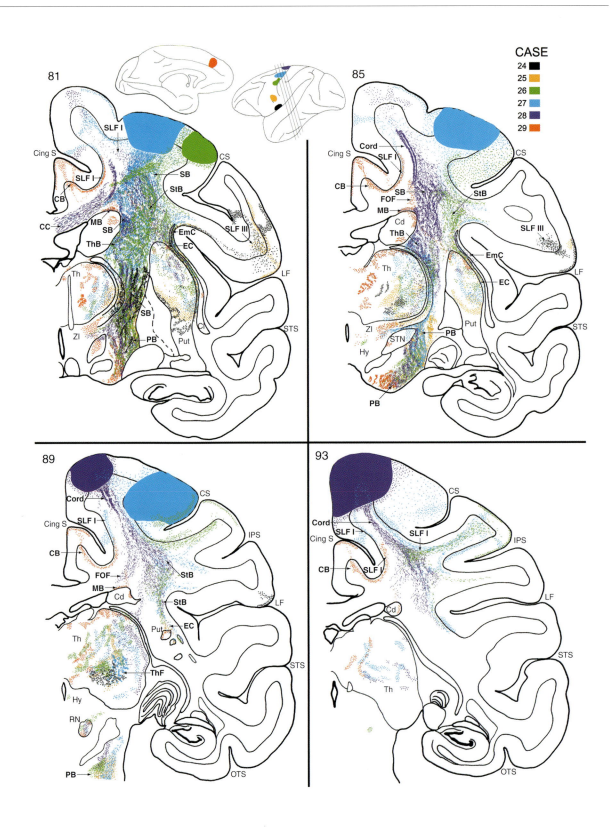

Figure 11-13 (continued)

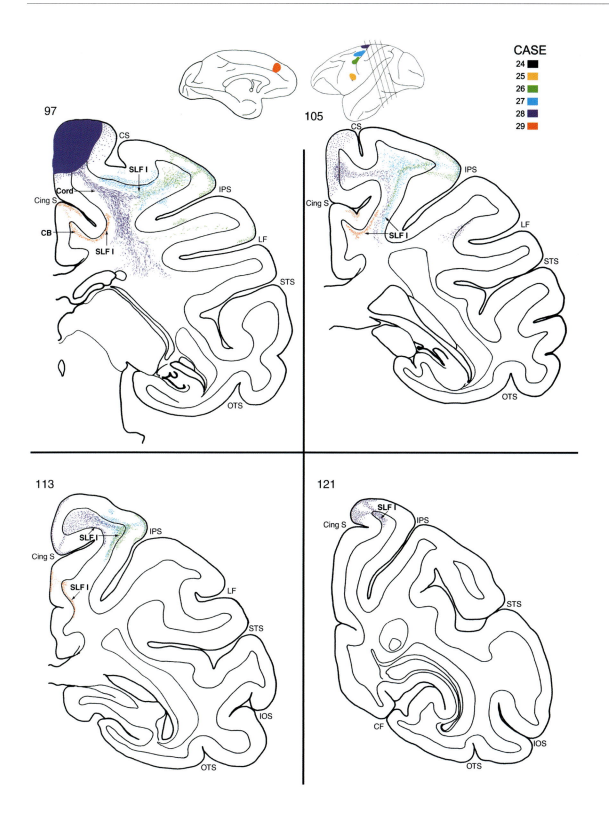

Prefrontal Cortex

In this chapter we describe the isotope injections that were placed in the prefrontal cortex of four rhesus monkeys and analyze the resulting association, striatal, commissural, and subcortical fiber trajectories, as well as the cortical and subcortical terminations. The injections were in the medial surface of the prefrontal cortex involving mainly area 32 (Case 30), above the midportion of the principal sulcus in area 46d (Case 31), the middle part of ventral area 46 in both the sulcal and gyral cortices (Case 32), and the orbital frontal cortex in the orbital part of area 47/12 (Case 33).

As in the previous chapters, the architectonic designations of the cortical terminations are described in the text but not identified on the coronal sections. Architectonic areas are labeled on external views of the hemisphere as well as in the coronal series of chapter 4. Terminations in the thalamus are shown and thalamic nuclei are referred to in the text, but the nuclei are not designated on the coronal sections. Pontine terminations are described in the text but not illustrated. Striatal terminations are illustrated and an overview of their termination patterns is presented in the text.

CASE 30

Isotope was injected in this case in the medial surface of the prefrontal cortex involving mainly area 32 (Scs. 20, 31). See figures 12-1 and 12-2.

Association Fibers

Local Association Fibers

Local fibers leave the injection site and travel dorsally and ventrally. The dorsally directed fibers arch upward around the depth of the cingulate sulcus and terminate in the depth of the sulcus and in medial area 9. Some fibers continue in the white matter of the superior frontal gyrus and terminate in a columnar manner with a first-layer emphasis in area 9 (Scs. 20, 31). The ventrally directed fibers give rise to terminations in area 14 at the medial wall of the hemisphere (Scs. 20, 31). Fibers leave this bundle and cross the white matter to lie within the white matter under the orbital cortex and terminate in area 14 at the orbital cortex in a columnar manner with a first-layer preference (Sc. 31).

Long Association Fibers

Caudally Directed Fibers

The caudally directed fibers are conveyed by three fiber bundles. Fibers that course ventrally from the injection site travel via the medial and ventral portion of the uncinate fasciculus (UF) and terminate in a columnar manner in area 25 and in the periallocortex at the caudal part of the orbital surface (Scs. 41, 49). Some of the fibers traveling within the uncinate fasciculus continue laterally and ventrally into the temporal lobe and terminate in the amygdala (Scs. 65, 73).

Other association fibers move laterally from the injection site and continue in the extreme capsule (EmC), lying in the white matter adjacent to the lateral orbital cortex. These fibers terminate in area 47/12 (Sc. 41). The orbital fibers continue further caudally in the extreme capsule and terminate in the insular proisocortex (Sc. 49).

A third group of fibers leaves the injection site and travels caudally, lying within the cingulum bundle. As these fibers progress caudally, they terminate near the injection site in area 24 (Scs. 41, 57). They continue caudally, lying within the most ventral part of the cingulum bundle, until they reach the splenium of the corpus callosum. Here they terminate within the dorsal part of the agranular retrosplenial cortex, area 30 (Scs. 105, 113). The fibers then descend and curve around the splenium, extending into the ventral part of the cingulum bundle. They terminate in the first layer of the ventral part of the agranular retrosplenial cortex situated in the upper bank of the calcarine sulcus (Sc. 113).

Rostrally Directed Fibers

Fibers leave the injection site and course rostrally in the white matter of the dorsal and medial prefrontal cortex. The fibers terminate dorsally in area 9 and medially in areas 32 and 14 (Scs. 20, 31). Some fibers can be traced laterally lying below the principal sulcus before terminating in ventral area 46 (Sc. 20).

Commissural and Subcortical Fibers

Apart from the association fibers that leave the injection site, there is a dense accumulation of fibers situated beneath the injection site (the cord). These fibers, destined for the opposite hemisphere and for ipsilateral subcortical sites, are distinguishable from medial to lateral into three fiber bundles.

An intensely labeled aggregate of fibers lies immediately beneath the injection site and moves caudally a short distance in this location until the genu of the corpus callosum. At this level (callosal sector CC1), the fibers move medially into the callosum, occupying its dorsal through ventral extents, and head toward the opposite hemisphere (Sc. 41).

A dense group of subcortical fibers (SB) located lateral to the head of the caudate nucleus enters the most rostral part of the anterior limb of the internal capsule, ICa-1 (Sc. 41), and descends gradually as the fibers progress caudally, in a medial position in the capsule, until they reach level ICa-6 (Sc. 73) just rostral to the genu. At this level, the subcortical bundle separates into a dorsal and a ventral component.

The dorsal component (ThB) penetrates directly into the most rostral aspect of the thalamus. These fibers terminate in most of the rostrocaudal extent of MDmc, as well as in the AV, AM, Pf, and midline thalamic nuclei (Scs. 81, 85, 89, 93).

The ventral group of fibers (PB) within the internal capsule continues into the rostral aspect of the posterior limb (ICp-1, Sc. 81) and first gives rise to terminations in the zona incerta and the hypothalamus (Scs. 81, 85). The bulk of these capsular fibers, however, continues to descend and enters the medial aspect of the cerebral peduncle at the level of the most rostral aspect of the LGN (Scs. 81, 85). These fibers terminate in the rostral third of the basis pontis in the paramedian and medial parts of the peripeduncular pontine nuclei.

Striatal Fibers

The striatal fibers leave the injection site and are located lateral and medial to the subcortical fiber bundle in the internal capsule. These fibers aggregate rostral to the appearance of the head of the caudate nucleus. At the appearance of the caudate nucleus, the fibers completely surround it, and result in intense terminations (Sc. 41). As the internal capsule starts to make its appearance, the striatal fiber system divides into two components.

The dorsal component (Muratoff bundle) occupies a position above the caudate nucleus and provides terminations to the medial part of the head and the rostrocaudal extent of the body of the caudate nucleus (Scs. 49, 57, 65, 73, 81, 85). The ventral component surrounds the caudate nucleus medially, ventrally, and laterally (within the external capsule), and these fibers provide terminations to the ventral part of the putamen (Scs. 49, 57). Some of the fibers in the external capsule provide terminations to the claustrum (Scs. 49, 57, 65, 73, 81), while others cross the claustrum to enter the extreme capsule. The fiber systems that constitute these dorsal and ventral striatal components are interconnected, mostly by fibers that cross the internal capsule from the Muratoff bundle to enter the external capsule.

CASE 30

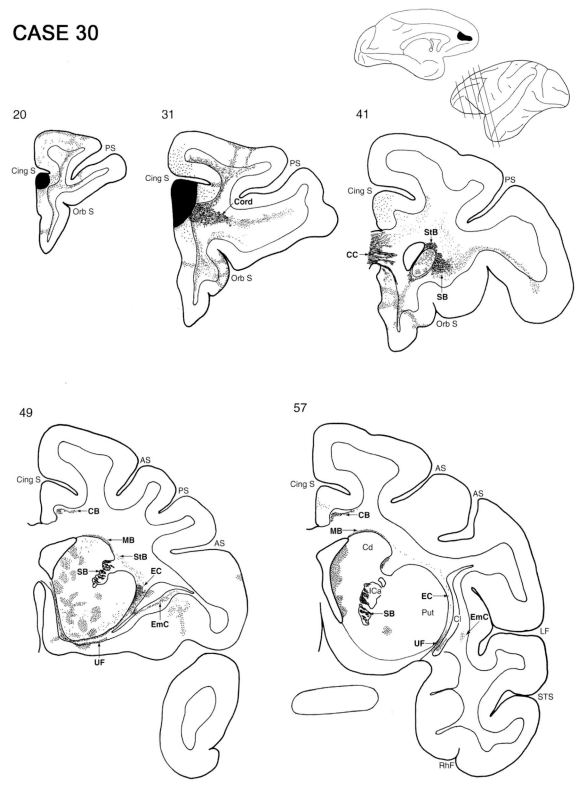

Figure 12-1

Schematic diagrams of 14 rostral–caudal coronal sections in Case 30 taken at the levels shown on the hemispheric diagrams above right, showing the isotope injection site in the medial surface of the prefrontal cortex involving mainly area 32 (black-filled area), the resulting trajectories of the cortical association, commissural, and subcortical fibers (dashed lines and dots) in the white matter, and the terminations in the cortex and subcortical regions (black dots). See list of abbreviations, page 617.

CASE 30

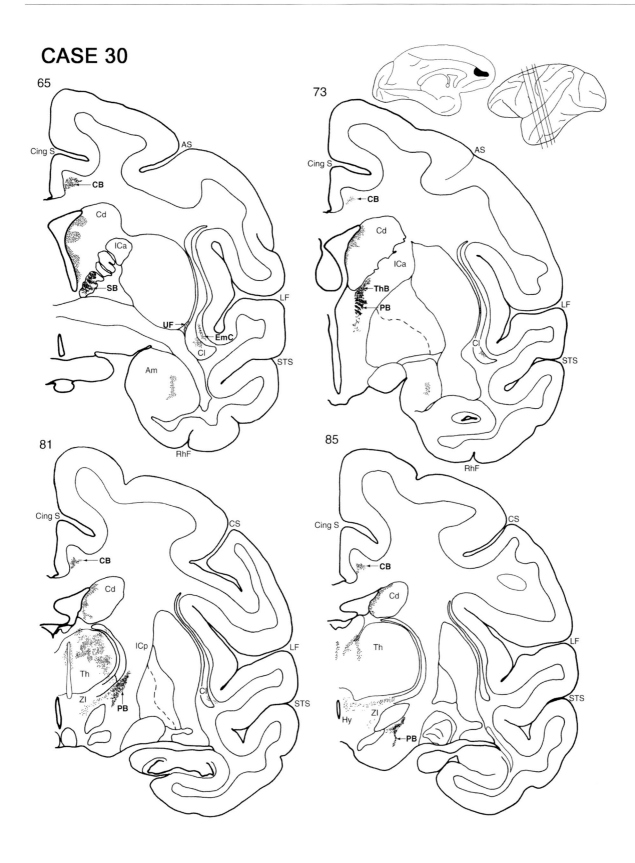

CASE 30

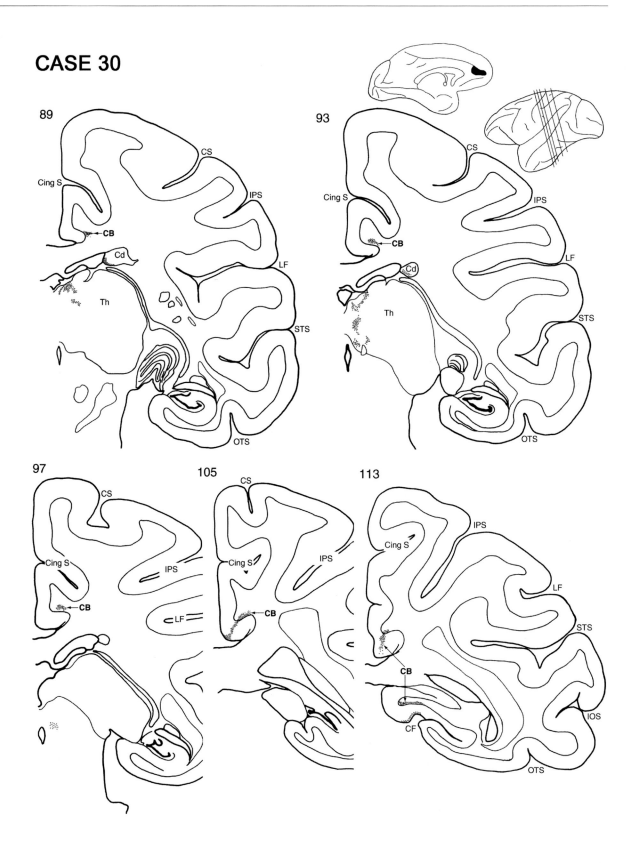

Figure 12-1 (continued)

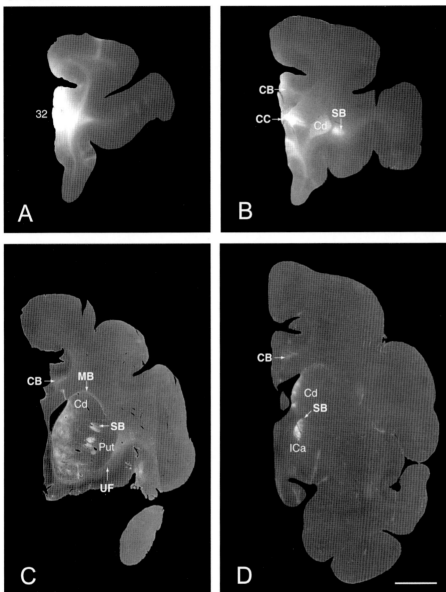

Figure 12-2

Photomicrographs of selected coronal sections of Case 30 showing the injection site in A and the resulting labeled fibers and terminations in A through D. A through D correspond to sections 31, 41, 49, and 65, respectively (Mag = 0.5×, bar = 5 mm).

CASE 31

Isotope was injected in this case in the prefrontal cortex above the midportion of the principal sulcus in area 9/46d (Sc. 41). See figures 12-3 and 12-4.

Association Fibers

Local Association Fibers

Local association fibers leave the injection site and travel dorsally toward the superior frontal gyrus, lying first within the white matter immediately beneath the cortex and then in the white matter of the superior frontal gyrus. They terminate in area 6 in a columnar manner and in area 8B in columns with an emphasis in the first layer (Sc. 41).

Long Association Fibers

Caudally Directed Fibers

The long association fibers from the injection site travel caudally and are distinguishable as four distinct fiber bundles: the superior longitudinal fasciculus (SLF) I, cingulum bundle (CB), SLF II, and fronto-occipital fasciculus (FOF).

Medially directed fibers leave the injection site and occupy a position in the SLF I that lies in the white matter of the superior frontal gyrus extending up to the depth of the cingulate sulcus. As the SLF I proceeds caudally, it lies within the white matter first of the superior frontal gyrus and then of the superior parietal lobule. In the frontal lobe, the SLF I provides terminations in area 6d in a columnar manner (Scs. 49, 57). In the parietal lobe, fibers within the medial aspect of the SLF I provide extensive terminations in a columnar manner with a first layer preference in area 31, and then in areas PGm and PO at the medial parietal convexity (Scs. 105, 113, 121, 129, 137, 145). Fibers within the lateral aspect of the SLF I terminate dorsally in area PEc, also in a columnar manner with a first-layer predominance (Scs. 129, 137).

Other medially directed fibers are situated in the cingulum bundle (CB) in the white matter of the cingulate gyrus, and they separate into two subdivisions. One group of fibers in the CB lies at the periphery of the cingulate white matter. These fibers travel caudally and terminate first in the cingulate gyrus in area 24 in a columnar manner with a first-layer preference (Scs. 57, 65, 73, 81, 85, 89). The remaining fibers proceed caudally in the upper part of the periphery of the cingulate white matter to the level of the caudal portion of the cingulate gyrus, where they provide columnar terminations to area 23 (Scs. 93, 105).

The other group of fibers in the CB is situated more deeply in the cingulate white matter beneath the cingulate gyrus. These fibers travel caudally to provide terminations in area 24 in the ventral part of the cingulate gyrus (Scs. 65, 73, 81, 85, 89, 93). Further caudally these fibers terminate in the retrosplenial cortex in the most ventral aspect of the cingulate gyrus in two locations: more laterally in retrosplenial granular cortex (area 29) and more medially in the retrosplenial agranular cortex (area 30) (Sc. 93). The fibers in the CB then continue further caudally, descend around the splenium of the corpus callosum, turn rostrally, and enter the ventral aspect of the CB that lies in the white matter of the calcarine fissure. In this location the fibers continue to progress rostrally and provide terminations to the first layer of area prostriata in the calcarine sulcus, and then to the superficial and deep layers of the caudal portion of the presubiculum (Scs. 105, 113).

A more laterally situated group of long association fibers leaves the injection site and is situated within the SLF II, lying deep to the principal sulcus and the arcuate concavity. Some of these fibers terminate in area 8Ad in the frontal lobe (Scs. 49, 57). Other fibers then progress caudally and lie in the white matter deep to the central sulcus. At the rostral aspect of the intraparietal sulcus, the SLF II fibers move laterally to occupy a position within the white matter of the inferior parietal lobule. In this location they provide terminations to the dorsal part of areas PFG and PG in a columnar manner with a first-layer preference (Scs. 93, 97, 105, 113). Further caudally the fibers terminate in the first layer of area POa as well as area Opt (Scs. 113, 121, 129). A small contingent of SLF II fibers courses ventrally to occupy the arcuate fasciculus (AF) from where fibers terminate in area TPO in the caudal portion of the superior temporal sulcus, and in area Tpt in the superior temporal gyrus, predominantly in the first layer (Scs. 105, 113).

Apart from the SLF I and SLF II fiber systems coursing caudally from the injection site, some fibers are noted also in the FOF that lies above the Muratoff bundle, and these FOF fibers course caudally until a level corresponding to the caudal end of the lateral geniculate nucleus (LGN). Fibers in the FOF have two quite separate destinations. A number of fibers descend from the FOF to enter the Muratoff bundle. In contrast, the fibers that lie within the dorsal aspect of the FOF appear to merge with those of the SLF I and II as they proceed caudally.

Rostrally Directed Fibers

Association fibers directed rostrally from the injection site course toward the frontal pole in the superior frontal gyrus and terminate in areas 46d and 9 in a columnar manner (Scs. 20, 31). Ventrally situated fibers travel within the white matter immediately beneath the lower bank of the principal sulcus and terminate in a columnar manner in area 10 and ventral area 46 (Scs. 20, 31).

Commissural and Subcortical Fibers

From the injection site a dense cord of fibers (Sc. 41) travels medially in the white matter. The most medial component of these fibers arches slightly upward and continues medially to enter the lateral aspect of the genu of the corpus callosum (sector CC1), where it courses in the dorsal part of the genu toward the opposite hemisphere (Sc. 41).

The remaining fibers in the cord enter the lateral aspect of the anterior limb of the internal capsule (level ICa-2) as multiple, intense discrete fiber bundles (subcortical bundle [SB]). These fiber aggregates descend medially within the capsule as they proceed caudally. At the genu of the internal capsule the SB fibers divide into two major constituents.

The more medial component (thalamic bundle [ThB]) is directed caudally to penetrate and terminate in the rostral aspect of the reticular nucleus of the thalamus before entering and terminating in the anterior thalamic nuclei (AV and AD), the parvocellular component of MD, the intralaminar nuclei (CL, Pcn, and Pf), and more caudally in the LP and PM nuclei (Scs. 81, 85, 89, 93).

Some fibers from the lateral component of the capsular system move medially below the thalamus to terminate in the zona incerta (ZI), as well as in the hypothalamus (Scs. 81, 85).

The bulk of the laterally situated capsular fibers (pontine bundle [PB]) descend sharply at the level of the genu and the most rostral part of the posterior limb of the internal capsule (ICp-1, Sc. 81) to enter the medial aspect of the cerebral peduncle at a level corresponding to the optic tract just anterior to the LGN (Scs. 81, 85). These fibers descend to terminate in rostral to caudal levels of the basis pontis but with a rostral predominance, situated within the paramedian and dorsomedial pontine nuclei and in medial aspects of the ventral and peripeduncular nuclei and the NRTP.

Striatal Fibers

From the injection site a prominent aggregation of fibers courses toward and surrounds the rostral aspect of the head of the caudate nucleus. Further caudally, at the level of the ICa, these striatal fibers can be seen in two locations, a dorsal group and a ventral group. The dorsal group of striatal fibers courses medially to enter the Muratoff bundle and travels caudally, immediately above the caudate nucleus. Fibers from the Muratoff bundle provide terminations throughout the head and body of the caudate nucleus (Scs. 41, 49, 57, 65, 73, 81, 85, 89). Some of the fibers in the Muratoff bundle are derived from the FOF, as mentioned above. The ventral group of striatal fibers enters the external capsule and terminates in the medial and ventral aspects of the putamen (Scs. 49, 57, 65, 73, 81, 85, 89).

Finally, some of the fibers within the SLF II and the Muratoff bundle descend into the external and extreme capsules and terminate in the claustrum, in its lateral aspect rostrally and in its ventral part more caudally (Scs. 49, 57, 65, 73, 81, 85, 89).

CASE 31

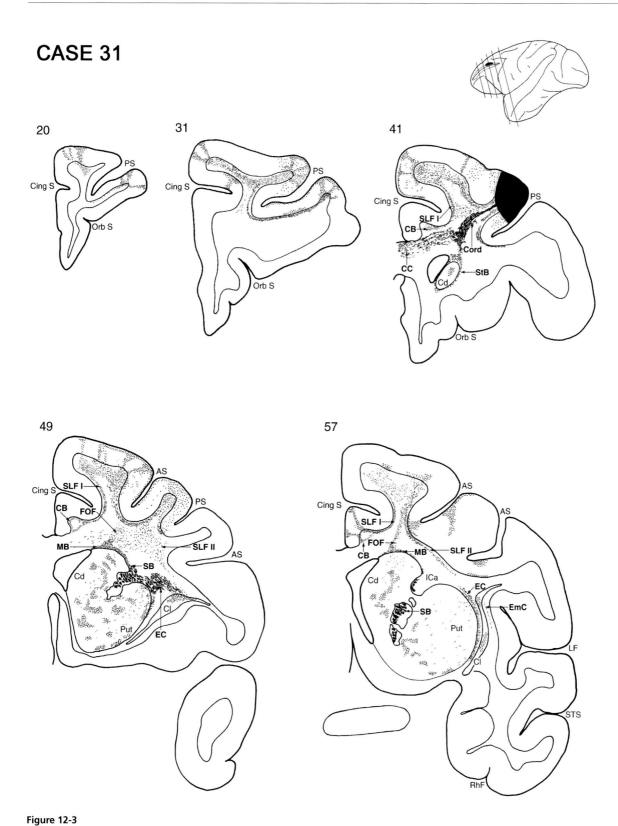

Figure 12-3
Schematic diagrams of 18 rostral–caudal coronal sections in Case 31 taken at the levels shown on the hemispheric diagram above right, showing the isotope injection site in the prefrontal cortex above the midportion of the principal sulcus in area 46d (black-filled area), the resulting trajectories of the cortical association, commissural, and subcortical fibers (dashed lines and dots) in the white matter, and the terminations in the cortex and subcortical regions (black dots).

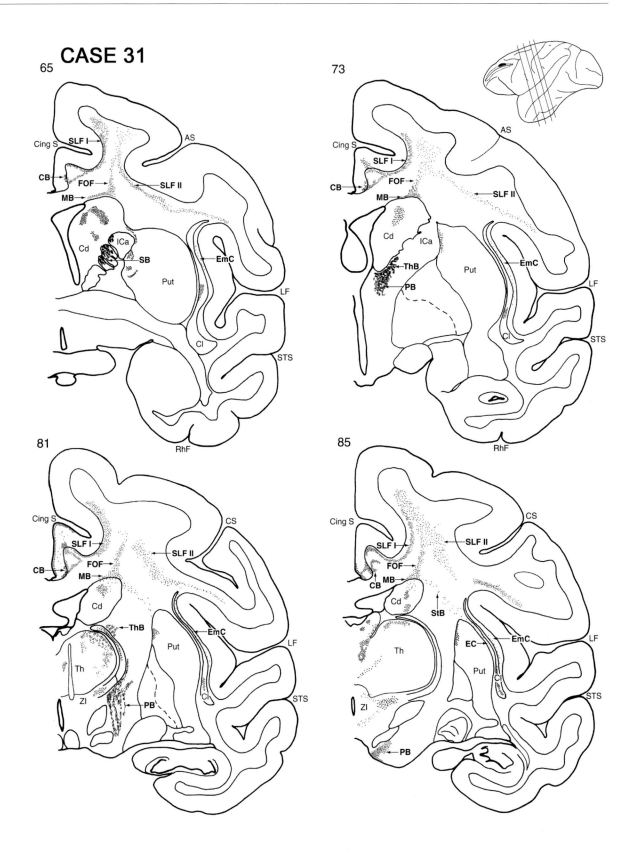

Figure 12-3 (continued)

CASE 31

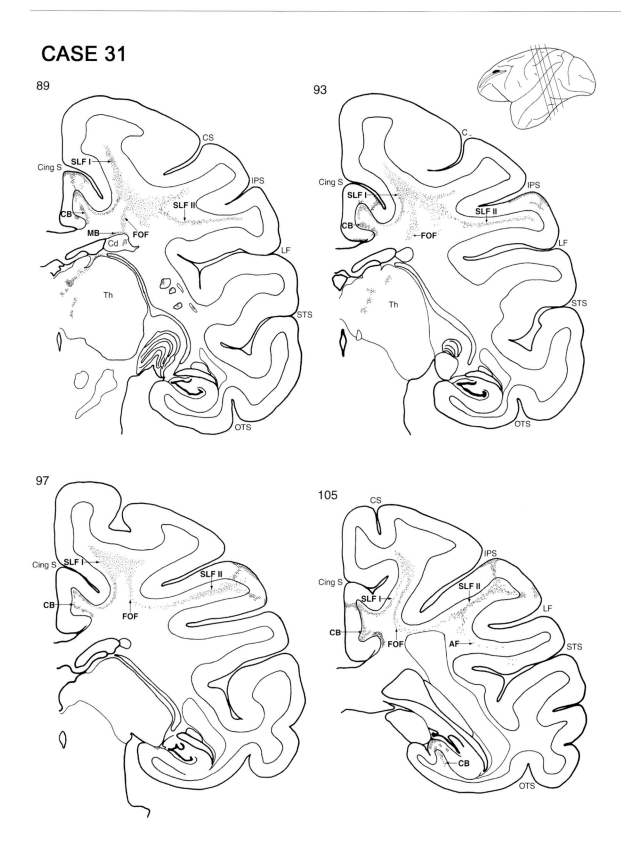

CASE 31

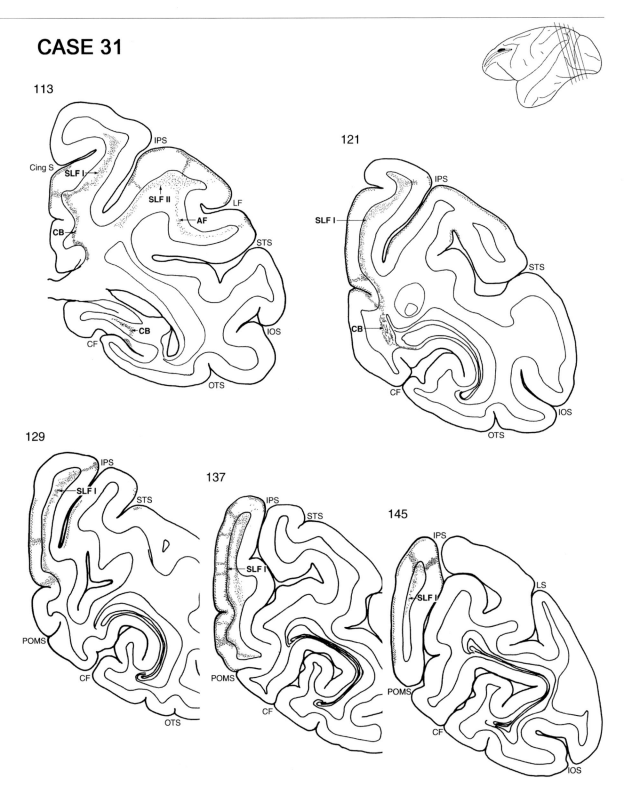

Figure 12-3 (continued)

CASE 31

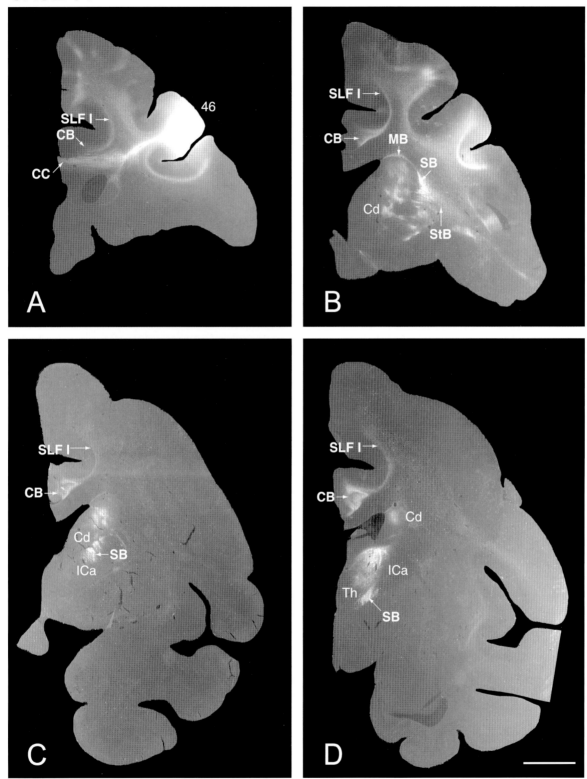

Figure 12-4

Photomicrographs of selected coronal sections of Case 31 showing the injection site in A and the resulting labeled fibers and terminations in A through E. A through D correspond to sections 41, 49, 65, and 81, respectively (Mag = 0.5×, bar = 5 mm). E is a high-power photomicrograph (section 89, Mag = 4×, bar = 0.5 mm) taken from the location indicated in the low-power photomicrograph above, showing caudally directed fibers in the cingulum bundle and the SLF I.

CASE 31

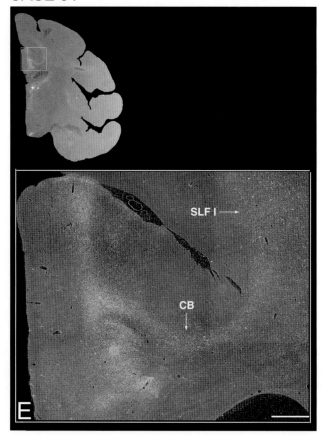

Figure 12-4 (continued)

CASE 32

Isotope was injected in this case in area 9/46v below the midcaudal portion of the principal sulcus (Scs. 31, 41). See figures 12-5 and 12-6.

Association Fibers

Local Association Fibers

Adjacent to the injection site, fibers travel beneath the cortex of the inferior frontal gyrus and terminate in area 47/12, as well as in area 11 in a columnar manner, and in the first layer in area 46v (Scs. 31, 41).

Long Association Fibers

Caudally Directed Fibers

From the injection site a prominent collection of fibers descends into the superior longitudinal fasciculus III (SLF III) lying within the opercular white matter and then progresses caudally in this location. Fibers leave the ventral aspect of this fiber bundle and provide terminations in area ProM in a columnar manner, and in area 6v in a columnar manner with an emphasis in the first layer (Scs. 49, 57, 65). At the dorsal aspect of the SLF III, fibers terminate in the cortex below the principal sulcus in area 8AV, and in area 45B in columns and in the first layer (Scs. 49, 57).

The bulk of the fibers in SLF III continue caudally, closely adjacent to the upper shoulder of the Sylvian fissure and the opercular white matter. As they progress caudally in this location, the SLF III fibers provide terminations to the gustatory area, area SII, and areas 1 and 3 in a columnar manner (Scs. 49, 57, 65, 73). The dorsally situated fibers of SLF III terminate in areas 44 and 6v in a columnar manner with a first-layer preference (Scs. 57, 65).

As the SLF III progresses caudally in the ventral part of the opercular white matter in the postcentral region, it continues to provide columnar terminations to SII cortex and first-layer terminations in area PF in the rostral part of the inferior parietal lobule (Scs. 73, 81, 85).

Upon entering the parietal lobe, the SLF III occupies the central part of the white matter of the inferior parietal lobule. From this location terminations are given off to the inferior parietal lobule in areas PF, PFG, and PG, both in a columnar manner and in the first layer (Scs. 89, 93, 97, 105, 113, 121).

A separate group of fibers travels medially from the injection site and descends to form two distinct bundles: a dorsal component lying in the extreme capsule (EmC) and a ventral contingent that continues in the uncinate fasciculus (UF).

Fibers in the extreme capsule provide columnar terminations to the dysgranular insula (Sc. 73).

The UF travels caudally from the injection site, traverses the limen insulae, and descends into the white matter of the temporal stem. Here the UF fibers are situated deep to the fundus of the superior temporal sulcus (STS) and then in the white matter of the inferior temporal gyrus. The fibers terminate in the fundus of the STS in area IPa, and in the ventral bank of the STS in areas TEa and TEm in a columnar manner and in the first layer, and in area TE1 in a columnar manner (Scs. 57, 73, 81).

Fibers destined for the cingulate cortex travel medially from the injection site. At the level of the rostral part of the head of the caudate nucleus they ascend obliquely to enter the CB. These fibers then travel caudally within the CB and terminate in columns in the rostral part of area 24 (Sc. 57).

Rostrally Directed Fibers

Fibers travel rostrally from the injection site within the white matter of the inferior frontal gyrus and terminate in columns and in the first layer in area 10 and in the first layer in area 46v (Sc. 20). Other fibers leave the injection site and travel medially, ventral to the cord of fibers, and enter the UF. These fibers progress rostrally and medially in a plate-like manner lying in the white matter beneath the orbital cortex and provide columnar terminations to the orbital proisocortex and more rostrally to areas 13 and 11 (Scs. 31, 41, 49).

Commissural and Subcortical Fibers

From the injection site a dense cord of fibers travels medially toward the rostral part of the head of the caudate nucleus (Sc. 41).

A prominent dorsal contingent of cord fibers ascends and courses medially toward the genu of the corpus callosum, enters the genu in the rostral part of sector CC1 (Sc. 41), and travels to the opposite hemisphere, mostly in the ventral part of the genu (Scs. 41, 49).

Other fibers within the cord traveling medially gather in multiple discrete bundles and descend obliquely into the rostral aspect of the anterior limb of the internal capsule (ICa-2, Sc. 49) before progressing caudally. Just rostral to the genu of the internal capsule in level ICa-6 (Sc. 73), the fibers in this subcortical bundle (SB) differentiate into two major components (Sc. 73).

A dorsomedial component of fibers (thalamic bundle [ThB]) aggregates anterior to the reticular nucleus (Sc. 73) and enters the thalamus. These fibers terminate in the intralaminar nuclei (Pcn, CL, and CM), as well as in the MD and PO nuclei (Scs. 81, 85, 89, 93).

The ventral and lateral component of fibers (pontine bundle [PB]) descends sharply in the capsule at level ICa-6 (Sc. 73) and courses toward the medial part of the cerebral peduncle. These fibers terminate in the medial and rostral parts of the basis pontis in the paramedian and dorsomedial pontine nuclei and in medial parts of the peripeduncular nucleus.

Striatal Fibers

The fibers destined for the striatum accumulate in the white matter of the inferior frontal gyrus between the striatum and the SLF III. From this location fibers can be seen heading in two directions.

Medially directed fibers travel above the ICa and enter the Muratoff bundle. These fibers then course caudally and provide terminations to the head of the caudate nucleus, concentrated in its lateral aspect (Scs. 49, 57, 65, 73, 81).

Ventrally directed fibers descend into the external capsule (EC), coursing caudally until they reach the most caudal aspects of the putamen. Throughout their course in the external capsule these fibers provide intense terminations to the putamen, predominantly in its ventromedial portions (Scs. 49, 57, 65, 73, 81, 85).

At rostral levels, fibers descending from the Muratoff bundle are situated at the most medial aspect of the head of the caudate nucleus. Here they come together with the fibers ascending medially from the external capsule (Scs. 41, 49). Some of the fibers from the extreme and external capsules terminate in the rostral part of the claustrum (Sc. 57).

CASE 32

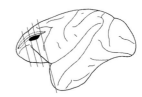

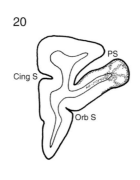

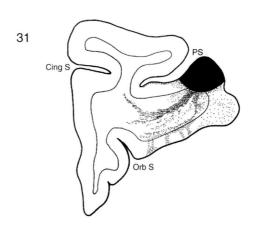

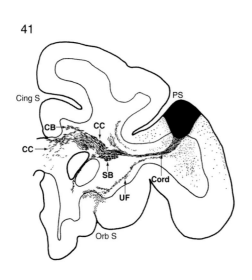

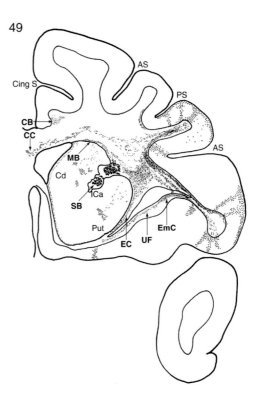

Figure 12-5

Schematic diagrams of 15 rostral–caudal coronal sections in Case 32 taken at the levels shown on the hemispheric diagram above right, showing the isotope injection site in the middle part of ventral area 46 in both the sulcal and gyral cortices (black-filled area), the resulting trajectories of the cortical association, commissural, and subcortical fibers (dashed lines and dots) in the white matter, and the terminations in the cortex and subcortical regions (black dots).

CASE 32

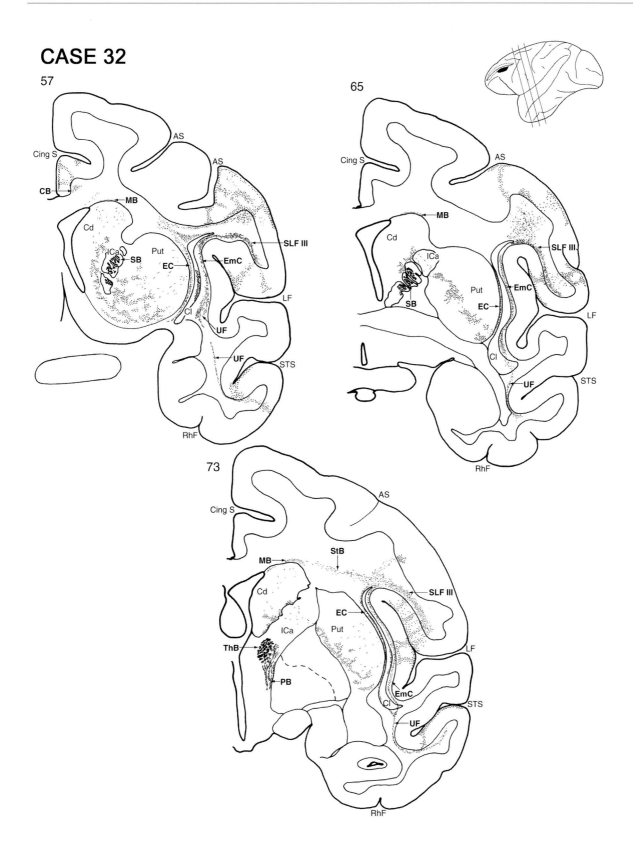

CASE 32

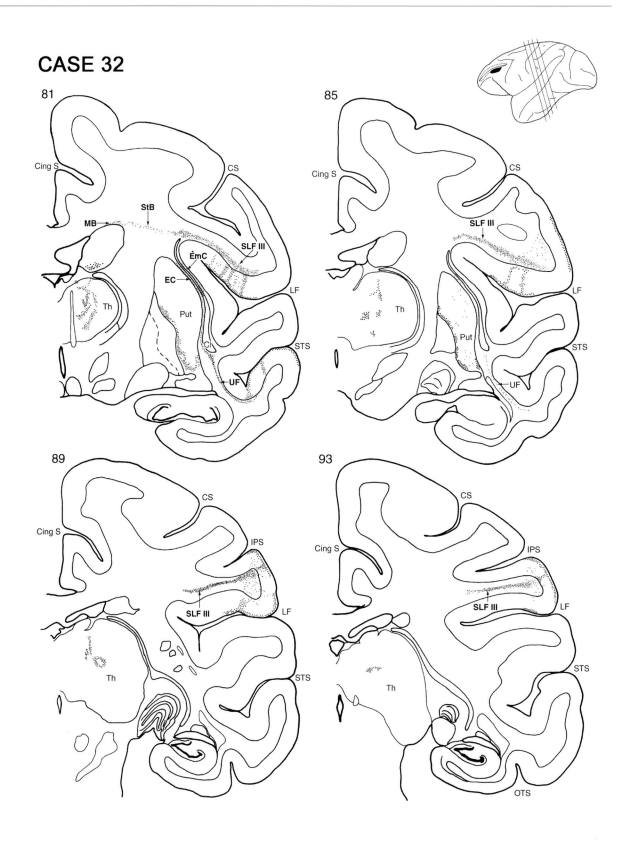

Figure 12-5 (continued)

CASE 32

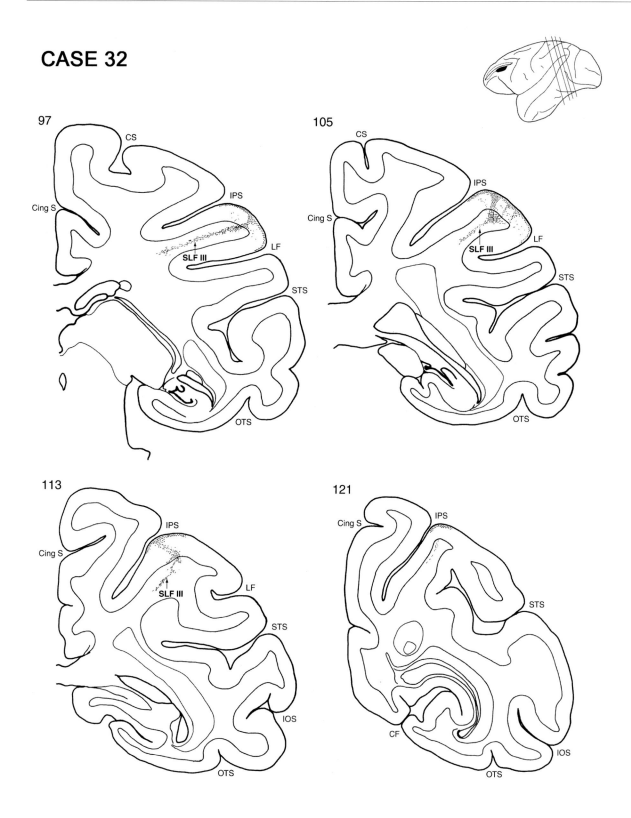

CASE 32

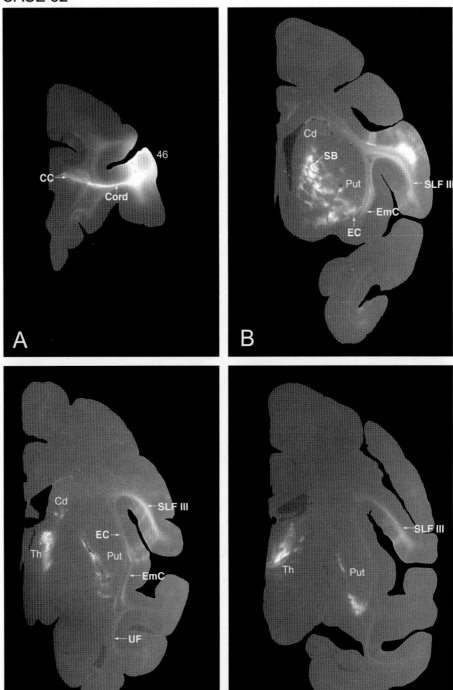

Figure 12-6

Photomicrographs of selected coronal sections of Case 32 showing the injection site in A with the injection halo in B, and the resulting labeled fibers and terminations in A through E. A through D correspond to sections 41, 57, 73, and 81 respectively (Mag = 0.5×, bar = 5 mm). E is a high-power photomicrograph (section 89, Mag = 4×, bar = 0.5 mm) taken from the location indicated in the low-power photomicrograph above, showing fibers in the SLF III terminating in the inferior parietal lobule, in the first layer of area PF.

CASE 32

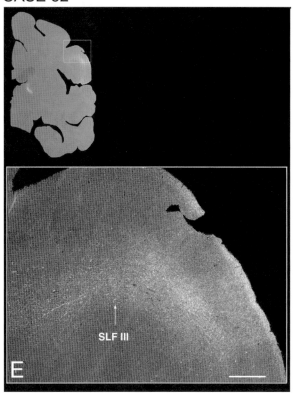

CASE 33

In this case the isotope was injected in the orbital frontal cortex in the orbital part of area 47/12, encroaching posteriorly on the insular proisocortex (Scs. 41, 49). See figures 12-7 and 12-8.

Association Fibers

Local Association Fibers

Locally directed fibers terminate in a diffuse columnar manner in the medial part of area 47/12 and in the ventral part of area 6, predominantly in the first layer (Scs. 41, 49).

Long Association Fibers

Caudally Directed Fibers

Association fibers from the injection site travel within four distinct fiber bundles: the extreme capsule, the SLF III in the opercular white matter, the CB, and the UF.

A distinct aggregate of long association fibers leaves the injection site and travels caudally deep to the insular cortex, lying within the extreme capsule (EmC) and occupying its entire dorsal to ventral extent. These fibers leave the EmC and terminate ventrally in the insular proisocortex, as well as in the middle and dorsal parts of the insula dysgranular cortex. The insular terminations are in a columnar manner, with a first-layer predominance (Scs. 65, 69, 73, 78, 81, 85). Fibers at the ventral part of the extreme capsule enter the middle longitudinal fasciculus (MdLF) in the white matter of the superior temporal gyrus and terminate in the rostral part of the cortex in the upper bank of the superior temporal sulcus (STS) in areas PGa and TPO, predominantly in the first layer (Scs. 78, 81, 85).

From the injection site fibers travel caudally in the SLF III lying in the opercular (Sylvian) white matter. Some fibers leave the SLF III and move laterally within the opercular white matter to terminate in the precentral portion of area 3 (Sc. 65). The remainder of the fibers lying within SLF III terminate in the cortex of the dorsal Sylvian operculum, rostrally within the gustatory cortex, and further caudally within SII, in the first layer (Scs. 57, 81, 85).

Other association fibers leave the injection site and course dorsally and medially, traversing the white matter above the internal capsule to enter the white matter of the cingulate gyrus, passing through the CB. These fibers terminate in the first layer of the cingulate gyrus in area 24 (Scs. 49, 57, 65, 69).

Another group of fibers emanating from area 47/12 courses medially and ventrally via the UF. These fibers descend in the temporal stem and provide terminations medial to the rhinal fissure, in the prorhinal and entorhinal cortices (Scs. 57, 65, 69, 73). Uncinate fibers also terminate in the amygdala (Scs. 57, 65, 69, 73). Some of the fibers of the UF terminate in lateral forebrain areas (Scs. 57, 65).

Rostrally Directed Fibers

Rostrally directed association fibers from area 47/12 course via four fiber bundles: the extreme capsule, SLF I, the CB, and the rostral segments of the UF.

Fibers that enter the extreme capsule proceed rostrally in the white matter deep to the orbital cortex and in the ventral bank of the principal sulcus. These fibers terminate predominantly in area 11 and in the first layer in the rostral part of ventral area 46 and in the ventral part of area 10 (Scs. 20, 31).

A medially directed fiber system courses deep to the principal sulcus and moves dorsally to lie within the SLF I, situated medially in the white matter of the superior frontal gyrus. These fibers proceed rostrally in this location and terminate in area 9, dorsal area 46, and dorsal area 10 (Sc. 31).

Fibers stream medially from the injection site and lie in the UF, which occupies the white matter immediately adjacent to the caudal part of the orbital cortex. These fibers, present in the lateral to medial extent of the UF, give rise to predominantly columnar terminations in the orbital cortex in areas 12, 13, 25, and 14 (Scs. 31, 41, 49).

Some fibers that ascend medially into the CB travel rostrally in this location deep to the cingulate gyrus and terminate in area 24, with an emphasis in the first layer (Sc. 31).

Commissural and Subcortical Fibers

A dense cord of labeled fibers penetrates the white matter and ascends medially from the injection site. From this cord of fibers one contingent continues dorsally and medially above the internal capsule and enters the genu of the corpus callosum. The fibers cross the callosum mostly in the ventral half of the genu (sector CC1) and enter the opposite hemisphere (Scs. 41, 49).

A small contingent of fibers runs caudally, lateral to the claustrum and above the UF, before passing medially to enter the anterior commissure and heading toward the opposite hemisphere (Sc. 65).

A major aggregate of fibers leaves the cord and is poised at the rostral and lateral aspects of the anterior limb of the internal capsule (ICa-1, ICa-2). These fibers then descend gradually in the ICa as they proceed caudally, occupying a middle and lateral position within the capsule. At the level of the genu (Sc. 78), the fibers in this subcortical bundle (SB) separate into distinct components. One contingent (thalamic bundle [ThB]) continues caudally as whorls of fibers that penetrate the thalamus and provide terminations to the ventral part of the MD nucleus throughout much of its rostrocaudal extent. Terminations are also present in the rostral part of the VA nucleus and in the midline and intralaminar thalamic nuclei (Scs. 78, 81, 85, 89, 93, 97).

The remaining fibers within the capsule (pontine bundle [PB]) descend at the level of the genu (Sc. 78) to lie in the most medial and rostral parts of the cerebral peduncle. They move medially at the level of the mammillary body and terminate in the lateral hypothalamic area (Scs. 78, 81).

Some fibers that emerge from the orbital cortex travel along with the UF as it moves medially and provide terminations to the basal forebrain. These fibers then continue medially, travel above the optic tract, curve around the ansa lenticularis, and then ascend in the inferior thalamic peduncle (ITP) before terminating in the hypothalamus and in the bed nucleus of the stria terminalis (Scs. 73, 78, 81).

Striatal Fibers

Fibers destined for the striatum ascend medially from the injection site. At the lateral aspect of the putamen they enter the external capsule (EC) and then terminate in the ventral putamen (Scs. 49, 57, 65, 69, 73, 78, 81, 85). Some of these fibers continue medially within the putamen, heading toward the ventral part of the head of the caudate nucleus, where they terminate (Scs. 49, 57, 65, 69, 73, 78, 81). Some fibers in the external capsule also terminate in the middle and ventral parts of the claustrum (Scs. 57, 65, 69, 78, 81, 85). A few striatal fibers ascend to lie within the Muratoff bundle, from where they contribute some terminations to the dorsal part of the head of the caudate nucleus (Sc. 49).

CASE 33

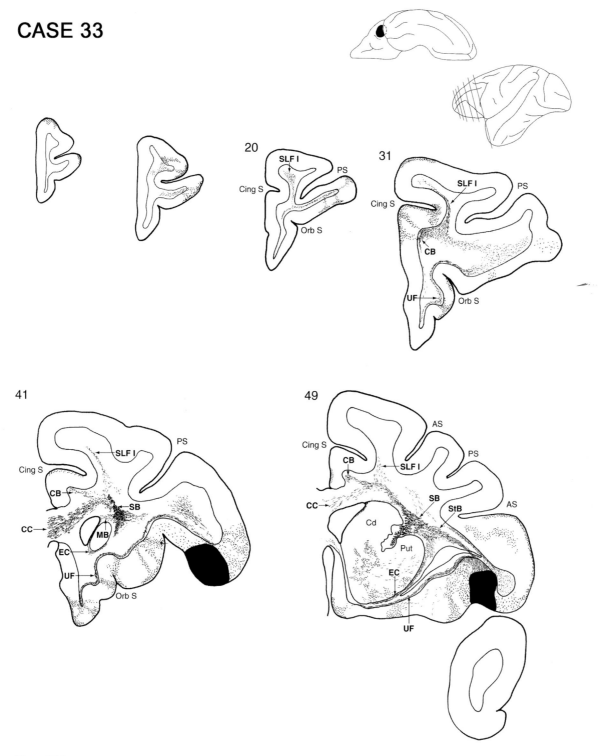

Figure 12-7
Schematic diagrams of 16 rostral–caudal coronal sections in Case 33 taken at the levels shown on the hemispheric diagrams above right, showing the isotope injection site in the orbital frontal cortex in the orbital part of area 47/12, encroaching posteriorly on the insular proisocortex (black-filled area). The resulting trajectories of the cortical association, commissural, and subcortical fibers in the white matter are shown (dashed lines and dots), as well as the terminations in the cortex and subcortical regions (black dots).

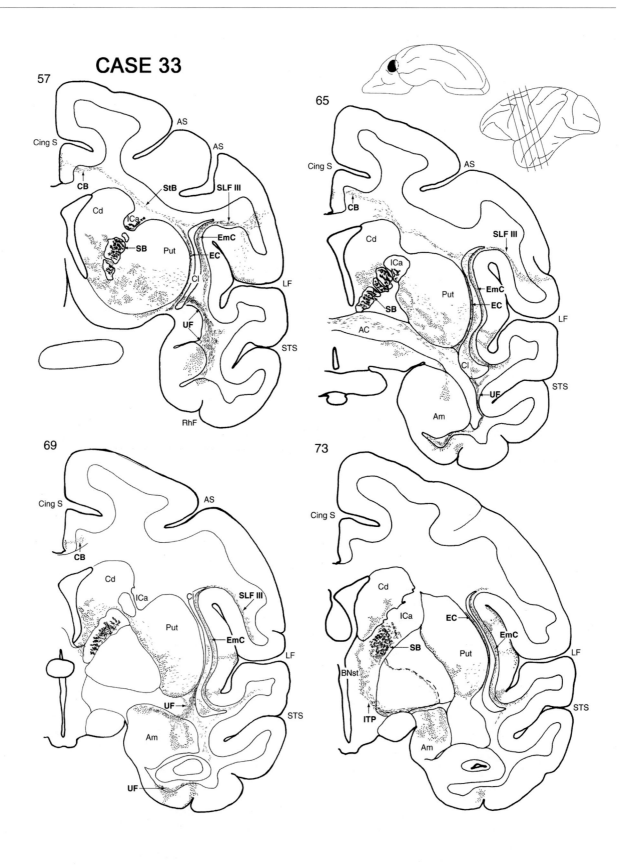

Figure 12-7 (continued)

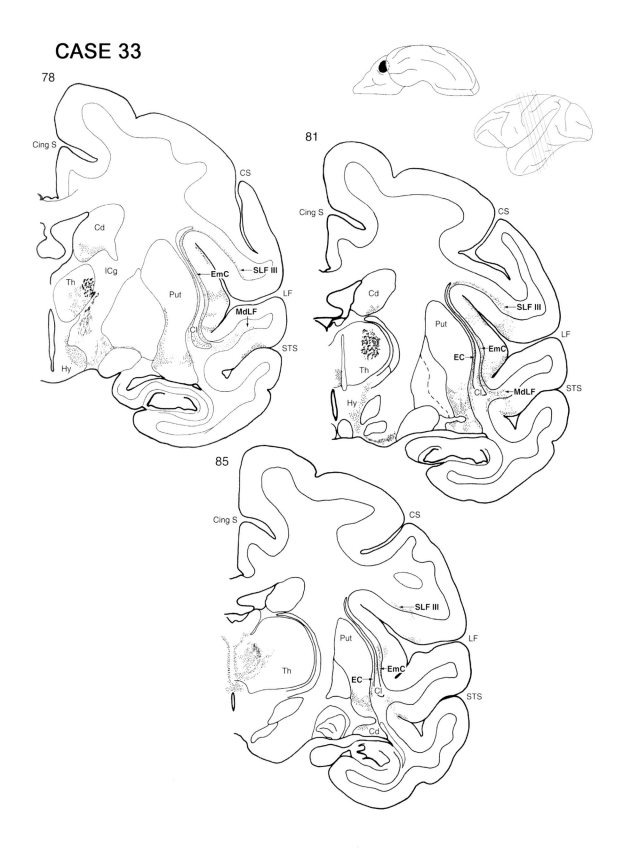

78

Cing S

CS

Cd

ICg

Th

Put

EmC

SLF III

LF

MdLF

Cl

STS

Hy

81

Cing S

CS

Cd

Th

SLF III

Put

LF

EC

EmC

Cl

MdLF

STS

Hy

85

Cing S

CS

Th

SLF III

Put

LF

EC

EmC

Cl

STS

Cd

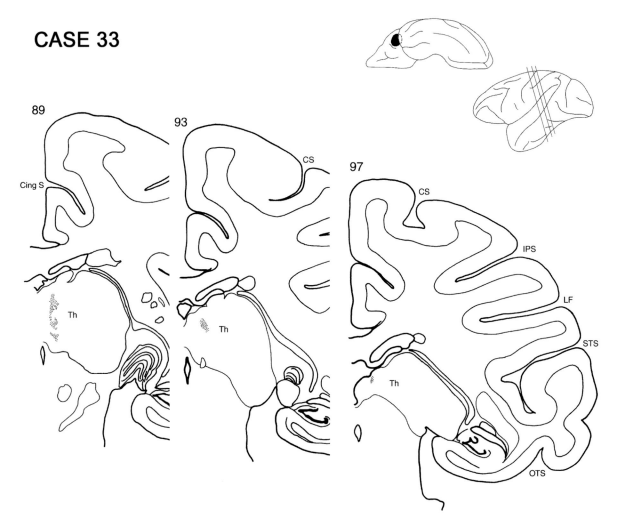

Figure 12-7 (continued)

CASE 33

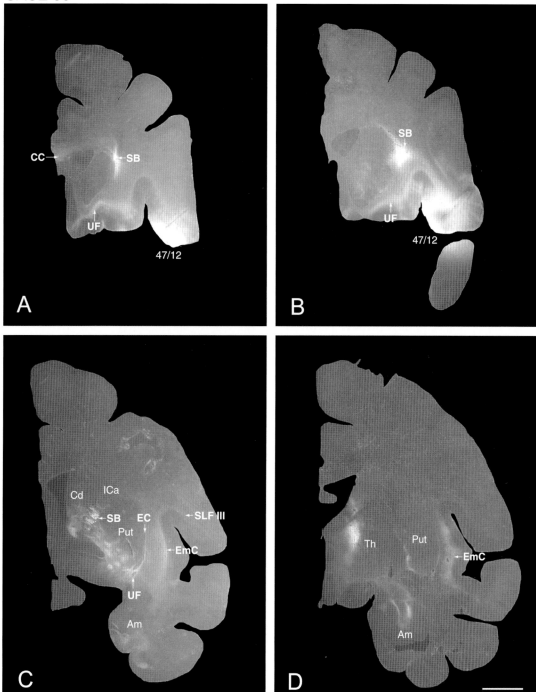

Figure 12-8

Photomicrographs of selected coronal sections of Case 33 showing the injection site in A and B and the resulting labeled fibers and terminations in A through D. A through D correspond to sections 41, 49, 57, and 73, respectively (Mag = 0.5×, bar = 5 mm).

Prefrontal Cortex Summary

Association Fibers

The prefrontal cortex sends long association projections to other cortical areas via the cingulum bundle, superior longitudinal fasciculus (subcomponents I, II and III), the fronto-occipital fasciculus, uncinate fasciculus, the extreme capsule, and the middle longitudinal fasciculus (figure 12-9).

Lateral Orbital Cortex

Two major association fiber bundles emerge from the orbital area: the uncinate fasciculus and the extreme capsule. Some fibers are also conveyed by the SLF III and the cingulum bundle.

1. Uncinate Fasciculus

The uncinate fibers course rostrally and medially through the orbital white matter and terminate in areas 12, 13, 25, and 14. Caudally directed fibers of the uncinate fasciculus course via the limen insulae and reach the temporal polar cortex, from where they terminate in the amygdala, perirhinal cortex (area 35), and entorhinal cortex.

2. Extreme Capsule

The rostrally directed fibers of the extreme capsule terminate in ventral area 46, area 10, and area 11. The caudally directed fibers of the extreme capsule terminate in the insular proisocortex and the dysgranular insula and via the middle longitudinal fasciculus to the multimodal areas in the rostral part of areas TPO and PGa in the upper bank of the superior temporal sulcus.

3. Superior Longitudinal Fasciculus III

Some fibers from area 47/12 are conveyed by the SLF III. These course through the frontal operculum and terminate predominantly in the rostral part of area SII, as well as in the precentral portion of area 3 and the gustatory area.

4. Cingulum Bundle

The cingulate fibers cross medially from the orbital cortex, gather in the cingulum bundle, and terminate in areas 32 and 24.

Ventral Area 46

The main association fiber bundles emerging from ventral area 46 are the uncinate fasciculus and the SLF III. Some fibers are also conveyed in the extreme capsule and the cingulum bundle.

1. Uncinate Fasciculus

Fibers from ventral area 46 course rostrally through the orbital white matter of the orbital cortex in the uncinate fasciculus and terminate in the orbital proisocortex and areas 13 and 11. Fibers traveling caudally in the uncinate fasciculus from ventral area 46 course via the limen insulae and reach the temporal pole. These fibers travel in the white matter deep to the superior temporal sulcus and terminate in the cortex of the lower bank of the STS, in areas IPa and TEm, and in area TE1.

2. Superior Longitudinal Fasciculus III

The SLF III fibers first travel via the white matter of the frontal operculum and terminate in ventral prefrontal and frontal areas 8AV, 45B, 44, 6v, gustatory area, and precentral areas 1 and 3. The fibers continue caudally in the parietal operculum and terminate in areas SII, PF, and PFop. Further caudally, the SLF III fibers course through the white matter of the inferior parietal lobule in the same location as those of the SLF II, and from this location they terminate in areas PFG, PG, and PGop.

3. Extreme Capsule

Some of the fibers from ventral area 46 course via the extreme capsule. Rostrally the fibers course laterally through the white matter of the inferior frontal gyrus and terminate in areas 10 and 46v. Caudally, the extreme capsule fibers terminate mainly in the dysgranular insula.

4. Cingulum Bundle

Some of the fibers from ventral area 46 course medially and continue in the cingulum bundle, from where they terminate in the rostral part of area 24.

Dorsal Area 46

The principal fiber pathways emanating from the dorsal part of area 46 are the SLF I, SLF II, cingulum bundle, and fronto-occipital fasciculus.

1. Superior Longitudinal Fasciculus I

The fibers in the SLF I that arise from dorsal area 46 move medially in the white matter of the superior frontal gyrus and terminate in the medial and dorsal parts of area 9. Further caudally in the frontal lobe, SLF I fibers terminate in dorsal area 6. The SLF I continues caudally, remaining primarily around the dorsal part of the cingulate sulcus, and it results in terminations in area 31 in the medial parietal cortex. These fibers then spread out in the caudal part of the white matter of the superior parietal lobule and terminate in areas PGm, PEc, and PO.

2. Superior Longitudinal Fasciculus II

The SLF II is located in the white matter of the superior frontal gyrus, closely adjacent to the arcuate and principal sulci. Rostrally it provides terminations to areas 8Ad, 46, and 10. Caudally, the SLF II courses around the caudal part of the arcuate sulcus and terminates in dorsal area 6. It continues through the white matter deep to the central sulcus and above the upper shoulder of the Sylvian fissure, and subsequently in the white matter of the inferior parietal lobule. At this level it provides terminations to areas PG and PGop. The fibers of the SLF II in the white matter of the inferior parietal lobule continue further caudally and terminate in areas PG, POa, and Opt. Some of the fibers of the SLF II arch around the caudal end of the Sylvian fissure and terminate in areas TPO and Tpt of the superior temporal region.

3. Cingulum Bundle

A distinct fiber system leaves dorsal area 46, moves medially in the white matter, and localizes discretely within the cingulum bundle. Some fibers terminate in area 24 and others continue caudally, remaining mainly in the white matter deep to the cingulate sulcus and in the periphery of the cingulum bundle, terminating in area 23. Further caudally, the fibers arch around the splenium of the corpus callosum and enter the ventral part of the cingulum bundle in the parahippocampal gyrus. These fibers terminate in area prostriata, the retrosplenial area in the banks of the calcarine sulcus, and the caudal part of the presubiculum.

4. Fronto-Occipital Fasciculus

A distinct fiber bundle that leaves area 46d occupies a position between the SLF I and SLF II fibers, being situated in the FOF in the white matter above the caudate nucleus, lateral to the corpus callosum and medial to the corona radiata. The FOF fibers course caudally and merge dorsally with the fibers of the SLF II. Because the FOF merges with the SLF II, it may share the terminations of the SLF II in the inferior parietal lobule. By virtue of FOF fibers entering the Muratoff bundle, the FOF may also contribute to the striatum.

Area 32 at the Medial Prefrontal Convexity

Rostrally directed fibers from area 32 in the prefrontal cortex course in three directions: dorsally, ventrally, and laterally. The dorsally running fibers course in the white matter of the superior frontal gyrus and terminate mainly in area 9. The ventral fibers descend along the medial wall of the prefrontal cortex and terminate in area 14. The lateral group of fibers runs in the white matter of the inferior frontal gyrus and terminates in area 46 in the lower bank of the principal sulcus.

The caudally directed association fibers from area 32 are conveyed in three separate fiber pathways: the cingulum bundle, uncinate fasciculus, and extreme capsule.

1. Cingulum Bundle

One component of association fibers occupies the CB. Some of these fibers terminate in area 24. The remaining fibers of the CB continue caudally as far as the splenium of the corpus callosum, where they provide terminations to the dorsal retrosplenial area, arch around the splenium, and terminate in the ventral portion of area 30 in the calcarine sulcus.

2. Uncinate Fasciculus

A second long association fiber system courses medially and ventrally and continues caudally as the UF. These fibers terminate in area 25 and the periallocortex before entering the temporal polar white matter, where they terminate in the amygdala.

3. Extreme Capsule

A laterally directed group of fibers emanates from area 32 and enters the extreme capsule. These fibers terminate in area 47/12 and the insular proisocortex.

Callosal Fibers

The fibers from the prefrontal cortices that course to the opposite hemisphere travel first with the fibers in the cord and then enter the genu and rostrum of the corpus callosum. They cross the midline at this level in callosal sector CC1. The fibers from dorsal area 46 and medial hemisphere area 32 course through the rostral part of the genu. The fibers from the ventral part of area 46 and the orbitofrontal cortex extend further caudally within the genu. Callosal fibers from the medial, ventral, and orbital prefrontal cortices are relatively ventral in location, whereas those from the dorsolateral prefrontal cortex are more dorsally situated in the genu. In addition, fibers arising from the orbital prefrontal cortex travel to the opposite hemisphere through the rostral and central parts of the anterior commissure.

Subcortical Fibers

Medial Prefrontal Area 32 (Case 30)

From medial prefrontal area 32, subcortical fibers in the form of a cord course laterally, and at the rostral pole of the caudate nucleus they occupy a position lateral to the caudate nucleus. These fibers proceed caudally, enter the rostral aspect of the anterior limb of the internal capsule (ICa), and descend obliquely. Rostral to the genu of the internal capsule these subcortical fibers divide into two groups. A dorsal contingent of fibers penetrates the rostral pole of the thalamus and terminates in most of the rostral to caudal extent of MDmc, as well as in the AV, AM, Pf, and midline thalamic nuclei. The more ventrally situated fibers descend in the genu of the capsule, provide terminations medially to the zona incerta and hypothalamus, and continue into the cerebral peduncle before terminating in the medially situated basilar pontine nuclei.

Dorsal Area 46 (Case 31)

The subcortical fibers in the form of a cord that arises from dorsal area 46 course medially through the white matter of the superior frontal gyrus. They travel ventrally and medially, aggregate in the medial part of the anterior limb of the internal capsule (ICa), and gradually descend as they are directed caudally. Immediately rostral to the genu of the internal capsule, the fibers divide into two components. At the genu, the dorsal component enters the dorsal segment of the external medullary lamina and terminates in the anterior thalamic nuclei (AV and AD), MDpc, the intralaminar nuclei (CL, Pcn, Pf), and more caudally in the LP and PM nuclei.

The ventral component continues to course caudally into the ventral aspect of the posterior limb of the internal capsule (ICp). Some fibers move medially and terminate in the zona incerta and the hypothalamus. The major strands of descending fibers enter the medial compartment of the cerebral peduncle and terminate in the medial pontine nuclei.

Ventral Area 46 (Case 32)

The subcortically directed fibers that emanate from ventral area 46 travel medially in the cord. At the level of the rostral pole of the caudate nucleus, the subcortical fibers enter the rostral aspect of the ICa. The fibers travel caudally while descending gradually within the ICa. At the caudal part of the ICa, the fibers divide into two components. The medial and dorsal segment penetrates the reticular nucleus at the rostral pole of the thalamus and terminates in the intralaminar nuclei (Pcn, CL, CM) and MD, and further caudally in the PO nucleus. The ventral and lateral segment of fibers continues to descend into the medial portion of the cerebral peduncle and terminates in the medial part of the rostral pons.

Orbital Prefrontal Cortex (Case 33)

From the orbital prefrontal cortex the subcortical fibers travel in the cord of fibers, ascend and move medially, and lie lateral to the anterior aspect of the ICa. These fibers then descend medially into the ICa and move caudally to the level of the genu. Some fibers at the genu continue caudally, penetrate the reticular nucleus of the thalamus, and travel within the thalamus, providing terminations to the ventral part of the MD nucleus throughout much of its rostrocaudal extent, as well to the VA, intralaminar, and midline nuclei. The remaining fibers in the genu of the internal capsule descend in the most rostral part of the ICp, enter the rostral and anterior aspect of the cerebral peduncle, move medially, and terminate in the lateral hypothalamic area.

Corticostriate Projections

The prefrontal cortex provides extensive projections to the head of the caudate nucleus, the nucleus accumbens, and the rostral putamen, with lesser input to the body of the caudate nucleus and minimal projections to the middle and caudal zones of the putamen.

Striatal fibers from area 32 course initially along with the subcortical fibers and surround the rostral pole of the head of the caudate nucleus. Further caudally, these striatal fibers divide into two components. The dorsal component courses caudally in the Muratoff bundle and terminates in patches throughout the medial sectors of the head and body of the caudate nucleus. The ventrally situated striatal fibers cross the anterior limb of the internal capsule (ICa), run in the external capsule, and terminate in the dorsolateral part of the putamen rostrally, the dorsal and medial regions of the putamen further caudally, and the midregion of the claustrum. Terminations in the rostral part of the ventral striatum are conveyed by the external capsule as it curves beneath the putamen, and by fibers that descend through the caudate nucleus from the Muratoff bundle.

The striatal fibers from dorsal and ventral areas 9/46 are first intermingled with the subcortical fibers in the cord, and they surround the rostral pole of the head of the caudate nucleus. At the most rostral aspect of the ICa, the striatal fibers divide into a dorsal and a ventral segment. The fibers from area 9/46d in the dorsal segment first course through the fronto-occipital bundle and then aggregate in the subcallosal fasciculus of Muratoff, travel caudally, and provide terminations to the intermediate and dorsal sectors of the head and body of the caudate nucleus. The ventrally situated striatal fibers from area 9/46d gather in the external capsule and are directed to the nucleus accumbens, the dorsal and medial sectors of the putamen, and the claustrum (dorsal part of the claustrum rostrally and ventral part caudally). The dorsal component of fibers from ventral area 9/46 enters the Muratoff bundle and gives rise to terminations in the ventral and lateral parts of the head and body of the caudate nucleus. The ventral component courses in the external capsule and results in substantial projections to the nucleus accumbens and to intermediate regions of the rostral putamen and medial and ventral parts of the caudal putamen. Fibers from area 9/46v travel through the external capsule to the middle and ventral regions of the claustrum.

The fibers destined for the striatum arising from the orbital cortex, area 47/12, ascend medially from the injection site and at the lateral aspect of the putamen they descend into the external capsule. The fibers curve ventrally and medially around the lateral part of the rostral putamen and provide extensive projections to the ventral and lateral parts of the rostral putamen, the ventral and lateral parts of the head of the caudate nucleus, and the nucleus accumbens. The external capsule fibers terminate further caudally in the ventral and lateral parts of the body of the caudate nucleus, the medial part of the caudal putamen, and the ventral region of the claustrum. Unlike other prefrontal regions, area 47/12 has projections to the caudally situated ventral putamen and the tail of the caudate nucleus.

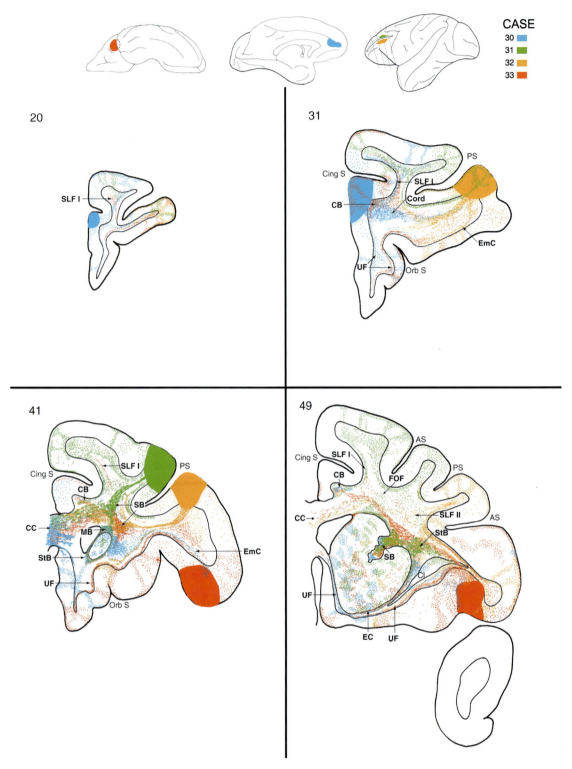

CASE
30 ■
31 ■
32 ■
33 ■

20

31

41

49

Figure 12-9

Schematic composite diagrams of the rostral–caudal coronal sections of the template brain, illustrating the four prefrontal cases (Cases 30 through 33). The injection sites and the association, commissural, and subcortical fibers, as well as the termination patterns, are color-coded for each case. The schematic diagrams of the basal, medial, and lateral surfaces of the cerebral hemispheres (at top) rep-

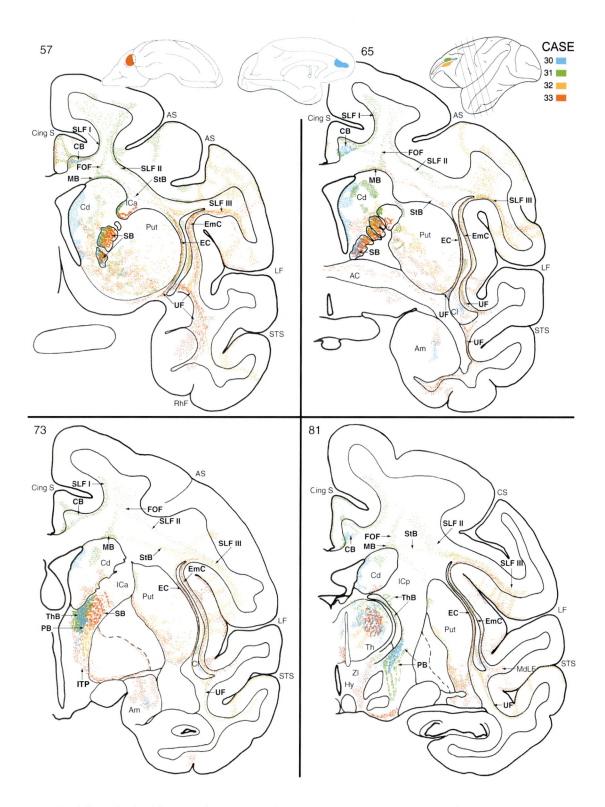

resent the different levels of the coronal sections and the injection sites. Color-coding is as follows: Case 30—blue, medial prefrontal convexity area 32; Case 31—green, area 46d above the midportion of the principal sulcus; Case 32—orange, area 46v below the midportion of the principal sulcus, involving sulcal and gyral cortices; Case 33—red, orbital frontal cortex, area 47/12.

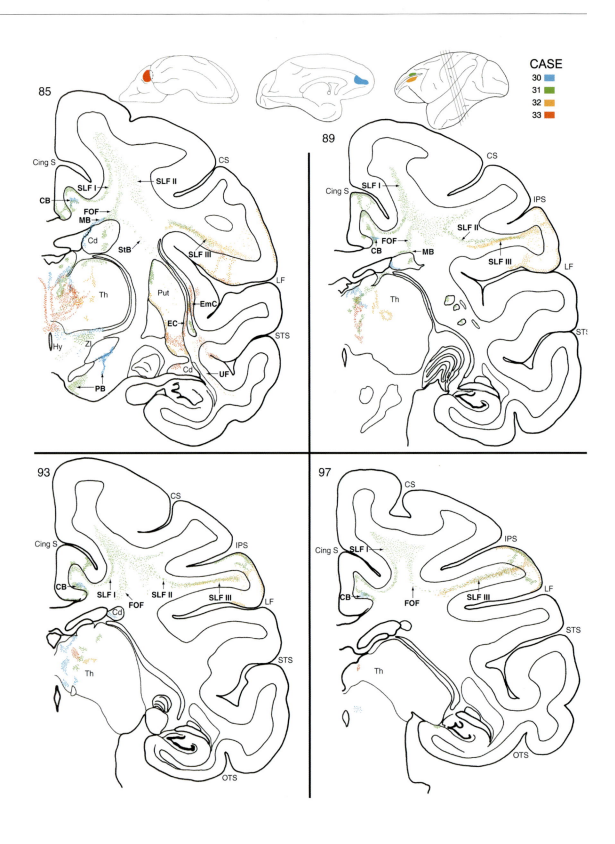

Figure 12-9 (continued)

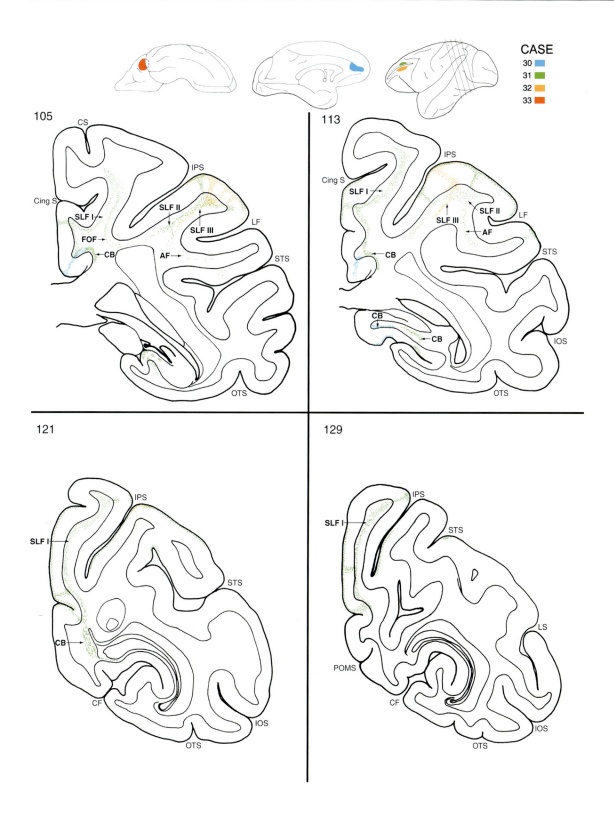

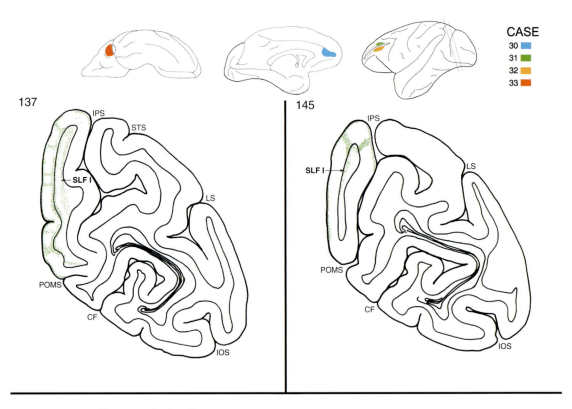

Figure 12-9 (continued)

Connectional Topography and Putative Functional Roles of Individual Fiber Bundles

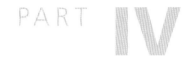

The descriptions of the fiber systems in the individual cases indicate that there are distinct association fiber pathways that course from the post-Rolandic regions to the frontal lobe and from the prefrontal cortex back to the post-Rolandic regions. In addition, the striatal, commissural, and projection fibers arising from each cortical area are also quite distinct. In this section we describe each fiber bundle in the light of the accumulated knowledge regarding its anatomic organization and its possible functional relevance.

Long Association Fiber Pathways

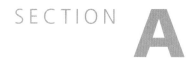

Superior Longitudinal Fasciculus and Arcuate Fasciculus

Separate Pathways With a Shared History

The superior longitudinal fasciculus (SLF) and the arcuate fasciculus (AF) have long been considered synonymous in the human, and these names have been used interchangeably. According to our observations in the monkey, however, they are separate entities. The SLF comprises three subcomponents (SLF I, II, and III) linking the parietal lobe association cortices with the frontal lobe. The AF, by contrast, appears to be separate and distinct from the SLF. Its fibers course adjacent to the SLF II but are distinguished from the SLF II by their location and by the fact that the AF links the caudal part of the superior temporal region with the dorsal prefrontal cortex. Because the SLF and the AF were considered a unitary entity, the historical account of these fiber bundles is presented together as we review the origins of the earlier notions, and how the understanding of these fiber bundles became embedded in neurological anatomy and perpetuated in current terminology.

The first report of what would become known as the AF/SLF system was that of Reil, who used gross fiber dissection in humans to describe an "intermediate myelinated substance . . . that runs from anteriorly to posteriorly, curves around the posterior wall of the [Sylvian] fissure in an arc-like fashion, and then expands in the gyri that occupy the lateral part of the brain as well as its lower border and its basal plane" (Reil, 1809d, pp. 202–203). In his 1812 works, Reil wrote:

> On the roof of the Sylvian fissure where the corpus callosum, the corona radiata of the crus cerebri and the external capsule meet, on the superior edge and on the radiation of the external capsule lies the intermediate myelin substance ("intermediaire Marksubstanz"). [The label "f" in his figure ("Tafel") XII is situated on the arcuate fibers.] It is most massive in the middle of the Sylvian fissure, runs backwards from there, curves concentrically around the ganglion [subcortical gray matter including basal ganglia] and disappears in the gyri of the occipital lobe. In contrast, the intermediate myelin substance is not present in the anterior part of the Sylvian fissure (Reil, 1812a, p. 98).

> [I]t seems to serve the connection of distant gyri (Reil, 1812b, p. 358).

Burdach acknowledged Reil's observations (Burdach, 1822, p. 371, annotation to paragraph 197) and provided a more comprehensive description. He reported (p. 153, paragraph 197) that a

> Bogenbündel (fasciculus arcuatus) is a massive sheath that radiates in the same direction as the cingulum, but unlike the cingulum it is situated in the lateral aspect of the hemisphere. It runs from the temporal lobe posteriorly and supe-

riorly into the occipital lobe and it circles around the Sylvian fissure through the parietal lobe into the frontal lobe. It therefore extends through all lobes and connects them longitudinally along their lateral surface by being situated initially adjacent to the corona radiata.

It arises from the lateral portion of the apex of the temporal lobe, lateral to the unciform fasciculus. Sometimes it appears as if it is connected with Ammon's horn. In the temporal lobe it runs in an oblique fashion posteriorly, superiorly and medially, and forms the gyri on the superior and lateral surface of this lobe.[1] Some of its fibers extend into the occipital lobe. The remaining portion ascends behind the gyri of the insula, curves anteriorly, and receives fibers from the superior portion of the lateral surface of the occipital lobe that run anteriorly in the horizontal plane without ascending in an arc-like fashion. The arcuate fasciculus continues anteriorly as two leaves. One, more medially situated, runs within the "Stammlappen"[2] towards the external capsule, and initially is adjacent to the claustrum where it forms the insula. The other, laterally situated leaf, forms the operculum. In the angle between the superior portion of the insula and the operculum another leaf consisting of longitudinal fibers merges with both these leaves. Above, those two leaves are conjoined, and the arcuate fasciculus then forms a broad and massive layer that runs anteriorly at the same height as the corpus callosum along the lateral surface of the corona radiata, occupies the lateral portion of the superior surface of the brain, and forms the gyri in this area. Anteriorly it passes far laterally into the frontal lobe through the central sulcus that is situated between the parietal and frontal lobes, and it expands at the lateral surface of the frontal lobe. In other words, a bundle runs from the anterior portion of the operculum to the lateral surface of the frontal lobe and forms its gyri. This bundle runs longitudinally but sends its fibers laterally, superiorly, and inferiorly.

The existence of this prominent aggregation of fibers was reaffirmed by later studies using the fiber dissection technique, such as those of Mayo (1827), Arnold (1838a), and Foville (1844). Wernicke (1897) commented on this bundle in his atlas of myelin-stained sections of the brain in the three cardinal planes. In volume I (coronal plane), he referred to the "superior longitudinal bundle, or arcuate bundle" (Tafel XII, comment on p. 20 of the accompanying text) that runs

around the lateral edge of the lentiform nucleus, and the corona radiata fibers that exit it, like the cingulum around the corpus callosum, or the bundle that courses around the caudate nucleus. It is a long association bundle of the cortical portion of the convexity that surrounds the Sylvian fissure and contains to a large extent medium length fibers, and only in part, in the deepest area, long fibers that encircle the Sylvian fissure at a distance.

Dejerine (1895, p. 756; see our figures 2-10B and 2-11A) recognized Burdach's previous observations and designated the

Superior Longitudinal Fasciculus or Arcuate Fasciculus, [as] the Arcuate Fasciculus of Burdach. The arcuate fasciculus is to the external aspect of the hemisphere what the cingulum is to the internal aspect. It is located at the base of the convolutions of the Sylvian operculum outside the fifth fibers of the corona radiata and at the level of the body of the corpus callosum. This fascicle, like the cingulum and uncinate fasciculus, has a curved shape that is open inferiorly and rostrally. On brain dissections the arcuate fascicle reveals a compact shape only in the region of the parietal operculum where the fascicles are parallel to the superior edge of the putamen. Its most inferior and superficial fibers reach the supramarginal sulcus of the insula, demarcate the superior edge of the claustrum, cover the lateral aspect of the fibers of the corona radiata, and contribute to form the superior part of the external capsule. At the level of the posterior edge of the Sylvian fissure, the arcuate fascicle exhibits a curve with the tip located rostrally, and the curve joins the posterior edge of the putamen. The fibers then cross those of the corona radiata and the radiation of the corpus callosum, and travel for some distance along the parietal-occipital temporal convolutions. The most superficial fibers travel rostrally and cover the lateral aspect of the uncinate fasciculus, radiating in the crest forming the anterior part of the first temporal convolution. Other fibers terminate in the posterior segment of the first and second temporal convolutions, crossing at this level the fibers of the corona radiata and the enlargement of the corpus callosum. Finally, the deepest fibers radiate within the crest of the supra-marginal gyrus, the angular gyrus [literally, "curved fold"] and the convolutions of the external aspect of the occipital lobe.

On coronal [literally, "vertical transverse"] sections of hardened brain, the shape of the arcuate fascicle is triangular. Its inferior and medial angle corresponds to the external capsule and courses between the external capsule and the claustrum. Its inferior and lateral angle corresponds to the convolution of the Sylvian operculum. Its superior angle fuses with the layer of neighboring fibers. It is poorly delineated laterally and in its lower aspect, where it fuses with the white matter belonging to the convolutions of the Sylvian operculum. The arcuate fasciculus is well delineated medially, where it lies at the foot of the corona radiata, and its fibers are in fact perpendicular to the main axis of the fibers of the corona radiata. At the level of the supramarginal gyrus, the arcuate fascicle curves rostrally and laterally to reach the temporal lobe. Posteriorly it cannot be distinguished from the other vertical fibers of the occipital and parietotemporal convexity that in fact are formed by the occipital fascicle of Wernicke.

On microscopic sections stained with the Weigart or Pal technique, the arcuate fascicle is lightly stained with hematoxylin and can barely be distinguished from the white matter found at the convolution of the Sylvian operculum. The mode of termination of the arcuate fascicle rostrally is greatly disputed. According to Meynert it terminates in the Rolandic operculum and in the operculum of the third frontal convolution, and forms the associative fascicle connecting the external aspect of the temporal occipital regions to the frontal lobe convexity. According to Schnopfhagen, in contrast, the arcuate fascicle does not terminate at the level of the third frontal convolution, but at this level would cross the fibers of the corona radiata, travel rostrally and medially towards the anterior part of the corpus callosum, cross the midline at the level of the genu of the corpus callosum and terminate in the frontal lobe of the opposite hemisphere. According to this author the arcuate fascicle belongs to the corpus callosal system and connects the temporal-occipital lobes from one side to the other. This question can be addressed only by studying the development of these regions or using secondary degeneration. The hypothesis of Schnopfhagen is not supported by cases of agenesis of the corpus callosum.

Dejerine continued (1895, p. 758):

> The arcuate fascicle does not appear to be composed only of short associative fibers allowing connection of two neighboring convolutions. The deep layers that are in contact with the external capsule contain some longer fibers that connect remote convolutions, but the arcuate fascicle does not appear to contain fibers that occupy its entire length and connect remote regions of two different lobes. We have been able to observe many times using the technique of serial sections that when the arcuate fascicle or superior longitudinal fascicle of Burdach is within an old cortical lesion, we cannot really follow degenerated fibers any further than the immediate neighborhood of the primary focus of the lesion.

Obersteiner (1896, translated by Leonard Hill) summarized the main features of the "fasciculus arcuatus (or longitudinalis superior)" as consisting of (p. 349) "sagittally-disposed fibres, beneath the inferior and middle frontal convolutions, running partly towards the occipital lobe and partly arching round towards the apex of the temporal lobe."

In his influential English language text, Lewellys Franklin Barker (1867–1943) described the SLF as being

> triangular in coronal sections of the brain, extend[ing] as a curved bundle in a sagittal direction, apparently between the frontal lobe and the occipital lobe. The cell bodies of the neurones, which give rise to the axones which constitute it, have not been well localized. It would appear that the axones of the bundle are of variable length, the majority of them not running through the whole extent of the fasciculus, but, as with so many of the association bundles, axones are ever entering and leaving this fasciculus. Among the axones in it are doubtless some extending between the gyrus temporalis superior and the inferior frontal gyrus. This bundle on the left side is therefore, in all probability, of the highest importance in connection with the functions of speech, since in the gyrus temporalis superior is located the center for word memories, while in the gyrus frontalis inferior is situated the center for memories of the movements concerned in the articulation of words (Broca's center). It is highly probable that axones run in both directions in the fasciculus longitudinalis superior (Barker, 1899, pp. 1063–1065).

Gordinier, too, referred to the SLF as passing

> through the centrum semiovale . . . beneath the lower border of the frontal and parietal convolutions, being situated above the level of the body of the corpus callosum. Beneath the supramarginal gyrus this fasciculus curves downward, backward, and then forward, its fibers spreading out fan-shaped and passing between the fibers of the corona radiata and corpus callosum, to terminate, according to Meynert, about the nerve-cells of the cortex of the convexity of the occipital and temporal lobes. In front it terminates in the convexity of the frontal lobe, the exact location of its anterior termination being still unsettled (Gordinier, 1899, p. 368).

These insights into the SLF/AF system were not advanced in the ensuing century, and subsequent investigators using the dissection method (Gluhbegovic and Williams, 1980; Heimer, 1983, 1995; Ludwig and Klingler, 1956; Türe et al., 2000), as well as contemporary anatomic texts (Brodal, 1981; Carpenter, 1976; *Gray's Anatomy*, 1995; Nieuwenhuys et al., 1978), also adopted these early notions. Thus, in the monograph by Crosby and Schnitzlein (1982), the SLF/AF occupies the same location described by Dejerine, coursing above the putamen, dorsal to the claustrum, and close to the internal capsule, and is said to extend from the frontal to the occipital poles, arching into the temporal region, and fanning out into the occipital area, being made up largely of short fibers that begin and end in cortical areas along its course.

The emerging techniques of white matter tractography using MRI have relied upon the conventional wisdom of earlier anatomical texts to guide the determination of fiber tracts *in vivo*. These studies in the human display diagrams of an SLF/AF system (Catani et al., 2002; Cellerini et al., 1997; Lazar et al., 2003), but as in the case of the blunt dissection technique, they do not convey a precise understanding of the origins and terminations of these fiber pathways.

The foregoing account establishes that the conventional notion regarding the SLF, from the earliest descriptions until the present time, is that it is a unitary entity, synonymous with the AF, and that it links the parietal, temporal, and occipital regions with the frontal lobe. The use of the autoradiographic tract-tracing technique to study Burdach's AF or SLF in the experimental animal is our response to Todd's (1845) admonition that the only way to remove the uncertainties regarding the course and composition of the fiber tracts of the brain is (p. 137) "by the successful application of extensive and patient microscopic analysis to the whole cerebral structure." This approach does indeed facilitate more detailed and accurate understanding of the SLF and the AF in terms of their origin, course, and terminations.

Superior Longitudinal Fasciculus

The autoradiographic technique was used by Petrides and Pandya (1984) to evaluate the posterior parietal projections to the frontal lobe in the monkey. They observed that there were three relatively distinct bundles of fibers leading from the parietal lobe to the frontal lobe. One led from the superior parietal lobule and medial part of the posterior parietal cortex, traveling in the white matter of the superior parietal and superior frontal gyri, to terminate in the dorsal and medial prefrontal cortices. A second bundle, arising from the caudal inferior parietal lobule, coursed in the white matter above the shoulder of the Sylvian fissure, leading to the dorsolateral prefrontal cortices. The third bundle emanated from the rostral part of the inferior parietal lobule and traveled through the white matter of the parietal and frontal operculum to the parietofrontal opercular cortices and the ventrolateral prefrontal cortices. Petrides and Pandya (1988) later showed that the AF is distinct from the SLF, as discussed further below.

Results of the Present Investigation

Our observations in the monkey confirm and extend the conclusions of Petrides and Pandya (1984) that the SLF consists of three separate components linking the parietal lobe with the frontal lobe. In Nissl-stained material we have been able to identify the stem portion of these three long association fiber bundles deep in the white matter of the parietal and frontal lobes, and these separate divisions of the SLF are observed in the experimental material.

Superior Longitudinal Fasciculus, Subcomponent I

The SLF I (figures 13-1 and 13-2) originates from the medial posterior parietal region (area PGm) and the caudal superior parietal lobule (areas PE and PEc). Caudally it is confined to the white matter of the superior parietal lobule, and it courses rostrally into the white matter of the superior frontal gyrus, adjacent to the medial wall of the hemisphere, remaining dorsal to the cingulate sulcus. In the frontal lobe the SLF I fibers project to the supplementary motor area (MII), dorsal area 6, and area 9. The SLF I also conveys information from these areas of the frontal lobe back to the parietal lobe cortices from which the rostrally directed projections are derived.

Superior Longitudinal Fasciculus, Subcomponent II

The SLF II (figure 13-3) arises from the caudal part of the inferior parietal lobule, areas PG and Opt, as well as from the cortex in the lower bank of the intraparietal sulcus, area POa. These fibers travel first within the white matter of the inferior parietal lobule. As they move rostrally, they are situated above the claustrum and the upper shoulder of the Sylvian fissure, dorsal and medial to the fibers of the AF (described below). Further rostrally the SLF II fibers intermingle in part with the corona radiata fibers near the level of the central sulcus, and in the frontal lobe they flatten into a plate of fibers located beneath the arcuate and principal sulci. From this position, the fibers terminate in dorsal areas 6, 8 (8Ad), 9/46, and 46. As with SLF I, this SLF II fiber pathway is also bidirectional.

Superior Longitudinal Fasciculus, Subcomponent III

The SLF III (figure 13-4) emerges from the rostral part of the inferior parietal lobule, area PF, and the parietal operculum, area PFop. It courses horizontally through the white matter of the parietal and frontal operculum and reaches the region of the arcuate sulcus, where fibers terminate in the ventral part of area 6, area 44 in the lower bank of the arcuate sulcus, and the ventral part of area 46. The SLF III also is reciprocal in nature.

These connections between the parietal and frontal regions that we identified are in agreement with the earlier findings (Barbas, 1988; Bullier et al., 1996; Cavada and Goldman-Rakic, 1989; Deacon, 1992; Godschalk et al., 1984; Jones and Powell, 1970; Leichnetz, 2001; Neal et al., 1990; Pandya and Kuypers, 1969; Petrides and Pandya, 1984).

Functional Notions

The prevailing notion that the SLF courses mainly above the Sylvian fissure thus needs to be revised. The SLF originates not only from the caudal inferior parietal lobule (that is, the angular gyrus) but it also receives contingents of fibers from the superior parietal lobule (SLF I) and the rostral part of the inferior parietal lobule (SLF III).

Superior Longitudinal Fasciculus I

The fibers in SLF I link the superior parietal region and adjacent medial parietal cortex in a reciprocal manner with the frontal lobe supplementary and premotor areas. Neurons of the superior parietal lobule code movement and position-related activities of the limbs (Duffy and Burchfiel, 1971; Johnson et al., 1996; Mountcastle et al., 1975;

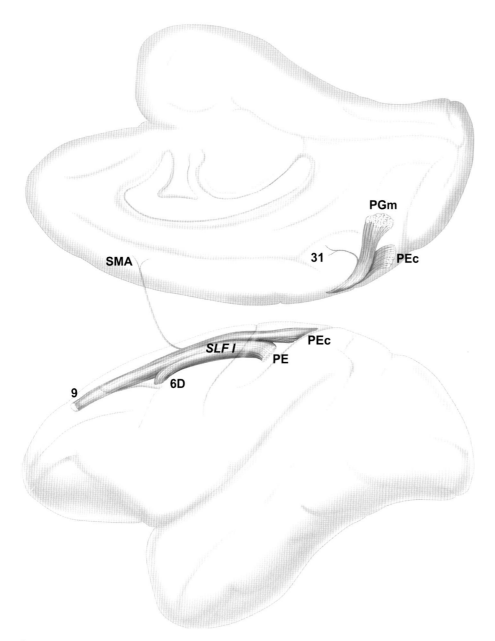

Figure 13-1

Summary diagrams of the course and composition of the SLF I in the rhesus monkey. The lateral view (below) and medial view (above) of the cerebral hemisphere show the trajectory of the SLF I and the cortical areas that are linked in a bi-directional manner by the fibers in this pathway.

Sakata et al., 1973) in a body-centered coordinate system (Ferraina and Bianchi, 1994). It thus seems likely that the SLF I conveys higher-order somatosensory and kinesthetic information regarding the trunk and limbs to the frontal lobe. The supplementary and premotor areas that receive input via the SLF I are also concerned with higher-order aspects of movement (Goldberg, 1987). Eccles (1982) proposed that the SMA contains the "inventory" and "addresses" of stored subroutines of learned motor programs and translates the mental act of intention into the intended movement (Eccles, 1982). This notion is supported by the finding in monkeys (Donchin et al., 1971) and humans of a

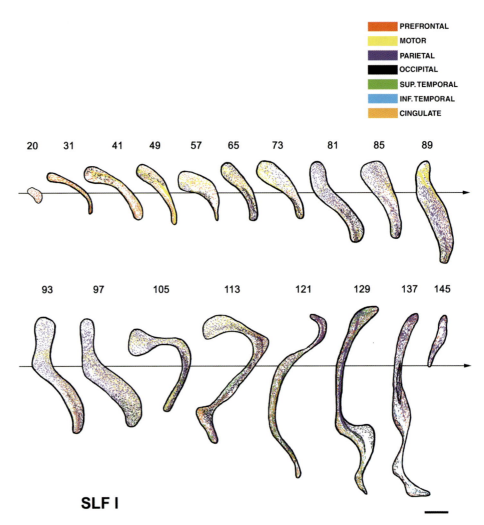

PREFRONTAL
MOTOR
PARIETAL
OCCIPITAL
SUP. TEMPORAL
INF. TEMPORAL
CINGULATE

SLF I

Figure 13-2

Summary diagrams of rostral to caudal coronal sections through SLF I extracted from the composite views of the hemisphere shown in chapter 27. The numbers refer to the sections of the template brain from which the fiber bundles are derived. The areas of origin of the fibers within the SLF I are color-coded according to the legend at top right. Bar = 2 mm.

"bereitschafts" (readiness) potential in the SMA (Deecke, 1987) and in the pre-SMA (Yazawa et al., 2000) prior to movement or activation of M1. Moreover, neurons in the premotor cortex are activated by the anticipation of predictable events in the environment (Mauritz and Wise, 1986). The SLF I may therefore play a role in the regulation of higher aspects of motor behavior that require information about body part location. In addition, by linking parietal regions with the SMA, the SLF I may contribute to the initiation of motor activity. This is exemplified by the observation that lesions of the target zone of the SLF I in monkeys, the rostral dorsal premotor area 6 (Halsband and Passingham, 1982; Petrides, 1982), or of the equivalent dorsolateral prefrontal region in humans (Petrides, 1985, 1997) produce severe impairments on conditional associative tasks in which different competing motor acts must be selected on the basis of appropriate conditional rules (Petrides, 1982, 1985; Petrides and Pandya, 2002a).

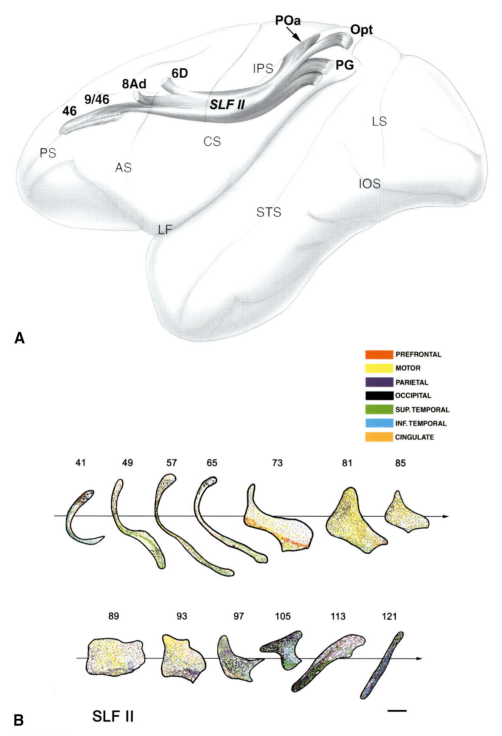

A

PREFRONTAL
MOTOR
PARIETAL
OCCIPITAL
SUP. TEMPORAL
INF. TEMPORAL
CINGULATE

41 49 57 65 73 81 85

89 93 97 105 113 121

B   **SLF II**

Figure 13-3

Summary diagrams of the course and composition of SLF II in the rhesus monkey. A, Lateral view of the cerebral hemisphere shows the trajectory of the SLF II and the cortical areas that are linked in a bidirectional manner by the fibers in this pathway. B, Rostral to caudal coronal sections through the SLF II extracted from the composite views of the hemisphere shown in chapter 27. The numbers refer to the sections of the template brain from which the fiber bundles are derived. The areas of origin of the fibers within the SLF II are color-coded according to the legend above right. Fibers from motor cortex (in yellow) in sections 73 through 93 are actually those of the corona radiata descending through the SLF II, but they do not course in a rostral–caudal direction between the cortical areas linked by the SLF II. Bar = 2 mm.

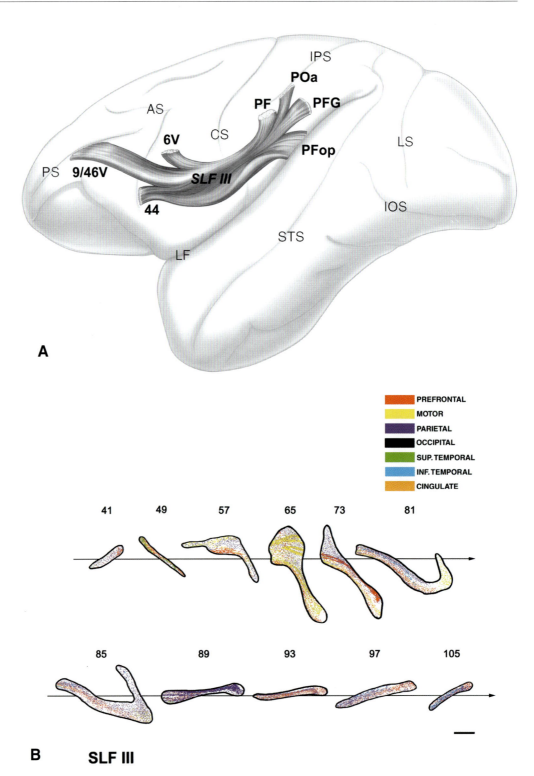

A

PREFRONTAL
MOTOR
PARIETAL
OCCIPITAL
SUP. TEMPORAL
INF. TEMPORAL
CINGULATE

B   **SLF III**

Figure 13-4

Summary diagrams of the course and composition of SLF III in the rhesus monkey. A, Lateral view of the cerebral hemisphere shows the trajectory of the SLF III and the cortical areas that are linked in a bidirectional manner by the fibers in this pathway. B, Rostral to caudal coronal sections through the SLF III extracted from the composite views of the hemisphere shown in chapter 27. The numbers refer to the section of the template brain from which the fiber bundles are derived. The areas of origin of the fibers within the SLF III are color-coded according to the legend above right. Bar = 2 mm.

Superior Longitudinal Fasciculus II

The SLF II fiber bundle that in part corresponds to the fiber tract traditionally recognized as the SLF links the caudal inferior parietal lobule (area PG/Opt, equivalent in the human to the angular gyrus) and the occipito-parietal area (area POa) with the posterior part of the dorsolateral prefrontal cortex and the mid-dorsolateral prefrontal cortex, areas 6, 8Ad, 9/46, and 46. The posterior parietal cortex is one of the cortical epicenters described by Mesulam (1998) that is involved in the integration of inputs from multiple modalities, a component of the network for spatial awareness that plays a major role in the visual and oculomotor aspects of spatial function (Blatt et al., 1990; Gnadt and Andersen, 1988; Goldberg and Segraves, 1987; Lynch et al., 1977). When the posterior parietal cortex is lesioned, patients and animals experience severe deficits of spatial attention, including trimodal neglect, and patients with angular gyrus lesions demonstrate unawareness of deficit, or anosognosia (Denny-Brown et al., 1952; Heilman et al., 1970, 1971; Heilman and Valenstein, 2003; Mesulam, 2000). Frontal lobe regions linked to the posterior parietal cortex by the SLF II are also important in the realm of spatial awareness. Premotor area 6 contains mirror neurons that respond to actions similar to those that they initiate (Rizzolatti et al., 1996), area 8Ad is important for spatial awareness and the orienting aspects of attention (Courtney et al., 1998; Lawler and Cowey, 1987), and area 46 is involved with spatial working memory (Levy and Goldman-Rakic, 2000). The SLF II pathway may thus provide the prefrontal cortex with information from the posterior parietal cortex concerning the perception of visual space and serve as the conduit for the neural system subserving visual awareness, the maintenance of attention, and engagement in the environment.

The SLF II fibers from the prefrontal cortex directed back to the posterior parietal cortex provide a means whereby the prefrontal cortex can regulate the focusing of attention within different parts of space (Petrides and Pandya, 2002a). This has been shown to be clinically relevant in patients with prefrontal lesions. Whereas healthy controls can use information provided in advance about the location of an impending stimulus to speed up their detection of it, patients with lateral prefrontal cortical lesions show impairments in this ability (Alivisatos and Milner, 1989; Koski et al., 1998).

Superior Longitudinal Fasciculus III

The fibers within the SLF III coursing in the parietal and frontal opercula link the rostral portion of the inferior parietal lobule (which in the human brain constitutes the supramarginal gyrus) and the adjacent opercular area, with the ventral premotor area 6, adjacent area 44 (equivalent in the human brain to the pars opercularis), the gustatory area in the frontal operculum, and the ventral part of area 46. This pathway is reciprocal. The rostral part of the inferior parietal lobule receives input from the ventral precentral gyrus, and its neurons exhibit complex somatosensory responses related to face, head, and neck (Andersen et al., 1990). Thus, SLF III provides the ventral premotor region and pars opercularis with higher-order somatosensory input. The firing of neurons in this frontal region is correlated with specific goal-related motor acts rather than with single movements, with different classes of neurons forming a vocabulary of motor acts (Rizzolatti et al., 1988). Furthermore, in the monkey this region contains "mirror neurons" that discharge both when the monkey makes a particular action and when it observes another individual (monkey or human) making a similar action (Rizzolati et al., 1996, 1999), indicating that these neurons are involved in computing information necessary for imitation. Mouth mirror neurons in the ventral premotor area discharge when a monkey observes another individual performing mouth actions involved with ingestive behavior, and they are triggered most effectively by observing communicative mouth gestures such as lip smacking (Ferrari et al., 2003).

In a functional imaging study these observations were extended to human subjects by Buccino et al. (2001), who showed that during action observations there is recruitment in a somatotopically organized fashion of the same premotor regions that would normally be involved in the actual execution of the observed action. In addition, during the observation of object-related actions, somatotopically organized activation was found in the posterior parietal lobe, indicating that concept of an action observation/execution matching system (mirror system) is not restricted to the ventral premotor cortex but involves several somatotopically organized interlinked circuits, including the parietal lobe.

Gestural impairments in the clinical syndromes of ideomotor and buccofacial apraxia result from lesions of the rostral part of the inferior parietal lobule or underlying white matter and from the premotor cortices in the frontal lobe (Alexander et al., 1992; Barbieri and De Renzi, 1988; Heilman and Valenstein, 2003; Kareken et al., 1998), and thus the interactions mediated by SLF III between the rostral inferior parietal lobule and ventral premotor region may be a prerequisite for gestural communication that in turn presages linguistic communication (Petrides and Pandya, 2002a).

The bidirectional connections between rostral IPL and ventral area 46 facilitated by SLF III may be crucial for monitoring orofacial and hand actions, since this part of the middorsolateral prefrontal region plays a critical role in monitoring information in working memory (Petrides, 1995; Petrides and Pandya, 2002a; Preuss and Goldman-Rakic, 1989).

Thus, it seems that in the larger context of the SLF fiber system, each component has a particular role to play. The SLF I may be involved in the initiation of motor activity, SLF II subserves visual spatial awareness and attention, and SLF III is engaged in phonemic and articulatory aspects of language.

A recent DT-MRI study reveals that these three SLF bundles are identifiable also in the human brain, occupying positions equivalent to those observed in the monkey (Makris et al., 2005). Further, this study revealed that the arcuate fascicle can also be distinguished from the SLF fiber fascicles as in the monkey (see below). The DT-MRI technique visualizes only the stem portion of each fiber pathway, and therefore the precise origins and terminations of these tracts as determined in the nonhuman primate are of great value in interpreting the newly available information in the human.

Arcuate Fasciculus

Dejerine (1895) adopted Burdach's designation of the AF/SLF, and both conceived of this fascicle as a unitary system of fibers connecting the parietal and temporal lobes with the frontal lobe. Based on his observations, and the findings of Meynert with regard to the connections subserved by this tract, Dejerine concluded that the "arcuate fascicle" carries fibers from the caudal superior temporal and middle temporal gyri to the inferior frontal gyrus. He remained skeptical, however, that it contained "fibers along its whole length connecting remote regions of two different lobes" because of his inability to "follow degenerated fibers any further than the immediate neighborhood of the primary focus of the lesion" (p. 758).

These notions—that the SLF and AF are synonymous and constitute one system, and that the AF links the caudal superior temporal region with the inferior frontal gyrus—persisted through more than a century of reformulations and re-explorations using the fiber-dissection technique. This has begun to be perpetuated and reinterpreted using the *in vivo* DT-MRI tractography technique that is heavily reliant on these pre-existent ideas. Furthermore, clinical investigators, including Wernicke (1874), Dejerine (1895), Barker (1899), Liepmann (see Brown, 1988), and Geschwind (1965a,b) relied on these anatomical descriptions of the AF to develop an understanding of brain systems that subserve language and the involvement of the AF in conduction aphasia.

Architectonic analyses and connectivity studies focusing on the frontal and temporal lobes shed light on the way different subdivisions of these areas are linked (Galaburda and Pandya, 1983; Jones and Powell, 1970; Pandya, 1995; Pandya et al., 1969; Pandya and Kuypers, 1969; Pandya and Sanides, 1973; Pandya and Yeterian, 1996; Petrides and Pandya, 1994; Rajkowska and Goldman-Rakic, 1995a,b). Chavis and Pandya (1976) showed that whereas the caudal portion of the superior temporal gyrus projects to the frontal periarcuate cortex, the middle portion of the superior temporal gyrus and the caudal inferotemporal cortex are linked predominantly with the prearcuate cortex; the rostral superior temporal gyrus projects primarily to the medial and orbital surface of the frontal lobe, while the rostral inferotemporal area projects principally to the orbital surface of the frontal lobe. Seltzer and Pandya (1989a) showed that the rostral polymodal cortex (area TPO) in the upper bank of the superior temporal sulcus is interconnected with ventral, medial, and lateral sectors of the frontal lobe, the midportion of TPO is linked with rostral subdivisions of lateral prefrontal cortex, and the caudal segment of TPO has reciprocal connections with caudal subdivisions of the lateral frontal lobe, including dorsal areas 6 and 46 and the dorsal part of area 8.

Petrides and Pandya (1999) later showed that area 8B in the frontal lobe can be differentiated from the more ventrally situated area 8Ad on the basis of distinct architectonic features and connections. They showed that after injection of fluorescent retrograde tracers into area 8Ad, large numbers of labeled neurons were identified in auditory-related areas in the caudal superior temporal gyrus in area Tpt, with some neurons in areas paAlt and area TS3, and in the caudal part of the upper bank of the superior temporal sulcus in areas TAa and TPO. Romanski et al. (1999a) determined that retrograde tracers placed in the dorsal periarcuate cortex in area 8A resulted in labeled neurons selectively in the most caudal region of the superior temporal gyrus, area Tpt. Further, whereas anterior parts of the superior temporal gyrus were reciprocally connected with the frontal pole (area 10), rostral principal sulcus (area 46), and ventral prefrontal regions (areas 12 and 45), more caudal temporal areas were connected mainly with the caudal principal sulcus (area 46) and area 8A (Romanski et al., 1999b).

Hackett et al. (1999) showed that projections from auditory cortices in the mid- and caudal-superior temporal regions are directed toward the dorsolateral prefrontal cortices—caudal regions project to the dorsal prearcuate area and rostral regions to the dorsal aspect of the principal sulcus. These patterns of long corticocortical projections are consistent with the notion that each sector of the auditory association area is connected with frontal lobe regions that have essentially similar architectonic features. Further, these findings provide support for the view that the architectonically similar interconnected temporal and frontal lobe regions may have evolved in concert with each other and may participate in similar functional domains (Pandya and Yeterian, 1985).

Isotope tract tracing helped further define the temporal lobe connections with the prefrontal cortex, facilitated analysis of the fiber systems conveying these projections, and elucidated the course of the AF and its relationship to the SLF (notably SLF II). Petrides and Pandya (1988) reported that the posterior part of the superior temporal gyrus (area Tpt) projects to the lateral frontal cortex (particularly area 8Ad), and whereas these projections are conveyed partly through the extreme capsule, they travel mostly via fibers in the AF that curve around the caudal end of the Sylvian fissure and occupy a position above and medial to the upper branch of the Sylvian fissure. The present results complement these earlier conclusions.

Results of the Present Investigations

According to our observations the AF is a distinct fiber system, separate from the SLF II both in terms of its location and trajectory and also with respect to the cortical areas that it links (figure 13-5). The AF originates in the caudal part of the superior temporal region—that is, caudal parts of the superior temporal gyrus (area Tpt) and superior temporal sulcus (area TPO). Its fibers arch around the caudal part of the depth of the Sylvian fissure and course first in the white matter of the ventral part of the parietal operculum. Further rostrally they remain above the extreme and external capsules and the claustrum but below and lateral to the SLF II fiber bundle. In the frontal lobe the AF fibers move dorsally into the white matter of the arcuate sulcus. From there the fibers project to the dorsal part of area 8 (area 8Ad), dorsal area 46, and the dorsal part of area 6. Our observations thus show the course of the AF and add to the weight of evidence that caudal parts of the superior temporal region are linked with the dorsal frontal lobe but not with the ventral prefrontal cortex.

Functional Notions

The AF is one of three distinct pathways that arise from the superior temporal gyrus and adjacent upper bank of the superior temporal sulcus and that lead to the frontal lobe (the other two are the uncinate fasciculus and the extreme capsule, discussed below).

A sophisticated understanding of the anatomy and functional properties of the temporal lobe has arisen out of architectonic parcellations and connectional studies in monkeys and architectonic analyses in humans, referenced above, along with physiological mapping studies in monkeys (Benson et al., 1981; Imig et al., 1977; Merzenich and Brugge, 1973; Rauschecker and Tian, 2000; Rauschecker et al., 1995, 1997; Romanski et al., 1999a,b; Tian et al., 2001). A central conclusion arising from this extensive body of research was summarized by Romanski et al. (1999a, p. 142):

> [T]he electrophysiological and anatomical evidence supports a view of the auditory cortical system as a series of concentric circles with a central core, the primary auditory cortex, surrounded by a narrow belt of secondary association areas located laterally and medially, and a parabelt auditory association cortex located on

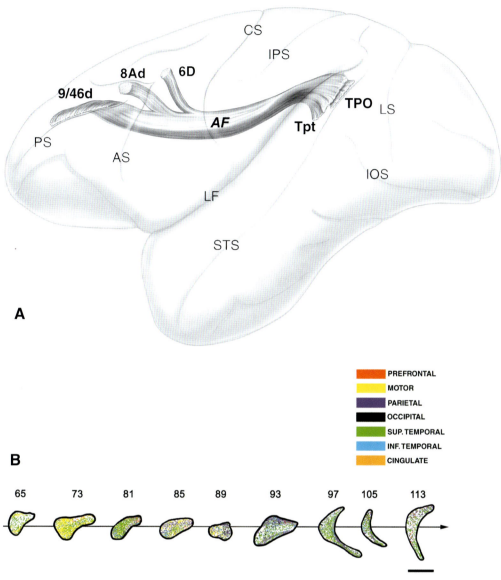

ARCUATE FASCICULUS

Figure 13-5

Summary diagrams of the course and composition of the AF in the rhesus monkey. A, Lateral view of the cerebral hemisphere shows the trajectory of the AF and the cortical areas that are linked in a bi-directional manner by the fibers in this pathway. B, Rostral to caudal coronal sections through the AF extracted from the composite views of the hemisphere shown in chapter 27. The numbers refer to the sections of the template brain from which the fiber bundles are derived. The areas of origin of the fibers within the AF are color-coded according to the legend above right. Bar = 2 mm.

the ventral gyral surface of the superior temporal gyrus just below the lateral belt, with successively higher areas processing increasingly complex stimuli.

Within this larger context of examining the role of the temporal lobe in auditory processing, physiological experiments in monkeys (Benson et al., 1981; Leinonen et al., 1980; Rauschecker and Tian, 2000), functional imaging studies in humans (Martinkauppi et al., 2000; Rauschecker and Tian, 2000; Wise et al., 2001), and clinical observations (Clarke et al., 2002; Clarke and Thiran, 2004) suggest that the caudal superior temporal gyrus (including areas Tpt and TPO) is particularly specialized for the localization of sound. Similar analyses of the frontal lobe in the monkey reveal that area 8Ad also is concerned with auditory spatial information. Neurons in the dorsolateral prefrontal area are activated by acoustic stimuli delivered in a restricted range of directions with respect to the animal's head (Azuma and Suzuki, 1984); neurons in monkey postarcuate area 6 and prearcuate areas 8 and 9 respond predominantly during active localization behavior (Vaadia et al., 1986), and lesions of the periarcuate region in monkeys have been shown to impair auditory discrimination (Gross and Weiskrantz, 1962). Differential temporal and parietal lobe inputs to area 8 suggested to Barbas and Mesulam (1981) that caudal area 8 may be involved in head and eye movements in response to visual stimuli, whereas the anterior subdivisions of area 8 may be involved in directing the head and eyes in response to auditory stimuli.

The AF that links the caudal temporal lobe (areas Tpt/paAc) with the frontal cortex (area 8Ad, dorsal area 6, and dorsal area 46) may therefore be viewed as an auditory spatial bundle: it provides the means whereby the prefrontal cortex can receive and influence spatial information in the auditory domain. The role of the arcuate fasciculus in the audiospatial domain may thus be viewed as equivalent to the role of the SLF II and the fronto-occipital fasciculus that subserve spatial awareness in the visual domain (as discussed elsewhere).

Is the Arcuate Fasciculus Really a Language Bundle?

Convention holds that the AF is a language bundle that links Wernicke's area in the posterior third of the superior temporal gyrus with Broca's area in the pars triangularis of the frontal operculum, and that destruction of the AF results in conduction aphasia. Lesion-deficit studies were predicated on this anatomical conclusion, but neuronography studies could not decipher the pathways involved in corticocortical connections, there are no published focal degeneration studies in humans in which the lesion responsible for conduction aphasia is confined exclusively to the AF, and there are no human studies showing that it is the AF that links these two language-related cortical areas. The results of the present investigation, together with those of Petrides and Pandya (1988) and other connectional studies (Hackett et al., 1999; Pandya and Yeterian, 1996; Petrides and Pandya, 1999, 2002b; Romanski et al., 1999a,b) are at odds with this understanding that the AF is a "language bundle" because it links area Tpt in the caudal part of the superior temporal region with area 8Ad in dorsolateral prefrontal cortex. Neither of these areas is homologous to the cortical areas in humans that are directly concerned with language. Indeed, the foregoing discussion suggests that the AF is important for the spatial attributes of acoustic stimuli and auditory-related processing, but that it is not related to language *per se*.

If not the AF, then, which fiber systems *do* subserve linguistic processing? As discussed above, the SLF III that links the supramarginal gyrus with area 44 (equivalent to the human pars opercularis) may be one component of this system, possibly involved in the phonemic aspects of language. According to our observations, the fiber bundles that may be particularly important substrates supporting nonarticulatory aspects of language are the extreme capsule and the middle longitudinal fasciculus. These are dealt with in the next sections.

Extreme Capsule

14

The early studies of Vicq d'Azyr, Reil, Gall and Spurzheim, Burdach, and others led to the definition of the major fiber bundles of the cerebral hemispheres, including the internal and external capsules, but the extreme capsule (EmC) was not recognized as a separate entity until much later. It was depicted on coronal and axial sections of the hemispheres lateral to the claustrum and medial to the insular cortex (see Barker, 1899; Gordinier, 1899; Obersteiner, 1896; Van Gehuchten, 1897). Dejerine (1895) concluded that the EmC receives a contingent of fibers from the external capsule and contains a large number of short association fibers.[1]

The fiber pathway contained within the EmC and the putative functional attributes of this tract have been somewhat elusive. Crosby et al. (Ariëns-Kappers et al., 1936; Crosby and Schnitzlein, 1982, p. 614) described the EmC as being situated between the claustrum and the insular cortex, conveying "many association fibers between frontal and temporal and parietal and temporal cortices and between these areas and the insular cortex . . . The extreme capsule has in it or accompanying it some projection fibers which end in the claustrum." Berke (1960) similarly determined that the EmC is primarily a cortical association bundle interconnecting frontal, insular, and temporal cortices, as well as linking parietal and temporal lobes.

The EmC seems inadvertently to have been relevant in the dissections of Trolard (1906) and Curran (1909). These authors identified the internal and external capsules and a fiber system they termed the "inferior occipitofrontal fasciculus." As discussed in chapter 18, contemporary tract-tracing studies provide no evidence in support of such a bundle, but Trolard and Curran's bundle has relevance here because it seems that it included part of what we now understand to be the EmC. The proposed "inferior occipitofrontal fasciculus" was deemed to have two components: a caudal horizontally oriented system in the temporal lobe white matter and a rostrally situated ascending limb passing from the temporal lobe to the frontal lobe. Together, these two limbs suggested to Curran (1909) the appearance of a bowtie. From our observations, the caudal, horizontal component of their "inferior occipitofrontal fasciculus" may actually comprise the horizontal limb of the inferior longitudinal fasciculus, and the middle longitudinal fasciculus running in the white matter of the superior temporal gyrus. In our material, the rostral, ascending limb of this supposed "inferior occipitofrontal fasciculus" actually corresponds to the EmC.

Results of the Present Investigation

According to our observations, the EmC is a compact bundle situated between the claustrum and the insular cortex. It occupies this position in the rostral-caudal direction from a level just behind the islands of the putamen until the frontal lobe (figures 14-1

409

and 14-2). At the point in the frontal lobe where the claustrum assumes a horizontal position, the fibers of the EmC divide into a superior and inferior ramus. The superior ramus lies in the white matter of the inferior frontal gyrus, and the inferior ramus lies beneath the claustrum, on the floor of the orbital cortex, laterally adjacent to the fibers of the uncinate fasciculus.

In our material, along with the observations of Petrides and Pandya (1988), it appears that the EmC is the principal long association fiber bundle of the middle part of the superior temporal region. Fibers leave the middle and rostral parts of the superior temporal gyrus, medial part of the supratemporal plane, and the cortex of the superior temporal sulcus, ascend into the EmC, and terminate first in the rostral insular cortex. They then proceed rostrally and separate into the superior ramus of fibers that terminates in the caudal part of the ventrolateral prefrontal cortex (area 9/46 ventral) and the inferior ramus that terminates in the caudal part of the orbital frontal cortex and in area 45 (equivalent to the pars triangularis of human). A contingent of fibers originates within the multimodal areas of STS and terminates in the frontal polar area 10. These medial and orbital prefrontal cortices in turn, as well as the rostral cingulate gyrus, send fibers that move caudally, descend obliquely in the EmC, and terminate in the rostral insula and in the rostral part of the superior temporal gyrus. The ventrolateral prefrontal cortices also commit backgoing fibers to the middle part of the superior temporal gyrus via this EmC pathway. Some fibers from the ventral prefrontal cortex travel caudally in the EmC within the white matter of the superior temporal gyrus and continue caudally within the fiber bundle termed the middle longitudinal fasciculus (MdLF) to terminate in multimodal area TPO in the superior temporal sulcus.

Thus, the EmC is the principal association pathway linking the middle superior temporal region with the caudal parts of the orbital cortex and the ventral—lateral prefrontal cortex.

In addition to carrying these long association fiber connections, the fibers destined for the claustrum from the parietal, temporal, and frontal lobes also traverse the EmC.

Functional Notions

The conclusion that the EmC is important for language is derived from the knowledge of the cortical areas that it links. Stimulation of areas 44 and 45 in the human results in speech arrest (Rasmussen and Milner, 1975), but in the monkey the afferents of these two cortical areas are quite different. Area 44 in the monkey receives afferents from the supramarginal gyrus via SLF III, leading to the suggestion, as discussed in chapter 13, that in the human the SLF III is involved in the higher-order articulatory control of speech.

In contrast, area 45 in the monkey is situated in the ventrolateral prefrontal cortex in the anterior bank of the lower lip of the arcuate sulcus and the cortex immediately anterior to it. It is the homologue in the monkey of the pars triangularis of the inferior frontal gyrus in the human, or Broca's area (Pandya and Yeterian, 1996; Petrides and Pandya, 1994, 2002b), that plays a major role in language processing. In monkey, areas paAlt, TS3, the parabelt region of the superior temporal gyrus, and area TPO in the adjoining part of the STS, have been shown through architectonic analysis to be homol-

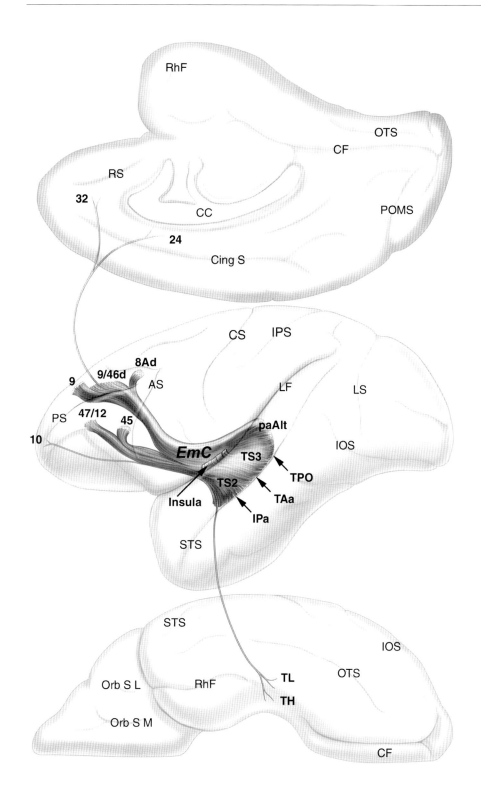

Figure 14-1

Summary diagrams of the course and composition of the EmC in the rhesus monkey. The lateral view of the cerebral hemisphere (middle diagram) shows the trajectory of the EmC and the cortical areas that are linked in a bidirectional manner by the fibers in this pathway. The medial view (above) and basal view (below) of the hemisphere are shown to represent other cortical areas that contribute to the EmC.

ogous to Wernicke's area in humans (Fullerton and Pandya, in preparation). These areas in the midportion of the superior temporal region of the monkey are linked with prefrontal area 45 by the EmC, and thus with all due caution it seems reasonable to postulate that the EmC is an important pathway in what Mesulam (1998) termed the language communication epicenter, linking Wernicke's area with Broca's area. Thus, in

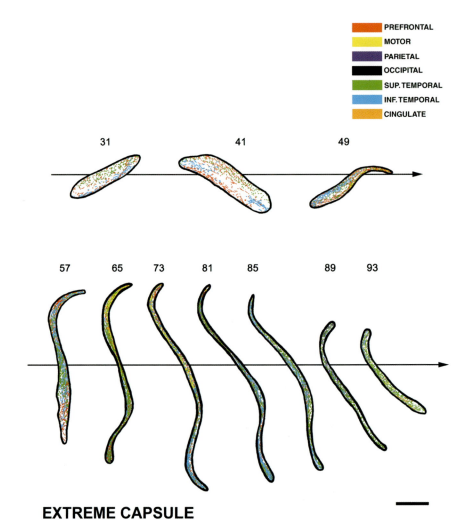

PREFRONTAL
MOTOR
PARIETAL
OCCIPITAL
SUP. TEMPORAL
INF. TEMPORAL
CINGULATE

EXTREME CAPSULE

Figure 14-2
Summary diagrams of rostral to caudal coronal sections through the EmC extracted from the composite views of the hemisphere shown in chapter 27. The numbers refer to the sections of the template brain from which the fiber bundles are derived. The areas of origin of the fibers within the EmC are color-coded according to the legend at top right. Bar = 2 mm.

contrast to the SLF III, which connects the supramaginal gyrus with the pars opercularis (area 44), the EmC, by virtue of its connections, may have a role in humans in the nonarticulatory control of linguistic functions such as syntax and grammar (Petrides and Pandya, 2002a).

These conclusions derived from the monkey have received support from recent observations in the human. Amunts et al. (2004) combined the analysis of functional language data in human subjects with an elastic warping tool and cytoarchitectonic maps of the human brain to determine that although both areas 44 and 45 in human participate in verbal fluency, they do so differentially. Whereas area 44 on the left is likely to be involved in high-level aspects of programming speech production, area 45 on the left is thought to be more involved in the semantic aspects of language processing.

In the monkey, both the EmC and area 45 that contributes to it are small. While there are gestural and perhaps elements of linguistic communication in the monkey, area 45 in the monkey is certainly not engaged in language to the extent that it is in the human, and therefore this cortical area (45) and the fiber bundle that links it with the temporal lobe (i.e., the EmC) are small in the monkey compared to the homologous areas that are thought to subserve language in the human.

The phenomenon of conduction aphasia is characterized by fluent, paraphasic conversational speech, normal comprehension, and repetition disturbance of a significant degree (Geschwind, 1974); it has been considered to result from disruption of the communication between posterior and anterior language cortices. The arcuate fasciculus has long been thought to mediate this link and thus has been implicated in this disorder since the descriptions of Wernicke (1874, 1908), Lichtheim (1885), Kleist (1962), Geschwind (Benson et al., 1973; Geschwind, 1974), and others. The present results suggest, however, that it is not the arcuate fasciculus that is responsible for the deficits of conduction aphasia but perhaps the EmC. The insular cortex itself has sometimes been implicated in the pathophysiology of conduction aphasia (Damasio and Damasio, 1980; Marshall et al., 1996), and this may be accounted for, at least in part, by the close proximity to the insula of the EmC.

Middle Longitudinal Fasciculus

15

In their study of the parietotemporal connections in the rhesus monkey, Seltzer and Pandya (1984) described for the first time a fiber bundle emerging from the caudal inferior parietal lobule (area PG/Opt) and coursing in the white matter of the superior temporal gyrus (STG). These fibers course toward the cortex of the superior temporal sulcus and terminate in areas TPO, PGa, and IPa. They termed this bundle the middle longitudinal fasciculus (MdLF). Barnes and Pandya (1992) have shown that the superior temporal sulcus region TPO and PGa projects back to the inferior parietal lobule, presumably by the same pathway.

Results of the Present Investigations

Our observations confirm the presence of the MdLF pathway that lies in the white matter of the STG and extends from the caudal end of the STG to the temporal pole (figures 15-1 and 15-2). In addition to the fibers within the MdLF that arise in the caudal inferior parietal lobule and terminate in the STG and the cortex of the superior temporal sulcus, we observed that the MdLF conveys fibers from the caudal cingulate gyrus and the middle sector of the parahippocampal gyrus toward the multimodal cortex (area TPO and PGa) in the upper bank of the superior temporal sulcus. Further, the MdLF links caudal with rostral sectors within the superior temporal region itself. In addition, fibers arise from the lateral and orbital prefrontal cortices and travel caudally first in the extreme capsule, and then within the MdLF to terminate in area TPO.

Functional Considerations

The MdLF running in the white matter of the STG thus is responsible for linking a number of high-level associative and paralimbic cortical areas. These include the inferior parietal lobule, the caudal cingulate gyrus, the parahippocampal gyrus, and the prefrontal cortex. It conveys information reciprocally between these high-level regions and the multimodal regions of the superior temporal sulcus as well as cortices in the STG.

The functional role of the MdLF remains to be ascertained. In view of these connections, however, it may be reasonable to speculate that in the human the MdLF plays a role in language. It may imbue linguistic processing with information dealing with spatial organization, memory, and motivational valence.

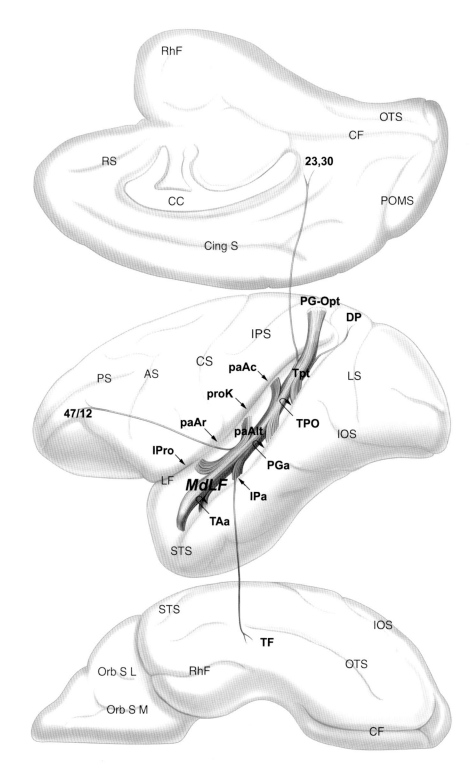

Figure 15-1

Summary diagrams of the course and composition of the MdLF in the rhesus monkey. The lateral view of the cerebral hemisphere (middle diagram) shows the trajectory of the MdLF and the cortical areas that are linked in a bidirectional manner by the fibers in this pathway. The medial view (above) and basal view (below) of the hemisphere are shown to represent other cortical areas that contribute to this fasciculus.

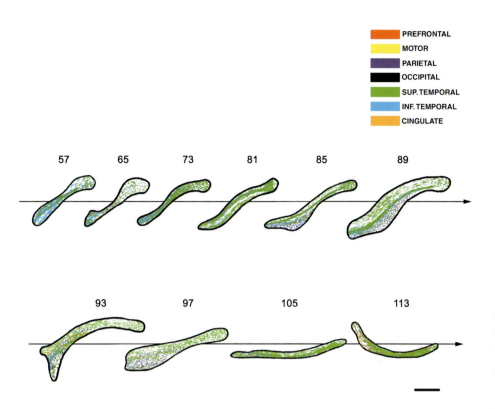

57   65   73   81   85   89

93   97   105   113

MIDDLE LONGITUDINAL FASCICULUS

Figure 15-2
Summary diagrams of rostral to caudal coronal sections through the MdLF extracted from the composite views of the hemisphere shown in chapter 27. The numbers refer to the sections of the template brain from which the fiber bundles are derived. The areas of origin of the fibers within the MdLF are color-coded according to the legend at top right. Bar = 2 mm.

Uncinate Fasciculus

The first description of the uncinate fasciculus (UF) was provided by J. C. Reil. From his fiber dissections he concluded that

> the unciform myelinated bundle connects the anterior [frontal] with the middle [temporal] lobe at the entrance to the Sylvian fissure (Reil, 1809a, p. 144). [It] originates from the gyri of the frontal lobe on which the root of the olfactory nerve lies, curves laterally around the lamina perforata, courses through the entrance of the Sylvian fissure in the temporal lobe, arcs forwards and descends into the superior surface of the apex of the temporal lobe [temporal pole]. This unciform fascicle therefore encircles the gap by which the frontal lobe is separated from the temporal lobe, and is constituted by the fan-like expansions of the central fibers of the gyri of the frontal and temporal lobes that aggregate from both sides in one stem (Reil, 1809d, p. 200).

Burdach (1822) recognized Reil's priority in designating a UF and elaborated upon the

> Häkenbundel (fasciculi unciformes). The radiations of the uncinate fasciculus terminate in the frontal and temporal lobes, although in the middle of their course they belong to the "Stammlappen" [see footnote 2, chapter 13] and in this manner they connect all three of these lobes to each other by running like arcs through them. These arcs circle around the Sylvian fissure, with their convex aspect pointing superiorly and posteriorly, while the concavity of the arc points anteriorly and inferiorly. The uncinate fasciculus begins in the most lateral corner of the superior area of the apex of the temporal lobe [temporal pole]. Converging fibers run posteriorly, superiorly and medially, reach the "Stammlappen," curve anteriorly, and run below the lentiform nucleus and the convergence point of the external capsule along the lateral side of the cribriform plate. The fibers then curve further laterally, reaching the frontal lobe where the unciform fasciculus radiates into its lateral areas as well as into the lateral portions of the basal areas (Burdach, 1822, p. 152, paragraph 195).

Later investigators confirmed the location of the UF (e.g., Obersteiner, 1896; Sachs, 1893), and Wernicke (1897, p. 16) reported that its fibers "come anteriorly from the orbital surface of the frontal lobe and run posteriorly towards the transition point between frontal lobe and temporal lobe . . . they then run downwards into the temporal lobe."

The UF was one of the five long association fascicles discussed by Dejerine (1895): "the cingulum, the arcuate fascicle or superior longitudinal fasciculus, the inferior longitudinal fasciculus, the uncinate fascicle, and the occipito-frontal fascicle." The UF (p. 753), also called the hooked fasciculus, and unciform fasciculus of Burdach, represents the shortest of the long association fascicles of the cerebral cortex. It connects the temporal pole to the orbital aspect of the frontal lobe, and occupies the edge of the insula where it spreads in a transverse orientation from the anterior perforated substance to the extreme capsule. Because the orbital aspect of the frontal lobe is very close to the temporal pole, the most medially situated fibers in this fascicle are as curved as the U fibers that cover the bottom of the sulci. This pronounced curvature gives rise to the name fasciculus uncinatus, but only the most medial fibers exhibit this accentuated curved shape. As one moves away from the anterior perforated substance the more laterally situated fibers of the fascicle become straighter with a less accentuated curvature so that these fibers not only become straight, but they appear to have an inverse curvature in the other direction. . . . On coronal slices it is very irregular and is found between the extreme capsule and the anterior perforated substance. Lateral to the region of the anterior commissure and at a level corresponding to the posterior marginal sulcus of the insula, the uncinate fasciculus intermingles with the inferior longitudinal fasciculus and separates the horizontal part of the claustrum. At the level of the frontal pole, the most inferior, medial and superficial fibers of the uncinate fascicle move rostrally and travel between the anterior perforated substance and the inferior aspect of the putamen. At the level of the olfactory surface they cross with the fibers of the genu of the corpus callosum, and then terminate in the most medial part of the first frontal convolution. Some of the fibers descend and terminate in the gyrus rectus, and others terminate in the orbital part of the first and third frontal convolution. The most laterally situated fibers become intermingled with the fibers of the genu of the corpus callosum and together they terminate in the crest of the orbital and external parts of the third frontal convolution. At the temporal pole, the fibers of the fascicle subdivide the gray matter that connects the claustrum to the amygdala and to the temporal cortex at the level of the anterior perforated substance. They intermingle with the inferior longitudinal fasciculus, but can be distinguished from this fasciculus in microscopic sections stained with Weigert or Pal because of their lighter staining. They radiate in the U or hook convolution in the temporal lobe and in the anterior part of the first and second temporal convolutions, and finally at this level they cross the superior longitudinal fasciculus. The uncinate fasciculus is often involved with lesions of the insula and the external capsule, and degenerated fibers can be traced in the temporal lobe and in the orbital part of the frontal lobe [see figure 2-11A, B].

Marchi degeneration (Mettler, 1935c) and strychnine neuronographic studies (MacLean, 1952; MacLean and Pribram, 1953; Pribram et al., 1950) subsequently revealed connections between rostral temporal and inferior frontal cortices. Nauta (1964) confirmed that it was the UF that linked the rostral part of the temporal lobe with the ventral prefrontal and orbitofrontal cortex in a bidirectional manner. This was also shown by Leichnetz and Astruc (1975), who observed degeneration coursing through the UF to the temporal and insular cortices after ablation of the orbitofrontal cortex of marmosets. Moran et al. (1987) showed input into the temporopolar cortex from the orbitofrontal and medial frontal regions. Petrides and Pandya (1988) used the autoradiographic technique and demonstrated that the UF links the temporal and orbitofrontal cortices. Ungerleider et al. (1989) noted that transections of the UF deprived the prefrontal cortex of virtually all input from area TE in the inferior temporal cortex.

Dissections in humans by Klinger and Gloor (1960) verified the findings of the earlier investigators regarding the course of the UF, while Ebeling and von Cramon (1992) showed it to have the form of a curved dumbbell, measuring 2 to 5 mm in height and 3 to 7 mm in width. These latter authors determined that the UF links the anterior three temporal convolutions and the amygdala with the gyrus rectus (area 11), medial retro-orbital cortex (area 12), and subcallosal area (area 25) and that it travels in the extreme and external capsule along the lateral and ventral circumference of the putamen toward the retro-orbital cortex and gyrus rectus. In a study of cholinergic pathways within the human brain, Selden et al. (1998) showed cholinergic fibers within the UF adjacent to the putamen and amygdala, some of which penetrated the amygdala while others continued into the temporal lobe.

Results of the Present Investigation

In agreement with earlier observations, the UF was seen to be a bidirectional pathway that preferentially links the anterior temporal lobe with the medial and orbital prefrontal cortex (figures 16-1 and 16-2). Fibers from the rostral part of the superior temporal gyrus (temporal proisocortex and area TS1) and the inferotemporal region (areas TE1 and TEa) ascend in the temporal stem, where they are positioned rostral to the most anteriorly situated fibers of the inferior longitudinal fasciculus. The uncinate fibers then aggregate lateral to the ventral part of the claustrum, situated medial to the insular cortex, and below and medial to the fibers of the extreme capsule. They then move medially through the limen insula into the white matter of the orbital cortex. Here they assume a plate-like formation as they move rostrally and medially in the frontal lobe. These fibers terminate in ventral prefrontal area 47/12 and in the orbital cortex in areas 11 and 13 and the orbital proisocortex. Some fibers move medially, ascend at the medial wall of the prefrontal cortex, and terminate in areas 14 and 32, and others terminate in the rostral cingulate gyrus, area 24. The fibers in the UF also originate from the rostral parts of the superior temporal sulcus (areas TEa and Ipa) and the parahippocampal gyrus (areas TF, TL, and TH), course to the frontal lobe, and terminate first in basal forebrain areas and then in areas 47/12, 13, 14, 10, and 25. As the UF courses from all these temporal lobe areas through the temporal stem toward the frontal lobe, it contributes projections also to the amygdala and to the temporal polar proisocortex and perirhinal region.

The uncinate bundle also contains reciprocal fibers leading from these orbital, ventrolateral, and medial prefrontal regions back to the temporal lobes. They lead to the rostral parts of the superior temporal gyrus, superior temporal sulcus, and inferotemporal region, as well as to the parahippocampal gyrus and the amygdala.

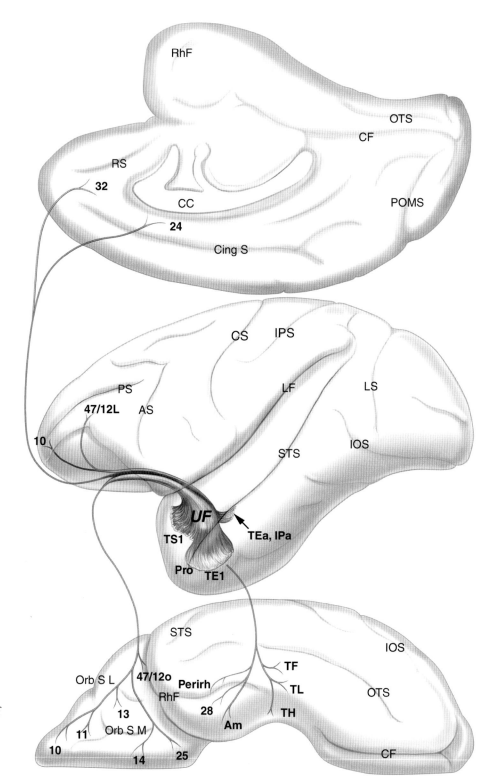

Figure 16-1

Summary diagrams of the course and composition of the UF in the rhesus monkey. The lateral view of the cerebral hemisphere (middle diagram) shows the trajectory of the UF and the cortical areas that are linked in a bidirectional manner by the fibers in this pathway. The medial view (above) and basal view (below) of the hemisphere are shown to represent other cortical areas that contribute to this fasciculus.

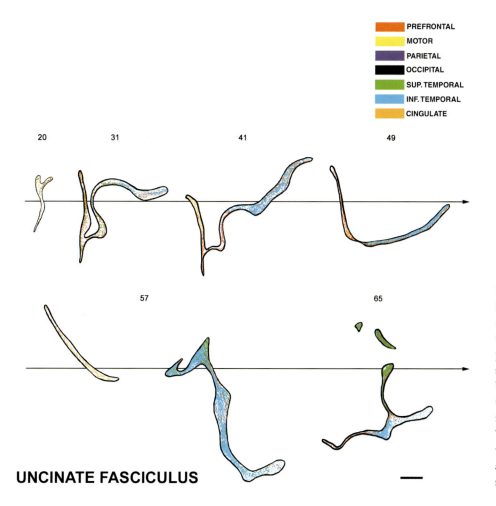

PREFRONTAL
MOTOR
PARIETAL
OCCIPITAL
SUP. TEMPORAL
INF. TEMPORAL
CINGULATE

20   31   41   49

57   65

UNCINATE FASCICULUS

Figure 16-2
Summary diagrams of rostral to caudal coronal sections through the UF extracted from the composite views of the hemisphere shown in chapter 27. The numbers refer to the sections of the template brain from which these images of the UF are derived. The areas of origin of the fibers within the UF are color-coded according to the legend at top right. Bar = 2 mm.

Functional Considerations

The UF has been considered part of a limbic ring on the medial surface of the hemisphere. In describing the cingulum bundle, Burdach (1822, p. 148) stated that "each cingulum forms a ring-like belt throughout the entire brain, except inferiorly and anteriorly, both ends of which come very close to each other, and through the unciform fasciculus are truly connected." Similarly, Yakovlev and Locke (1961b, p. 392) were impressed by the interdigitation of the cingulum bundle with the UF and regarded these two tracts as "a circular system of fibers running through the entire circumference of the limbus of the hemisphere from its dorsomedial (cingulate) sector through the inferomedial (parahippocampal) sector to the basolateral (insular) and the anterior (orbital) sectors, thus closing the limbic ring."

This is an appealing notion; however, our observations are in agreement with those of Dejerine (1895), Ariëns-Kappers et al. (1936), and Whitlock and Nauta (1956), indicating that the cingulum bundle and the UF are two separate and distinct limbic association pathways. The cingulum bundle is a dorsal limbic pathway connecting the frontal, parietal, cingulate, and ventral temporal cortices, whereas the UF is a ventral limbic pathway connecting the rostral temporal, inferotemporal, and ventral temporal regions with the medial and orbital frontal cortices. It appears that there is no direct link between these two fiber tracts. Further, although both the cingulum bundle and the UF are limbic pathways at the medial border of the hemisphere and both are strongly cholinergic (Selden et al., 1998), they appear to have distinctly different functional attributes. The functional roles attributed to the cingulum bundle have been in the domains of spatial and working memory, motivation, pain perception, avoidance behavior, response selection, and error detection (see chapter 17). The putative functions of the UF, in contrast, appear to be somewhat different, as may be inferred from a consideration of the cortical areas that it links.

The *rostral part of the superior temporal gyrus* and the superior temporal proisocortex have been shown to be involved in sound recognition and in memory for acoustic information (see Colombo et al., 1996). These areas give rise to fibers that run in the UF and terminate in areas 13, 47/12, and 11 in the orbitofrontal cortex, which are important for behavioral responses to emotionally salient stimuli (see Angrilli et al., 1999; Frey et al., 2000), and in areas 14, 25, and 32 in the medial prefrontal cortex. The UF, therefore, that connects these temporal and prefrontal areas may be a crucial component of the system that regulates emotional responses to auditory stimuli.

The UF also conveys fibers to the frontal lobe from regions of the *rostral part of the inferotemporal cortex* (area TE1 and the ventral part of inferotemporal proisocortex), which are concerned with object-related visual information, to orbitofrontal cortex areas 47/12 and 11. As in the auditory domain, by transmitting object-related visual information from the temporal lobe to the orbitofrontal cortex, the UF makes it possible to attach emotional valence to visual information and to facilitate appropriate responses.

Another contingent of fibers within the UF leads from the *parahippocampal* region (entorhinal, perirhinal, parahippocampal gyrus, areas TF, TH, and TL) to the orbitofrontal cortex. Some of these fibers terminate in medial forebrain areas, while the major component of the fibers terminates in areas 13, 47/12, 11, and 10. Some fibers from the posterior parahippocampal gyrus terminate also in the rostral cingulate cortex area 24. The parahippocampal gyrus receives input from modality-specific association areas, multimodal regions of the parietotemporal cortices, the prefrontal cortex, and the cingulate gyrus. Recognition memory has been shown to be dependent upon the medial temporal region (Mishkin, 1982; Squire and Zola-Morgan, 1991; Suzuki et al., 1993) as well as the orbitofrontal cortex (Bachevalier and Mishkin, 1986). Therefore, the UF association system that links these two cortical regions is likely to be an important component of the circuit underlying recognition memory.

Thus, the UF links temporal lobe areas that contain highly processed modality-specific information, multimodal information, and limbic/emotional processing with frontal lobe areas that regulate behaviors and emotions. The modality specific inputs are auditory, rostral superior temporal gyrus; visual, rostral inferotemporal region; and somatosensory and gustatory, rostral insular opercular cortex. The multimodal information in the UF is derived from the rostral superior temporal sulcus, and mnemonic information from parahippocampal areas. The amygdala connections with the medial prefrontal and caudal orbital regions (also shown in detail by Barbas and De Olmos, 1990, and Ghashghaei and Barbas, 2002) that are carried by the UF have relevance for the processing of information about the emotional significance of stimuli and the generation of emotional expression.

The orbitofrontal regions that are linked by the UF with these temporal cortices are involved in emotion (Butter et al., 1970), self-regulation (Levine et al., 2002), recognition memory (Bachevalier and Mishkin, 1986), and decision-making (Bechara et al., 1994). The UF also links the amygdala with the temporal pole and the inferior temporal cortices. It may therefore be crucial in facilitating optimal responses to the prevailing external as well as internal milieu and consequently may play a crucial role enabling what Nauta (1971) regarded as the nervous system's need to ensure "stability in time and space." Further, this tract appears to be critical in what Barbas regards as a triadic network consisting of the orbitofrontal cortex, anterior temporal visual and auditory association cortices, and the amygdala, which may be recruited in cognitive tasks that are inextricably linked with emotional associations (Ghashghaei and Barbas, 2002).

The potential clinical relevance of the UF has received attention in recent years. Damage to the UF produces disruption of temporal–frontal connections, and it is conceivable that this may result in disordered behaviors. Levine et al. (1998) described a patient who was densely amnesic for experiences predating an injury causing damage to the right ventral frontal cortex and underlying white matter, including the UF. This patient showed impairment of autonoetic awareness (i.e., awareness of oneself as a continuous entity across time), which supports the formulation of future goals and the implementation of a behavioral guidance system to achieve them. The authors concluded from this case that this form of self-regulation is dependent upon the right ventral frontal lobe and the UF that links the frontal and temporal lobes.

In a DTI study of schizophrenia, Kubicki et al. (2002) determined that there is greater anisotropy in the left UF compared to the right, indicating a higher number and/or density of fibers on the left. Highley et al. (2002) also used DTI to conclude that asymmetry of the UF in humans is normal: in 80% of individuals it is 27% larger on the right and contains 33% more fibers. Further, they found that in patients with schizophrenia this asymmetry is preserved. The normal morphometry of the UF and its relationship to psychiatric disease will need to be studied further.

The UF may be relevant in consideration of the interictal personality disorder of temporal lobe epilepsy. Temporal lobectomy lowers seizure frequency by excision of the epileptic focus (e.g., Glaser, 1980; Rasmussen, 1980). It also improves psychosocial outcome and aggressive and antisocial behavior in some children and adults (Ettinger, 2004; Helmstaedter et al., 2003; Hill et al., 1957; Nakaji et al., 2003), and it is conceivable that this represents the beneficial effect of a temporal–frontal disconnection syndrome because components of the UF may be damaged along with the anterior temporal lobectomy (e.g., Sindou and Guenot, 2003). As a consequence, perhaps, the UF can no longer convey pathologic information from the temporal lobe to the decision-making regions of the medial and orbitofrontal cortex, thereby promoting clinical improvement. This would be analogous to the beneficial effects of cingulotomy (e.g., Ballantine et al., 1987; Cosgrove and Rauch, 2003). This hypothesis remains to be tested by performing clinical studies in patients and by taking advantage of the chemical specificity of the UF that has been shown using acetylcholine staining (Selden et al., 1998) in the study of surgical and autopsy specimens.

Cingulum Bundle

The cingulum bundle (CB) was among the first of the major fiber systems of the brain to be recognized and depicted, and its precise anatomy and possible functional importance have excited interest and speculation from the outset. Vicq d'Azyr (1786) "noted the anterior origin of the cingulum and designated it the 'pedunculi corporis callosi' that runs from the corpus callosum posteriorly in a diverging arc to the cribriform plate" (Burdach, 1822, p. 370, annotation to paragraph 194). Reil (1809a) "examined the cingulum bundles in their entire extent, and in the greatest detail" (Burdach, ibid.), identified their close proximity to the corpus callosum and their circumferential course and sagittal orientation resembling that of the fornix, and concluded that they link the orbital cortex anteriorly with the hippocampus posteriorly.[1]

The CB was one of the four major long association systems clearly described by Burdach (1822, p. 148, paragraph 194), the others being the arcuate, unciform, and inferior longitudinal fasciculi.[2] According to Burdach (1822, p. 148, paragraph 194):

> The cingulum bundle is the most prominent white matter system and it is the most easily peeled off from the cortex. The cingulum bundles are situated on both sides of the midline on the peripheral surface of the corpus callosum as a pair of round bundles consisting of longitudinal fibers and fibers that radiate into their own gyri, in which, on occasion, one finds a gray tract in cross-section. Extending from the cribriform plate of the 'Stammlappen' [see footnote 2, chapter 13] they run anteriorly to the basal surface of the frontal lobe then ascend superiorly, run backwards through the parietal lobe, bend and run within the temporal lobe anteriorly to its pole. In this manner each cingulum forms a ring-like belt throughout the entire brain, except inferiorly and anteriorly, both ends of which come very close to each other, and through the unciform fasciculus are truly connected. In the largest part of its course the cingulum bundle is situated on the peripheral surface of the body of the corpus callosum on its lateral border and enveloped by the callosal radiations that take their origin here. By encircling the body of the corpus callosum like the hub of a wheel from which the spokes radiate, the direction of its fibers cross the callosal fibers.[3]

> They [the cingulum bundles] form the larger portion of the gyri on the medial surface of the hemispheres and are situated on both sides of the midline. Where they are attached to the corpus callosum they are close to the midline, but where they separate from the corpus callosum they run more laterally so that both ends are furthest away from the midline. In their course they form an arc that is convex superiorly and posteriorly, and that corresponds to the

ventricle. In this manner their relationship to the external surface of the brain is roughly analogous to that of the fornix to the interior of the brain.[4]

The prevailing notion at the turn of the 20th century was that the cingulum contained short arcuate fibers that enter and leave the bundle, as well as association fibers linking distant parts of the cerebral cortex (Broca, 1878; Foville, 1844; Huguenin, 1879; Obsersteiner, 1888, translated into English 1896; Quain, 1882; Schwalbe, 1881; von Kölliker, 1894).[5]

In Charles Beevor's (1891) evaluation of the CB in the Marmoset monkey using the myelin stains of Weigert and Pal, he sectioned the brain in the three cardinal planes to obtain "a mental image of the structure in the three dimensions of space" (Beevor, 1891, p. 138). He described the cingulum (p. 153) as "a comma or pear-shaped bundle of fibres with the concavity towards the middle line, and with its general axis directed downwards and outwards, presenting the distinct appearance of fibres cut transversely." Like the earlier investigators, Beevor noted that the cingulum does not vary in size throughout its course above the corpus callosum, even though it "continually gives off fibres upwards into the centrum ovale along its whole horizontal course" (p. 155). Consequently, he reasoned, the "fibres must be reinforced by continual additions, and it is suggested that these additions are received from the gyrus fornicatus [cingulate gyrus]" (p. 155). "To facilitate the description of the cingulum" (p. 159) he divided it into three parts. Beevor's description of these three components is presented *verbatim* here (1891, pp. 159–160), and Dejerine's (1895, pp. 752–753) helpful précis of Beevor's observations is in brackets:

> The horizontal part extends from the isthmus of the gyrus fornicatus behind to the anterior part of the corpus callosum in front [thus originating in the frontal lobe, traveling along the superior aspect of the corpus callosum, and linking the different regions of the cingulate gyrus] . . . The anterior part of the cingulum in front and below the genu of the corpus callosum appears in sagittal sections to consist of fibers, which arising from the most anterior part of the centrum ovale, pass downwards and backwards and thence into the internal root of the olfactory nerve [thus linking the hippocampal convolution within which it lies, with the lingual lobule, fusiform lobule, and the convolutions of the temporal lobe] . . . The posterior part of the cingulum extends from behind the splenium of the corpus callosum to the anterior part of the temporosphenoidal lobe [linking the anterior perforated substance, and particularly the internal olfactory root, with the inferior aspect of the frontal lobe].

Beevor did not observe fibers in the cingulum to reach the hippocampus or amygdala. In collaboration with Sir Victor Horsley (1857–1916) who "completely severed" (p. 161) the cingulum in a monkey so that the consequent degeneration could be studied, Beevor concluded that the cingulum "does not degenerate forwards, but any change takes place in a posterior direction." Complete section of the cingulum did not result in degeneration of all its fibers, and this served to "confirm the opinion that the cingulum does not contain fibres running through its whole length, but is made of relays of fibres which are continually leaving it. [Further, the fibers of the cingulum] "end deeply in the centrum ovale, and are not part of the superficial connecting fibres of the cortex." (Beevor, 1891, p. 162).

Dejerine (1895, p. 749) referred to the cingulum as the "cingulum bundle of Burdach, also called the fornix periphericus of Arnold [1838a,b] and the longitudinal fasciculus of the gyrus fornicatus." He regarded it as "the long association fascicle of the rhinencephalon; an arcuate fascicle with a sagittal orientation located on the internal aspect of the hemisphere, that contributes to the white matter of the first and second limbic convolutions." The earlier contributions of Burdach regarding the CB in the human were refined by Dejerine's description (Dejerine, 1895, p. 750; see figures 2-10B,C and 2-11C):

> The cingulum is easy to dissect on a brain hardened in either alcohol or bichromate after removing the cortex and the U fibers of the first limbic convolution [cingulate gyrus]. This tract is apparent in the form of an arcuate fascicle that courses around the rostrum, genu, trunk and enlargement [splenium] of the corpus callosum, then the isthmus of the limbic lobe, and spreads out and becomes broad at the level of the hippocampal convolution, moving towards the ventral and rostral portion of the anterior cruciate convolution . . . On coronal section . . . the cingulum appears as a . . . clearly delineated, pyriform fascicle, which occupies the inferior half of the first limbic convolution. Its base lies on the corpus callosum at the level where the corpus callosum penetrates the white matter of the centrum ovale. Its tip corresponds to the front of the first limbic convolution. Its medial aspect is concave and abuts the taenia tecta and the gray matter of the first limbic convolution from which it is separated only by short association fibers. Its lateral or convex aspect is in contact with the fibers of the centrum ovale, and it is distinct from callosal fibers that travel to the superior edge of the hemisphere and to the convolutions of the medial aspect . . . Behind the enlargement of the corpus callosum, the cingulum is interrupted by fibers of the forceps major coursing to the cuneus and lingual lobule. At the level of the precalcarine fissure a portion of the cingulum is in contact with the most anterior fibers of the stratum calcarinum that cover the common branch of the parieto-occipital and calcarine fissures. In the hippocampal convolution the cingulum is comprised of sagittally oriented fibers that are darkly stained with hematoxylin and that cover the medial extremity of the vertical subiculum.

In addition to describing the location of the CB in more detail, Dejerine's

> [d]issections indicate[d to him] that the cingulum is not formed by fibers that travel along the whole length of the fascicle, but rather is formed progressively of short fibers that curve at their extremities in order to reach the white matter of neighboring convolutions, and at some point in their trajectory these constitute the Cingulum of Burdach. This fascicle receives and contributes fibers to the first frontal convolution, the paracentral lobule, the precuneus, the cuneus, the lingual lobule, the fusiform lobule, and the temporal pole. The large number of afferent and efferent fibers explains why the thickness of the cingulum is constant along the superior aspect of the corpus callosum. The cingulum narrows only at the level of the pre-calcarine isthmus (Dejerine, 1895, p. 750).

In his further discussion of the cingulum, Dejerine reviewed some of the other contemporary controversies regarding the anatomy and functions of the CB.[6]

Cajal reported three types of fibers within the CB itself (Cajal, 1901, 1955 translation, p. 111; 1909–1910, 1995 translation, p. 666). The axons were seen to arise from pyramidal neurons of the cingulate gyrus. Some traveled caudally, others rostrally, and a third group, which constituted the majority, bifurcated and gave rise to both caudally and rostrally directed fibers. Caudal fibers were directed toward the occipital pole, whereas rostrally directed fibers terminated in the septum or were "lost" in the corpus striatum. Further, according to Cajal (1955, p. 117; 1995, p. 669), there were three kinds of "exogenous fibers . . . in the white matter of the interhemispheric cortex." These were "conductors of projection destined for inferior centers which are still unknown; conductors of association for distant regions which embrace areas rather far from the interhemispheric region; and long conductors of association terminating in the subiculum and Ammon's horn."

Following Beevor and Horsley's experiments in the monkey, connectional studies were performed by Probst (1903), who lesioned the cingulum in cat and observed Marchi granules extending anteriorly and posteriorly, with degenerating fibers reaching the hippocampus. The cortical and subcortical connections of the cingulate gyrus were further evaluated during the era of strychnine neuronography (e.g., Bailey et al., 1944; MacLean and Pribram, 1953; Pribram et al., 1950), but these studies did not provide information regarding the fibers in the CB itself. Degeneration studies performed by Mettler (1935b) determined that in contrast to Beevor's earlier assertion, fibers in the CB travel in both directions, and Adey (1951) determined in the rabbit that lesions of the anterior cingulate and adjacent frontal cortex produced degeneration in the CB fibers leading to the presubiculum of the hippocampus. Adey and Meyer (1952) then performed ablation degeneration studies in green monkey (*Cercopithecus sebaceus*) and determined, using the Glees (1946) technique, that lesions of the anterior cingulate area result in degenerating fibers in the cingulum leading to the posterior cingulate area and the presubiculum; lesions of the posterior cingulate lead to a smaller number of degenerating fibers leading to the retrosplenial cortex and the presubiculum; and lesions of the medial aspect of the prefrontal cortex led to a greater number of degenerating fibers in the cingulum than from either the anterior or posterior cingulate lesions, terminating in the presubiculum and the adjacent entorhinal area.

Showers (1959) used the Marchi method in rhesus monkey to evaluate the CB and the sensorimotor, visceral, and autonomic phenomena associated with electrical stimulation of the cingulate gyrus. She determined that there are intracingulate paths linking rostral and caudal cingulate regions, as well as "cingulofrontal and cinguloparietal tracts [that] occupy a lateral and dorsal position in the cingulum and swing across the medial edge of the corona radiata to ascend medially in the radiation path up to the superior convolution" (p. 270). Cingulate projections were directed to all areas of the frontal lobe (precentral gyrus, superior frontal gyrus, inferior frontal gyrus, and frontal operculum), as well as to medial and lateral regions of the parietal lobe (postcentral gyrus, inferior parietal lobule, and medial and lateral cortices of the superior parietal lobule). Cingulate projections to the caudate nucleus, globus pallidus, thalamus, hypothalamus, and brainstem were also identified.

Yakovlev and Locke (1961b) evaluated the connections of the cingulate gyrus in rhesus monkey following focal ablations of the cingulate gyrus and the CB. They studied the pattern of gliosis with the aid of the Loyez stain for myelin and the cresyl violet stain for Nissl substance. Cajal's earlier observations regarding the supracallosal white matter influenced the terminology adopted by Yakovlev and Locke, who thus referred to the white matter of the cingulate gyrus as the medullary core; within this core region they identified an area of compact and homogeneous appearance that they termed the cingulum proper, or the ground bundle of the cingulum. They regarded the cingulum proper as a system of efferent fibers, including association, projection, and commissural systems. The remaining area of the medullary core, the neuropil of finely medullated fibers, they regarded as conveying thalamic afferent fibers.

They reiterated Cajal's notion (referring to his figure 521, reproduced in the 1995 translation) that the cingulum comprises fibers arising from neurons in the cingulate gyrus that course anteriorly, posteriorly, or bifurcate, and concluded that "[t]he bulk of the fibers of the cingulum originates . . . from the 'pyramids' of the limbic cortex" (Yakovlev and Locke, 1961b, p. 389).[7] They also believed that the branching of fibers seen emanating from the cingulate gyrus represented divergence into multiple directions of the axons of single neurons.[8]

Further, Yakovlev and Locke ascertained that the "cingulum consists of very long fibers encompassing the entire circumference of the medial limbus of the hemisphere and receiving all along its anteroposterior course a constant accession of shorter fibers" (1961b, p. 376). In its course around the corpus callosum, they concluded (Yakovlev and Locke 1961a,b) that the CB consists of five "more or less" discrete components:

1. The dorsal radiation traverses the medullary core of the cingulate gyrus and provides short association projections (U–fibers) to the medial aspects of the frontal, parietal, occipital, and temporal lobes.

2. The lateral radiation emerges from the medullary core into the centrum semi-ovale, where it enters the internal capsule. These authors credit Showers (1959) with the notion that these fibers also reach the putamen, pallidum, and external capsule.

3. The ventral radiation traverses the callosal fibers in short arcs, turns ventrally medial to the internal capsule, and enters the subcallosal fasciculus of Mu-ratoff.

4. The medial stream comprises fibers that turn medially from the cingulum and course in the dorsal lamina of the corpus callosum to head to the opposite hemisphere. The authors also noted that some of these callosal fibers enter the septum.

5. The perforant radiation comprises fibers nearest the floor of the cingulate sulcus that turn sharply medially, perforate the cortical plate in the floor of the sulcus, and enter the tenia tecta and the rudimentary cortex of the indusium griseum.

Streams 1 and 5 were Cajal's "associational" (i.e., corticocortical) fibers, whereas fiber streams 2, 3, and 4 were Cajal's "projectional" fibers to the thalamus, pallidum, zona incerta, subthalamic region, and substantia nigra (Yakovlev and Locke, 1961a, p. 391; see their figure 6A reproduced here in Notes, figure N–2).

Like Burdach, Yakovlev and Locke were impressed with the interdigitation of the CB with the uncinate fasciculus at both the orbital frontal cortex and the temporal pole. This suggested to these authors that (1961b, p. 391): "[t]he cingulate and the uncinate bundles form thus a circular system of fibers running through the entire circumference of the limbus of the hemisphere from its dorsomedial (cingulate) sector through the inferomedial (parahippocampal) sector to the basolateral (insular) and the anterior (orbital) sectors, thus closing the limbic ring."

In an isotope tract-tracing study to elucidate the course and composition of the CB in the rhesus monkey, Mufson and Pandya (1984) determined that the CB consisted of subcortical and association fibers. Thalamic fibers were derived from the anterior and lateral dorsal thalamic nuclei and occupied the ventral sector of the CB. Those from the anterior thalamic nucleus terminated in area 23 and the retrosplenial cortex, whereas fibers from the lateral dorsal nucleus reached the retrosplenial cortex as well as the parahippocampal gyrus and presubiculum. Efferent fibers from the cingulate gyrus itself occupied the dorsolateral sector of the CB. Those derived from anterior cingulate area 24 were directed to premotor and prefrontal regions, as well as to area 23 and the retrosplenial cortex. Fibers in the CB derived from posterior cingulate area 23 extended rostrally to the prefrontal cortex and caudoventrally to the presubiculum and parahippocampal gyrus. Association fibers within the CB, originating mainly from the prefrontal cortex and the posterior parietal region, were in a dorsal and lateral position in the periphery of the cingulate white matter. Cingulum bundle fibers from the prefrontal cortex extended up to the retrosplenial cortex, whereas those from the posterior parietal cortex extended caudally to the parahippocampal gyrus and presubiculum and rostrally up to the prefrontal cortex.

Results of the Present Investigation

Our observations regarding the location and course of the CB are in general agreement with the conclusions of earlier investigators (Baleydier and Mauguiere, 1980; Morecraft and Van Hoesen, 1998; Morecraft et al., 2004; Morris et al., 1999a,b; Pandya et al., 1973b, 1981; Vogt et al., 1979, 1987; Vogt and Pandya, 1987). The CB stretches from the frontal lobe around the rostrum and genu of the corpus callosum, extends caudally above the corpus callosum lateral to the cingulate gyrus, curves ventrally around the splenium, and then lies in the white matter of the ventral part of the temporal lobe—the parahippocampal gyrus (figures 17-1 and 17-2). The confusing nomenclature used to designate the various components of the CB appears to be a result of the complexity of the white matter tracts conveyed within and through it. The CB may be conceptualized in the same manner as the white matter underlying any other cortical region in that it conveys long association, short association, striatal, subcortical (including thalamic and pontine), and commissural fibers. It may be helpful to outline the constituents of the CB in the following manner.

Association Fibers

The efferent long association fibers of the CB originate from the rostral cingulate cortex area 24, the caudal cingulate cortex area 23, and the retrosplenial cortex areas 29 and 30. These fibers travel rostrally or caudally to provide projections to distant cortical areas. Fibers directed rostrally terminate in the mid-dorsolateral prefrontal cortex, in areas 9 and 46. Some fibers are also directed toward the orbitofrontal cortex, area 11, as

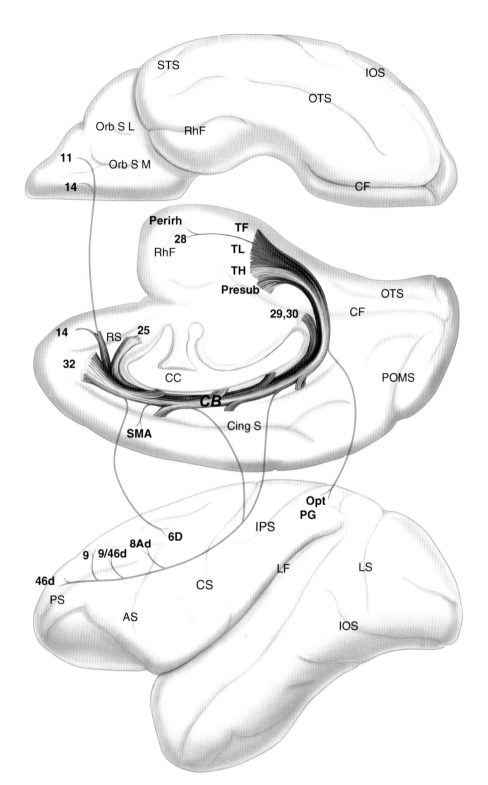

Figure 17-1

Summary diagrams of the course and composition of the CB in the rhesus monkey. The medial view of the cerebral hemisphere (middle diagram) shows the trajectory of the CB and the cortical areas that contribute axons to this fasciculus. The lateral view (above) and basal view (below) of the hemisphere are shown to represent other cortical areas that are linked in a bidirectional manner by the fibers in this pathway.

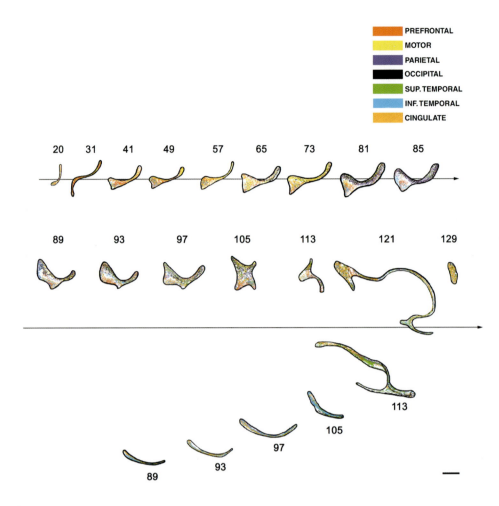

PREFRONTAL
MOTOR
PARIETAL
OCCIPITAL
SUP. TEMPORAL
INF. TEMPORAL
CINGULATE

CINGULUM BUNDLE

Figure 17-2
Summary diagrams of rostral to caudal coronal sections through the CB extracted from the composite views of the hemisphere shown in chapter 27. The numbers refer to the sections of the template brain from which these images of the CB are derived. The areas of origin of the fibers within the CB are color-coded according to the legend at top right. Bar = 2 mm.

well as to area 32 on the medial surface of the frontal lobe. Caudally directed fibers lead to the parietal cortex (area PG/Opt), retrosplenial cortex, and ventral temporal lobe (presubiculum, parahippocampal gyrus, and entorhinal cortex).

The afferent fibers to the cingulate gyrus traveling in the CB are derived from the same prefrontal, parietal, and temporal regions to which the efferent fibers from the cingulate gyrus are relayed.

These long association fibers travel in the periphery of the CB and may be viewed in the same manner as the other long association fascicles in the cerebral white matter.

In addition to the long association fibers, there are also short association fibers within the CB that link the various cingulate regions with each other in a bidirectional manner.

Another long association fiber system emanating from the cingulate cortex penetrates laterally through the CB and collects in the fronto-occipital fasciculus located above the Muratoff bundle. These fronto-occipital fibers course rostrally and terminate in dorsal area 6, dorsal area 8, and area 9 (see chapter 19).

Striatal Fibers

Fibers destined for the striatum originate from the cingulate gyrus and retrosplenial areas, course laterally through the CB, move ventrally, and collect in a compact bundle above the head and body of the caudate nucleus (i.e., the subcallosal fasciculus of Muratoff, the Muratoff bundle). From this position, the fibers terminate throughout the entire length of the body and head of the caudate nucleus. Some of the striatal fibers move further laterally, either directly from the CB or via the Muratoff bundle, cross the corona radiata or the internal capsule, and then descend in the external capsule before terminating in the claustrum and putamen.

Cord System

Another group of fibers originating from the cingulate gyrus aggregates in a dense cord, moves laterally through the CB, and immediately divides into two components, commissural and subcortical. The commissural fibers course ventrally to become incorporated into the callosal fibers that pass to the opposite hemisphere. The subcortical fibers progress laterally into the corona radiata and enter the internal capsule. One group of fibers terminates in the thalamus, and the other continues into the cerebral peduncle as it courses to the pons.

Thus, the CB is a composite fiber structure consisting of association fibers, striatal fibers, commissural fibers, and subcortical fibers. The fibers in the CB are topographically organized with some degree of overlap. The association fibers generally course through the periphery of the CB, whereas the subcortical (commissural and subcortical) fibers tend to occupy a more ventral and central position. The subcortical, commissural, striatal, and some association fibers that emanate from any region of the cingulate gyrus have a characteristic radiating appearance in the coronal plane. Yakovlev and Locke (1961b) termed this arrangement the "Indian war bonnet" (see figure N-2 in Notes).

Functional Notions

Although the CB was demonstrated and its anatomy described by Reil, Burdach, Beevor, Dejerine, and others, more detailed investigations into its anatomy and connections were prompted by new hypotheses regarding the functional role of the cingulate area. Papez (1937) proposed that the cingulate gyrus and CB were integral components of the circuitry subserving emotion, and MacLean incorporated them into his conception of the "visceral brain" (MacLean 1949, 1952; see Vogt and Gabriel, 1993).

Anatomical Insights

Early indications of the possible functional roles of the CB were derived from neuronographic studies of the cortical areas that it links (e.g., Bailey et al., 1944; Dunsmore and Lennox, 1950; Lennox et al., 1950; Pribram et al., 1950). Ablation-degeneration studies further explored these connections. Yakovlev and Locke (1961a, pp. 385–386) showed that

> the corticocortical connections of the cingulate gyrus are mainly with the cortical areas of the medial wall of the ipsilateral hemisphere, and . . . these ipsilateral corticocortical fibers arise mainly from the cingulum. They form a parasagittal sheet of subcortical arcuate fibers of Arnold . . . Fanning as far posteriorly as the parastriate area OA [nomenclature of von Bonin and Bailey, 1947] in the precuneus, these fibers appear to radiate from the respective anteroposterior sectors of the anterior cingulate gyrus, anteriorly into areas FL, FF, and FD in the medial wall of the frontal lobe, dorsally into the medial fields of areas FC, FB, and FA in the superior frontal gyrus, posteriorly into area LC [nomenclature of von Economo and Koskinas, 1925] in the posterior cingulate gyrus, and into areas PC and PE in the medial wall of the superior parietal gyrus, and around the splenium of the corpus callosum into the medial (parahippocampal) lip of the temporal lobe.

Considerable detail is available from more recent anatomical studies in the rhesus monkey using contemporary retrograde and anterograde tracing techniques (e.g., Baleydier and Mauguiere, 1980; Morecraft and Van Hoesen, 1998; Morecraft et al., 2004; Morris et al., 1999a,b; Pandya et al., 1973b, 1981; Vogt et al., 1979, 1987; Vogt and Pandya, 1987), and these are summarized as follows. Area 24 is reciprocally linked with the premotor region (areas 6 and 8), the orbitofrontal cortex (area 12), the rostral part of the inferior parietal lobule, the anterior insular cortex, the perirhinal area, and the laterobasal nucleus of amygdala. Area 23, by contrast, is linked with the dorsal prefrontal cortex (areas 9 and 46), the rostral orbitofrontal cortex (area 11), the posterior part of the inferior parietal lobule and associative regions in the superior temporal sulcus, the parahippocampal gyrus (areas TH and TF), the retrosplenial region, and the presubiculum. These connections are bidirectional. In addition, area 30 of the retrosplenial cortex has reciprocal connections with adjacent areas 23, 19 and PGm, with the mid-dorsolateral part of the prefrontal cortex (areas 9, 9/46 and 46) and its medial extension (medial areas 9 and 9/32), with multimodal area TPO in the superior temporal sulcus, as well with posterior parietal cortical areas PG and POa, and the posterior parahippocampal cortex, presubiculum, and entorhinal cortex.

In monkey and human, areas 24 and 23 are both linked with the "limbic" thalamic nuclei: anteromedial, anteroventral, and lateral dorsal nuclei (Baleydier and Mauguiere, 1980; Locke et al., 1961; Morris et al., 1999b; Vogt et al., 1987; Yakovlev et al., 1960). Area 24 has, in addition, connections with intralaminar, mediodorsal, and ventral anterior thalamic nuclei, as well as the amygdala, and the nucleus accumbens septi; and area 23 is also interconnected with the medial pulvinar. Area 30 has bidirectional connections with the lateral posterior thalamic nucleus, as well as with the LD and AV limbic thalamic nuclei.

In addition to conveying association fibers of the cingulate gyrus itself, the CB contains association fibers arising from other cortical regions, as well as fibers linking the cingulate gyrus with subcortical structures, including the thalamus, striatum, and pons, and commissural fibers to the opposite hemisphere.

The results of the present investigations, together with the observations of the earlier studies, indicate that the cortical connections of the cingulate gyrus that run in the CB may be grouped into three broad categories based on their functional affiliations. These are isocortical areas that include the association cortices; proisocortical or paralimbic cortices; and periallocortical or limbic regions (Mesulam, 2000). The functional roles of the CB may thus be viewed in the light of the properties that characterize these cortical areas that it links.

Isocortical Connections

The isocortical connections of the cingulate gyrus are with the higher-order association areas in the frontal, parietal, and temporal regions. These areas are multimodal or polysensory because they receive input from parasensory association cortices in the visual, auditory, and somatic sensory domains. Specifically, the cingulate gyrus connections with the frontal lobe are with dorsolateral areas 8, 9/46 and 10, orbitofrontal area 11, medial prefrontal area 32, and premotor area 6. The connections with the parietal lobe are with the lateral (area PG/Opt) and medial (area PGm) regions of the posterior parietal lobule. The cingulate gyrus connections with the temporal lobe are with the caudal superior temporal gyrus area Tpt, with area TPO in the upper bank of the superior temporal sulcus, and with the parahippocampal gyrus. In addition, unlike the primary motor cortex, the cingulate motor areas (Morecraft and Van Hoesen, 1993; Picard and Strick, 1996) have widespread connections with sensorimotor regions, as well as with cortical association areas.

Proisocortical Connections

The CB enables cingulate gyrus connections with proisocortical areas, including the retrosplenial cortex, parahippocampal gyrus, and perirhinal area. These proisocortical areas are linked with cortical association areas on the one hand and with limbic structures on the other, such as the amygdala and the hippocampal formation.

Periallocortical Connections

Cingulate gyrus connections with the limbic or periallocortical areas include the presubiculum and the entorhinal cortex.

It is likely that the connections conveyed in the CB facilitate the behavioral properties attributed to this fiber system in lesion and behavioral studies in humans and animals. This includes such processes as autonomic phenomena (Kaada et al., 1949; Showers, 1959; Talairach et al., 1973); complex motor behaviors (Showers, 1959; Talairach et al., 1973); the emotional coloring of sensation and nociception (MacLean, 1949, 1952); attention toward sensory stimuli with affective valence and visual spatial attention (Watson et al., 1973, 1978); facial movements that convey emotional expression (Morecraft et al., 2001; Showers, 1959); avoidance behavior (Pribram and Fulton, 1954); motivation, drive, will, and exploratory behavior (Stuss and Benson, 1986); and working memory and self-monitoring (Morris et al., 1999b). In the memory domain, the CB may contribute to different aspects of mnemonic processing. Thus, declarative memory invokes the hippocampal connections (Mishkin, 1982; Squire and Zola-Morgan, 1991; Suzuki et al., 1993); spatial memory and spatial attention draw on parietal and hippocampal systems (Kolb et al., 1994; Nadel, 1991); working memory is supported by its links with the dorsolateral prefrontal cortex (Goldman-Rakic, 1999; Goldman-Rakic et al., 1984; Mufson and Pandya, 1984; Pandya et al., 1981; Petrides, 1995); and episodic memory may be dependent upon area 10 in the frontal pole (Lepage et al., 2000).

A distinct component of the CB comprises fibers relayed in an anatomically precise manner via the Muratoff bundle to the caudate nucleus, nucleus accumbens, and putamen. The striatum has been considered crucial for the initiation of motor, cognitive, and emotional behaviors, and these functional properties are differentially arranged. The caudate nucleus is implicated in the pathophysiology of obsessive-compulsive disorder and decreases in size in patients after treatment of this condition with cingulotomy (Rauch et al., 2000). It is possible, therefore, that fibers passing through the CB are linked with striatal regions that play a role in initiating the expression of affective behavior and motor responses.

A strong bidirectional fiber tract passes through the CB as it links the thalamus with the cingulate gyrus. The thalamic nuclei include those regarded as "limbic," namely the anterior nuclear group (AV, AM, AD), and the LD and intralaminar nuclei, as well as limbic regions of the PM and MD (MDdc) and the VA nucleus. The functions of thalamic nuclei have generated considerable interest. Johnson and Ojemann (2000) concluded that thalamus provides a "specific alerting response" (Ojemann, 1983), increasing the input to memory of category-specific material while simultaneously inhibiting retrieval from memory. Crosson's analysis (1999) of patients with focal thalamic lesions led to the conclusion that thalamus contributes a "selective engagement mechanism" (Crosson, 1985; Nadeau and Crosson, 1997) to cortical areas required to perform a cognitive task while maintaining other areas in a state of relative disengagement. The defects of emotional expression and affective regulation that occur following lesions of the limbic thalamus (see Schmahmann, 2003) may result in part from destruction of these thalamocingulate connections that travel in the CB.

Finally, a contingent of fibers that penetrates laterally through the CB contributes to the feed-forward limb of the cerebrocerebellar pathway by linking the cingulate gyrus with nuclei in the basis pontis (Vilensky and Van Hoesen, 1981). The cingulopontine projections have been implicated in the investigations of patients who show impairments of cognitive and affective behaviors following cerebellar lesions (Levisohn et al., 2000; Schmahmann and Sherman, 1998). Likewise, patients with selective infarction of the rostral basis pontis have been described who display emotional blunting and pathologic laughter and crying (Bassetti et al., 1996; Kim et al., 1994; Schmahmann et al., 2004a). This would suggest that cingulate gyrus projections that travel through the CB to the basilar pons may be relevant in the modulation of these behaviors in the normal individual.

Clinical Insights

The crucial role of the CB in the regulation of emotional processing is underscored by historical and contemporary accounts of the effects of lesion and stimulation experiments in animals and patients.

Marked behavioral changes in monkeys were noted following ablation of the anterior cingulate region, including tameness and loss of fear (Glees et al., 1950; Smith, 1944, 1945; Ward, 1948). Autonomic phenomena in monkeys (Showers, 1959; Smith, 1944, 1945) and humans (Tailarach et al., 1973) are elicited by electrical stimulation of the anterior cingulate cortex, and more complex behavioral responses, including fear, anxiety, and pleasure, have been recorded in humans following stimulation of the CB itself (Meyer et al., 1973).

Cingulotomy was introduced as a treatment for depression and psychosis (Egaz Moniz, 1937; Freeman, 1948; Freeman and Watts, 1942) based largely on the theory of Papez (1937) and experimental observations in the monkey (Fulton, 1949; see Pressman, 1988). Glees et al. (1950) noted little change following localized ablation of this area in patients with advanced psychosis, but there was considerable improvement in those with obsessive-compulsive behaviors. Adey and Meyer (1952) believed that the therapeutic effect of prefrontal leucotomy lay in its interruption of fibers in the cingulum arising from areas 9 and 10 of the prefrontal cortex. Cingulectomy (LeBeau, 1954) and subsequently bilateral stereotaxic cingulotomy have achieved the status of established management for certain forms of neuropsychiatric illness, such as obsessive-compulsive disorder, and for intractable pain (Ballantine et al., 1967, 1987; Cosgrove and Rauch, 2003; Foltz and White, 1962; Hitchcock et al., 1972; Jenike et al., 1991; Price et al., 2001; Spangler et al., 1996). The heterogeneous composition of the CB, containing association, commissural, subcortical, and striatal fibers, indicates that, as Mufson and Pandya (1984) stated, "disrupting the cingulum bundle, whether for clinical or experimental purposes, must necessarily involve extensive disconnections among various cortical, subcortical, and limbic structures."

Inferior Longitudinal Fasciculus

Historical Accounts

There has been persistent uncertainty regarding the existence, course, and composition of the inferior longitudinal fasciculus (ILF) since its description by Burdach. Early investigators were unsure of its location and whether it was an association system linking the occipital lobe with other cortical areas, or whether it was a projection system between the occipital cortex and subcortical structures, including the thalamus and basal ganglia. It appears that this lack of clarity resulted from a combination of reliance on the gross dissection methodology and terminological confusion between the sagittal stratum, the optic radiation, and the ILF. In reviewing the history of the observations and ideas leading up to the present investigation, it is necessary to report what earlier authors wrote in regard to the "inferior longitudinal fasciculus," even though it appears that almost without exception these earlier works confused the sagittal stratum with the system that we now know to be a true inferior longitudinal fasciculus association system. This historical overview therefore serves to introduce both systems: the true inferior longitudinal fasciculus and the sagittal stratum.

In the earliest studies using gross dissection in alcohol-hardened brain, Reil (1809b, p. 166) noted "a layer of longitudinal fibers that runs from the apex of the temporal lobe continuing towards the apex of the occipital lobe that merges with the crus cerebri system within the occipital lobe." In a critique of Reil's statement, Burdach (1822) found it "obvious that the lower longitudinal bundle only abuts the lower part of the corona radiata, but does not transition into it, and furthermore it has a different orientation. Only when one peels it off can one find the true corona radiata" (p. 371, annotation to paragraph 196).

The term that Burdach uses to denote an ILF, however, more clearly applies in much of its course to what we now conceive of as the sagittal stratum. Thus (p. 152):

> In each hemisphere the lower long bundle (untre Längenbündel, fasciculus longitudinalis inferior) forms the foundation of the corona radiata, and has a span reaching from the occipital pole through the temporal lobe to the frontal pole in uninterrupted continuity, forming a prominent eminence on the under surface of the brain. In its longitudinal direction it is slightly curved; laterally it is slightly convex; and medially it is slightly concave. It also forms a slight arc in its vertical direction, and like the external capsule but unlike the unciform fasciculus, it is slightly convex inferiorly, and slightly concave superiorly. It originates in the occipital pole (apex of the occipital lobe) and runs anteriorly in the lateral aspect of the floor of the temporal horn [of the lateral ventricle]

(Unterhorns). In the temporal lobe it runs slightly more laterally, becomes the foundation of the lateral wall of the temporal horn of the lateral ventricle, or the most lateral portion of its floor, and cradles (trägt) the Ammon's horn. It forms a groove in which the corona radiata progresses. It is bounded medially by the tapetum and the cingulum. It is bounded laterally by the arc-like bundles that ascend deep to the lateral gyri of the temporal lobe.[1] A part of it runs in an oblique fashion anteriorly below the unciform fasciculus and in the apex of the temporal lobe. The remaining portion curves anteriorly and medially, reaches the 'Stammlappen'[2] below the lentiform nucleus, and forms the floor of the external capsule. It curves slightly laterally, enters the frontal lobe where it courses above the unciform fascicles, and extends to the lateral aspect of the frontal pole.

Burdach's description of this bundle within the occipital and temporal lobes appears to correspond to the sagittal stratum. One wonders, however, whether his "arc-like bundles that ascend deep to the lateral gyri of the temporal lobe" situated lateral to the "inferior longitudinal fasciculus" bundle may indeed be equivalent to the ILF that we describe in detail in the present study. In addition to these fiber systems, Burdach also described an internal basal bundle, although it is unclear to which system he refers.[3]

Following Burdach's observations, other investigators described fiber systems of the occipital lobe and offered different, and often conflicting, interpretations. Gratiolet performed gross dissections of the monkey brain and showed a projection fiber system that he designated the "optic radiation," linking the thalamus to the occipital lobe (Leuret and Gratiolet, 1839). In 1892, Sachs introduced the term sagittal stratum (SS) for the system that Gratiolet labeled optic radiation, and he divided the SS into two layers, the external and the internal. He concluded that afferent fibers leading to the cerebral cortex traveled in the external segment (SSe), whereas efferent fibers from the cerebral cortex were situated within the internal segment (SSi). Further, Sachs believed that there was an inferior longitudinal bundle situated within the external segment of the sagittal stratum that was "a fasciculus of association fibers originating within the occipital lobe and terminating within the temporal lobe, especially in the first and second temporal convolutions" (quoted and translated in Davis, 1921, p. 371). Wernicke recognized an ILF and named it the "sagittal layer of the occipital lobe," whereas Charcot and Ballet concluded that it conveyed sensory fascicles to the occipital lobe.

Dejerine provided a masterful account of what was considered at the time to be the ILF. His descriptions and accompanying illustrations of this "ILF" correspond to what we now understand to be the external component of the sagittal stratum (see figures 2-10D and 18-1). His careful study of the topic reflects the prevailing confusion regarding the identity, nomenclature, and constituents of the misnamed "ILF."[4] Ultimately unable to resolve the conflicting data from anatomical and lesion-degeneration studies, Dejerine concluded that the ILF was both a projection system and an association system. The lower part was associative, extending from the occipital pole to the rostral part of the temporal lobe, almost near the area giving origin to the uncinate fascicles. It contained fibers connecting the occipital lobe with the hippocampal convolutions (parahippocampal gyrus), fusiform lobule, and third temporal convolution. Fibers destined for pulvinar, medial geniculate, globus pallidus, and cerebral peduncle merely pass through

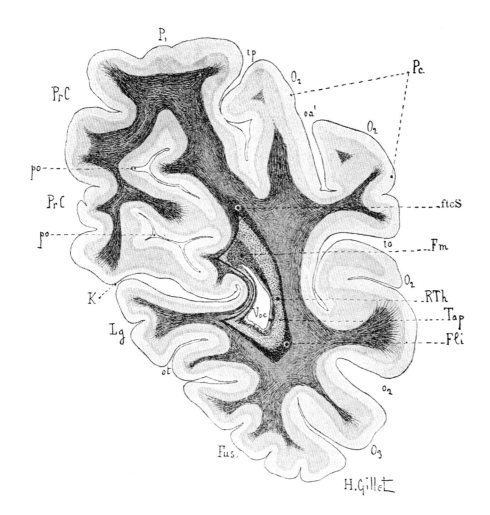

Figure 18-1
Reproduction of figure 384 from Dejerine (1895, p. 768), a myelin-stained coronal section of the human brain in the parieto-occipital region. This figure illustrates the notion prevailing at that time that the "inferior longitudinal fasciculus" (labeled Fli in Dejerine's diagram) was synonymous with what is now identifiable as the external component of the sagittal stratum, SSe. The "radiations optiques de Gratiolet," labeled RTh by Dejerine, are identical with what is considered, since the work of Sachs, to be the internal component of the sagittal stratum, SSi. Also in this diagram the superior aspect of the SS is labeled ftcS, the "faisceau transverse du cunéus de Sachs," which our observations suggest is analogous to the dorsal occipital bundle and distinct from the sagittal stratum. For further discussion of the sagittal stratum, see chapter 25.

the ILF to reach the thalamic radiations. The upper part, in contrast, was a projection system, intimately united with the retrolenticular segment of the internal capsule, containing fibers destined for subcortical centers, including the thalamus, LGN, and globus pallidus.

Flechsig's (1896) myelination studies had a significant impact on this discussion. He identified the fasciculus in question as a subcortical system, observed that it linked the occipital lobe with the thalamus, and regarded it as a bundle of the corona radiata constituting a part of Gratiolet's visual radiation.[5] Based on these observations indicating that the ILF, as then defined, was a subcortical projection system, he opposed Sachs' notion that it could carry associative fibers.[6]

Polyak (1957) summarized this debate (p. 178): "The visual radiation identical with the inferior longitudinal fascicle of Burdach was, according to Flechsig, not a system of association fibers connecting the visual centers of the occipital lobe with the speech centers of the temporal lobe as it was considered by Wernicke, Sachs, Edinger, Monakow, Dejerine and many others, but a constituent of Reil's corona radiata."

The conclusions reached in the present work regarding the association system that we term the ILF are not at variance with Flechsig's conclusions about the projection fibers contained within the fascicles identified at that time as the ILF. The bundles that

Felchsig studied were the "primary optic radiation" conveying fibers from the pulvinar and lateral geniculate to the occipital lobe (termed the geniculo-calcarine tract by Archambault, 1905, 1909; now the SSe) and the "secondary optic radiation" (now the SSi) conveying fibers from occipital lobe to the thalamus. Flechsig's myelination studies thus provided the accurate observation that the bundle we now term the sagittal stratum (after Sachs) was exclusively a projection system. Meyer (1907) later concluded, from a case of cerebral softening, that the SSe conveyed projection fibers from the thalamus to the occipital lobe, in agreement with the conclusions of Flechsig and Sachs that the primary optic radiation (the SSe) conveys information to the cortex from the thalamus.

After Flechsig differentiated the projection system situated within the SS from the occipital association system (now the ILF), it remained unclear as to precisely where this ILF association system was anatomically located. Niessl von Mayendorf (1903, 1919) concluded that the ILF was identical with the primary optic radiation of Flechsig (the SSe), although he also deduced that the sagittal stratum was a purely subcortical projection system containing thalamocortical fibers in the SSe and corticothalamic fibers in the SSi. Probst (1901b) similarly observed fibers within what he regarded as the ILF, traveling from the thalamus to the temporal and occipital lobes, as well as from these cortical areas to the cerebral peduncle, and Redlich (1905) regarded the ILF as a subcortical system within the optic radiation as well. Archambault's papers dealing with the ILF (1905, 1909) delineate the presence of thalamocortical fibers in the "fasciculus geniculocalcarinus," occupying a portion of the SSe (and SSi) in the temporal lobe, and the SSe in the occipital lobe. Edinger's (1904) clinicopathological observations of the course of degenerated fibers in a case of ablation of the temporal cortex were at odds with these findings, however, and he believed the ILF to be an association system situated within the SSe. Review again of Dejerine's monograph, and in particular the diagrams that illustrate his text, makes it clear that his ILF was identical to the SSe.

Thus, at the beginning of the 20th century, "much confusion exist[ed] as to the exact anatomy of the inferior longitudinal fasciculus" (Davis, 1921). The notion that the ILF was an association system (Burdach, Sachs, Dejerine, Edinger) competed with the conclusion that it was a purely projection system (Flechsig, Probst, Niessl von Mayendorf, Redlich, and Archambault). All these investigators were correct in part, and the mix-up seems to have arisen from a consideration of two separate systems as one (the SS on the one hand, and the ILF, as we know it now, on the other).

More recently, Tusa and Ungerleider (1985) used blunt dissection and autoradiographic tract tracing to challenge the existence of an ILF. They concluded that their data were "consistent with previous anatomical work suggesting that Burdach's ILF is nothing more than a portion of the geniculostriate pathway that has been mislabeled. Specifically, this fiber bundle corresponds to the ventral portion of the geniculostriate pathway in the occipital lobe and to Meyer's loop in the temporal lobe" (p. 587). In monkey and human brains "[t]he only long fiber bundle common to both the occipital and temporal lobes is the geniculostriate pathway (i.e., optic radiations), located within the external sagittal stratum" (p. 583). Further, these investigators determined that (p. 583) "the pathway from the occipital to the temporal cortex in monkeys consists of a series of U fibers that course beneath the cortical mantle to connect adjacent regions in striate, prestriate, and inferior temporal cortex" and suggested that a similar situation exists in the human. They proposed that the term "inferior longitudinal fasciculus" be replaced with the term "occipitotemporal projection system." The existence of U fibers linking adjacent cortical areas in the occipitotemporal region is consistent with the general organizing principles of neural connectivity. It appears, however, as shown in the current analysis, that the presence of an ILF long association pathway can no longer be disputed.

Our observations in monkey are supported by *in vivo* analyses in humans using DT-MRI. This novel approach has indicated that in humans an ILF association fiber tract within the inferior aspect of the occipitotemporal region is separate and distinct from the SS (Catani et al., 2002, 2003). Like the monkey material, the human *in vivo* studies show that the ILF links the ventral aspects of the extrastriate occipital cortex (areas V2 and V4) with anterior temporal structures (lateral temporal cortex, parahippocampal gyrus, and amygdala). The experimental monkey material provides the details of this pathway and of the cortical connections that the DT-MRI analysis cannot reveal.

Identification of an Apparently Nonexistent "Inferior Fronto-Occipital Tract" and its Confusion with the ILF

Another area of conflict that has persisted into the current literature relates to a putative "inferior fronto-occipital tract." The actual fronto-occipital fasciculus (FOF) situated above the subcallosal fasciculus of Muratoff is discussed in the following chapter, but the notion of an inferiorly situated bundle linking the occipital lobe with the frontal lobe is directly relevant to the discussion of the ILF.

In Burdach's original description of the ILF based on gross dissection, he observed that some fibers course beneath the uncinate fasciculus, "form the floor of the external capsule . . . and enter the frontal lobe where they course above the uncinate fasciculus and extend to the external side of the frontal pole" (excerpt from Burdach, 1822, p. 152 [see above], and as quoted also in Davis, 1921, p. 371). Davis thus concluded that "Burdach has very accurately described the fasciculus occipitofrontalis inferior." In 1906, using the blunt dissection method, Trolard concluded that the ILF, as described by Dejerine, formed a part of the "faisceau fronto-occipital" (p. 446). This idea was further developed by Curran (1909), who described the inferior fronto-occipital tract as (pp. 651–652)

> a new association tract . . . a long association bundle of fibres uniting the oc-
> cipital lobe with the frontal, and taking a course to the external side, and very
> close to the base of the lenticular nucleus, and in immediate relation with the
> anterior commissure as it enters the temporal lobe . . . It also contains fibers
> which join the frontal lobe with the posterior part of the temporal and parietal
> lobes . . . From all parts of the frontal lobe the fibers of this fasciculus can be
> traced converging to a single bundle which swings round the lower external
> side of the nucleus lentiformis, at which place it appears as a distinct bundle.

This bundle proposed by Trolard, Curran, and Davis supposedly originated in the occipital lobe, led into the temporal lobe, and continued uninterrupted into the inferior aspect of the frontal lobe. Davis further believed that (1921, pp. 380–381)

> [s]uch purely occipitotemporal fibers of association as may exist do not form
> any compact bundle which can properly be termed the inferior longitudinal

fasciculus; [that t]here exists a long fronto-occipital tract of association, which medially, represents the fibers spoken of by Dejerine and others, as the inferior longitudinal bundle and which, externally, represents the fasciculus occipitofrontalis inferior of Curran; [t]hat the term "inferior longitudinal fasciculus" should be dropped . . . as it refers to no anatomic entity . . . and the term "fasciculus occipitofrontalis inferior" should be used to describe this long association tract.

Subsequent gross dissections performed and depicted by Ludwig and Klingler (1956) and Heimer (1983, 1995) have helped solidify the notion that such a major ventrally situated association pathway links the occipital lobe with the frontal lobe.

Set against this observation derived from gross dissection in the human, and incompatible with it, are the observations from experimental studies in the rhesus monkey. Investigations using older techniques, as well as new and more sensitive anterograde and retrograde connectional neuroanatomical techniques, over the past four decades have failed to show substantial direct anatomical connections between the inferior aspect of the occipital lobe and the ventral prefrontal cortex. In the absence of such anatomical connections, the existence of an inferior fronto-occipital tract linking these areas is implausible. This is substantiated by reference to our material in the monkey in which we have been unable to confirm the existence of such an "inferior fronto-occipital fasciculus."

This matter is not of historical interest alone. Contemporary neuroimaging techniques using DT-MRI use conventional anatomical teaching as their road map to develop *a priori* hypotheses concerning the pathways that the mathematical modeling inherent in their technique requires. Consequently, the apparently spurious "inferior occipito-frontal fasciculus" is now making its way into a new generation of studies (e.g., Kier et al., 2004), although this probably nonexistent bundle seems to owe its existence to artifact embedded within the gross dissection method.

So what, then, were the investigators using the gross dissection method referring to when they concluded that there is a ventrally situated fiber system directly linking the occipital lobe with the frontal lobe? This bundle was reported and depicted as lying ventral to the lenticular nucleus, close to the ventral region of the claustrum, and above the uncinate fasciculus. This is precisely the location occupied by the uncinate fasciculus and the ventral component of the extreme capsule. In retrospect, it is likely that the gross dissection method led to the erroneous conclusion that these two separate fiber systems (uncinate fasciculus and extreme capsule) that lead into the frontal lobe were the rostral extension, of and continuous with, the true inferior longitudinal fasciculus and thus constituted an uninterrupted "inferior occipito-frontal" system. As has been seen in the connectional analysis and the fiber pathway study in this work, there is no longer justification for the perpetuation of this notion of an "inferior occipitofrontal fasciculus."

Summary

There are therefore a number of contentious and unresolved issues surrounding the understanding of the ILF. Is the ILF part of the SS, or is it entirely separate and distinct from it? Does the ILF contain fibers of projection as well as association fibers, or is it only associative? Is there indeed such a structure as the ILF? Is it possible that there is actually no such entity, and instead it is identical to Davis's proposed inferior occipitofrontal fasciculus? Alternatively, is the putative absence of an ILF accounted for by the possibility that occipital lobe efferents are conveyed to the temporal lobe exclusively through sequential short U-fibers, as Tusa and Ungerleider suggested? Finally, which pathways are involved in conveying information from the occipital lobe to the frontal lobe?

In the light of these persistent uncertainties, in the ensuing discussion we describe the course and composition of the ILF. The experimental material in the monkey has allowed us to clarify the earlier findings regarding the nature and course of the occipital and temporal long association fibers running in the ILF. This has made it possible to differentiate these fibers definitively from the SS, the anatomic and connectional details of which are considered later.

Results of the Present Investigation

According to our observations, the ILF is a long association fiber system that runs in the white matter of the parietal, occipital, and temporal lobes (figures 18-2 and 18-3). It is the preeminent fiber tract that conveys information in a bidirectional manner between the occipital lobe (preoccipital gyrus) and the temporal lobe. For most of its course this fiber bundle lies in the occipito-parietal region and the ventral part of the temporal lobe. It comprises a vertical limb and a horizontal limb. In the occipital-parietal region, the ILF fibers run vertically in the white matter. This vertical limb is bounded medially by the SS and laterally by the local U-fiber systems of the parietal, occipital, and temporal lobes. It can be discerned as a separate bundle in Nissl-stained material by noting that the orientation of the glial matrix is distinctly different from that of the SS and the local U fibers. In myelin stain preparations this bundle is also identifiable lateral to the SS.

The experimental material shows that in the occipito-parietal region, the ILF fibers are vertically oriented. At the ventral aspect of the occipital–temporal lobe junction, the ILF fibers change direction, separate into medial and lateral components, and course horizontally along the rostrocaudal axis of the temporal lobe within the white matter of the inferotemporal region and parahippocampal gyrus. The horizontal limb of the ILF continues rostrally within the temporal lobe up to the point of origin of the uncinate fasciculus, approximately at the level corresponding to the rostral end of the lateral geniculate nucleus. The location of the stem portion of the ILF, as determined in our Nissl and myelin preparations, is confirmed by the experimental material, which also allows the determination of the connections conveyed by the ILF.

Ventral-lateral and ventral preoccipital areas (areas V4D, V4, V4V, and V3V) give rise to fibers that travel within the ILF in topographically arranged locations in the temporal lobe white matter, leading to three main destinations within the temporal lobe:

1. Fibers traveling rostrally within the vertical limb of the ILF terminate in the cortex in the depth and the lower bank of the superior temporal sulcus (areas V4T, MST, MT, and FST, as well as areas TEa and IPa). One segment of fibers courses dorsally and terminates in area POa within the lower bank of the intraparietal sulcus.

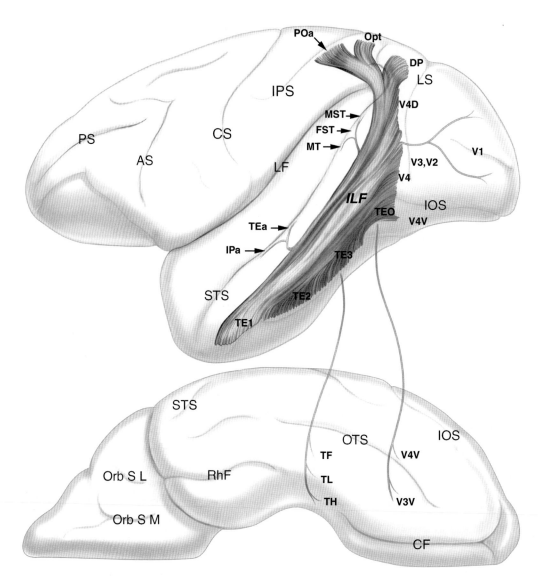

Figure 18-2
Summary diagrams of the course and composition of the ILF in the rhesus monkey. The lateral view of the cerebral hemisphere (upper diagram) shows the trajectory of the ILF and the cortical areas that are linked in a bidirectional manner by the fibers in this pathway. The basal view of the hemisphere (below) is shown to represent other cortical areas that contribute to this fiber pathway.

2. Fibers lying ventrally within the horizontal limb of the ILF in the temporal lobe white matter move lateral to the occipitotemporal sulcus and terminate in the inferior temporal gyrus (areas TEO, TE3, TE2, TE1).
3. ILF fibers that move medially within the white matter of the parahippocampal gyrus terminate mainly in areas TF, TH and TL, as well as in more caudally located transitional areas TFO, THO, and TLO.

In addition to the fibers from the occipital lobe, the vertical limb of the ILF also carries some fibers from the caudal part of the cingulate gyrus, the inferior parietal lobule (see also Seltzer and Pandya, 1984), and the superior temporal gyrus. These fibers lead to the parahippocampal gyrus.

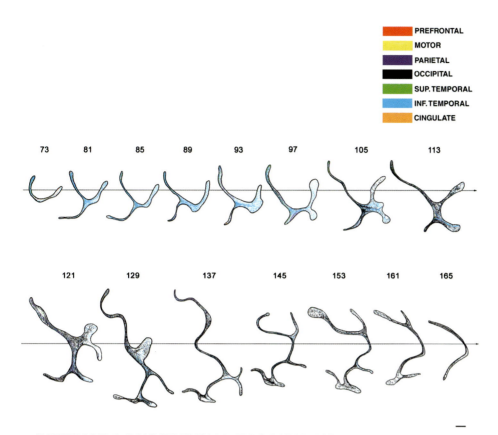

INFERIOR LONGITUDINAL FASCICULUS

Figure 18-3

Summary diagrams of rostral to caudal coronal sections through the ILF extracted from the composite views of the hemisphere shown in chapter 27. The numbers refer to the sections of the template brain from which these images of the ILF are derived. The areas of origin of the fibers within the ILF are color-coded according to the legend at top right. In this view, as in the composite summary diagrams in chapter 27, the lateral and superior limits of the ILF are liberally placed to include the fibers that leave or enter the ILF from the cortex of the posterior regions of the temporal, parietal, and occipital lobes, thus accounting for the lateral protuberances appended to the otherwise inverted L-shaped ILF. Note also that the most caudal fibers within the ILF (color-coded black here for their origin in the occipital lobe) merge with the intrinsic occipital lobe fibers termed the "occipital vertical fibers" by Wernicke. Bar = 2 mm.

Further, the connections conveyed in the ILF are reciprocal. The ILF carries information leading from extrastriate regions in the lower bank of the superior temporal sulcus back to the preoccipital region and from the parahippocampal gyrus and inferotemporal cortices to the preoccipital region, as well as the caudal inferior parietal lobule.

The ILF and the Intrinsic Occipital Lobe Fiber System

The caudal segment of the ILF is adjacent to and merges with the intrinsic fiber systems of the occipital lobe. Dejerine's synopsis of the intrinsic occipital lobe fiber systems in human is remarkably detailed and compares well with the intrinsic occipital lobe connections seen in our experimental material in the monkey. He summarized and described these "intrinsic fibers in the occipital lobe, organized as five fascicles that are more or less clearly delineated" (Dejerine, 1895, pp. 780–783; see figure 2-11D):

1. "The occipito-vertical fascicle, or perpendicular occipital fascicle of Wernicke, also called stratum proprium of the convexity of Sachs, constitutes a thick layer of fibers intrinsic to the occipital lobe and connects the superior aspect of this lobe to its inferior surface." We have observed that fibers that are caudally situated in the vertical component of the ILF link the dorsal and ventral aspects of the occipital lobe and are equivalent to this vertical occipital system of Wernicke.

2. "The occipital transverse fascicle of the cuneus (the transverse stratum of the cuneus of Sachs) connects the cuneus to the convexity of the occipital lobe and to its inferior lateral aspect. Its fibers originate . . . from the superior lip of the calcarine fissure, move transversely, . . . curve upward and . . . radiate within the cortex of the occipital convexity and its inferior external aspect. The most anterior fibers move slightly obliquely, rostrally, and laterally, and radiate in the superior parietal lobule and the angular gyrus." The system that we have termed the "dorsal occipital bundle" and that links medial and lateral parts of the dorsal occipital lobe is equivalent to this transverse fascicle of the cuneus of Sachs.

3. "The occipital transverse fascicle of the lingual lobule of Vialet is to the lingual lobule what the previous fascicle is to the cuneus. Described by Sachs, and studied further by Vialet, this fascicle takes origin from the inferior lip of the calcarine fissure, moves transversely laterally . . . and radiates into the cortex of the occipital convexity and its inferior lateral aspect. It connects the inferior lip of the calcarine fissure to the convexity of the hemisphere, and according to Vialet, represents the inferior half of the associative system." According to our observations, the transverse fibers in the ILF that lie within the ventral parts of the occipital and temporal lobe and that link the lateral cortices with the medial cortices are equivalent to the transverse fascicle of the lingual lobule of Vialet.

4. "The stratum proprium of the cuneus of Sachs . . . is a layer of short associative fibers intrinsic to the cuneus, [comprising] . . . vertical fibers . . . that take their origin from within the superior lip of the calcarine fissure . . . and radiate in the cortex of the superior aspect of the hemisphere." Fibers within the superior parietal lobule and dorsal occipital white matter caudal to SLF I link area PGm with area PO and perhaps are equivalent to this intrinsic fascicle of the cuneus of Sachs.

5. "The stratum calcarinum . . . or fringed blade of the cuneus of Brissaud, is a thick layer of vertical fibers, which . . . connects the superior lip of the calcarine fissure to its inferior lip . . . and represents the U-fiber layer of the calcarine fissure. The shortest and most superficial fibers connect the deep parts of the two lips of the calcarine fissure; the longest fibers connect the internal aspect of the cuneus to the inferior internal aspect of the lingual lobule." Dejerine emphasized that this stratum calcarinum of Brisaud is not a true association fiber system but rather represents the U-fiber system intrinsic to the pri-

mary visual cortex. We have also observed this fiber tract in the white matter of the calcarine sulcus.

Speculations on Earlier Confusion Regarding the ILF

The earlier uncertainty and confusion regarding the ILF are understandable now in the context of current knowledge and appear to have been a consequence of the material and techniques available for study at that time. The principal problem was that the gross dissection method led to the conclusion that the ILF was part of Gratiolet's optic radiation, or what Sachs termed the sagittal stratum (SS). Early investigators could not distinguish anatomically between the SS projection system and the ILF association system and thus considered them a unitary entity. This lack of distinction between the association fiber system (the ILF) and the projection fiber system (the SS) has led to a legacy of confusion in the analysis, interpretation, and discussion of the association pathways of the occipital and temporal lobes. Having observed the external layer of the SS (the SSe) that they regarded as the ILF, the early investigators witnessed conflicting patterns of degeneration following damage to this structure. Degeneration in other cortical areas implied that the ILF was associative, but degeneration was present in subcortical structures as well, indicating that this tract also contained projection fibers. Thus, was the ILF/SSe a cortical association bundle, as most thought, or was it a purely subcortical system, as Flechsig insisted? This ongoing uncertainty as to whether the tract under investigation was an association or a projection system may have been inevitable. What was described originally by Burdach as the ILF association system may have been, at least in part, the optic radiation projection system described later by Gratiolet.

The ILF as we understand it now (i.e., a long association fascicle) lies in close proximity to the medially situated SSe (the afferent projection system from subcortical structures to the cerebral cortex) and to the laterally adjacent U-fiber system. The ILF cannot readily be isolated from the SSe using gross dissection methods, and it is likely to be damaged in lesions that affect this area. Without recognizing that the ILF was a separate association system, there was no identifiable anatomic substrate other than the SSe/ILF to account for the distant cortical degeneration following lesions of the occipital or temporal cortices. The quandary may have persisted into the microscopic era in part because of the continuing terminological confusion of the ILF with the SSe, a troublesome legacy of the gross dissection method. It is relatively simple to identify the SS on gross dissection, but separating the ILF from the SSe with this approach appears to have been impossible. The ILF can be seen as a distinct entity with the Nissl stain by relying on the orientation and packing density of the glia. Moreover, the experimental isotope tract-tracing technique has further identified and clarified its location and connections.

Functional Notions

The demonstration in the monkey of the anatomic features of the ILF and the cortical areas that it links provides a vantage point from which to view its possible functional roles. These conclusions are bolstered by the observations in humans using magnetic resonance tractography (Catani et al., 2003) of the presence of an ILF that corresponds to that observed in the monkey. The monkey experimental material, however, provides the microscopic connectional details that the human material cannot yet identify. The ILF conveys information from the ventrolateral prestriate cortices to the inferotemporal region, areas TEO, TE3, TE2, and TE1. The ventral part of the occipital lobe subserves central vision (Boussaoud et al., 1991) and the functional attributes of the occipitotemporal cortices are encapsulated in the concept of the ventral visual pathway (Ungerleider and Mishkin, 1982). In this view, the occipitotemporal visual stream, the "what" pathway, is concerned with the recognition and identification of visually perceived objects, as opposed to the occipital-parietal dorsal visual stream, the "where" pathway, devoted to the spatial attributes of visual perception. This notion was elaborated upon by Goodale and Milner (1992), who suggested that the ventral stream/what pathway/perceptual system is involved in constructing perceptual representations of the visual environment and the objects within it. In contrast, they proposed, the dorsal stream/where pathway/action system facilitates visual control of actions that involve those objects. Functional imaging studies document the importance of the ventral temporal and ventral occipital cortices in the process of object recognition (Haxby et al., 2001; Ishai et al., 2000). The ILF that links these areas may therefore facilitate object identification, discrimination, and recognition.

The contingent of ILF fibers directed toward the parahippocampal gyrus terminates predominantly in area TF and to some extent in areas TL and TH. Whereas the inferotemporal segment of the ILF is likely to be involved with object recognition, fibers leading to the parahippocampal gyrus may facilitate that region's role in associating together sensory inputs within and across sensory modalities (Murray et al., 2000), as occurs in object–place associative memory (Malkova and Mishkin, 2003).

Fibers in the ILF that lead to the lower bank of the superior temporal sulcus may contribute to the analysis of visual motion with which this cortical area is engaged (Geesaman et al., 1997; Logothetis and Schall, 1989). Fibers in the ILF that lead to area POa in the parietal lobe may help facilitate visual-spatial and motion analysis (Leinonen et al., 1979; Motter et al., 1987), as well as the attentional mechanisms (Goldberg et al., 2002; Yin and Mountcastle, 1978) that characterize these parietal areas. These feedforward components of the ILF thus also provide a means of communication between areas involved in central vision and those involved with visual-spatial analysis.

By virtue of the feedback system to the first layer, the ILF also links occipitotemporal areas with earlier stages in the visual processing stream. Thus, preoccipital areas project back, through the ILF, to primary visual cortex V1. Rostral temporal areas, including the parahippocampal gyrus and amygdala, project back through the ILF to visual areas involved in early stages of visual perception. These feedback connections to the occipital lobe from inferotemporal cortices, and to both these areas from the amygdala (Amaral and Price, 1984; Amaral et al., 2003), may play a role in attention, memory retrieval, and visual matching. Finally, synthesis within the visual system may be subserved by the intrinsic fiber fascicles of the occipital lobe.

Hypotheses concerning the functions subserved by the various components of the ILF are supported by clinical studies in patients with lesions of the inferotemporal, parahippocampal, and ventral parastriate cortices. In his exposition of disconnection syndromes in animals and man, Geschwind (1965a,b) discussed visual agnosia as a manifestation of damage to the occipitotemporal association cortices and the fiber systems that link the occipital lobe with the temporal lobe. Visual form agnosia is the inability to identify objects by inspection that can be correctly identified through nonvisual domains such as touch and sound (Geschwind, 1965a,b; James et al., 2003). The functions of the ventral pathway are thus dependent upon the integrity of the inferior occipital and inferotemporal cortices and of the connections that link them, and are likely to be among the principal attributes subserved by the ILF.

A functional specialization within the realm of object identification subserved by the ventral stream is the recognition of faces, a crucial skill in emotional and social cognition. According to Haxby et al. (2002), face perception is mediated by a distributed neural system consisting of multiple bilateral regions. The system is organized into two major components. The invariant, or core aspect, is the basis for recognizing individuals and is distributed in extrastriate visual areas (inferior or lateral occipital cortex) and the inferotemporal areas, including the fusiform gyrus. The changeable or extended system perceives gaze, expression, and lip movement, acts in concert with the core system to extract meaning from faces, and is distributed in the face-responsive region of the cortex within the superior temporal sulcus (Haxby et al., 2000; Perrett et al., 1992) and in the amygdala (Haxby et al., 2002). The social/emotional component of perception thus requires feedback to occipital cortices from limbic-related regions in rostral temporal structures, including the fusiform face area (Rossion et al., 2003) and the amygdala, pathways also subserved by the ILF. Prosopagnosia, the loss of ability to recognize faces, results from bilateral lesions of the occipitotemporal region (Damasio et al., 1982), involving the fusiform face area and the occipital face area (Clarke et al., 1997; Joubert et al., 2003; Rossion et al., 2003). These areas, and the cortex in the superior temporal sulcus and the amygdala are all interconnected via the ILF. The ILF therefore appears to be the crucial white matter tract linking the anatomical regions that constitute the distributed neural system involved in face recognition.

The ILF may thus be viewed as the long association system of the ventral visual pathways in the occipitotemporal cortices. These putative functional conclusions are bolstered by the nature of the clinical impairments that occur following damage to these cortical areas and to the ILF that links them.

Fronto-Occipital Fasciculus

The Fronto-Occipital Fasciculus and the Subcallosal Fasciculus of Muratoff: Separate Pathways with a Shared History

19

The fronto-occipital fasciculus (FOF), also known as the occipitofrontal fasciculus, is one of the long association systems of the dorsal visual stream. Like the inferior longitudinal fasciculus (ILF) that subserves the ventral visual stream in the occipitotemporal region, the existence, course, and composition of the FOF have long been mired in controversy. The confusion surrounding the FOF, as well as the probably spurious "inferior fronto-occipital fasciculus" (see chapter 18), has persisted in current anatomical texts and is being propagated in contemporary DTI literature. The subcallosal fasciculus of Muratoff that links the cerebral cortex with the caudate nucleus was mistaken for the FOF, and this conceptual and terminological confusion continues to the present day. The tapetum is the extension into the hemispheres of the corpus callosum, lying adjacent to the ventricular ependyma. This is not dealt with in detail in our work but is included in this historical review because it featured prominently in earlier discussions as a part of the FOF. In the text that follows the FOF and Muratoff bundle are discussed individually, but the historical accounts of these bundles and also of the tapetum are so interwoven that it is useful first to consider them together to understand the difficulties encountered by earlier anatomists.

"Sachs-Probst Bundles" Mistaken for the FOF

The initial misidentification of the FOF arose as a consequence of a frank error in logic while studying the fiber tracts in brains of individuals with agenesis of the corpus callosum. The subsequent clear understanding of the FOF was also hampered by the methodologies available to earlier investigators. Congenital absence of the corpus callosum was first described by Reil (1812b) and in later subsequent reports, all of which contained scant clinical and pathological information (see Bruce, 1887-1888). In 1875, Knox studied such a brain and described a medially situated "lamina of white matter of considerable thickness, apparently having no attachment to corpus striatum." This observation was replicated by Eichler (1878) and Urquhart (1880).

In 1881 Forel presented a report on a case of agenesis of the corpus callosum to the Assembly of German Natural Scientists and Physicians in Salzburg. The contribution of Forel's student, Onufrowicz, in 1887 is of considerable historical as well as contemporary interest.[1] He presented a clinical account of this patient's course[2] before describing the anatomical features of the brain. The preservation of the brain was suboptimal,[3] but Onufrowicz was nevertheless able to describe its anatomic features:

55

Figure 19-1

Reproductions of the original diagrams showing the longitudinal callosal bundle in cases of callosal agenesis that were misidentified as an association fiber tract linking the frontal and occipital lobes. The misplaced callosal fibers (the correct identification of which may be attributed to Sachs and Probst) are shown in A, figure 5 from Onufrowicz's (1887) original paper, a coronal section in which he labeled the callosal fibers the "Ass. occ. front" (*arrow*). B, Figure 7 from Onufrowicz (1887) as reproduced by Dejerine (1895), in which "OF" points to the aberrant callosal fibers in a more caudal coronal section of the same brain (*arrow*). C, Coronal section of figure IX from the brain studied by Kaufmann (1888), who also misidentified the Sachs-Probst callosal fibers as the FOF (*arrow* and *asterisk*).

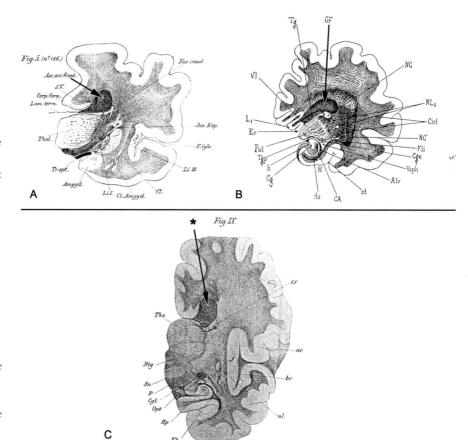

The septum pellucidum borders directly on the medial aspect of the cortex as well as the hemispheric white matter. The latter, i.e., the hemispheric white matter, forms at this location, a peculiar, massive, pear-shaped structure, sharply delineated in coronal section (the occipital frontal association system) which instead of the corpus callosum, forms the dorsal wall of the anterior horn of the lateral ventricle. The dorsal as well as the ventral leaf of the corpus callosum is missing completely (Onufrowicz, 1887, p. 316; figure 19-1A,B).

In addition to our fiber bundle, we recognized here the projection fibers of the occipital lobe in the posterior part of the internal capsule (optic radiations of Gratiolet/bundle H of Flechsig/projection tracts). We also see the well-developed inferior longitudinal fasciculus (association fibers of the temporal lobe to the occipital lobe). [See chapter 18 for discussion of the inferior longitudinal fasciculus. Onufrowicz here refers to what we now understand to be the sagittal stratum.] Furthermore, the comparison of coronal sections of a normal brain with those of our case of agenesis of the corpus callosum leads us to recognize that the tapetum of the corpus callosum in the normal brain is in fact the direct continuation of our occipital frontal association bundle, and the tapetum certainly does not belong to the callosal fibers (Onufrowicz, p. 318).

Despite the complete absence of the corpus callosum, the tapetum of the corpus callosum and the lateral appendix of the forceps of the corpus callosum have not disappeared, rather they are strongly developed, while the actual forceps of the corpus callosum is missing completely. This is clear evidence that the fibers in the tapetum of the corpus callosum do not belong to the corpus callosum, but to the longer association fiber systems of the hemisphere. We have thus seen that the part of the tapetum of the corpus callosum positioned close to the posterior horn seems to transition into the forceps, and in fact belongs to our occipital frontal association bundle. Because the radiation of the corpus callosum into the corona radiata is missing, a massive association system of the frontal lobe to the occipital lobe is clearly seen, isolated with utmost clarity. In the normal brain, this structure is intermingled with callosal fibers so that it cannot be distinguished from the other diffuse fibers of the corona radiata, and for this reason, it has been overlooked until the present time. In the occipital lobe, this bundle is represented by the so-called tapetum of the corpus callosum and the lateral continuation of the forceps of the corpus callosum, which gradually diminishes caudally. This fiber tract should best be termed the frontal occipital association bundle or the true superior longitudinal fasciculus. The genius Burdach recognized this fiber tract, or more accurately, he probably guessed it, and called it the arcuate fasciculus or the superior longitudinal fasciculus. But neither his nor Meynert's descriptions of this bundle are clear, and the fact is that it is impossible to see it in a normal brain. We were able to recognize its location between the fibers of the corpus callosum only after comparison with our experiment of nature, in the case of agenesis of the corpus callosum (Onufrowicz, p. 322).

Eduard Kaufmann (1887, 1888) concurred with Onufrowicz. He sectioned the brain of a patient with callosal agenesis (1888, p. 229):

in the frontal plane. Special consideration was given to the previously discussed association systems of the gyrus fornicatus [cingulate gyrus]. It soon became clear that the initial interpretation of this system, which seemed to be obvious before frontal cuts were performed, was incorrect, and in fact, this is a massive bundle that courses from the frontal lobe to the occipital lobe, that we together with Onufrowicz, would like to call the "frontal occipital association bundle" or true superior longitudinal fasciculus (see figure 19-1C).

Heinrich Hochhaus (1893) joined the fray (p. 92):

On the coronal sections we see medial to the sparse callosal fibers as initially described by Onufrowicz, the association bundle that on all cuts is clearly visible, as well as the tapetum of the posterior horn. There is almost no doubt about the accuracy of this interpretation by Onufrowicz, and possibly Burdach has interpreted it the same way. It is a long fiber system that mainly connects the frontal and occipital lobes, and in our case it also seems without doubt that the tapetum is very nicely preserved, and that it is in fact part of the association fiber bundle.

This confusion was confounded by Bruce (1887–1888), who described a "marginal arch" in his own case of agenesis but found untenable the view of Onufrowicz and Kaufman that (p. 338) "the fibers occupying its [marginal arch] position belong to the system of fronto-occipital association fibres . . . [and] that they are, in fact, the fibres of the cingulum of Burdach, no longer concealed by the fibres of the corpus callosum."

Thus, some 65 years after Burdach's lucid descriptions, a series of investigators became thoroughly muddled in their conceptions of the arcuate fasciculus, the superior longitudinal fasciculus, the cingulum bundle, and the tapetum and the displaced callosal fibers that they mistakenly thought was an association system linking the frontal lobe with the occipital lobe (i.e., a fronto-occipital fasciculus).

Callosal agenesis is a complex condition that is wholly unsuitable for deriving conclusions regarding normal brain anatomy because it may be associated with a number of morphological and clinical aberrations (Aicardi and Chevrie, 1994; Andermann and Andermann, 1994; Geoffroy, 1994; Hyndman and Penfield, 1937; Probst, 1973; Sauerwein and Lassonde, 1994). The obvious fallacy inherent in this approach was recognized within a few short years by astute investigators of the time.

Heinrich Sachs (1892), who was consistently and remarkably accurate in many of his observations, concluded that Onufrowicz's system was nothing more than a heterotopia, entirely lacking in normal brains, and consisting of callosal fibers "transformed into a sagittal bundle which does not leave the hemisphere in which the fibres belong" (translated and quoted in Barker, 1899, p. 1067). Carl Wernicke (1897) concurred with Sachs and emphatically denied that the subcallosal fascicle of Forel and Onufrowicz was an association system. He termed it the "longitudinal callosal bundle" and regarded it as carrying fibers of the corpus callosum radiating into the frontal lobe.

Dejerine Describes the Fronto-Occipital Fasciculus

Dejerine (1895) attempted to reconcile the findings of Forel, Onufrowicz, and others with his own observations (Dejerine, pp. 758–765):

> Forel and Onufrowicz identified [their] fascicle as the superior longitudinal fasciculus or arcuate fasciculus of Burdach, and their position was accepted by Kaufman and Hochhaus. We cannot agree with this opinion. Indeed . . . the superior longitudinal fasciculus of Burdach is located lateral to the corona radiata, and its more inferior fibers cover the lateral aspect of the external capsule. The occipital frontal fascicle, on the other hand, is located medial to the corona radiata and contributes to the formation of the roof of the lateral ventricle. We think that the occipital frontal fascicle of Forel and Onufrowicz is part of a sagittally oriented fascicle that runs, in a normal hemisphere, along the external angle of the lateral ventricle. This fascicle is located medial to the corona radiata, above the caudate nucleus, below and lateral to the corpus callosum, and it is separated from the ventricular cavity by sub-ependymal gray matter.
>
> [T]he occipital frontal fascicle is a sagittally oriented long association fascicle located between the cingulum and the arcuate fascicle or superior longitudinal fascicle of Burdach. It is separated from the cingulum by the whole thickness of the corpus callosum, and from the superior longitudinal fascicle by the foot of the corona radiata . . . It exhibits a curved shape open rostrally and ventrally, and is covered along its entire length by ependymal lining and by sub-ependymal gray matter, where it gives off numerous fibers. The fascicle then runs along the external angle of the lateral ventricle, located above the

caudate nucleus, medial to the corona radiata below the U, or the hook, that the callosal fibers make around the external angle of the lateral ventricles. On coronal section its surface is pyriform and about half a centimeter thick at its base . . . Clearly delineated at the level of the head and body of the caudate nucleus, this fascicle is in part dissociated at the level of the tail of the caudate, or separated by the fibers of the corona radiata and by the callosal fibers. Rostrally the occipital-frontal fascicle originates from the whole frontal lobe—external aspect, frontal pole, and orbital aspect. It receives a large number of fibers from the superior border of the hemisphere and from the external aspect of the convolutions. These fibers travel through the callosal fibers and through the fibers of the corona radiata. [A] large number of fine, lightly stained fibers leave the principal fascicle, move dorsally and medially, and completely fill the clear space situated between the fibers of the corona radiata and the corpus callosum that surrounds the lateral ventricle. Other fibers cross the sub-ependymal gray matter, and rostral to the frontal horn they cross the fibers of the corpus callosum and corona radiata and radiate within the anterior part of the extremity of the frontal lobe. From the base of the occipitofrontal fascicle some fibers leave in the ventral and lateral direction. They cross the foot of the corona radiata and enter the main part of the external capsule [see figures 2-10B,C and 2-11B].

Dejerine noted that the occipitofrontal fascicle degenerates following lesions of the occipital lobe, and (ibid.)

only partially following lesions of the temporal lobe and the convexity of the hemisphere . . . The occipito-frontal fascicle therefore constitutes a long associative fascicle that connects the temporo-occipital lobe to the frontal lobe, to the convexity of the hemisphere, and to the insula (through the fibers going to the external capsule). This fascicle is formed by fibers of different lengths that belong to the occipitofrontal fascicle only for a portion of their path. The occipitofrontal fascicle can thus be distinguished from other long association fascicles because it is more deeply located and is sub-ependymal, and because it is located medial to the projection system whereas the other long associative fascicles are more eccentric with regard to this system.

Dejerine thus rejected both arguments of Forel and Onufrowicz: that the FOF linking the occipital and frontal lobes was in the location they described, and that it was equivalent to the arcuate fasciculus of Burdach. He provided the first detailed account and illustrations of the location of the true FOF, described its shape and dimensions, and placed it medial to the corona radiata, whereas the arcuate fascicle of Burdach is lateral to the corona radiata. Further, Dejerine's FOF was not nestled immediately adjacent to the ventricle and the cingulum bundle, as Forel and Onufrowicz indicated, but rather it was ventral and lateral to the callosum, at some distance from the white matter of the cingulate gyrus. In attempting to reconcile his conclusions with those of Forel and Onufrowicz, however, as well as those of Meynert and Wernicke,[4] Dejerine concluded that the true FOF was identical to the subcallosal fasciculus of Muratoff.[5] By conflating these two fiber tracts (the FOF and the Muratoff subcallosal fasciculus), confusion regarding their course and composition persisted for over a century. Like many of his contemporaries, Dejerine also believed, incorrectly, that the FOF was continuous with the tapetum.[6]

Schröder (1901) provided a withering critique of Onufrowicz's conclusions.[7] As to the assertion that the FOF represents the superior longitudinal fasciculus, Schröder (1901, p. 83) acknowledged that it was Sachs who exposed the folly of this conclusion and who "first proved that this statement is untenable by pointing out that Burdach's fasciculus longitudinalis superior was situated lateral to the corona radiata, between the short association fibers of the cortex and the corona radiata, whereas Onufrowicz's fasciculus fronto-occipitalis lies medial to the corona radiata, and in the frontal lobe even medial to the ventricle, adjacent to the cingulum." He added his own interpretation based on volume I of Wernicke's (1897) atlas to which he contributed (Schröder, 1901, p. 81): "A number of association fiber bundles that connect distant parts of the cortex are an established fact. Among those, a new bundle has recently established a new place, the so-called fronto-occipital association bundle. The literature on this fiber tract is a reflection of our knowledge of the brain fiber tracts in general: imprecise descriptions, misunderstanding of earlier descriptions of other authors, hasty generalization and precipitate physiological application of the results play a role here." Schröder disapproved of the methods and conclusions of Onufrowicz, Kaufmann, and Hochhaus and lamented the fact that investigators were trying to determine the location of the fronto-occipital bundle in normal brain without first asking whether a fronto-occipital bundle in the sense of Onufrowicz exists. He dismissed Onufrowicz's claims in total and instead identified a region lateral and superior to the subcallosal fasciculus/fasciculus of the caudate nucleus, that he labeled "area r." He equated this area, at least in part, with the region that Dejerine identified as the location of the FOF. Schröder disputed Dejerine's claim, however, that this location contained association fibers traveling between the frontal and occipital lobes. Rather, Schröder agreed with Sachs that this area was part of the corona radiata.[8]

Moriz Probst (1901a) provided a definitive understanding of Onufrowicz's robust myelinated bundle in the agenesis brain that reflected precisely what Sachs had suggested almost a decade earlier. Probst regarded it as misplaced callosal fibers, which, being unable to cross to the opposite hemisphere, were directed in the rostral–caudal plane instead. He adopted the same term used by Wernicke (the "longitudinal callosal bundle") and observed that it "forms, anteriorly as well as posteriorly, a similar forceps-like continuation as does the normal corpus callosum" (translated and referenced in Probst FP, 1973, p. 13). These misdirected callosal fibers, subsequently termed the bundles of Probst, can be visualized on MRI (Kuker et al., 2003) and have been studied in the mutant mouse model of callosal agenesis (Wahlsten and Ozaki, 1994). They are not present in the normal brain. The nature of these misplaced bundles was first clearly articulated by Heinrich Sachs almost a decade earlier, and it therefore seems appropriate to refer to the longitudinal callosal bundles in cases of agenesis of the corpus callosum as the bundles of Sachs and Probst, or the Sachs-Probst bundles.

Thus, the fiber bundle that Forel and Onufrowicz described was not what is now known to be the FOF. Although there is indeed a fiber system linking the occipital and frontal regions, this is not what Forel and Onufrowicz observed. The proximity of Dejerine's FOF to the Sachs-Probst bundle is a matter of serendipity, and the resulting confusion is well demonstrated in these conflicting accounts in the original contributions above, as well as in authoritative texts of the time (Barker, 1899, pp. 1067–1069; Gordinier, 1899, pp. 369–370).

Dejerine's identification of an FOF that carried association fibers between the frontal and occipital lobes was not universally adopted, as reflected in the analysis of Schröder (1901).[9] Obersteiner and Redlich (1902), who surveyed the literature and compared it with their own experience, were also unable to agree with Dejerine in the determination of the FOF as an association fascicle. They concluded instead that the area in their work that corresponded to the location of Dejerine's FOF is a corticocaudate fascicle.[10]

Thus, despite Dejerine's attempt to define the anatomical features of the FOF, his findings remained a matter of debate, and several problems persisted, particularly regarding its differentiation from the tapetum and the Muratoff bundle.

The Tapetum

Forel and Onufrowicz stated that their medially lying system was the occipitofrontal fascicle and that the "tapetum" was a part of that (FOF) bundle, because both the FOF and the tapetum were preserved in their case of callosal agenesis. Bechterew (1899, 1900) agreed that the tapetum, being preserved in callosal agenesis, was not a callosal system but was the caudal extension of the medially lying system. Dejerine, too, believed that (p. 763) "[w]hen it reaches the confluence of the ventricles, this [FOF] fascicle curves ventrally and rostrally and its fibers spread over the inferior and external wall of the sphenoid (temporal) horn, forming the tapetum of previous authors" (see figure 2-11B, "OF[Ta]"). Muratoff (1893a, p. 722) reviewed the literature "to develop a consensus on the term 'tapetum of the corpus callosum' [and was able to] convince [him]self that the subcallosal fasciculus and the tapetum are one and the same, an anatomically indivisible system."[11] According to Schröder (1901, p. 90), von Monakow thought that the "tapetum and superior longitudinal fasciculus [constitute] a continuous fiber system that runs through the normal brain in its entire length and corresponds to the fronto-occipital bundle of brains without a corpus callosum."[12] Obersteiner and Redlich (1902) described the uncertainties at the turn of the 20th century concerning the tapetum, the FOF, and the subcallosal fasciculus of Muratoff[13] and concluded that (p. 307) "it appears more correct to abandon the term tapetum, which only is of historical significance, and designate the single layer that lines the lower horn according to its significance, as stratum subcallosum, callosal layer etc."

All these authors would have been well advised to pay closer heed to Burdach (1822, p. 148, paragraph 193), who wrote the following regarding the

> posterior portion of the corpus callosum and the splenium. The tapetum is the lateral extension of the lower layer of the body that lies above the anterior portion of the splenium and the extension of the anterior portion of the splenium itself . . . The tapetum is a fiber layer ½ to 1 Line thick that extends to cover part of the lateral wall of the lateral ventricle, where it is lined by epithelium [ependyma]. It runs posteriorly in an oblique fashion on each side of the corpus callosum within the roof of the entrance to the lower horn [temporal horn of the lateral ventricle], lateral and inferior to the posterior lateral corner of the thalamus. It then curves forwards, runs in the lateral wall of the lower horn, leaning towards the inner surface of the corona radiata along the lateral side of Ammon's horn and parallel to it, anteriorly and inferiorly to reach the apex of the temporal lobe.

These observations of Burdach have been repeatedly confirmed and validated by subsequent investigators (Ariëns-Kappers et al., 1936; Brodal, 1981; Carpenter, 1976; Cipolloni and Pandya, 1985; Crosby and Schnitzlein, 1982; Demeter et al., 1985, 1990; Rockland and Pandya, 1986; Seltzer and Pandya, 1983; Tusa and Ungerleider, 1988), and the confusion over the tapetum has abated. It is now known that the tapetum is a thin rim of bidirectional callosal fibers derived from and leading to the temporal and occipital lobes, lying laterally adjacent to the ependymal lining of the inferior and posterior horns of the lateral ventricles. There is no controversy today about these callosal fibers, and the tapetum is not dealt with further in detail in this work. Perhaps what was seen in agenesis of the corpus callosum were the tapetal fibers of the corpus callosum not crossing to the opposite hemisphere but remaining connected with the aberrant callosal fibers (not the FOF fibers), precisely as postulated by Sachs and Wernicke.

The Confusion Surrounding the Subcallosal Fasciculus of Muratoff

In 1893, Wladimir Muratoff (Muratoff, 1893a,b; Muratow, 1893) described a bundle of fibers situated directly above the caudate nucleus and beneath the corpus callosum. Uncertain as to whether the bundle he observed was an occipital frontal association system or a projection system, Muratoff designated this fiber bundle by its anatomic location and called it the subcallosal fasciculus. Muratoff's discussion set the stage for the debates that followed, as well as the persistent uncertainties.

Muratoff followed the tradition of investigators at the time and performed physiologically defined anatomic experiments in dogs with excitation and ablation of the motor cortex.[14] He noted degenerated fibers in the lesioned left hemisphere in the cortical U-fibers or arcuate fibers, in the corona radiata, and in the corpus callosum. In addition, Muratoff (1893b, p. 98) observed that

> below the corpus callosum one sees a transected nerve fiber bundle bordered superiorly by the corpus callosum. On our cuts it appears to be crescent shaped. It begins at the midline with its narrow end, enlarges in circumference in the middle portion, and is situated in the angle which is formed by the corpus callosum superiorly, the corona radiata laterally and by the caudate body inferiorly. At this location, the bundle broadens and its terminations cover the caudate nucleus. This bundle has been designated as "fasciculus fronto-occipitalis" by Onufrowicz [see below]. I will call it subcallosal fascicle.[15] I chose the name "fasciculus subcallosus" because the term of Onufrowicz "fasciculus fronto-occipitalis" is anatomically incorrect. These fibers by no means represent a particular fronto-occipital association tract. Fibers from different areas of the cortex run in it, for example from the suprasylvian gyrus, and these run only sagittally in the fronto-occipital direction. The mid-portion of this bundle is occupied by fibers from the cortical motor area. The designation "fasciculus subcallosus" has the advantage that it refers only to the anatomical position of this system without making implications regarding its function.

In a later publication devoted to the pattern of secondary degeneration following transection of the corpus callosum, Muratoff noted that the corpus callosum actually contains two systems. He wrote (Muratoff, 1893a, p. 721) that

One system of transverse fibers proceeds from right to left in the frontal plane. Another system consists of longitudinal fibers that lie in the rostrocaudal direction; in my last work [Muratoff, 1893b] I called this system the "subcallosal fasciculus". . . . We will further see that this system contains fibers of different significance. On the anterior frontal cuts, one can separate the system into three components. A superior horizontal part is positioned below the corpus callosum; a laterally placed descending part fills the angle between the corona radiata and the corpus callosum; and a lower part is adjacent to the basal ganglia.[16]

Muratoff's observations led him to conclude that his subcallosal bundle did not convey fibers between the frontal and occipital lobes.[17]

The elucidation of the subcallosal fasciculus by Muratoff based on the location of the bundle and the degeneration within it following motor cortex lesions is thus clear and comprehensive. Unfortunately, and perhaps inescapably, the description is then intermingled and conflated with the fiber systems of the corpus callosum, including the tapetum, and the elusive FOF. Despite Muratoff's use of the innovative experimental approach that combined clinical deficit with the anatomic study of the degeneration following lesion placement, it was still not possible to state with certainty what fiber system the subcallosal fasciculus conveyed. Muratoff's conclusions were as accurate as the contemporary understanding would permit, and in the end he cautiously named the bundle for its location rather than its constituents.

Sachs (1893) named the bundle that Muratoff observed the "fasciculus nuclei caudati," or fasciculus of the caudate nucleus. He correctly concluded that the fasciculus of the caudate nucleus, situated in the same location as Muratoff's subcallosal fasciculus, was not a frontal-occipital association bundle but rather an important fiber system linking the cerebral cortex with the corpus striatum.[18] Dejerine recognized the existence of the subcallosal fasciculus of Muratoff, but he equated it in terms of the fibers it conveys with his FOF.[19] Flechsig, by contrast, viewed the Muratoff bundle as part of the corona radiata.[20] Meynert (1865) and Bechterew (1900), like Sachs, viewed this fasciculus as a corticostriatal bundle, the "fasciculus nuclei caudati," but Meynert perpetuated the terminological difficulties by calling the FOF the "corona radiata of the caudate nucleus" (see Dejerine, p. 760). Anton and Zingerle (1902, p. 160) also regarded the subcallosal fasciculus as synonymous with the fronto-occipital fiber bundle, named it the medial longitudinal fasciculus, and concluded that it linked the posterior portion of the temporal lobe with the frontal lobe. Niessel von Mayendorf (1919) later concluded that the medial longitudinal fasciculus was not identical with the FOF, and that neither of these bundles was an association system.

Oskar Vogt (1895) accurately identified the two fiber systems adjacent to the caudate nucleus. He recognized the narrow fascicle covering the caudate nucleus, which he regarded as an association system of this nucleus. The other fascicle he believed to be a long association fiber system. Vogt's anatomic observations were hampered by the use of incorrect terminology—that is, he called the long association fiber system the subcallosal fascicle, whereas it should have been called the FOF; and he had no name for the corticocaudate system that should have been termed the subcallosal fascicle.[21]

In his evaluation of the earlier literature concerning the FOF and subcallosal fasciculus of Muratoff, Schröder (1901) acknowledged the accuracy of Muratoff's descriptions, distinguished it from the corpus callosum, and concluded that it was "the analog of the fasciculus nuclei caudati that has been described by Sachs." However, Schröder continued,

> Muratoff goes one step further by identifying his subcallosal fascicle with Sachs' fasciculus nuclei caudati, and he also unscrupulously identifies it with the fronto-occipital association bundle of Onufrowicz . . . This was crucial for the further development of the question regarding the fronto-occipital bundle—the fronto-occipital bundle was therefore found also in the normal brain [and not only in the callosal agenesis brain]. But if one takes a closer look, Muratoff's bundle has nothing more in common with the bundle postulated by Onufrowicz for the normal brain than its sagittal orientation.

Schröder proceeded to argue eloquently for the subcallosal fascicle as a striatal bundle. He marshaled three anatomic observations to support his contention: the intimate relationship in terms of location and size of the subcallosal fasciculus to the caudate nucleus; the morphologic appearance of the subcallosal fasciculus itself, which was unlike the other long association tracts; and the low probability of a long association tract diving deep into the periventricular region.[22]

Obersteiner and Redlich (1902, p. 289) noted Muratoff's view that "according to pathological findings on the human brain, the construction of the subcallosal fasciculus in the human is identical with the one in the dog," but they declared the direct comparison between dogs and humans to be

> completely illegitimate. . . . Muratoff's statements will also need correction in many other aspects. Unfortunately Muratoff's short descriptions and his sparse illustrations do not allow exact verification of his statements on the degeneration of this system after extirpation of cortex, especially pertaining to its association with the cortex. If one considers how difficult it is to create circumscribed lesions in the cortex, the lack of detailed descriptions carries especially heavy weight.

In their ablation–degeneration experiments, Obersteiner and Redlich found no evidence to support the assertion that the subcallosal fasciculus conveyed fibers from the frontal lobe to the occipital lobe, and they differentiated the subcallosal fasciculus from a "stratum zonale" that was more closely adjacent to the caudate nucleus.[23] Further, they made the prescient observation that (p. 300)

> Muratoff . . . includes the subcallosal fascicle among the association fiber systems. (If one considers the subcallosal fascicle as a connection between cortex and caudate nucleus, the designation association bundle seems more correct, as the caudate nucleus can be considered modified cortex, and this would mean that the subcallosal fascicle would represent a connection between two cortical areas, therefore representing association fibers).[24] One could also regard those fibers that apparently leave the subcallosal fascicle and break through the corona radiata as evidence that the subcallosal fascicle represents an association fiber system between cortex and caudate nucleus . . . An ultimate decision regarding this question cannot be made in our opinion. It is our speculation that collaterals of fibers of neighboring systems are also embodied here, including fibers from the corona radiata that enter the caudate nucleus and possibly also the lentiform nucleus and the thalamus.

In Rosett's (1933) paper provocatively entitled "The Myth of the Occipitofrontal Association Tract," he described his work based on microscopic sections prepared from flattened gross dissections. He concluded (p. 1257)

> that the subcallosal bundle is not an occipitofrontal association system, a radiation of the caudate nucleus or a contingent of the corpus callosum . . . [T]he mesial and more superficial portion of this bundle [are] made up of thalamic fibers. Its deeper and more lateral portion is made up of fibers which proceed from the prefrontal and frontal and perhaps the anterior portion of the parietal regions of the cerebral cortex to contribute to the formation of the pes pedunculi of the midbrain. They are, in other words, corticospinal and corticopontile fibers.

This reinterpretation by Rosett of the earlier work dealing with the subcallosal fasciculus was wholly fallacious. One subsequent study that included an appropriate notion of the subcallosal bundle was that by Yakovlev and Locke (1961a). This work, based on careful anatomic analysis using the ablation–degeneration technique, showed that the anterior cingulate gyrus gives rise to ventrally directed fibers that traverse the corpus callosum, travel in the stratum subcallosum, and enter the capsule of the caudate nucleus.

Authoritative sources in the more contemporary literature have perpetuated the uncertainty in their consideration of the FOF and Muratoff bundles. Riley (1960, p. 672) based his comments regarding the Muratoff bundle in large part on the investigations of Mettler and concluded that "its constituents are not clear." Crosby and Schnitzlein (1982) postulated two separate fronto-occipital fiber systems, one superior and one inferior. We have been unable to find evidence in support of the existence of an inferior FOF, as discussed in chapter 18. As there is no "inferior FOF," the qualifying "superior" adjective is superfluous when describing the actual FOF. Further, Crosby equated the "superior fronto-occipital fasciculus" with the subcallosal bundle and perpetuated the initial misconception by describing the FOF (not the Muratoff bundle) as conveying primarily frontocaudate fibers. Relying on previous anatomic studies for validation, the DT-MRI literature has already continued this conflation of the two bundles (e.g., "the superior fronto-occipital [subcallosal] fasciculus" in Catani et al., 2002).

Summary of Historical Accounts

Burdach provided clear descriptions, later elaborated upon, regarding the cingulum bundle, the arcuate fasciculus/superior longitudinal fasciculus, the corona radiata, and the tapetum and other components of the corpus callosum.

The paper by Onufrowicz and others purporting to describe a new association fiber bundle in cases of callosal agenesis that linked the frontal lobe directly with the occipital lobe threw the contemporary understanding of these systems into disarray. The "fronto-occipital fasciculus" of Forel and Onufrowicz was, in fact, an aberrant bundle present only in cases of callosal agenesis that contained misdirected callosal fibers oriented in the sagittal plane. Sachs, Dejerine, Wernicke, and Probst recognized this error. We elect to refer to these aberrant fascicles as the bundles of Sachs and Probst.

The dissection technique and even the lesion-degeneration studies comprehensively and carefully performed by some of the preeminent scientists of the day were unable to disentangle the FOF, the subcallosal fasciculus of Muratoff, and the tapetum that is a part of the corpus callosum. Dejerine described and illustrated the FOF, which he believed to be a long association fiber tract. However, he thought it was identical with the subcallosal fasciculus of Muratoff situated above the caudate nucleus, while Flechsig regarded the FOF as part of the corona radiata. The descriptions of a spurious and probably nonexistent "inferior fronto-occipital fasciculus" have led to the actual FOF being misnamed *post hoc* as the "superior fronto-occipital fasciculus."

It took considerable effort to disentangle the cingulum bundle and the arcuate fasciculus/superior longitudinal fasciculus from confusion with these other fiber pathways. Even straightforward issues such as distinguishing the ependymal lining of the ventricle from the subcallosal fasciculus met with mixed results.

Investigators using contemporary DT-MRI methodology have inadvertently incorporated some of the earlier imprecise concepts and terminologies in the belief that the classical neuroanatomy was established and incontrovertible. The foregoing account details the limitations inherent in the earlier discussions. In the present investigation, we have attempted to resolve the question as to whether the two bundles (FOF and Muratoff) are one and the same, or whether they are separate.

Results of the Present Investigation

Our observations in the monkey confirm the existence of the FOF where Dejerine located it in the human, and provide compelling evidence that it is a true association fasciculus linking parieto-occipital regions with the dorsolateral premotor and prefrontal areas. Moreover, the present study also adds detail to the understanding of its location and to the origin and termination of its fibers.

The FOF is a triangular bundle bounded laterally by the corona radiata and medially and superiorly by the corpus callosum; ventrally its base rests on the subcallosal fasciculus of Muratoff that separates the FOF from the body and head of the caudate nucleus. The FOF is formed by fibers that coalesce at a level just anterior to the atrium of the lateral ventricle, and the fasciculus continues rostrally into the frontal lobe until the frontal horn of the lateral ventricle (figure 19-2).

Rostrally directed fibers in the FOF are derived from the medial preoccipital area PO, lateral-dorsal preoccipital area DP, medial parietal area PGm, caudal cingulate gyrus, and area PG/Opt in the caudal inferior parietal lobule. The fibers of the FOF terminate in the frontal lobe in dorsolateral area 6, area 8Ad, area 8B, caudal area 46 dorsally, and area 9. Some fibers from the inferior parietal lobule pass through the SLF II before entering the FOF, where they travel rostrally into the frontal lobe.

Like the other long association fiber systems, the FOF also conveys reciprocal fibers from the frontal lobe into caudal sectors of the hemisphere. The caudal parts of the dorsolateral prefrontal cortex (area 8Ad and dorsal area 46) contribute fibers to the FOF that terminate caudally in area PGm and possibly also in area PO along with fibers from the SLF I, and in area PG/Opt along with fibers from the SLF II.

Our findings indicate that the FOF and the subcallosal fasciculus of Muratoff (Muratoff bundle) are two separate entities. The Muratoff bundle is a compact and distinct fiber tract that carries fibers from the occipital lobe, parietal lobe, cingulate gyrus, and temporal lobe,

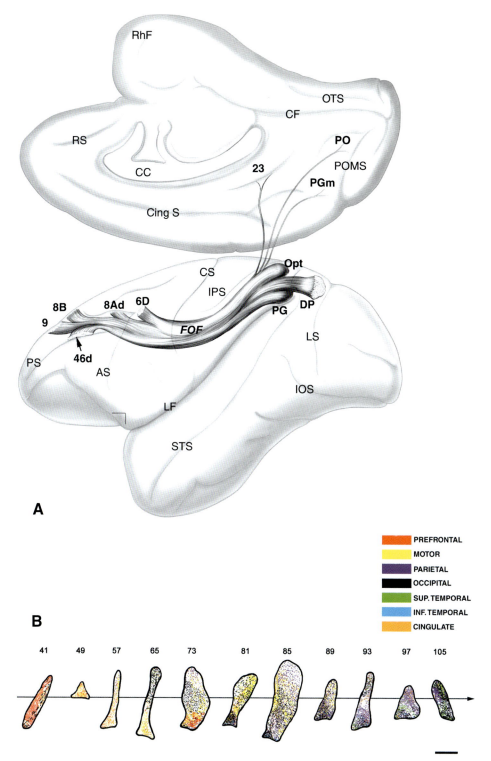

A

RhF
OTS
CF
RS
PO
CC 23 POMS
PGm
Cing S

Opt
CS
IPS
8B 8Ad 6D PG DP
9 FOF
46d LS
PS AS
IOS
LF
STS

B

■	PREFRONTAL
■	MOTOR
■	PARIETAL
■	OCCIPITAL
■	SUP. TEMPORAL
■	INF. TEMPORAL
■	CINGULATE

41   49   57   65   73   81   85   89   93   97   105

FRONTO-OCCIPITAL FASCICULUS

Figure 19-2
Summary diagrams of the course and composition of the FOF in the rhesus monkey. A, The lateral view of the cerebral hemisphere (lower diagram) shows the trajectory of the FOF and the cortical areas that are linked in a bidirectional manner by the fibers in this pathway. The medial view of the hemisphere (above) is shown to represent other cortical areas that contribute to this fiber pathway. B, Schematic diagrams from rostral to caudal coronal sections through the FOF extracted from the composite views of the hemisphere shown in chapter 27. The numbers refer to the sections of the template brain from which these images of the FOF are derived. The areas of origin of the fibers within the FOF are color-coded according to the legend above right. Bar = 2 mm.

as well as the frontal lobe, and these fibers terminate in the head, body, genu, and tail of the caudate nucleus. The Muratoff bundle is therefore strictly a corticostriatal bundle (see chapter 20). The FOF, in contrast, is an association bundle, although it does contribute some fibers to the Muratoff bundle, which then terminate in the striatum.

Functional Notions

The cortical regions from which the FOF originates (medial preoccipital area PO, lateral-dorsal preoccipital area DP, medial parietal area PGm, caudal cingulate gyrus, and caudal inferior parietal lobule area PG/Opt) are involved in the processing of visual information regarding the peripheral visual field. The FOF conveys this information predominantly to the dorsal premotor (area 6) and dorsal prefrontal (areas 8Ad, 8B, dorsal area 46, and area 9) cortices concerned with higher-order aspects of motor behavior and attention.

Ungerleider and Mishkin's (1982) concept of the dorsal visual stream (occipitoparietal cortices subserving spatial perception and projecting to dorsal regions of the frontal lobe) has been further subdivided (Rizzolatti and Matelli, 2003) into two components. This approach has relevance for the discussion of the putative functional properties of the FOF. In this view, the parietal lobe comprises two systems. The dorsal–dorsal stream is formed by areas V6, V6A, and MIP of the superior parietal lobule. Its major functional role is the control of actions "on line," and damage to these parietal areas leads to optic ataxia. The ventral–dorsal stream, in contrast, is formed by area MT and visual areas of the inferior parietal lobule; it is responsible for action organization and plays a crucial role in space perception and action understanding.

The FOF may be the fiber system of the dorsal–dorsal component of the dorsal visual stream. If the dorsal parieto-occipital and medial parietal areas, including area PO or V6, are engaged in the control of actions (Rizzolatti and Matelli, 2003), then their projection to motor-related regions via the FOF suggests a role of the FOF in the awareness and use of visual information for the purpose of guiding movements and in the preparation and release of reaching–grasping arm movements (Rizzolatti et al., 1990). Further, the FOF-mediated projections in dorsal frontal areas, including the supplementary eye field in area 9 (Schlag and Schlag-Rey, 1987), as well as in areas 6 and 8, which have been shown to be necessary to maintain vigilance (Rizzolatti et al., 1983), may be relevant for spatial aspects of attention.

The FOF also conveys reciprocal connections from dorsolateral prefrontal regions back to the parieto-occipital areas, and it is therefore the conduit by which the posterior dorsal prefrontal cortex (mainly area 8) may influence visual spatial processing within the occipital and caudal parietal cortices.

Thus, the FOF is the long association fiber pathway of the dorsomedial aspects of the dorsal visual stream, and it appears to be an important component of the anatomical substrates involved in peripheral vision and the processing of visual spatial information. It is distinguished from the SLF II, which subserves the ventral–dorsal component of the dorsal visual stream. It also stands in contrast to the ILF, the long association pathway of the ventral stream, which arises in part from the ventrolateral part of the extrastriate visual area and is engaged in processes subserving feature detection and object knowledge and memory.

Striatal Fibers

Corticostriatal fibers to the caudate nucleus, putamen, and claustrum are conveyed mainly by two fiber bundles: the subcallosal fasciculus of Muratoff and the external capsule. Striatal fibers emanate from the cerebral cortex and have a characteristic trajectory that distinguishes them from the intense cord of fibers contained within the core of the white matter that carries callosal fibers and the subcortical bundle. Whereas the striatal fibers are also distinct from the short and long association pathways once they have entered the Muratoff bundle or external capsule, early in their course from the cortical region of origin they are often intermingled with the association fiber systems.

Subcallosal fasciculus of Muratoff

External capsule

Muratoff Bundle (Subcallosal Fasciculus) and the External Capsule

Muratoff Bundle (Subcallosal Fasciculus of Muratoff)

The confusion surrounding the Muratoff bundle(MB) was discussed in detail along with the history of the fronto-occipital fasciculus (FOF, see chapter 19). Using the technique of ablation degeneration in dogs, Muratoff (1893a,b; Muratow, 1893) observed a compact fiber bundle situated above the caudate nucleus and beneath the corpus callosum. He was uncertain whether these fibers constituted an occipital frontal association system or a subcortical projection system and accordingly designated the tract by its anatomical location, calling it the subcallosal fasciculus. The uncertainty as to the precise nature of this bundle that Muratoff described has persisted for over a century into the present era. The origins and terminations of the fibers conveyed in the tract that lies just above the caudate nucleus have not been established.

Results of the Present Investigation

The MB is a semilunar, compact, fiber bundle located immediately above the head and body of the caudate nucleus, below and medial to the FOF. Both the MB and the FOF are situated beneath the corpus callosum and medial to the corona radiata. The MB is present caudally from a level corresponding to the atrium of the lateral ventricle to the most rostral part of the head of the caudate nucleus. In caudal regions at the level of the genu of the caudate nucleus, the Muratoff fibers are situated between the ependymal layer of the lateral ventricle and the tapetum. In coronal section it has a distinct appearance that led Dejerine to name it the "substance grise sous-ependymaire." It is differentiated on Nissl-stained section from the superiorly adjacent FOF, which is less compact.

The MB contains densely packed, horizontally running fibers leading to the caudate nucleus. These fibers arise from the dorsolateral and dorsomedial prefrontal region, the supplementary motor area, cingulate gyrus, posterior parahippocampal gyrus, medial and dorsal superior parietal lobule, and the caudal inferior parietal lobule, caudal superior temporal gyrus, and the medial and dorsal preoccipital region. Thus, the MB may be conceived of principally as a corticostriatal system from association and limbic areas. It also conveys fibers to the body of the caudate nucleus from the dorsal part of the motor cortex corresponding to the foot and trunk representations. The fibers destined for the caudate nucleus run parallel with the fronto-occipital fibers, aggregate in the subcallosal fascicle, and then terminate in the head and body of the caudate nucleus.

The MB continues its close approximation to the caudate nucleus caudally as it arches into its genu situated lateral to the confluence of the lateral ventricle. Therefore, a component of the MB (which we have called the ventral MB) lies ventral to the genu of the caudate nucleus, adjacent to the ependymal lining of the posterior horn of the ventricle. This ventrally situated small segment of the MB continues rostrally, just lateral to the tail of the caudate nucleus, and it conveys striatal fibers from caudal occipitotemporal cortices into the tail of the caudate nucleus.

External Capsule

The external capsule was recognized in the writings of the early investigators. Reil refers to it (1812a, p. 98), and Burdach provided an extensive description. (Burdach, 1822, p. 130, paragraph 180): "On the lateral surface of the lentiform nucleus and on the medial surface of the insular gyri, the external capsule is situated as a vertical myelinated layer that sends its radiating fibers anteriorly, superiorly and posteriorly. The converging point of its radiations is situated somewhat lower than the lentiform nucleus in the middle of the diameter of its basal plane . . . From there its fibers broaden and ascend like a fan that is loosely attached to the lentiform nucleus . . . It leans somewhat medially in its superior part but stands more vertically in its entirety, in contrast to the internal capsule that ascends in a more oblique fashion laterally. Both capsules then converge and meet at the superior well-demarcated border of the lentiform nucleus at an acute angle where they transition into a common radiation. . . . The external capsule is covered laterally by the longitudinal fibers of the arcuate fasciculus at the insula and the operculum. Anteriorly it runs medially in front of the lentiform nucleus and merges with the internal capsule between the striate and the lentiform nucleus, and posteriorly it merges with the radiations that run posterior from the thalamus. Superiorly its external layer arches laterally and enters the operculum."

The conception of the basal ganglia, and relationship of the cerebral white matter, cerebral peduncle, and the internal and external capsules was still in its infancy at the time of Burdach, and this is reflected in his attempt to understand the constituents of the external capsule. He believed that it arose from the fiber system of the tegmentum originating in the olivary bundle, and that along with the globus pallidus, the external capsule was continuous with the thalamus.[1]

In Dejerine's 1895 account, the location of the external capsule corresponded to the description provided by Burdach, and Dejerine concluded that it contained commissural, associative, and projection fibers.[2] The fibers in the medial aspect of the external capsule "probably" originated from the occipitofrontal fascicle and the medial aspect of the corpus callosum, the anterior fibers from the uncinate fasciculus, and the posterior fibers from the inferior longitudinal fasciculus, the anterior commissure, and the temporal fibers of the uncinate fasciculus. Moreover, he believed that it contained short association fibers terminating in the insular cortex and projection fibers destined for the claustrum and the inferomedial thalamic peduncle.

According to Crosby et al. (Ariëns-Kappers et al., 1936; Crosby et al., 1962; Crosby and Schnitzlein, 1982), the external capsule carries corticolenticular fibers from various cortical areas to the putamen and globus pallidus, provides corticotegmental fascicles to the ansa system, and carries associative fibers between frontal, parietal, and temporal areas. Berke (1960) concluded that the external capsule conveys principally corticotegmental fibers from frontal, temporal, anterior parietal, and insular cortices to the region around the red nucleus, with a few cortical association fibers present as well.

The name given to the external capsule, and the understanding that it is located between the putamen and claustrum, has remained constant since the time of Burdach. Many textbooks, including contemporary works, have based their descriptions of the external capsule on the conclusions reached by Burdach, Dejerine, and later Crosby et al. (e.g., Barker, 1899; Brodal, 1981; Carpenter, 1976; Gordinier, 1899; Heimer, 1995; Obersteiner, 1896). Despite this uniformity of agreement, the precise nature of the fiber constituents of this bundle are still uncertain, as these early observations were not based on a comprehensive study of experimental material using definitive tract-tracing techniques.

Results of the Present Investigation

In the material analyzed in this work, the external capsule appears to be strictly a corticostriatal fiber system. It conveys fibers from the ventral and medial prefrontal cortex, ventral premotor cortex, precentral gyrus, the rostral superior temporal region, and the inferotemporal and preoccipital regions. These fibers terminate in a topographic manner mainly in the putamen and also in the head, genu, and tail of the caudate nucleus. It conveys projections from many cortical areas to the claustrum. Projections conveyed by the external capsule from the primary motor cortex are directed exclusively to the putamen (as are those from the postcentral primary sensory cortex; Flaherty and Graybiel, 1991, 1993; Jones et al., 1977; Künzle, 1977), whereas those from the supplementary motor area and association cortices terminate in the caudate nucleus as well as in the putamen.

The striatal fibers that lie within the MB and the external capsule are not isolated from each other but are linked by cross-connections. Some fibers from the external capsule cross through the internal capsule and join the MB; similarly, some of the fibers of the MB cross through the internal capsule and join those fibers in the external capsule.

Functional Commonalities between the Muratoff Bundle and the External Capsule

The fact that the MB and external capsule are both striatal systems is reflected in their anatomical organization. Rostrally the striatal fibers form a shell around the head of the caudate nucleus (see figures 12-9, Sc. 41 and 27-1, Sc. 41). These encircling fibers are separated by the incoming fibers of the anterior limb of the internal capsule so that the dorsal striatal fibers continue over the head and body of the caudate nucleus as the MB, whereas the lateral, ventral, and medial striatal fibers constitute the external capsule. Thus, just as the corpus striatum (caudate and putamen) is divided into two parts by the internal capsule, so are the striatal fibers (the MB and the external capsule) also divided by the internal capsule. This is not to say that these two fiber tracts are totally independent; rather, the present observations provide evidence for cross-connections between the external capsule and the subcallosal fascicle at a number of levels. These may be seen in the individual cases and in the composite summary diagrams in figure 27-1 (Scs. 49–97), in which striatal fibers (StB) travel between the MB and the external capsule. These observations are in line with those of Showers (1959) and Yakovlev and Locke (1961b), who noted that corticostriate fibers arising in the cingulate gyrus travel via the subcallosal fasciculus of Muratoff to the caudate nucleus, while some fibers course through the internal capsule into the external capsule on their way to terminate in the lateral striatum, or putamen.

A notable feature of both the MB and the external capsule is that they lie in close proximity to cortical association pathways. The fibers of these striatal bundles at times intermingle with those of the association tracts. The MB is closely adjacent to the more dorsally situated fibers of the FOF, and in some instances fibers leave the FOF to pass through the MB before terminating in the striatum. Similarly, the external capsule is closely adjacent to the fibers of the extreme capsule. In some cases, extreme capsule fibers traverse the superior aspect of the claustrum to run in the dorsal component of the external capsule. These fibers then cross over the internal capsule in the striatal bundle, join the MB, and terminate in the caudate nucleus.

Corticostriate Connections

The functional importance of the two striatal fiber fasciculi (MB and external capsule) can be inferred from the pattern of corticostriate projections and findings from behavioral and clinical studies. Earlier investigations have revealed that projections from primary sensorimotor cortices are directed almost exclusively to the putamen (Flaherty and Graybiel, 1991, 1993; Jones et al., 1977; Kemp and Powell, 1970; Künzle, 1977), whereas those from the supplementary motor area and association and paralimbic cortices terminate in the caudate nucleus, as well as in the putamen, in a topographically organized manner (Cavada and Goldman-Rakic, 1991; Divac and Öberg, 1979; Nauta and Domesick, 1984; Saint-Cyr et al., 1990; Yeterian and Pandya, 1991, 1993, 1995, 1998; Yeterian and Van Hoesen, 1978). See footnote 3 for further discussion of corticostriate projection patterns derived from earlier observations.[3]

Certain principles of organization of the corticostriate projections have become established through these earlier studies. Kemp and Powell (1970) showed that the termination patterns in the striatum are topographically arranged according to the site of origin in the cerebral cortex, and Yeterian and Van Hoesen (1978) defined a principle by which areas of the cerebral cortex that have reciprocal corticocortical connections project in part to one and the same region of the caudate nucleus. The topographic arrangement of the corticostriate projection was confirmed by Goldman and Nauta (1977), who also showed that terminations in the head of the caudate nucleus arising from the prefrontal cortex are segregated into circular or elliptical clusters, suggesting that the caudate nucleus is organized as an anatomical and functional mosaic. Graybiel et al. extended this mosaic principle and have used histochemical and connectional studies to define a striosome and matrix pattern of organization of the striatum in animals as well as in humans (Graybiel and Ragsdale, 1978; Holt et al., 1997; Malach and Graybiel, 1986; Ragsdale and Graybiel, 1981).

As detailed in the earlier chapters, our observations are in general agreement with these previous studies and reveal that the corticostriate projections are conveyed by the MB and/or the external capsule, depending on their site of origin in the cortex. The MB conveys fibers predominantly from dorsal association areas to the head, body, and genu of the caudate nucleus. The external capsule, on the other hand, conveys fibers mostly from ventral association areas to the putamen and tail of the caudate nucleus. There is some interchange of fibers between these two striatal tracts, and the fibers from all areas reach the claustrum at least in part by way of the external capsule. The cortical afferents in the striatum are arranged in multiple discrete patches, each cortical area giving rise to a unique set of terminations. There appears to be interdigitation of projections from the different cortical areas, but some overlap is noted as well.

Functional Notions

The marked degree of topography within the pattern of corticostriate projections helped advance the realization that there are important functional divisions within the striatum, and that the striatum is a critical node in the distributed neural systems that participate not only in sensorimotor functions (Denny-Brown, 1962) but also in the domains of cognition and emotion (Alexander et al., 1986, 1990; Goldman-Rakic and Selemon, 1990; Nauta and Domesick, 1984; Saint-Cyr, 2003; Yeterian and Pandya, 1991). Further, the specificity of the corticostriate projections indicates that different regions of the striatum have behavioral specializations that are similar to those of the cortical areas from which they receive their major cortical input (Mesulam, 2000). An early indicator of differential contributions of striatum to cognitive operations was derived from maze-learning studies in rats, in which the nature of the learning impairments differed according to the location of the lesion in the caudate nucleus (Dunnett and Iversen, 1981). It now appears that the striatum is involved in the acquisition and retention of procedural knowledge, or habit learning, that is acquired incrementally and is dependent upon stimulus–response associations, and this differentiates it from medial temporal lobe structures that support declarative knowledge (Knowlton et al., 1996; Mishkin, 1982; Packard and Knowlton, 2002; Phillips and Carr, 1987; Squire, 1986, 1998). The caudate nucleus is important for motor skill learning in humans (Doyon et al., 2003), and the tail of the caudate that is anatomically linked with the inferior temporal lobe is necessary for visual habit formation in monkeys (Fernandez-Ruiz et al., 2001). The differential connectivity of the caudate nucleus is reflected also in different attributes of working memory, such that the head of the caudate, preferentially interconnected with the dorsolateral prefrontal cortex, participates in spatial working memory tasks in humans as determined by positron emission tomography, whereas the caudate body, more strongly interconnected with the temporal lobe, is activated in tasks of delayed object alternation (Levy et al., 1997). The precise nature of the striatal contribution to learning is a matter of ongoing study. It has recently been suggested that it is involved in fundamental aspects of attentional control used to guide the early stages of reinforcement-based learning and encoding strategies in explicit paradigms (Saint-Cyr, 2003). Graybiel (1998) conceptualized the striatal role as recoding cortically derived information to "chunk" the representations of motor and cognitive action sequences so that they can be implemented more efficiently as performance units. Learning and memory functions are thus seen as "core features of the basal ganglia influence on motor and cognitive pattern generators" (Graybiel, 1998, p. 119).

The associative functions of the striatum have direct clinical relevance. Observations in patients with extrapyramidal disorders such as Parkinson's disease, Tourette syndrome, Huntington disease, and progressive supranuclear palsy, in whom the burden of disease is in the basal ganglia, led to the notion of subcortical dementias (Albert et al., 1974; Growdon and Corkin, 1987; Heilman and Gilmore, 1998; Rauch and Savage, 1997; Savage, 1997; Turner et al., 2002), and focal lesions from stroke have emphasized the role of the caudate nucleus in language, neglect, and attention (Caplan et al., 1990).

A fundamental functional dichotomy has been suggested by anatomical studies of striatal connections with the cerebral cortex, as well as with subcortical structures. This distinction is between the dorsal striatum, which is linked with the dorsolateral prefrontal and posterior parietal cortices, and the ventral striatum, or nucleus accumbens, which is linked with limbic and paralimbic regions, including the orbitofrontal cortex, hippocampal formation, and amygdala, and is more involved in emotionally relevant behaviors. The notion that the striatum is involved with repetitive behaviors or habits that take place without true conscious awareness assumes particular significance when these habits are emotionally charged. This has been shown to be relevant in rats in which infusions of dopamine into the ventral striatum enhance conditioned reinforcement of formerly motivationally neutral stimuli (Robbins et al., 1989), and lesions of the accumbens impair aspects of response control related to affective feedback (Christakou et al., 2004). In monkeys, tonically active striatal neurons are involved in detecting motivationally relevant stimuli (Ravel, 2001). Studies of the role of the ventral striatum in reward, motivation, and addiction in humans have revealed insights into the functions of the basal ganglia and the pathophysiology of major addictive behaviors (Everitt et al., 1999; Gerdeman et al., 2003; Koob, 1999). The behaviors that characterize obsessive-compulsive disorder have also been shown to reflect dysfunction of the striatum, particularly its ventral component (Rauch et al., 1997; Stein et al., 2000), and preliminary evidence suggests that patients with this disorder can improve clinically following deep brain stimulation applied to the ventral striatum (Aouizerate et al., 2004). The role of dopamine in motor control regions of the basal ganglia is well understood from the study of Parkinson's disease and related disorders, and it appears that dopamine plays an important role also in these affective behaviors, possibly through associative binding of reward to cue salience and response sequences (Saint-Cyr, 2003).

The cortical connections to the striatum that are conveyed by the MB and the external capsule have thus been pivotal in advancing the knowledge of the role of the basal ganglia in motor and cognitive-affective performance, have enhanced understanding of the organization and functions of distributed neural circuits, and have deepened the appreciation of clinical manifestations of basal ganglia disorders. These insights into anatomy and pathophysiology have potential significance for future approaches to treatment.

Commissural Fibers

The dense cord of fibers that emanates from each cortical area and courses into the subjacent white matter comprises two major elements. One segment is destined for subcortical structures (see Section D), and the other, discussed here, comprises the commissural fibers directed toward the opposite hemisphere. A distinct topography is present within the corpus callosum, and to a lesser extent within the anterior commissure as well. Ventromedial temporal areas also send projections across the hemispheres in the forniceal commissures.

Anterior Commissure

The anterior commissure (AC) was first described by Riolani as a "funiculus transversus" similar to the optic nerve in color and caliber (Riolani, 1658, p. 254). It was also noted by Vieussens (1684), Vicq d'Azyr (1786), and a number of other early anatomists.[1] Gall and Spurzheim (1810; see also Gordon, 1817) concluded that it contains fibers that originate in the anterior part of the temporal lobe and the inferior part of the frontal lobe. Reil (1812a) observed the AC as a transversely running fiber bundle that passes through the basal ganglia and starts and ends in the anterior part of the temporal lobe, situated below the fornix medially and the uncinate fascicle laterally.[2]

Burdach (1822) also provided a comprehensive description of the course of the AC fibers and suggested that the bundle connects not only the temporal lobe but also parts of the occipital lobe between the two hemispheres.[3] He detailed its measurements and location within the hemisphere, predating by 150 years the AC-PC line measures used in current anatomical and functional neuroimaging studies (Tailairach and Tournoux, 1988).

Dejerine (1895) drew attention to the passage of the anterior commissure through the putamen and referred to this as "Gratiolet's canal." He noted that Meynert (1865) reported two components to the AC, one olfactory and the other hemispheric, and he summarized the views of contemporary authors about which areas give rise to fibers passing through it to the opposite hemisphere. These included the occipital and temporal lobes, cingulate gyrus, insula, lingual lobule, fusiform lobule, cuneus, rhinencephalon, hippocampus, amygdala, and anterior perforated substance. Dejerine concluded from his own material that it served principally to link the rhinencephalon across the two hemispheres. Indeed, Dejerine and Dejerine (1897) concluded that the AC "radiates into the hippocampal gyrus, including the uncus and the isthmus of the limbic lobe" (translated in Fox et al., 1948, p. 266). The temporal lobe contribution to the AC was convincingly implicated in lesion degeneration studies in the monkeys and baboons (Bucy and Klüver, 1940; Rundles and Papez, 1938) in which temporal lobectomy produced complete demyelination in the AC, and using the Marchi technique in monkeys Sunderland (1940b) observed degenerated fibers in the AC following a lesion of the rostral and mid-aspect of the superior temporal gyrus. Strychnine neuronography studies in the monkey (McCulloch and Garol, 1941) and chimpanzee (Bailey et al., 1941) further revealed that interhemispheric firing to the opposite middle temporal gyrus (area 21) consequent to the local strychninization of area 21 is abolished after sectioning the AC but persists after lesioning the corpus callosum. Fox and Schmitz (1943) found a prominent olfactory contribution to the AC in the cat, and Brodal (1948) observed bilateral degeneration in the olfactory tubercle of the rat following transection of the AC, but it transpired that there were important species differences between these

21

animals and the monkey. Fox et al. (1948) studied degeneration in the hemispheres after severing the AC in the monkey. They concluded that it consisted of a minute anterior limb distributed in the opposite hemisphere to the olfactory tubercle, anterior olfactory nucleus, and olfactory bulb and a sizable posterior limb distributed predominantly to the middle temporal gyrus. These authors questioned whether there was involvement of the inferior temporal gyrus as well, but the Marchi technique limited their ability to reach this conclusion with certainty.

In their study of subcortical projections of the temporal lobe in the monkey, Whitlock and Nauta (1956) reported a massive contralateral association of the middle temporal gyrus through the AC. Karol and Pandya (1971) sectioned the corpus callosum but not the AC, and with the Fink-Heimer modification of the Nauta-Gygax silver impregnation technique they observed resulting degeneration in widespread areas of the cerebral hemispheres. In contrast, there was sparing of the anterior third of the supratemporal plane, superior temporal gyrus, cortex of the superior temporal sulcus, temporal pole, and rostral and middle half of the inferior temporal gyrus, as well as the anterior part of the parahippocampal regions, and the orbital frontal cortex. Slight degeneration was seen in the middle third of the superior temporal region. These authors (Pandya et al., 1973a) then induced lesions in the AC of squirrel monkeys using focused ultrasound and studied the resulting degeneration in the hemispheres. They reported the bulk of the degeneration in and around layer IV in those areas spared in their previous study of the corpus callosum, namely the rostral fourth of the superior temporal gyrus and the adjoining depth of the superior temporal sulcus, and the rostral third of the inferotemporal area (i.e., the middle and inferior temporal gyrus). Fibers were also derived from the perirhinal area, the parahippocampal gyrus up to the rostral end of the occipitotemporal sulcus, the lateral surface of the temporal pole, and the rostral portion of the lower bank of the Sylvian fissure, and the claustrum. Some fibers in the AC were also derived from the amygdala and the orbital frontal surface.

In a subsequent lesion-degeneration study using the Wiitanen (1969) modification of the Fink-Heimer technique, Zeki et al. (1973) sectioned the AC of rhesus monkey brain and showed that fibers within this structure arise not only from the rostral part of the inferotemporal region but from the caudal part of the inferotemporal cortex as well.

In a study combining corpus callosum commissurotomy with massive injections of horseradish peroxidase in the entire temporal lobe of one hemisphere of rhesus monkey brain, Jouandet and Gazzaniga (1979) observed labeled fibers traversing the AC. Labeled neurons were seen in layer III from the temporal pole to the occipitotemporal border and from the inferior half of the insular cortex to the parahippocampal gyrus.

The contribution of the caudal orbital frontal cortex to the AC in rhesus monkeys was confirmed by the autoradiographic study of Barbas and Pandya (1984). Cipolloni and Pandya (1985) determined that the rostral thirds of the supratemporal plane and superior temporal gyrus send commissural connections through the ventral sectors of the AC; the midportion of the superior temporal region sends interhemispheric fibers through both the AC and the corpus callosum; and the caudal portions of this region, including the primary auditory area, send interhemispheric connections via the caudal part of the corpus callosum only (see also Pandya and Rosene, 1985; Pandya and Seltzer, 1986). Demeter et al. (1990) also showed that the AC conveys fibers from virtually the entire temporal lobe, including the temporal pole, the superior and inferior temporal gyri, and from the parahippocampal gyrus, as well as orbitofrontal area 13, the frontal and temporal divisions of the prepiriform cortex, and the amygdala. Temporal lobe projections through the AC were derived predominantly from the anterior part, and whereas the posterior part of the temporal lobe was observed to send some of its fibers through the AC, they were more heavily directed through the splenium of the corpus callosum.

Results of the Present Investigation

The gross anatomic features of the AC were portrayed with remarkable accuracy by Reil and Burdach and further elucidated by Ariëns-Kappers et al. (1936) and Fox et al. (1948). According to our observations, the AC traverses the midline as a compact and prominent fiber bundle located immediately in front of the anterior columns of the fornix, situated above the basal forebrain and beneath the medial and ventral aspect of the anterior limb of the internal capsule. In the hemisphere it moves caudally and passes laterally through the ventral aspect of the globus pallidus, constituting what Dejerine (1895) termed "Gratiolet's canal." It continues laterally beneath the putamen and descends lateral to the amygdala into the temporal stem. Further caudally, the AC is located lateral to the ventral aspect of the putamen and the tail of the caudate nucleus and medial to the ventral aspect of the claustrum. Earlier accounts placed this part of the AC in the external capsule (e.g., Demeter et al., 1990; Fox et al., 1948), although it appears from our material that although the AC abuts the ventral part of the external capsule, it is quite distinct and separate from it.

A survey of the origins of the projections in the AC in our material is in general agreement with the results of the earlier investigations. Fibers conveyed through the AC arise from and terminate in the caudal part of the orbital frontal cortex, the temporal pole, the rostral superior temporal region, the major part of the inferotemporal area, and the parahippocampal gyrus.

Fox et al. (1948, p. 267) reported that "the posterior limb [of the anterior commissure] undergoes torsion so that the rostral fibers in the commissure are maintained superiorly and the posterior fibers go inferiorly. A corollary of this is that the superior commissural fibers in the external capsule [see our comment above] distribute posteriorly in the hemisphere and the inferior commissural fibers in the external capsule distribute anteriorly in the hemisphere." Our material was not able to assess this pattern specifically, but by mapping the commissural fiber trajectories onto a single template we were able to discern a degree of topographic organization in the distribution of the commissural fibers in the midsagittal plane. The caudal orbital frontal lobe fibers travel through the rostral and central part of the AC. The fibers from the rostral part of the superior temporal gyrus run in its ventral aspect. The rostral inferotemporal region fibers occupy the dorsal and caudal part, and the fibers from the rostral superior temporal sulcus occupy its central and caudal sectors (figures 21-1 and 21-2).

The olfactory contribution to the AC was described by Meynert (1865) and Fox et al. (1948), and Lamantia and Rakic (1990a) considered it to be the archicortical compo-

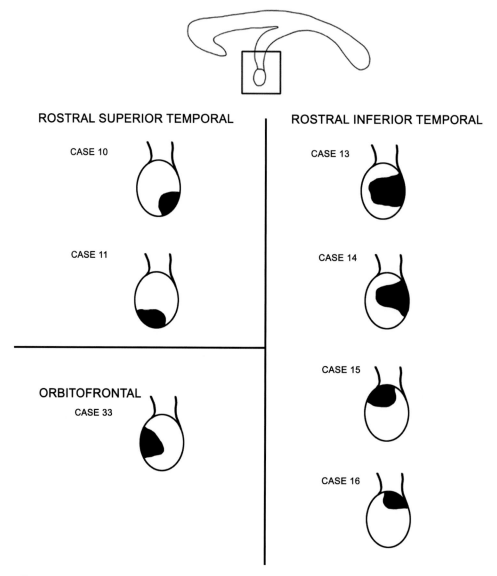

Figure 21-1
Schematic diagrams depicting the location within the midsagittal plane of the anterior commissure in the rhesus monkey of interhemispheric fibers (shaded black) derived from rostral regions of the temporal lobe and the orbitofrontal cortex. The location of the anterior commissure with respect to the corpus callosum is shown in the top figure.

nent they referred to as the "basal telencephalic commissure." This forms a small crescent at the anterior margin of the AC. The interhemispheric connections of olfactory regions were not evaluated in our study. However, we have observed fibers from the rostral aspects of the parahippocampal gyrus, superior temporal gyrus, inferotemporal region, and superior temporal sulcus coursing beneath the ventral aspect of the AC and leading to the ipsilateral basal forebrain (Cases 11, 13, 14, 15).

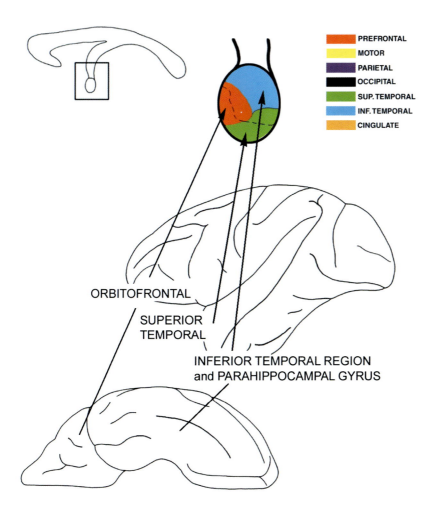

PREFRONTAL
MOTOR
PARIETAL
OCCIPITAL
SUP. TEMPORAL
INF. TEMPORAL
CINGULATE

ORBITOFRONTAL

SUPERIOR
TEMPORAL

INFERIOR TEMPORAL REGION
and PARAHIPPOCAMPAL GYRUS

Figure 21-2

Composite summary diagram of the topography in the midsagittal plane of interhemispheric fibers within the anterior commissure of the rhesus monkey. The location of the anterior commissure with respect to the corpus callosum is shown at top left. The lateral and basal views of the cerebral hemisphere are shown to depict the region of origin of the fibers traversing the anterior commissure, color-coded according to the legend at top right.

Functional Notions

Quantitative electron microscopic analysis reveals that the AC contains 3.3 million ±0.5 million axons in the adult rhesus monkey, mostly small myelinated axons with 30% unmyelinated axons (Lamantia and Rakic, 1990a, 1994). This number was reported to be relatively invariant from age 3 months to adulthood and reflected substantial elimination of mostly unmyelinated axons from a total of 11 million present in the AC at birth (Lamantia and Rakic, 1994). By virtue of quantitative differences between the AC and the corpus callosum in the magnitude and timing of axon overproduction and elimination, LaMantia and Rakic (1990b) postulated that there may be specific modulation of the development of each commissure, reflecting differences in the developmental history and functional identity of the cortical regions that give rise to them. Further, they argued, this process of overproduction and elimination of AC axons during postnatal development in primates might contribute to individual variations in AC size, correlated with a wide range of physical and behavioral differences. These notions are of interest in the light of the observations of Sandell and Peters (2003) that there are changes in the AC with age that are correlated with cognitive performance. These authors reported that 90% to 95% of the AC fibers are myelinated, and that their number decreases from 2.2 million in young and middle-aged monkeys to 1.2 million in old monkeys.

The functions of the AC remain elusive, but information available about the areas that it links provides insight into its possible roles. In non-mammalian species such as the marsupial, the AC is the principal conduit between the two hemispheres (e.g., Heath and Jones, 1971). The role of the AC, however, is more restricted in the higher scale of phylogeny, including the primate, and most of the neocortex is connected interhemispherically by the corpus callosum. Most of the areas connected by the AC in non-human primates are proisocortical regions—that is, the rostral part of the auditory, visual, and somatosensory cortices, as well as the olfactory and the parahippocampal regions. The role of the interhemispheric connections via the AC of the amygdala seems to be less important in the higher primate. These anatomical features lead to the suggestion that in the non-human primate, the AC is the pathway concerned with functional coordination across the hemispheres of highly processed information in the auditory and visual domains, particularly when imbued with mnemonic and limbic valence.

These anatomically derived conclusions are bolstered by observations from behavioral and physiological experiments in split-brain monkeys in which the AC was preserved but the optic chiasm and corpus callosum were sectioned. In these animals, the AC was shown to be involved in the interocular transfer of visual discrimination, particularly when there was a reward contingency (Sullivan and Hamilton, 1973a). Further, the AC was shown in this model to facilitate the interhemispheric transfer of memory in the visual domain (Sullivan and Hamilton, 1973b). This included interocular transfer of two-choice discrimination, memory for two-choice discrimination, comparison and discrimination of visual stimuli, including color, shape, and orientation, and transfer of matching-to-sample discrimination.

The human AC may carry axons from a wider territory than is the case in the monkey. Using the Nauta stain in patients with focal lesions, Di Virgilio et al. (1999) observed anterograde degenerating axons arising from the inferior part of the temporal and occipital lobes, the occipital convexity, pericentral region, and prefrontal convexity. As in the monkey, the inferior aspect of the temporal lobe provided the largest contingent of axons in the AC, situated mostly in its inferior part, directed toward homotopic targets, as well as heterotopic sites, including the amygdala and orbitofrontal cortex. The mnemonic components of visual memory have been studied in patients with agenesis of the corpus callosum and AC (Bayard et al., 2004). As discussed in chapter 22, connections between the hemispheres from more caudal regions of the temporal lobe are facilitated also by the splenium of the corpus callosum, and so these two major commissures (splenium and AC) appear to have complementary roles, at least in visual processing and perhaps in other domains as well. Olfactory functions in the monkey and human are vestigial in comparison to rodents, and the component of the AC in the monkey that transmits olfactory information between the hemispheres is correspondingly quite minor in comparison to these lower species.

In the clinical context, interhemispheric kindling of seizure discharges is most commonly propagated across the corpus callosum, although in some instance the AC is also implicated (Wada, 1991). There is some support for this observation from experimental studies in the rat in which interamygdala propagation of after-discharge is blocked by the combined sectioning of the anterior corpus callosum and the AC (McIntyre, 1975).

Corpus Callosum

The corpus callosum (CC) is the major interhemispheric commissure that connects most of the neocortical areas. It was named by Galen and described for the first time in humans by Vesalius (1543), who recognized that it linked the two halves of the brain and was continuous with the white substance of the cerebral hemispheres. Its anatomical features were elucidated in detail by Reil, who recognized the "beak" as the most rostral aspect of the genu (1809a, p. 144; 1809c); Alexander Monro, Tertius, who described it as a "broad white medullary plate, extending horizontally across the brain, and which unites its hemispheres" (Monro, 1813, p. 126); and Burdach, who regarded it as the largest and most evolved of all brain structures (1822).[1] Gall and Spurzheim (1813) concluded, with remarkable accuracy, that fibers from the upper part of the convolutions of the brain form the body of the corpus callosum, those from the lower convolutions of the anterior lobes form the genu, and those from the lower convolutions of the occipital lobe form the splenium.

It is perhaps surprising that essential anatomical details of the CC were not established until relatively recently (see Cummings, 1970; Tomasch, 1954). Indeed, Tomasch (1954), whose axon-counting study determined that there were 190 million axons traveling through the CC, was "amazed about the divergence of opinion on most of the important questions and problems related to it" (p. 119), including knowledge of the origins, course, and destination of its fibers. (Lamantia and Rakic [1990a] determined the number of fibers in the callosum to be considerably lower than that given by Tomasch—on the order of 56.0 million ±3.8 million axons.[2])

In the earliest studies, Hamilton (1886) concluded that the CC constituted a decussation of a great part of those fibers derived from the cerebral cortex that do not decussate at a lower level, and that its fibers pass from one hemisphere to the other, continuing into the external and internal capsules, ending in the thalamus and caudate nucleus. This view was supported by the degeneration studies of Ranson (1895), Bianchi and D'Abundo (1886), Gaddi (1871), Mellus (1904), Schnopfhagen (1909), Van Valkenberg (1911), and Milch (1932). These conclusions were soundly dismissed, however, by the investigations of human fetal material of Beevor (1886), who declared the CC an interhemispheric commissure; by the study of brains with callosal agenesis (Bruce, 1889); and as a consequence of stimulation experiments in monkey (Mott and Schaeffer, 1890). Subsequent anatomical studies, starting with Mettler (1935a–d) and Combs (1949), laid to rest the erroneous claim that callosal fibers were principally a decussation into subcortical and brainstem structures of the opposite hemisphere.

The nature of the origin of the callosal fibers, their precise termination in the opposite hemisphere, and their topography within the callosum itself were more intractable problems. Tomasch (1954), like Mingazzini (1922) before him, considered the fibers in the callosum to be either direct axis-cylinders of cells in the cortical gray matter, or formed below the cortex as collaterals or direct branches of the descending projection fibers or association fibers in the centrum ovale. It has subsequently been shown that callosal projections arise predominantly from neurons in cortical layer III and terminate in a columnar fashion in and around layer IV of the target zone (Jacobson and Trojanowski, 1974; Jones et al., 1975, 1979). Further, callosal fibers terminate both in homotypical cortical areas in the opposite hemisphere (i.e., in the same cortical areas from which the projections arise), as well as in heterotypical areas (i.e., in cortical areas of the opposite hemisphere that are not identical with the cortical area of origin). Heterotypical commissural projections are usually homotypical to intrahemispheric projection areas, however (Hedreen and Yin, 1981; Jacobson and Trojanowski, 1977; Mettler, 1935a–d; Pandya et al., 1969; Pandya and Seltzer, 1986; Pandya and Vignolo, 1968). Degeneration studies in monkey and human brains indicate that there are projections to the contralateral striatum from the cingulate gyrus (Locke et al., 1964), and anterograde and retrograde studies using horseradish peroxidase reveal crossed projections to the striatum from motor and premotor cortices (Fallon and Ziegler, 1979; Jones et al., 1977), as well as from all regions of the posterior parietal cortex (Cavada and Goldman-Rakic, 1991). Thus, it appears from these earlier studies that callosal projections do indeed terminate in selected subcortical areas of the opposite hemisphere, as Hamilton (1886) concluded, but these sites are not the principal destinations of callosal fibers, and no contemporary studies have identified fibers crossing within the callosum leading to the contralateral cerebral peduncle.

Whereas the early studies showed the callosal connections of various cortical regions, they did not evaluate the relative position that the commissural fibers occupy within the CC itself. Beevor (1891) credits Quain (1882) and Schwalbe (1881)[3] as identifying the splenium as the location of temporal and occipital lobe fibers within the callosum in human. A more reliable indication of intracallosal topography was derived from the Marchi study of Sunderland (1940b), who showed that in the monkey, frontal lobe fibers occupied the genu and the anterior third of the body of the CC; frontal, parietal, and temporal lobe fibers were in the middle third of the body; parietal, temporal, and occipital fibers were in the posterior third of the body; and the splenium contained fibers exclusively arising in the occipital lobe. This question of callosal topography was subsequently evaluated in a series of studies (Barbas and Pandya, 1984; Cipolloni and Pandya, 1985; Pandya et al., 1971; Pandya and Seltzer, 1986; Rockland and Pandya, 1986), the findings of which are summarized as follows:

> The rostral half of the CC carries fibers from various subdivisions of the
> frontal lobe. Prefrontal areas send interhemispheric fibers through the genu and
> the rostralmost portion of the body of the CC, while fibers from the premotor
> and motor areas cross more caudally, but still in the rostral half of the body.
> Anterior insular and anterior cingulate fibers appear to overlap with those
> coming from the premotor and motor areas. The caudal half of the CC carries
> fibers originating in the parietal, temporal, and occipital lobes. At the rostral-
> most level, just behind the motor cortex fibers, are fibers emanating from the
> primary and second somatosensory area. Posterior parietal "association" fibers
> are found more caudally in the body, with superior parietal fibers located more

dorsally and inferior parietal lobule fibers ventrally. Overlapping these posterior parietal fibers are commissural fibers coming from the caudal superior temporal gyrus. Fibers from the primary auditory area also cross within the caudal part of the body. Fibers from the posterior insular and posterior cingulate gyrus overlap those coming from the parietal and temporal lobes. Also in the caudal part of the body of the CC, immediately behind the parietal and superior temporal lobes, is the trajectory of interhemispheric fibers originating in the caudal portion of the inferotemporal region, but these fibers also extend into the splenium. Finally, fibers from the occipital lobe travel through the splenium, with fibers from area 18 and the juxtastriate region located ventral to those from area 19. Fibers from the lateral and caudal portions of the parahippocampal gyrus also pass through the splenium. Thus the CC contains topographically organized fibers coming from different cortical regions. However, there is some overlap in the fiber trajectories of the different zones and this is especially true for fibers originating in the posterior superior temporal, insular, and cingulate regions (Pandya and Rosene, 1985, pp. 32–35; figure 22-1).

Some more recent attempts have been made to determine the topography of callosal fibers in the human. In a study correlating the distribution of Wallerian degeneration in the CC with the anatomical sites of focal cortical lesions, de Lacoste et al. (1985) concluded that the topographical organization of fibers in the human CC appears to be fairly similar to that found in the rhesus monkey. In their cases, fibers from the inferior frontal and anterior inferior parietal regions course through the rostrum and genu of the CC, whereas those from the temporo-parietal-occipital region course through the splenium and caudal portions of the body. In a patient with infarction of the splenium and posterior body of the CC, however, Degos et al. (1987) observed degeneration in the occipital lobe and superior parietal lobule but not in the temporal lobe, raising the possibility that the human and monkey callosum are not identical with respect to their topographical organization. The callosal topography in humans is likely to be further established by the new and evolving neuroimaging techniques. Using diffusion tensor tractography, Abe et al. (2004) have already shown that, as in the monkey, the interhemispheric connections between the orbital frontal cortices are conveyed through the rostrum and those from the caudal temporal lobe through the ventral part of the splenium.

Elucidation of the topographical location of the callosal fibers in the midsagittal plane is important for understanding the organization of this preeminent interhemispheric system. It is directly relevant also in a number of clinical situations, including the epilepsies, partial or complete callosal disconnection, and callosal agenesis.

Results of the Present Investigation

Fibers destined to traverse the CC and travel to the opposite hemisphere leave the cortex of any given cortical area as part of the dense cord of fibers lying in the central part of the white matter. Callosal fibers are sometimes identifiable as distinct from the subcortical bundle that forms the other major component of the cord, but more usually they are indistinguishable from them early in their course. As the cord fibers leave the

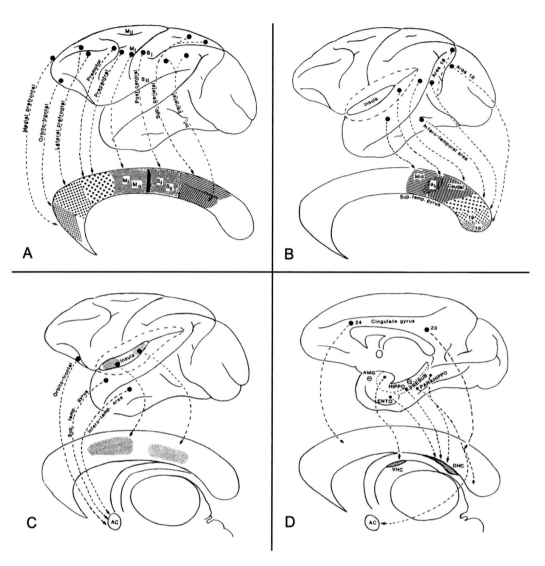

Figure 22-1

Schematic diagrams of the cortical origins of interhemispheric fibers passing through the midsagittal plane of the corpus callosum of the rhesus monkey. This diagram is from Pandya and Rosene (1985) and summarizes the observations recorded in Barbas and Pandya (1984), Cipolloni and Pandya (1985), Pandya et al. (1971), Pandya and Seltzer (1986), Rockland and Pandya (1986), and Seltzer and Pandya (1983).

white matter of the gyrus, they separate into two major components—the commissural fibers course medially to enter the CC, and the subcortical fibers take a course unique to each cortical area. Callosal fibers from the different parts of the cerebral cortex gather above and lateral to the lateral ventricle, enter the CC, and course medially in a compact bundle in a topographical manner to reach the opposite hemisphere. We concentrate here on the topography of the fibers within the CC itself rather than describing the patterns of termination in the opposite hemisphere, as this has been described previously, as reviewed above.

For descriptive purposes, we have segmented the CC into five approximately equal sectors (CC1 through CC5), from rostral to caudal. In the template brain, the callosum

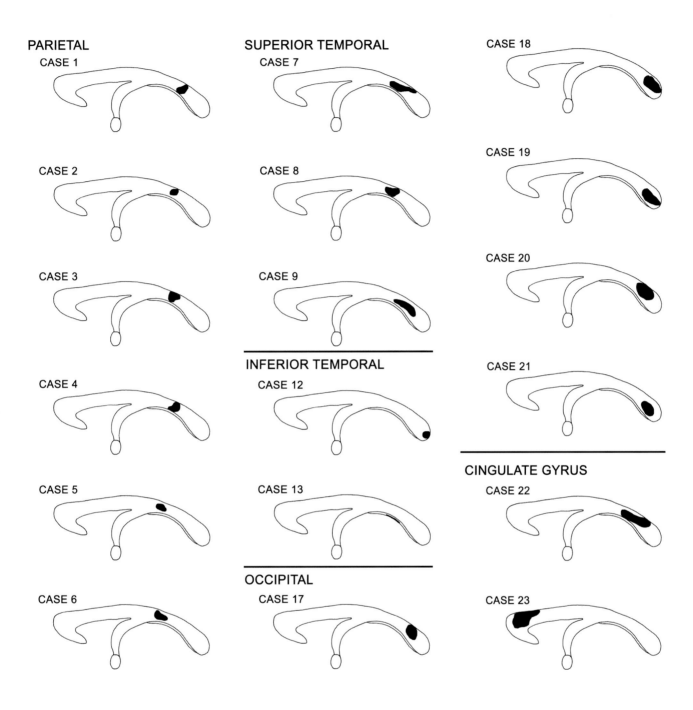

Figure 22-2
Schematic diagrams depicting the location of interhemispheric fibers (shaded black) within the mid-sagittal plane of the corpus callosum derived from the different cortical areas in the rhesus monkey.

(Figure continued on page 490)

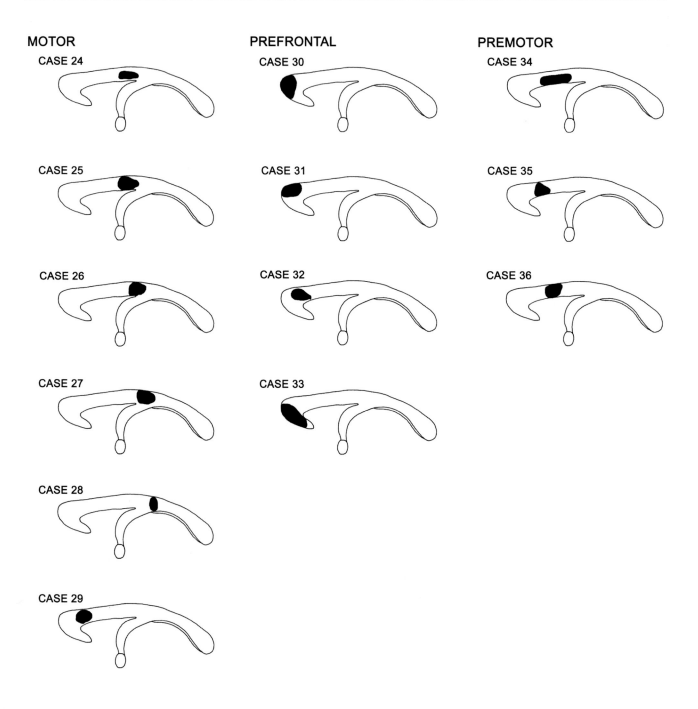

Figure 22-2 (continued)

extends from coronal section 38 rostrally to 113 caudally. Thus, sector CC1 is present in sections 38 to 51, CC2 in sections 52 through 66, CC3 in sections 67 through 82, CC4 in sections 83 through 97, and CC5 in sections 98 through 113. This parcellation proved to be convenient for expressing the topography of the fibers arising from the different cases. The results of the present work are summarized in figure 22-2, which shows the location of callosal fibers at the midline for each case studied, and in figure 22-3, a

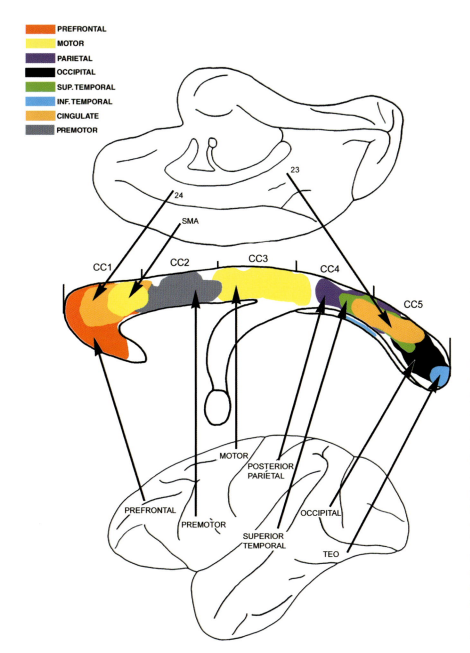

Figure 22-3

Composite summary diagram of the topography in the midsagittal plane of the corpus callosum of axons derived from the major lobar regions of the cerebral hemisphere of the rhesus monkey. The lateral view of the cerebral hemisphere (below) and the medial view (above) depict the region of origin of the fibers traversing the corpus callosum, color-coded according to the legend at top left. The designations CC1 through CC5 refer to the five rostral to caudal sectors of the corpus callosum described in the text. The detail of the topography within the callosum of fibers derived from the individual cases is represented in the preceding figures.

color-coded composite diagram that also shows the division of the CC into five rostral to caudal sectors. In human material, a similar approach was adopted by de Lacoste et al. (1985), who also divided the callosum into sectors I through V,[4] and Witelson (1989), who segmented the human CC into seven regional subdivisions.[5]

As shown in the midsagittal views of the CC in figures 22-2 and 22-3, the anterior sector (CC1) comprises the genu and rostrum of the CC. Most of the prefrontal fibers course through this sector. The fibers from dorsal area 46 and the medial hemisphere area 32 course through the rostral part of the genu. The ventral part of area 46 and the orbitofrontal cortex extend further caudally within the genu. The medial and orbital cortices are relatively ventral in location compared to the dorsolateral cortex, which is more dorsally situated. Just caudal to the prefrontal fibers are those that arise from the supplementary motor area (MII). The callosal fibers of the rostral cingulate gyrus travel through the dorsal part of the rostrum and the genu as well.

The next sector of the corpus callosum, CC2, is situated between the caudal portion of the genu and the rostral limits of CC3. In the material derived from the cases that we have studied, there is a gap in the callosal topography in sector CC2—that is, between the fibers in CC1 arising from the prefrontal, supplementary motor, and rostral cingulate cortices, and those in CC3 that arise from the motor cortices. An earlier study suggested that this CC2 area is most likely related to the fibers that arise from the dorsal premotor area (Pandya et al., 1971). We therefore examined the callosal projections from premotor areas in three additional experimental cases. Callosal fibers from area ProM (Case 34) and from area 6d (Case 35) are confined to sector CC2, and those from area 6v (Case 36) are present in the rostral part of CC2, as well as in the caudal part of CC1.

CC3 lies above the fornix in the midportion of the CC and contains interhemispheric fibers from the motor cortex. Fibers from the ventral premotor and face representation are most rostral. These are followed sequentially by those from the hand and then the foot regions, with essentially no overlap between these two. Fibers from the trunk representation, however, have a more extensive rostral–caudal dimension, and they overlap with the fibers from the other motor regions.

The CC caudal to CC3 is divided roughly into two sectors: CC4 rostrally, and CC5 caudally that includes the splenium.

CC4 conveys fibers that originate mostly in the parietal lobe. The gap in our material in the rostral part of CC4 is most likely occupied by fibers emanating from the postcentral gyrus SI, and SII cortices (Pandya et al., 1971; Seltzer and Pandya, 1983). Within CC4, crossing fibers from the posterior parietal cortices are topographically arranged. The parietal opercular and rostral inferior parietal lobule fibers cross most rostrally, followed by the superior parietal lobule fibers, which are mostly dorsal in location. The caudal inferior parietal and medial parietal fibers course in the caudal half of this sector, those from the inferior parietal region situated dorsal to those from the medial convexity.

The caudal fifth of the corpus callosum (CC5), which includes the splenium, conveys fibers from the temporal and occipital lobes. The rostral part of CC5 contains fibers from the caudal half of the superior temporal gyrus and the adjacent parts of the caudal superior temporal sulcus. The caudal part of CC5 conveys fibers from the caudal aspect of the inferotemporal region and from the preoccipital gyrus. The dorsal and medial preoccipital fibers travel dorsally, and those from the ventral preoccipital gyrus are situated ventrally in this sector. The lateral preoccipital fibers course caudal to those from the medial and ventral occipital cortices. The caudal aspect of the splenium conveys fibers from the juxtastriate (V2) and properistriate (V3) cortices (Pandya et al., 1971; Rockland and Pandya, 1986).

The fibers from the caudal part of the cingulate gyrus course through the callosum at the junction of CC4 and CC5, intermingling with those from the posterior parietal and superior temporal regions.

Thus, the rostral fifth of the CC transmits fibers from various parts of the prefrontal cortex, rostral cingulate region, and supplementary motor area. The second fifth contains fibers from the premotor cortex. The third fifth carries fibers from the ventral pre-motor region and the motor cortex. From the motor cortex there is topography such that fibers from the face representation are most rostral, followed by the hand and the leg. The fibers from the postcentral gyrus are most likely situated behind the motor fibers, followed in the fourth sector by those from the posterior parietal cortex. In the caudal fifth, the superior temporal region fibers are found rostrally, and the inferotemporal and preoccipital fibers are caudal. These comments regarding the topography of commissural fibers are applicable only to the midsagittal plane of the CC.

Functional Notions

The role of the CC has excited speculation since antiquity. Whereas the callosum was initially regarded as a mechanical bridge uniting the two hemispheres, it received a more elevated status in the 1600s. Willis regarded it as the site of imagination, Lancisi saw in it the merging of all senses and thus concerned with imagination, deliberation and judgment (hence the seat of the soul), and La Peyronie regarded it as the seat of intellectual abilities (see chapter 2). Burdach considered it to be the structure that imbued one with a sense of self, essential to mental activity, and the organ of reason.[6]

Increasingly accurate anatomical depictions of the callosum became evident from the time of Vesalius, particularly in the works of Vicq d'Azyr, Mayo, Arnold, Gall and Spurzheim, and Foville (see chapter 2), but knowledge concerning its functions remained entirely theoretical. Whereas some clinicians concluded, based on anecdotal observations, that "whether the defect in the corpus callosum be primary or secondary, there is no disturbance of mobility co-ordination, general or special sensibility, reflexes, speech or intelligence" (Bruce, 1889), by the late 1930s the callosum was generally "looked on as hallowed ground" (Van Wagenen and Herren, 1940, p. 741). Callosal lesions (mostly tumors) were said to result in higher-order motor and sensory impairments (e.g., apraxia and astereognosis), incontinence, and disturbances of memory, reason, and intellect. It was thus with great caution that surgeons sectioned the callosum to interrupt interhemispheric transmission of seizure discharges in intractable cases of generalized epilepsy (Erickson, 1940; Van Wagenen and Herren, 1940; see Proctor, 1965). The physicians who studied these patients were surprised to find that when tested using the methods available at that time, patients seemed entirely unaffected from the perspective of motor and sensory performance, as well as psychological and higher mental function (e.g., Akelaitis, 1941a,b; 1942; Akelaitis and Smith, 1942; Van Wagenen and Herren, 1940). Geschwind (1965b) offered two explanations for the failure to detect deficits in the callosal section patients. First, the long-standing nature of the deficits (the seizure disorder itself) in these individuals was likely to lead to functional reorganization, and second, the presence of severe epilepsy itself made it highly possible that the seizures could lead to learning of new pathways.

Geschwind's prescient observations were borne out by the observations of Myers and Sperry (1953), who showed in cats that there was a failure of transmission of interocular transfer of information after sectioning of both the CC and the optic chiasm. The early experimental studies in split-brain animals also evaluated the effects of callosal section on interhemispheric transfer of somesthetic information in cats (Stamm and

Sperry, 1957) and on eye–hand coordination in monkeys (Gazzaniga, 1964). The approach of callosal sectioning was used in an innovative manner by Mishkin (Mishkin, 1966; Semmes and Mishkin, 1965), who severed the callosal connections between parastriate areas to evaluate the connections and visual functions of the temporal and occipital lobes within the individual hemispheres. Further studies of interhemispheric communication in split-brain cats (Myers, 1965) determined that the transmission of visual experiential information between the hemispheres has limitations in its capacity. Direct sensory stimulation predominates over transcallosal transmission of information, and initial performance on the untrained eye is always at a lower level than the immediately preceding performance as tested through the trained eye. In the monkey, Myers observed that the callosum plays a prime role in tactual discrimination learning, which is crucial to producing a well-developed memory trace system in the opposite hemisphere. Whereas information transmitted from one hemisphere to the other becomes degraded in its passage through the callosum, this interhemispheric transfer is nevertheless essential for the optimal performance of the opposite hemisphere. Trevarthen (1965) found that a spilt-brain monkey may simultaneously acquire two conflicting memories of visual pattern associated with a reward and retain these memories separately in the two halves of the cerebrum. It was as though the brain had been divided into two complete and independent mechanisms of visual perception, cognition, and memory. In the higher primate such as the chimpanzee, Black and Myers (1965) determined that more complex functions (such as latch-box solving skills) were transferred across the hemispheres by the forebrain commissures (the CC and anterior commissure).

According to Doty (1989), the role of the callosum in interhemispheric suppression was first noted in dogs by investigators in Pavlov's laboratory. This was further established in cats by Kaas et al. (1967), who demonstrated an engram for auditory discrimination in the hemisphere opposite the trained ear, but if the CC was sectioned prior to training, then the engram was present bilaterally. Doty et al. (1973) then demonstrated this phenomenon in monkeys trained to respond to electrical stimulation of the striate cortex. With the callosum intact, animals responded to excitation of the striate cortex in the opposite untrained hemisphere. After the callosum was transected by use of a snare previously placed around the splenium, however, responses could be obtained only from the trained hemisphere. This led Doty et al. (1973) to conclude that the callosum provides a path by which each hemisphere has access to memory traces laid down in the other hemisphere, and that the callosal system prevents the same memory trace from being laid down in both hemispheres—a mechanism to double the storage capacity of the brain, which accounts also for hemispheric specialization and dominance for particular sets of engrams, including language (Doty, 1989; Lewine et al., 1994).

The first description of a clinically relevant lesion of the CC in humans was that of Dejerine (1892) in his report of alexia without agraphia. In this circumstance, a lesion of the left occipital lobe prevents visual information from accessing the language area in the left posterior temporal lobe, and a lesion of the splenium of the CC prevents visual input from the intact right occipital lobe from reaching the language area in the left hemisphere. This syndrome was later emphasized by Geschwind and Fusillo (1964) and Geschwind (1965a,b). Hugo Liepmann is credited by Geschwind (1965a) as providing the first description of the effects of callosal disconnection on motor function (Liepmann and Maas, 1907). It was over half a century later before descriptions of a number of intriguing deficits of complex behavior resulting from lesions of the CC helped establish the disconnection syndromes as an important clinical entity and validated the clinical relevance of the white matter pathways linking cerebral association areas. Geschwind and Kaplan (1962; also Geschwind, 1965b) described apraxia and "tactile aphasia" in a patient who had undergone excision of a left frontal lobe tumor and suffered infarction of the CC at the time of surgery. Their patient could not name objects (with the left hemisphere) that were held in the right hand, although he could name them when the objects were held in the left hand. These authors interpreted this observation as reflecting a failure of somesthetic stimulation to cross to the opposite hemisphere by virtue of the infarcted corpus callosum.

Unlike the conclusions reached by earlier investigators, more modern studies of patients with agenesis of the CC have revealed difficulties with bimanual coordination, stereoscopic vision, and transfer of learning between the hemispheres (Jeeves, 1965, 1991). The effective use of callosotomy for the treatment of a variety of intractable seizure disorders (Devinsky and Laff, 2003; Harbaugh et al., 1983; Maehara and Shimizu, 2001; Mamelak et al., 1993; Reutens et al., 1993) has provided a unique opportunity to study the effects of disconnection of the hemispheres. A comprehensive program of examination of these patients over the past few decades has revealed that the commissures are responsible for transferring information concerning specific sensory modalities (Gazzaniga et al., 1975), that specific kinds of information are carried by subgroups of callosal fibers (Funnell et al., 2000; Gazzaniga et al., 1989), and that the callosum is the primary interhemispheric pathway by which sensory and high-level cognitive integration is achieved (Seymour et al., 1994). Callosal section has been used also to provide new insights into the functional specialization of the hemispheres (Gazzaniga, 1967; Gazzaniga and Sperry, 1967; Gazzaniga et al., 1977) and the complex mosaic of mental processes that participate in human cognition (Gazzaniga, 2000). Sperry (1982, p. 1224) stated that by 1967, "the collected observations on the commissurotomy subjects were being taken to uphold the conclusion (Sperry et al., 1970) that each of the disconnected hemispheres, not only the left, has its own higher gnostic functions. Each hemisphere in the lateralized testing procedures appeared to be using its own percepts, mental images, association and ideas." These studies on callosal patients showed that whereas the left hemisphere was engaged in linguistic and analytical tasks, the right hemisphere specialties were "nonverbal, nonmathematical, nonsequential . . . spatial and imagistic, the kind in which a single picture or mental image is worth a thousand words" (Sperry, 1982, p. 1225).

The range of possible functional roles of the corpus callosum prompted some recent studies of the morphology of the CC in cadaver brains and using MRI in a search for morphologic differences according to gender, handedness, and age. Some investigators have suggested that there are definable and regional anatomical differences that correlate with these parameters, although the findings are not always consistent and are sometimes contradictory (Dubb et al., 2003; Hopper et al., 1994; Oppenheim et al., 1987; Witelson, 1985, 1989; Witelson and Nowakowski, 1991). Further population-based investigations will be required to establish reproducible patterns.

As to its function, Gazzaniga (2000) believes that the corpus callosum has enabled the development of specialized systems in each hemisphere. In this view, the callosum serves as the great communication link between redundant systems in the two hemispheres, thus allowing the reworking of existing cortical areas while preserving existing function. In other words, a preexisting system could be jettisoned as new functions develop in one hemisphere, while the other hemisphere continues to perform the previous functions for both half-brains.

The results of this body of innovative studies have thus led to deeper and novel insights into the anatomical underpinnings of perception, attention, memory, language, and reasoning and have provided insights into such elusive concepts as consciousness, self-awareness, and creativity (Bogen and Bogen, 1988; Gazzaniga, 1967, 2000; Sperry, 1964, 1968, 1982, 1984). Attempts to understand the functions of the CC and the mechanisms by which "the normal unity of experience is synthesized from the potentially independent processes in the two hemispheres" (Doty, 1989, p. 2) continue to drive investigations of normal animal models and human subjects, as well as individuals with neuropsychiatric diseases and disorders of the corpus callosum, including stroke (e.g., Chrysikopoulos et al, 1997; Degos et al., 1987), tumors (e.g., Christiaens and Blond, 1998), and toxins such as alcohol (Marchiava–Bignami disease; e.g., Heinrich et al., 2004).

The newer notions of the functions of the CC as a whole, the importance of its regional topography for a variety of specific high level processes, and the relevance of callosal function for such elusive human qualities as consciousness and sense of self are at once intriguing and reminiscent of earlier conversations in neuroscience. The apparently fanciful notions of Lancisi, Peyronie, Burdach, and others are now being reconsidered in the light of new observations using contemporary terminology. Interhemispheric communication subserved by the corpus callosum appears to be essential to some of the most highly developed aspects of human experience. Knowledge of the precise topography of the callosal fibers within the midsagittal plane is thus of great importance both for the understanding of the functions of the corpus callosum in the normal brain as well as in the clinical context of callosal section for the control of seizures.

Hippocampal Commissures

23

In addition to the corpus callosum and anterior commissure, there are three other fiber systems that link the ventral limbic and paralimbic regions across the hemispheres. In the present work, only Case 13 resulted in fibers in one of these commissures (the dorsal hippocampal commissure; see figure 8 3, Scs. 89, 93, 97, and 105, and figure 22-2, Case 13). Figure 22-1D summarizes the cortical areas using the hippocampal commissures, and the following limited discussion is derived from the analyses of Demeter et al. (1985, 1990; figure 23-1).

There are two hippocampal commissures and a hippocampal decussation:

1. The ventral hippocampal commissure lies at the transition between the body and anterior columns of the fornix in the vicinity of the subfornical organ and the interventricular foramina of Monro. It contains interhemispheric fibers arising from the most anterior subdivisions of the hippocampal formation— the uncus and the genu. (The remainder of the hipocampal formation in non-human primates is devoid of commissural connections.)
2. The dorsal hippocampal commissure lies inferior to the posterior end of the body of the corpus callosum. It contains fibers from the presubiculum, entorhinal cortex, and posterior parahippocampal gyrus (see Case 13). Despite its name, this commissure actually contains no fibers arising from the hippocampal formation.
3. The hippocampal decussation lies between the ventral and dorsal hippocampal commissures. It conveys fibers from the hippocampal formation that cross the midline to join the contralateral fornix and continue rostrally to terminate in the contralateral septal nuclei.

There is little information concerning the functional attributes of these commissures in humans or experimental animals. It is reasonable to suppose, however, that their role may be related, at least in part, to declarative learning and memory, which have been shown to depend on the integrity of structures in the medial temporal lobe that are linked by these commissures (e.g., Scoville and Milner, 1957; Mishkin,1982; Squire, 1986; Hyman et al., 1990; Squire and Zola-Morgan, 1991; Suzuki et al., 1993; Milner, 2003, 2005). The dorsal hippocampal commissure is sizable in the human brain, and it has been suggested that the fibers it conveys between the parahippocampal gyri of the two hemispheres may be relevant in the phenomenon of pure amnestic seizures (Palmini et al., 1992; Gloor et al., 1993). Patients with lesions of the splenium of the corpus callosum develop selective impairment of memory. This has been attributed to a fornix disconnection syndrome (Rudge and Warrington, 1991). The dorsal hippocampal commissure linking the presubiculum, entorhinal cortex, and parahippocampal gyrus across the two hemispheres is also directly affected by this invasive lesion of the splenium of the corpus callosum, however, and thus may be relevant in the pathophysiology of the anterograde amnesia.

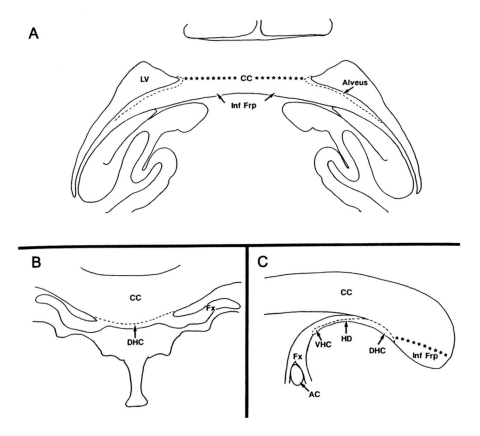

Figure 23-1

Schematic diagrams reproduced from Demeter et al. (1990) showing the location of the hippocampal commissures in the rhesus monkey. A, Coronal view through the splenium of the corpus callosum. B, Coronal section through the caudal part of the body of the corpus callosum showing the relation to the dorsal hippocampal commissure. C, Midsagittal view of the caudal part of the corpus callosum showing its relation to the hippocampal commissures. Stars in A and C represent the approximate boundary between the dorsal component of the splenium of the corpus callosum and the ventral component (the inferior forceps). Abbreviations: AC, anterior commissure; CC, corpus callosum; DHC, dorsal hippocampal commissure; Fx, fornix; HD, hippocampal decussation; Inf Frp, inferior forceps; LV, lateral ventricle; VHC, ventral hippocampal commissure.

Projection Fibers
(The Subcortical Fiber Bundle)

The fibers that make up the other major segment of the cord emanating from each cortical area form distinct subcortical fiber bundles destined for the thalamus, nuclei of the basis pontis, other brainstem and diencephalic structures, and spinal cord. These cortico-subcortical fibers are conveyed to their destinations via the internal capsule (anterior and posterior limbs) and the sagittal stratum. Each fiber bundle differentiates further as it progresses in the white matter into two principal components, one destined for the thalamus and the other for the brainstem and spinal cord. The rostral part of the temporal lobe also gives rise to a ventral subcortical bundle that conveys fibers destined purely for the thalamus, and this is considered along with the thalamic peduncles.

SECTION

Internal capsule

Sagittal stratum

Thalamic peduncles

Internal Capsule

The history of the study of the internal capsule is long and illustrious, and it has received close scrutiny by many of the major figures in neuroscience. The internal capsule was first depicted by Vesalius (1543), while Vieussens (1684) described and named the centrum ovale and showed that it was continuous with the internal capsule, cerebral peduncle, and pyramidal tracts in the pons and medulla. These anatomical relationships were emphasized by Reil (1809a–d), who named the radiating fibers in the centrum ovale the "corona radiata." A number of other early investigators studied the internal capsule in the latter part of the 19th century.[1] These studies, along with those cited below, contributed greatly to the understanding of the anatomy and clinical neurology of this fiber tract.

The detailed investigation into the topographic organization of the internal capsule was prompted by the new appreciation arising from lesion experiments in the monkey (Ferrier and Yeo, 1884; Schäfer, 1883) that the precentral cortex itself was topographically arranged. The demonstration in 1870 by Fritsch and Julius Eduard Hitzig (1838–1907) that electrical excitation of the cerebral cortex evoked focal movements of cranial, trunk, and extremity musculature enabled the detailed exploration of the topographical arrangement of the precentral motor cortex by electrical stimulation in the monkey (Beevor and Horsely, 1887, 1888, 1894; Horsely and Schäfer, 1888) and higher primates—orangutan, chimpanzee, and gorilla (Beevor and Horsely, 1890b; Leyton and Sherrington, 1917).

The study by Beevor and Horsely (1890a) of the "arrangement of the excitable fibres of the internal capsule of the bonnet monkey" must rank among the great and enduring early contributions to experimental neuroscience. As such, a synopsis of the work is presented here before summarizing the results of the present investigations. A number of subsequent studies have refined the understanding of the capsule, but the original work of Beevor and Horsely defined the major concepts, and established principles of organization that remain valid.

The authors lamented the "unfortunately misleading title of the *internal capsule*" and believed that "when the destination and function of these fibres is fully known, this term will be abandoned with great advantage for a specific topographic nomenclature. At present, however, we must use the old expression in default of a better one" (pp. 49–50). This nomenclature has, of course, not changed, but then neither have the major findings of this early study. They noted that the term *internal capsule* was applied to

> the descending and ascending fibers of the *corona radiata*, while passing between the basal ganglia; consequently [they] assume[d] that the term [was] only applicable to the fibres as long as they are passing between the two following

24

levels . . . the superior level is seen to be a plane directed slightly obliquely downwards and outwards, and resting on the upper surfaces of the caudate and lenticular nuclei. The lower level is . . . inclined upwards and backwards in a line with the upper surface of the optic tract and drawn from the optic chiasm backwards and upwards to the . . . pulvinar . . . Of course, these levels are purely arbitrary divisions of the fibres of the pyramidal tract, separating a part of them from the centrum ovale above and the crus cerebri below.

The bundles of fibers in the internal capsule were arranged like the rays of a fan, with the handle in the crus cerebri, and the rays corresponding (in the sagittal dimension) to the anterior-inferior and posterior-superior borders of the capsule. In horizontal section, the capsule was limited by lines drawn at right angles to the anterior and posterior extremities of the lenticular nucleus. The fibers in the capsule were classified according to the region of cortex with which they were connected. Arranged from anterior to posterior, these were prefrontal; excitable, pyramidal or frontoparietal; temporal; occipitotemporal; and occipital.

The Beevor and Horsely study was designed to determine whether there were bundles of fibers emanating from the cerebral foci (meaning "the point where the movements of any given segment are most intensely represented") that conveyed the functional impulses that originated in those foci, and whether those fibers were arranged "in an order similar to that which prevails on the surface of the cortex" (p. 50). They applied electrical stimulation to the fibers of the internal capsule as exposed in eight dorsal-to-ventral horizontal sections of the hemispheres of the anesthetized animals. The rostrocaudal measurement of the capsule was fairly consistent at all levels in the posterior limb, whereas the anterior limb became smaller in ventral level ("Group") VII and was no longer detectable at ventral level VIII (figure 24-1).

The anterior limb contained horizontal fibers as well as superior-descending and inferior-ascending fibers. Those from the prefrontal cortex, including the frontal pole, ran horizontally in the anterior limb, situated in the middle of the anterior limb in the horizontal plane, and passed backward through the genu to the thalamic region. These were electrically inexcitable with respect to motor activity. The anterior limb also contained inexcitable fibers from the medial surface of the hemisphere in the anterior third of the marginal (cingulate) gyrus and neighboring gyri, located medially in the horizontal plane. A group of electrically excitable fibers situated laterally in the anterior limb was derived from the "so-called motor cortex" at the external aspect of the hemisphere in the opercular region.

The posterior limb contained the excitable fibers that constitute the pyramidal tract (fibers to limbs, trunk, and cranial muscles grouped together). The anterior and posterior limits of the excitable fibers were defined for each body representation. The extent of excitable (motor) and inexcitable fibers in the posterior limb varied according to the level of the capsule. In the superior two (of eight levels), the posterior limb was excitable in its whole length, whereas in level III, the caudal 10% ("9/100ths") was not excitable, and the inexcitable portion steadily increased in more ventral levels so that in levels VI through VIII the caudal limit of the excitable (motor) fibers was at the "hinder limit of the middle zone." Thus, Beevor and Horsely concluded that the already "classical dictum" of Carville and Duret (1875) and Charcot (1878, 1883) that the sen-

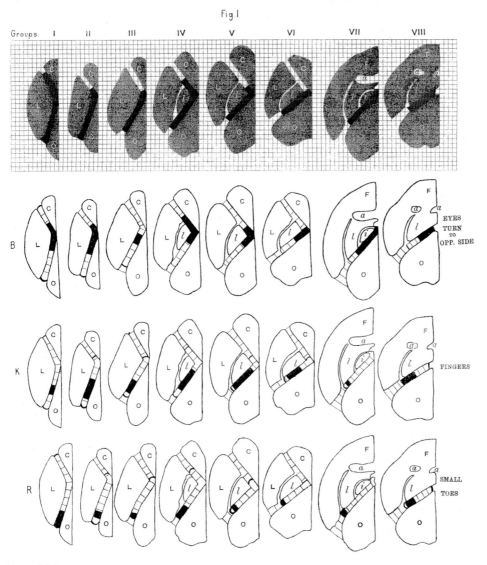

Figure 24-1

Schematic diagrams of the internal capsule from the work of Beevor and Horsely (1890), plate 5, figure 1. "This figure [top panel] consists of a number of drawings of the internal capsule and basal ganglia of the left side in horizontal section, corresponding to the eight different levels into which we have grouped our observations . . . [The diagrams below are] tracings of the outlines of fig. 1, [on which are shown] the limitation of the fibres [indicated by black shading], excitation of which produced a particular movement, the character of which is indicated in the margin . . . [Abbreviations:] a–anterior commissure, C–caudate nucleus, F–the point of fusion of the lenticular and caudate nuclei in the basal grey matter, i–inner zone of the lenticular nucleus, l–middle zone of lenticular nucleus, L–outer zone of lenticular nucleus or putamen, O–optic thalamus" (p. 87). Three representative diagrams (B, K, and R) of the 18 diagrams in Beevor and Horsely's original report are reproduced here in the lower three panels, reflecting locations in the internal capsule associated with movement of the eyes, fingers, and toes.

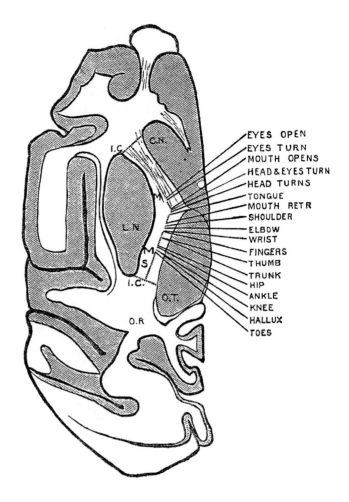

Figure 24-2

Diagram from Charles Edward Beevor's textbook *Diseases of the Nervous System* (1898, figure 5, p. 15), reflecting his conception of motor topography within the internal capsule of the monkey. Abbreviations: "C.N.–caudate nucleus, L.N.–lenticular nucleus of the corpus striatum, O.T.–optic thalamus, I.C.–internal capsule, M.–excitable or motor part, S.–sensory part, O.R.–optic radiations."

sory fibers are contained in the posterior third of the posterior limb of the internal capsule holds good only for the lowest levels of the capsule.

The anteroposterior direction of the excitable fibers in the capsule determined the nature of the motor response and, by corollary, the cortical area from which the fibers were derived. Further, the motor cortex topography was reflected in the organization of the capsule. Eye movements and eyelid opening were situated most anteriorly in the motor cortex and in the capsule, followed sequentially by movements of the head, upper limbs, trunk, and lower limbs. (See Beevor's [1898] figure 5, reproduced here as figure 24-2.)

With the development of improved lesion-degeneration techniques and contemporary tract-tracing methods applied to the study of internal capsule fibers derived from motor and nonmotor areas (e.g., Crosby et al., 1962; Fries, 1993; Schmahmann and Pandya, 1992, 1994), sophisticated *in vivo* structure–function correlations in patients with focal capsular lesions (Chukwudelunzu et al., 2001; Wenzelburger et al., 2005), and newer notions of motor areas outside the precentral gyrus in both monkeys and humans (Muakkassa and Strick, 1979; Picard and Strick, 1996), the understanding of the anatomy of the internal capsule has become further refined, but nevertheless still within the general framework defined by Beevor and Horsely and other investigators over a century ago. This is exemplified by the recent investigation by Morecraft et al. (2002) of fibers derived from the various motor areas governing arm representation in the precentral gyrus (MI), ventral lateral and dorsolateral premotor, supplementary motor (MII), and cingulate motor areas (M3 rostrally and M4 caudally). Fibers from each of these cortical areas have a distinct and separate trajectory in the corona radiata as they converge on the internal capsule. Within the capsule, the fibers are widespread, topographically organized, and partially overlapping. At superior levels fibers from M3 course through the middle and posterior portion of the anterior limb, those from MII in the posterior aspect of the anterior limb and the genu. Ventral premotor fibers travel through the genu and anterior portion of the posterior limb, dorsal premotor fibers through the anterior portion of the posterior limb, those from M4 in the midportion of the posterior limb, and MI fibers are caudal to M4. Consistent with the observations regarding the MI fibers by Flechsig, Dejerine, Beevor and Horsely, and the more recent fiber dissections of Ross (1980), among others, all the fibers studied by Morecraft et al. moved caudally into the posterior limb as they descended, with overlap of fibers derived from the different arm representation areas seen more prominently at ventral regions.

Limits and Subdivisions of the Internal Capsule

The internal capsule is bounded by the putamen–globus pallidus laterally, the head and body of the caudate nucleus anteriorly, and the thalamus posteriorly. The dorsal-lateral and ventral-medial boundaries of the capsule were defined by Beevor and Horsely (1890a,b), and these are somewhat arbitrary. The dorsal-lateral limit is an imaginary line joining the lateral and dorsal aspect of the caudate nucleus with the most superior and medial aspect of the putamen. In the anterior limb the "natural" ventral-medial boundaries are the caudate nucleus, nucleus accumbens, and anterior commissure. The hypothalamus lies at the ventral-medial border of the capsular genu. The ventral aspect of the rostral posterior limb is distinguished from the cerebral peduncle below it by an imaginary horizontal line joining the ventral part of the globus pallidus with the subthalamic nucleus. Caudal parts of the posterior limb (Dejerine's "retrolenticular capsule") located caudal to the striatum are bounded ventrally by the reticular nucleus of thalamus as it arches over the lateral geniculate nucleus and further caudally by the sagittal stratum.

Results of the Present Investigation

Anterior Limb of the Internal Capsule (ICa)

The ICa begins lateral to the head of the caudate nucleus, anterior to the appearance of the putamen. It progresses caudally, bounded medially by the head of the caudate nucleus, laterally by the putamen, and ventrally by the nucleus accumbens and then the anterior commissure. Caudally, this fiber system extends until the appearance of the thalamus, flanked by the head of the caudate nucleus medially and the putamen and globus pallidus laterally. The subcortical fibers in the ICa descend obliquely as they course caudally within the capsule.

The anterior limb of the internal capsule can be divided into six segments, from rostral to caudal. ICa-1 is the most rostral segment, present anterior to the appearance of the putamen, and it commences at template level 41. ICa-2 starts at section 49 at the rostral tip of the putamen. ICa-3 is noted from section 57 at the level of the limen insulae. ICa-4 begins at section 65 at the level of the crossing of the anterior commissure. ICa-5 is from section 69 at the level of the appearance of the globus pallidus. ICa-6 begins at section 73 and is the most caudal end of the anterior limb of the internal capsule. Immediately behind ICa-6 is the genu of the internal capsule, seen in section 78, which is defined by the presence of the most rostral part of the thalamus.

Genu of the Internal Capsule (ICg)

The genu of the internal capsule separates the anterior from the posterior limbs. It is a narrow segment at the level of the most rostral part of the thalamus (the reticular nucleus). In our template brain, the ICg is seen in section 78.

Posterior Limb of the Internal Capsule (ICp)

The ICp is bounded anteriorly by the genu of the internal capsule. It is demarcated medially by the reticular nucleus of the thalamus and by the head and body of the caudate nucleus. Laterally it is bounded by the putamen and globus pallidus until the retrolenticular segment, at which point it is bounded first by the islands of the putamen and the external capsule and further caudally by striatal fibers and the inferior longitudinal fasciculus. Its superior aspect is defined by the head and body of the caudate nucleus and by the striatal fibers situated between the Muratoff bundle and the putamen/external capsule. Its ventral limit corresponds to the ventral aspect of the thalamus rostrally, the upper aspect of the lateral geniculate nucleus in its midsector, and the sagittal stratum posteriorly. The caudal end of the ICp is demarcated by the full extent of the sagittal stratum at a level corresponding to the most caudal end of thalamus.

The ICp can be divided into five segments from rostral to caudal. ICp-1 is seen at template section 81, just caudal to the genu. ICp-2 starts in section 85, corresponding to the first appearance of the LGN. ICp-3 begins in section 89, at the midportion of the LGN, and the islands of the putamen. ICp-4 commences at section 93, at the caudal end of the geniculate, and is the first of two retrolenticular segments. ICp-5, the remaining retrolenticular segment, is present in section 97 and corresponds to the caudal end of the body of the caudate nucleus (immediately rostral to the genu of the caudate nucleus and the full extent of the sagittal stratum that are found in section 105).

Internal Capsule Fibers from the Posterior Parietal Cortex

The *medial part of the superior parietal lobule* (area PGm) sends its subcortical bundle of fibers into the ICp via the dorsal part of the sagittal stratum (figures 24-3 and 24-4). They enter the dorsal aspect of ICp-5, and at ICp-4 the thalamic contingent separates and provides terminations to the thalamus. The other part of the subcortical bundle (the pontine bundle) continues rostrally as it descends in the capsule. At the level of the midportion of the LGN (ICp-3) the pontine bundle starts to descend sharply toward the cerebral peduncle, and the most rostral contingent of these descending pontine fibers is present in ICp-2.

PARIETAL

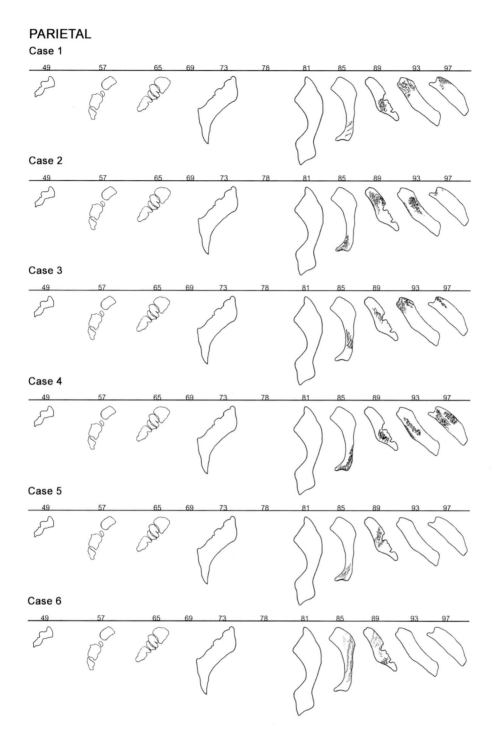

Figure 24-3
Schematic diagrams depicting the location of subcortical fibers within the internal capsule of the rhesus monkey derived from the different cortical areas. The internal capsule boundaries are derived from the composite summary diagrams shown in chapter 27. The fibers shown are derived from the diagrams in each case. The internal capsule is seen in sequential rostral to caudal levels in the coronal plane, and the level of the coronal section is identified by the number above the diagram for each case.
Figure continues on page 508–511

The fibers from the *superior parietal lobule* (areas PE and PEc) leave the cord and traverse the rostral part of the sagittal stratum before entering the superior aspect of the caudal part of the posterior limb of the internal capsule, in ICp-5. These fibers descend gradually as they travel rostrally. A thalamic contingent of these capsular fibers terminates in the thalamus at the levels of ICp-4 to ICp-2. The other contingent of capsular fibers continues rostrally until they take a sharp descent into the cerebral peduncle at levels ICp-3 and ICp-2.

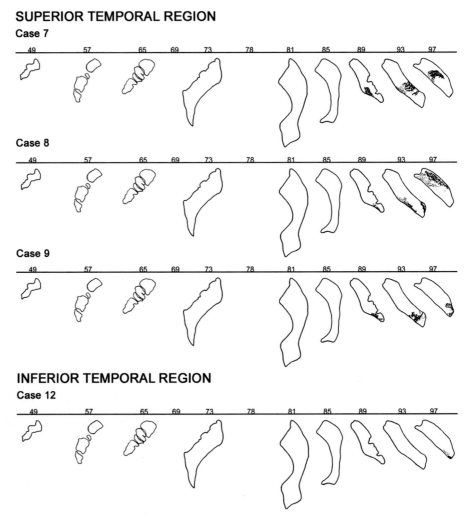

Figure 24-3 (continued)

The subcortical fibers from the *caudal part of the inferior parietal lobule* (area PG/Opt) leave the cord of fibers and traverse the dorsal segment of the sagittal stratum before continuing rostrally to enter the posterior limb of the internal capsule at level ICp-5. The thalamic contingent terminates at levels ICp-5, 4, and 3. The pontine fibers separate from the thalamic bundle at ICp-5 and descend gradually as they course rostrally until ICp-2, at which stage they dive sharply down into the cerebral peduncle.

The subcortical fibers from the *rostral part of the inferior parietal lobule* enter the posterior limb of the internal capsule at level ICp-4, move rostrally into ICp-3, and provide terminations to thalamus at this level. The caudally adjacent *parietal opercular fibers* enter the internal capsule at levels ICp-2 and 3 and descend in these levels and ICp-4 before terminating in the thalamus. The pontine contingents from both the rostral and the opercular parietal regions descend from the capsule into the cerebral peduncle at ICp-2.

OCCIPITAL
Case 17

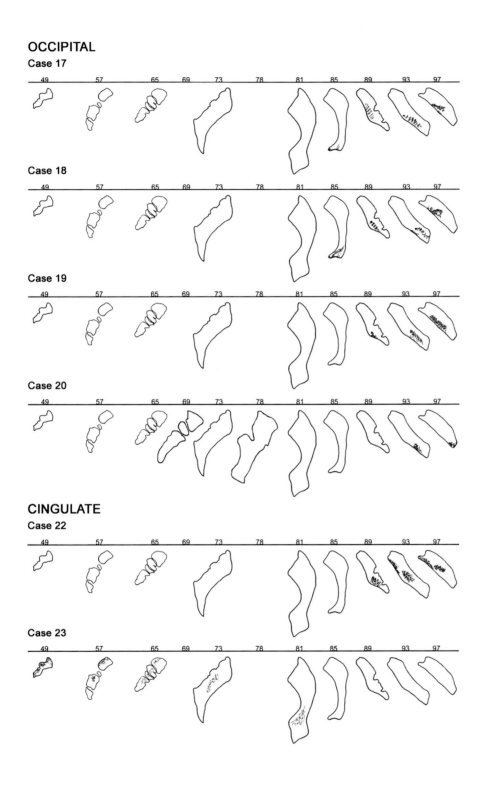

Case 18

Case 19

Case 20

CINGULATE
Case 22

Case 23

Figure 24-3 (continued)

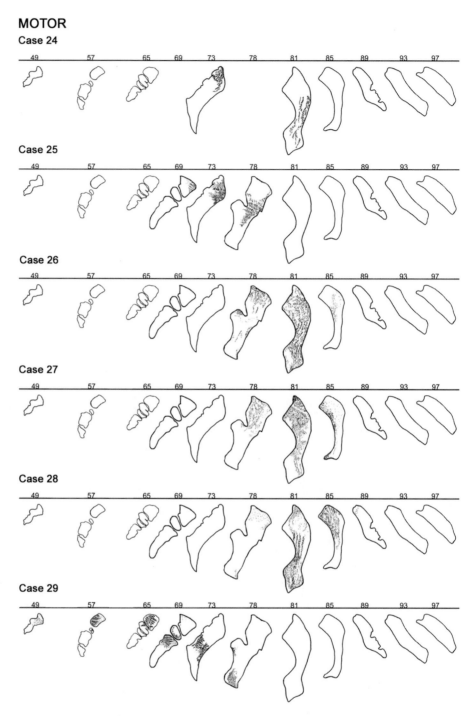

Figure 24-3 (continued)

Internal Capsule Fibers from the Superior Temporal Region

The subcortical bundle arising from the *caudal region of the superior temporal gyrus* separates from the cord of fibers, travels rostrally in the dorsal sector of the sagittal stratum, and enters the posterior limb of the internal capsule at level ICp-5 (see figures 24-3 and 24-4). A medially situated thalamic bundle enters and terminates in the thalamus at lev-

PREFRONTAL

Case 30

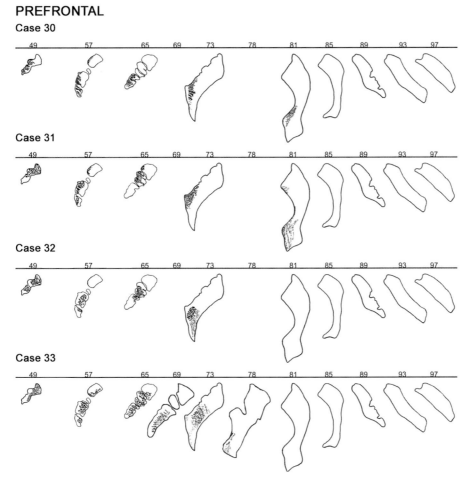

Case 31

Case 32

Case 33

Figure 24-3 (continued)

els ICp-5 and 4, whereas the pontine bundle continues to proceed rostrally until its sharp vertical descent into the cerebral peduncle at level ICp-3.

The *caudally adjacent superior temporal sulcal region* sends the subcortical bundle into ICp-3, 4, and 5. Fibers penetrate thalamus at ICp-4 and 5, and the pontine fibers descend into the cerebral peduncle at ICp-3.

Fibers from the *middle part of the STG* leave the cord of fibers and aggregate in the most ventral aspect of the posterior limb of the internal capsule at levels ICp-4 and 3. Thalamic fibers penetrate the thalamus at level ICp-4, and the pontine bundle continues rostrally before descending into the cerebral peduncle at level ICp-2.

The subcortical fibers from the *most rostral part of the superior temporal gyrus* destined for the thalamus and brainstem travel in the ventral subcortical bundle (see below) and avoid the internal capsule entirely.

Internal Capsule Fibers from the Inferior Temporal Region

The inferior temporal region does not commit fibers to the internal capsule, with the single exception of the caudal inferotemporal region, area TE3, which has a few fibers in the ventral aspect of ICp-5 as they proceed rostrally from the sagittal stratum on their way to terminate in the thalamus (see figures 24-3 and 24-4).

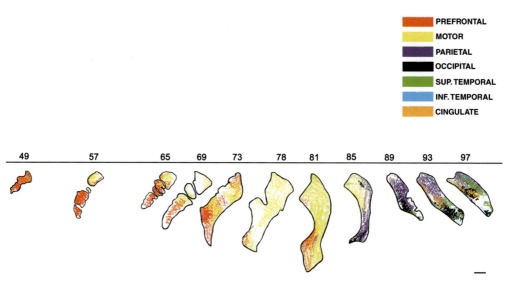

PREFRONTAL
MOTOR
PARIETAL
OCCIPITAL
SUP. TEMPORAL
INF. TEMPORAL
CINGULATE

49   57   65   69   73   78   81   85   89   93   97

INTERNAL CAPSULE

Figure 24-4

Summary diagram of the locations within the internal capsule of the rhesus monkey of the fibers derived from the major lobar areas of the cerebral hemisphere. The internal capsule boundaries are derived from the composite summary diagrams shown in chapter 27. The fibers within the internal capsule are color-coded according to the legend at top right. Sections 69 and 78 show prefrontal fibers from the orbital cortex (Case 33) only. Bar = 2 mm.

Internal Capsule Fibers from the Parastriate Occipital Cortices

The subcortical fibers from the *medial preoccipital region* leave the cord of fibers and travel rostrally in the sagittal stratum before entering the internal capsule at level ICp-5. Here the fibers are distinguishable as two separate components, a thalamic and a pontine bundle (see figures 24-3 and 24-4). The thalamic fibers enter the thalamus at levels ICp-5 and 4, whereas the pontine bundle continues rostrally as it gradually descends until it cascades into the cerebral peduncle at, and just caudal to, level ICp-2.

The subcortical fibers from the *dorsal preoccipital gyrus* also leave the sagittal stratum to enter the internal capsule at level ICp-5. Fibers enter the thalamus at levels ICp-5 and 4, whereas the pontine bundle continues its gradual descent as it moves rostrally until level ICp-2. The fibers that descend into the cerebral peduncle at ICp-2 lie above those from the medial preoccipital gyrus.

The fibers from the *midpreoccipital gyrus* enter the internal capsule from the midportion of the sagittal stratum at level ICp-5, at which stage one contingent of fibers enters the thalamus. The pontine bundle continues rostrally at the ventral aspect of the posterior limb of the internal capsule until it arches over the LGN at levels ICp-3 and ICp-2 to enter the cerebral peduncle.

The subcortical fibers from the *ventral preoccipital gyrus* do not travel in the internal capsule but rather move directly from the sagittal stratum into the thalamus.

Internal Capsule Fibers from the Cingulate Cortex

The subcortical fiber bundle from the *rostral cingulate cortex*, area 24, leaves the cord of fibers and enters the precapsule component of the anterior limb of the internal capsule, ICa-1 (see figures 24-3 and 24-4). The fibers course caudally with a gently descending slope in the medial aspect of the ICa until the genu. At this level one contingent of fibers enters the thalamus, whereas the other (pontine contingent) descends in the capsule toward the cerebral peduncle at level ICp-1.

The *caudal cingulate cortex*, area 23, sends its subcortical fibers via the dorsal sector of the sagittal stratum into level ICp-5 of the internal capsule, as two distinct bundles. The thalamic bundle enters the thalamus at this level and further rostrally at ICp-4. The pontine bundle continues its rostral course, descending as it goes, toward level ICp-3. It arches over the LGN, and below the internal capsule it enters the cerebral peduncle at a level corresponding to ICp-2.

Internal Capsule Fibers from the Motor Cortices

The subcortical fibers ascend dorsally and medially from the *opercular cortex of the precentral gyrus* (see figures 24-3 and 24-4). A prominent contingent of fibers descends in an almost perpendicular manner from the cord of fibers and enters the anterior limb of the internal capsule at ICa-6. These fibers progress caudally, and at the level of ICp-1 the medially placed fibers enter the thalamus, move caudally, and terminate. The laterally situated strands of fibers in ICp-1 descend vertically toward the cerebral peduncle.

Subcortical fibers from the *face motor area* leave the cord of fibers and enter the lateral aspect of the anterior limb of the internal capsule at ICa-5. In this position the fibers travel caudally, descending gradually into the genu. As the fibers pass into the posterior limb of the internal capsule, some enter the thalamus in ICp-1, while the remaining fibers in ICp-1 continue a sharp descent toward the cerebral peduncle. At the level of ICp-2, the fibers aggregate medial to the rostral part of the LGN before continuing caudally in the middle third of the cerebral peduncle.

Subcortical fibers emanating from the *hand motor area* cascade vertically down from the cord of fibers into the posterior limb of the internal capsule at level ICp-1. Fibers situated dorsally and medially enter the thalamus, terminate at that level, and continue caudally within the thalamus before terminating in its more caudal sectors. The remaining fibers in the internal capsule form vertical strands that continue to descend and move caudally to enter the cerebral peduncle, where they occupy its middle third. At the level of the genu (rostral to the main descending system), some fibers descend from the cord and approach the capsule from above, while a few fibers are seen within the capsule itself. Caudally in ICp-2, a small amount of fibers enter the thalamus through the external medullary lamina superiorly, while fibers descending in the peduncle are seen inferiorly.

Subcortically directed fibers from the *trunk motor area* cascade down from the cord of fibers in a thick bundle and enter the internal capsule. These fibers are also anteriorly bowed, such that fibers enter the capsule at the level of the genu and the rostral part of the posterior limb, ICp-1; they are evident in the midportion of the capsule at ICp-1 and descend from the capsule into the cerebral peduncle at ICp-1 and ICp-2. A substantial component of fibers in the capsule enters the thalamus in its rostral part. Some of these fibers terminate at rostral thalamic levels, but a sizable component of fibers continues caudally within the thalamus itself to terminate in its more caudal sectors. The remaining fibers that descend vertically into the midportion of the cerebral peduncle lie medial to the anterior part of the LGN.

Subcortical fibers from the *leg motor area* move rostrally in the white matter of the precentral gyrus. Some fibers enter the posterior limb of the internal capsule at level ICp-3 and proceed directly into the thalamus. The majority of fibers, however, enter more rostrally at ICp-2 and rain down in the medial part of the capsule in the form of dense bundles, with an anterior bowing, such that fibers reach rostrally into ICp-1. Some dorsally situated fibers within the capsule continue to pass through the external medullary lamina to enter the thalamus. Most fibers descend vertically to enter the midportion of the cerebral peduncle at levels ICp-1 and ICp-2.

The *supplementary motor area* (SMA) subcortical fibers gather around the anterior part of the internal capsule and enter the capsule at ICa-2. These fibers occupy a dorsal position at first and then descend gradually as they proceed caudally, coming to lie in two distinct bundles in the ventral part of ICa-6. The dorsal contingent continues caudally to terminate in the thalamus. The ventral component descends in the genu into the cerebral peduncle, remaining in the second quarter (from medial) of the peduncle.

Internal Capsule Fibers from the Prefrontal Cortex

The fibers from the *medial prefrontal cortex*, area 32, enter the most anterior part of the ICa, rostral to the appearance of the putamen (ICa-1) (see figures 24-3 and 24-4). They travel caudally, situated ventrally and medially within the capsule. The fibers remain in this position as they continue caudally, and they aggregate in the ventral and medial aspect around the genu of the internal capsule. From this location some of the fibers continue caudally to terminate in the thalamus, whereas the others descend in the rostral part of the posterior limb of the internal capsule (ICp-1) and enter the cerebral peduncle at a level corresponding to ICp-2.

From the *dorsolateral prefrontal region*, the subcortical fibers enter the internal capsule at the level of ICa-2, behind the fibers from the medial prefrontal region. They travel caudally within the capsule, situated medially and at times dorsal to the medial prefrontal fibers. At the level of the genu, the dorsal contingent of the fibers continues caudally into the thalamus, while the ventral contingent descends into the cerebral peduncle immediately behind the genu, rostral to the fibers from the medial prefrontal cortex, at a level corresponding to ICp-1.

Fibers from the *ventral prefrontal region* enter the ICa at the level of the rostral part of the putamen (ICa-2). The fibers occupy a central and lateral position as they travel caudally through the anterior limb of the capsule. Rostral to the genu, at about the level of ICa-6, a lateral and ventral contingent of fibers descends into the cerebral peduncle. The remaining aggregate of fibers continues through the genu to terminate in the thalamus.

The *caudal orbital prefrontal cortex* fibers enter the internal capsule at the most rostral aspect, ICa-1, situated lateral to those derived from the medial prefrontal cortex. These fibers course caudally within the ICa, remaining in a lateral and central position within the capsule. At the level of ICa-6 and the genu, a major contingent of fibers courses posteriorly and terminates in the thalamus. The remaining ventrally situated fibers descend at the genu and course medially to enter the hypothalamus.

Thus, the medial prefrontal and caudal orbitofrontal fibers enter the anterior limb of the internal capsule at its most rostral aspect (ICa-1), those from the medial prefrontal cortex lying medial to those from the orbital surface. The fibers from dorsal and ventral area 46 enter the rostral part of the anterior limb at ICa-2. Within the anterior limb, the medial and dorsal prefrontal fibers travel predominantly in its medial part, the orbital fibers occupy the most lateral position, and the ventrolateral prefrontal fibers occupy a central position. The ventral prefrontal fibers descend into the cerebral peduncle at the level of the caudal part of the anterior limb (ICa-6); the caudal orbital fibers enter the peduncle at the genu; the dorsal prefrontal fibers descend into the peduncle at the level of the rostral part of the posterior limb, ICp-1; and the medial prefrontal fibers start to leave the capsule at ICp-1 but descend into the peduncle at the level of ICp-2.

Functional Notions

The direct clinical relevance of the internal capsule in focal neurological deficit has long been recognized, and stroke in the internal capsule as a consequence of occlusion or rupture of the lenticulostriate (e.g., Marinkovic, 2001), anterior (Hupperts et al., 1994), and posterior choroidal arteries (Helgason et al., 1986) is common. Beevor and Horsely (1890a) were impressed by the report of Hughes Bennett and Campbell (1885), who described paralysis of the left arm from hemorrhage located at the junction of the first and second quarters of the posterior limb of the internal capsule. The entity of lacunar infarction, or small deep strokes, was recognized in 1901 by Pierre Marie (1853–1940) and further examined meticulously by C. Miller Fisher in patients with stroke in the brainstem and internal capsule (Fisher, 1967, 1978; Fisher and Cole, 1965; Fisher and Curry, 1965), leading to a greater understanding of the sensory and motor consequences of focal lesions of the capsule. The location of the lesion in the rostral-caudal dimension in the posterior limb of the internal capsule is important in determining the nature of the deficit (e.g., Shelton and Reding, 2001). The dorsal-ventral location of the infarct within the capsule is also relevant both for the nature and severity of the deficit and also for the extent of recovery. As a consequence of crowding together of motor fibers in the ventral portions of the internal capsule, lacunes in the ventral part of the capsule (Beevor and Horsley's levels VI through VIII) affect fibers from a wider cortical motor distribution, thus producing a deeper and more persistent hemiparesis than occurs after strokes in a more dorsal location in the capsule (Fries et al., 1993; Morecraft et al., 2002). Correlation analysis of clinical features with MRI lesion location in stroke patients has been used to determine the topographical organization of the human basis pontis (Schmahmann et al., 2004a), and it will be interesting to apply this approach in a similar manner to help refine the understanding of the organization of the internal capsule. Anterograde and retrograde fiber tract degeneration can be visualized on MRI following strokes in the internal capsule (Danek et al., 1990), and these approaches have the potential to be particularly informative if combined with white matter tractography, which can identify the cortical origin of the fibers that are infarcted in the normal individual as well as in a particular stroke patient (e.g., Kunimatsu et al., 2003). The recently available technology should make it possible to characterize the human internal capsule with a degree of precision that matches the experimental studies in the monkey.

In addition to the focal motor and sensory deficits that follow infarction of the posterior limb, complex behavioral syndromes resulting from lesions of the genu and the anterior limb of the internal capsule have been recognized (Chukwudelunzu et al., 2001; Schmahmann, 1984; Tatemichi et al., 1992). Deficits include fluctuating alertness, inattention, memory loss, apathy, abulia, and psychomotor retardation, with neglect of contralateral space and visual-spatial impairment from lesions of the genu in the right hemisphere. Severe verbal memory loss follows genu lesions on the left. The anatomical basis of this presentation is likely a result, at least in part, of disconnection of the reciprocal thalamocortical fibers in the anterior limb of the internal capsule that link the dorsomedial and anterior thalamic nuclei with the prefrontal cortex and anterior cingulate region. If the lesion is ventral enough, it may interrupt the inferior thalamic peduncle that links the anterior thalamic nuclei with the orbital cortex and the amygdala. Behavioral effects of anterior capsular lesions may not be the result of disruption of the thalamocortical interaction exclusively. The anterior limb and genu of the internal capsule also convey descending prefrontal input to the cerebrocerebellar system. A cerebellar cognitive affective syndrome (Schmahmann and Sherman, 1998) has been observed following lesions of the cerebellar posterior lobe reciprocally linked with the prefrontal cortex (Middleton and Strick, 1994; Schmahmann, 1991; Schmahmann and Pandya, 1995, 1997a,b), and so the behavioral effects of anterior capsular lesions may thus also reflect loss of cerebellar incorporation into the distributed neural circuits that subserve high-level processing. Mild motor deficits are also noted following anterior capsular lesions (e.g., Chung et al., 2000), likely reflecting damage to fibers leading to spinal cord from the SMA and M3 motor areas (Biber et al., 1978; Morecraft et al., 2002; Muakkassa and Strick, 1979).

The anterior limb of the capsule has received further attention in recent years as a locus where deep brain stimulation, pioneered by Irving S. Cooper (1922–1985) (Cooper et al., 1980, 1982; Rosenow et al., 2002), is being applied with some success in cases of obsessive-compulsive disorder (Anderson and Ahmed, 2003) and relief of intractable pain (Kumar et al., 1997). Lesions of the anterior limb have also previously been used with varying degrees of success for psychiatric indications (López-Ibor Aliño and Burzaco, 1972).

Sagittal Stratum

A legacy of uncertainty surrounds the definition of the sagittal stratum (SS), the nature of its constituent fibers, and the distinction between it and the neighboring fiber systems. This was discussed in chapter 18 devoted to the inferior longitudinal fasciculus (ILF), the fiber bundle most frequently confused with the SS. The reader is referred to that section for comprehensive treatment of this issue.

Historical events led to the controversy regarding the SS and the inferior longitudinal fasciculus. A number of investigators contributed to this discussion, among whom the following are perhaps most notable. Reil (1809b) identified a fiber system in the human occipital and temporal lobes that Burdach (1822) subsequently named the inferior longitudinal fasciculus and regarded as an association fiber system. In 1832 Gratiolet described a tract linking the thalamus with the occipital lobe in the monkey and named it the optic radiation. Heinrich Sachs (1892) observed the sizable parasagittally oriented white matter fiber bundle in posterior regions of the hemisphere and termed this the sagittal stratum. According to Sachs, the SS comprised an external segment (SSe) that conveyed corticopetal fibers from the thalamus to the occipital lobe and an internal segment (SSi) that conveyed corticofugal fibers from cortex to the thalamus. He concluded that the inferior longitudinal fasciculus that conveyed association fibers from the occipital to the temporal lobes was also situated within the SSe. Dejerine (1895) thought that the lower part of what he regarded as the ILF was associative (linking occipital regions with the temporal lobe), whereas the upper part was a projection system intimately united with the retrolenticular segment of the internal capsule. In describing what he regarded as the ILF, Dejerine actually provided a detailed gross anatomical description of the external layer of the SS. Based on his myelination studies in human brain, Flechsig (1896) concluded that the SS was purely a projection system, and therefore the ILF (widely regarded then to be synonymous with the SSe) was also a projection system.

Steven Polyak (1889–1955), in his authoritative account of the visual system (Polyak, 1957), was unable to fully resolve the factual and terminological disparities that had arisen regarding the relationship of the SS to the ILF. He determined that (p. 400) "the visual radiation, the most external of the three sagittal strata of Sachs, identical with Burdach's 'inferior longitudinal fascicle', is found lateral to the posterior horn of the lateral ventricle."[1] He nevertheless provided a lucid description of the gross anatomy of the SS (p. 394): "The shape of these particular fibrous sagittal layers varies from plane to plane, usually somewhat resembling an irregular horseshoe. The two ends of the horseshoe point toward the medial face of the hemisphere, the horseshoe enclosing in its concavity the more or less collapsed posterior horn of the lateral ventricle." Polyak recognized the anatomical relationship of the SS to the visual radiation (the geniculocalcarine tract) and the detour of the geniculocalcarine fibers into the temporal lobe that was described by Flechsig (Flechsig's knee, later identified by Meyer and named Meyer's loop). Indeed, Polyak identified the optic tract as but one part of the SS.[2]

The SS is still generally thought of as being synonymous with the optic radiation, however, and the question as to whether the SS is a projection system, an association pathway, or both, is not yet settled. Important details regarding the organization and functional relevance of the SS have thus remained unresolved until the present time.

Results of the Present Investigation

According to our observations, the SS is a major fiber system visible on gross inspection of coronal section of the hemispheres, and readily identifiable using conventional Nissl and myelin staining techniques. Its prominence in the occipital lobe and its long-identified role in linking the lateral geniculate nucleus with the calcarine cortex has led to its becoming synonymous with the optic radiations, although this is a misnomer. The SS is a major corticosubcortical white matter bundle that conveys fibers from the parietal, occipital, cingulate, and temporal regions to subcortical destinations in the thalamus, the nuclei of the basis pontis, and other brainstem structures. It also conveys afferents principally from the thalamus to the cortex. It may therefore be viewed as equivalent to the internal capsule in that it is a major subcortical fiber system and not exclusively a fiber tract linking the lateral geniculate nucleus with the calcarine cortex.

The SS comprises two distinct segments that can be visualized using Nissl staining by the differential arrangement of the glia. The internal segment consists mainly of corticofugal fibers efferent from the cortex, whereas the external segment contains incoming corticopetal fibers. However, fibers arising from different parts of the post-Rolandic cortices pass through the corticopetal external segment as they course toward the tapetum on their way to the opposite hemisphere, and to the SSi as they lead to their subcortical destinations.

Around the ventricle, the SS is bounded medially by the tapetum. For much of its course, it is bounded laterally, and sometimes superiorly and ventrally, by the inferior longitudinal fasciculus.

In our template brain the SS extends from the midpoint of the LGN until the occipital pole. We have divided the SS into four approximately equal segments from rostral to caudal. The most rostral division, SS-1 (Scs. 89, 93, and 97), is situated ventral to the posterior limb of the internal capsule, and its rostral end lies in the white matter of the temporal lobe, at a level corresponding to the midpoint of the LGN. This rostral and ventral sector of the SS is largely equivalent to the Flechsig-Meyer loop of the visual radiation. In the next division, SS-2, the SS reaches its broadest extent both dorsoventrally and mediolaterally at the level of, and just caudal to, the splenium of the corpus callosum (Scs. 105, 113, and 121). The third division, SS-3 (Scs. 129, 137, and 145), forms a semilunar arc around the rostral part of the calcarine fissure. The most caudal segment confined to the occipital lobe, SS-4 (Scs. 153, 161, and 165), is restricted in width and surrounds the internal aspect of the calcarine fissure.

Sagittal Stratum Fibers Arising from the Posterior Parietal Cortex

The parietal lobe fibers that course through the SS arise from the medial and caudal aspects of the superior parietal lobule and from the caudal aspect of the inferior parietal lobule (figures 25-1 and 25-2). The subcortical fibers from the *medial parietal cortex* enter the most dorsal and medial portion of the sagittal stratum at mid-SS-2 and travel rostrally into the dorsal and medial aspects of rostral SS-2 before entering the posterior limb of the internal capsule as they course toward the thalamus and basilar pons. Some

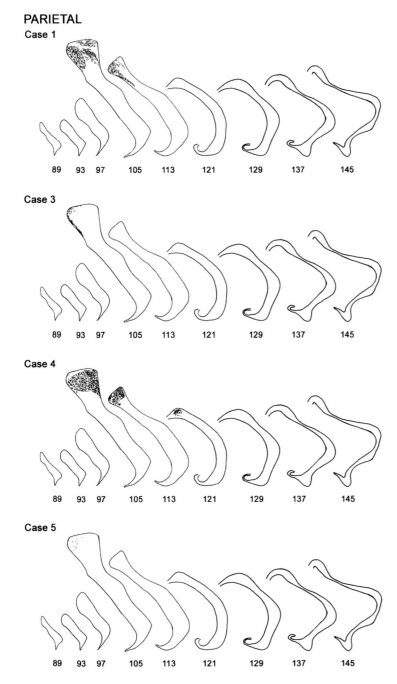

PARIETAL

Case 1

89 93 97 105 113 121 129 137 145

Case 3

89 93 97 105 113 121 129 137 145

Case 4

89 93 97 105 113 121 129 137 145

Case 5

89 93 97 105 113 121 129 137 145

Figure 25-1

Schematic diagrams depicting the location of fibers within the SS of the rhesus monkey derived from the different cortical areas. The SS boundaries are derived from the composite summary diagrams shown in chapter 27. The fibers shown are derived from the diagrams in each case. The SS is seen in sequential rostral to caudal levels in the coronal plane, and the levels of the coronal sections are identified by the numbers below the diagrams for each case. The rostral three (of four) sectors of the SS are shown: SS-1 comprises sections 89, 93, and 97; SS-2 sections 105, 113, and 121; and SS-3 sections 129, 137, and 145.

Figure continues on pages 520–521

Figure 25-1 (continued)

SUPERIOR TEMPORAL
Case 7

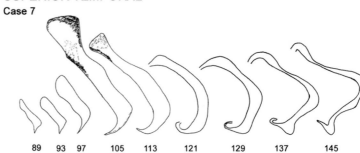

89   93   97   105   113   121   129   137   145

Case 8

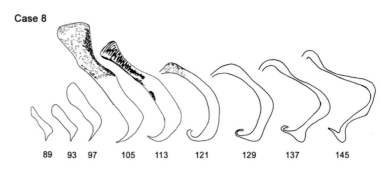

89   93   97   105   113   121   129   137   145

Case 9

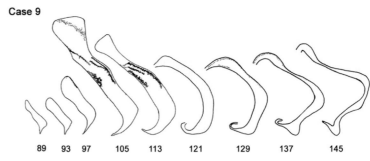

89   93   97   105   113   121   129   137   145

INFERIOR TEMPORAL
Case 12

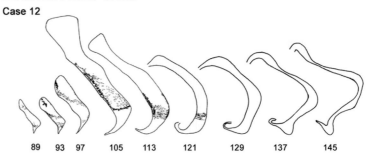

89   93   97   105   113   121   129   137   145

CINGULATE
Case 22

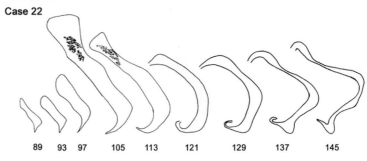

89   93   97   105   113   121   129   137   145

OCCIPITAL

Case 17

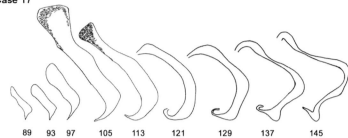

89 93 97 105 113 121 129 137 145

Case 18

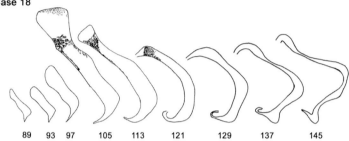

89 93 97 105 113 121 129 137 145

Case 19

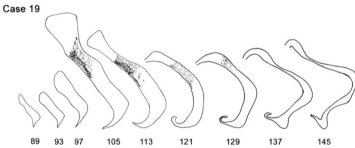

89 93 97 105 113 121 129 137 145

Case 20

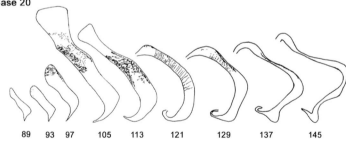

89 93 97 105 113 121 129 137 145

Case 21

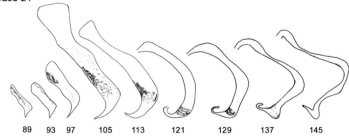

89 93 97 105 113 121 129 137 145

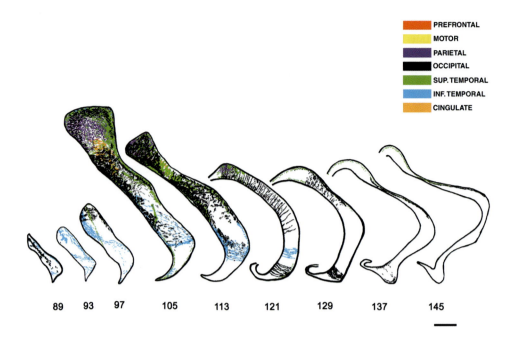

PREFRONTAL
MOTOR
PARIETAL
OCCIPITAL
SUP. TEMPORAL
INF. TEMPORAL
CINGULATE

89 93 97   105   113   121   129   137   145

SAGITTAL STRATUM

Figure 25-2
Summary diagram of the location within the SS of the fibers derived from the major lobar areas of the rhesus monkey cerebral hemisphere. The SS boundaries are derived from the composite summary diagrams shown in chapter 27. The fibers within the SS are color-coded according to the legend at top right. As with the previous diagram, the rostral three (of four) sectors of the SS are seen in sequential rostral to caudal levels in the coronal plane, and the levels of the coronal sections are identified by the numbers below the diagrams for each case. Bar = 2 mm.

fibers from the *caudal aspect of the superior parietal lobule* pass through the dorsal and medial sector of rostral SS-2, although the majority of the subcortically directed fibers enter the dorsal aspect of the posterior limb of the internal capsule at level ICp-5. The cord fibers arising from the *caudal inferior parietal lobule* give rise to fibers that descend and enter the dorsal aspect of caudal SS-2. These fibers progress rostrally in SS-2, occupying the dorsal aspect of the SS. The fibers are grouped into two identifiable constituents—a lateral component destined for the basilar pons, and a medial contingent that leads to the thalamus.

Sagittal Stratum Fibers Arising from the Superior Temporal Region

The caudal aspects of the superior temporal region give rise to subcortical fibers that travel in the sagittal stratum. Fibers from the *caudal region of the superior temporal gyrus* enter the dorsal aspect of the caudal part of SS-2. The fibers occupy the dorsal part of the SS-2 further rostrally, aggregating laterally before moving toward its medial aspect. Further rostrally, the fibers course in the ICp. Striatal fibers that arise from the midcaudal sectors of the upper bank of the superior temporal sulcus traverse the rostral part of SS-2 before terminating in the genu of the caudate nucleus, but the subcortically directed fibers from this cortical area are more rostrally situated within the ICp.

Sagittal Stratum Fibers Arising from the Inferior Temporal Region

The subcortically directed fibers from the most caudal part of the inferior temporal region enter the ventral sector of SS-2 and travel rostrally and caudally. Rostrally directed fibers ascend at the border of SS-1 and SS-2 and divide into a dorsal and a ventral component. The dorsally situated fibers in SS-1 divide into two parts. One contingent penetrates the retrolenticular ICp and terminates in the thalamus; the other contingent continues rostrally in the dorsal aspects of SS-1, lies adjacent to the lateral aspect of the ventral part of the putamen, and enters the anterior commissure. The ventrally situated fibers in SS-1 move medially and ventrally through the ventral subcortical bundle and terminate in the thalamus. Caudally directed fibers are destined for the corpus callosum. They travel caudally in the ventral part of the junction of SS-2 and SS-3 and course medially into the tapetum before they ascend, travel rostrally again, and enter the splenium of the corpus callosum before coursing to the opposite hemisphere.

Sagittal Stratum Fibers Arising from Parastriate Regions of the Occipital Lobe

The subcortical fibers from the medial preoccipital gyrus enter the most dorsal part of the sagittal stratum at the midpoint of SS-2. These fibers travel rostrally in SS-2 before entering the posterior limb of the internal capsule on their way to the thalamus and basilar pons. The subcortical fibers emanating from the dorsal preoccipital gyrus enter the dorsal aspect of caudal SS-2 and move rostrally in this location confined to SS-2, ventral to the fibers from the medial preoccipital gyrus, before entering the posterior limb of the internal capsule. The fibers from the lateral part of the preoccipital gyrus enter the middle aspect of the SS at the junction of SS-2 and SS-3 and move rostrally in this location into the medial and rostral parts of SS-2 before entering the ICp. The ventral preoccipital gyrus commits subcortical fibers to the most ventral part of the SS at the border of SS-2 and SS-3. These fibers proceed rostrally, within the internal segment of the SS. At the level of the caudal part of SS-1, some fibers move medially to terminate in the thalamus, whereas others continue rostrally within the ventral subcortical bundle before terminating in the thalamus.

Thus, subcortically directed fibers arising from sectors within the parietal, occipital, and temporal lobes travel in a topographically arranged manner within the second quarter of the SS. Here, fibers from the medial and dorsal preoccipital region, the medial and caudal SPL and caudal IPL, and the caudal STG all travel within the dorsal part of the SS. Fibers from the dorsolateral portion of the preoccipital gyrus travel via the middle sector of the SS. Those from the ventral preoccipital and caudal inferotemporal regions occupy the ventral portion of the SS.

As may be seen in figures 25-1 and 25-2, which show the location of the fibers within the SS, the caudal region SS-4 is devoid of labeled fibers in our material. The same is true for most of the ventrally situated rostral sector, SS-1, as well as parts of SS-2 and SS-3 ventrally. Our cases do not include injections within the striate cortex of the occipital lobe. It is therefore probable that these "empty" areas of the SS in the present series reflect those regions that convey the visual radiations. Thus the rostral sector, SS-1, corresponds to the anteriorly reflected fibers of the Flechsig-Meyer loop, while the ventral parts of SS-2 and SS-3 contain the optic radiations that Gratiolet described, in addition to the thalamic fibers of the caudal inferior temporal and occipitotemporal areas. The reciprocal links between the lateral geniculate nucleus and the visual cortex in the occipital pole are wholly contained within the SS. This was the view held by Flechsig (although the terminology of the time was contradictory: "the 'inferior longitudinal fasciculus' is therefore nothing more than a part of the optic radiation of Gratiolet" [Flechsig, 1896]), and it was also Polyak's (1957) position. The visual radiations therefore constitute one distinct component of the fiber bundles within the SS.

Functional Notions

This analysis helps clarify some of the uncertainties regarding the SS that have persisted until now. The SS is unrelated to the association fibers in the superior and inferior longitudinal fasciculi. It is strictly a corticosubcortical projection system. It contains the Flechsig-Meyer temporal loop in its rostral sector, and the optic radiation of Gratiolet in its ventral region in the temporal lobe and in its caudal position in the occipital lobe. It conveys fibers from the parietal, temporal, and occipital lobes in a topographically arranged fashion to the thalamus and brainstem, including the nuclei of the basis pontis. It is likely a bidirectional fiber system conveying corticopetal fibers from the thalamus back to these cortical areas, as judged by the geniculocalcarine pathway that also traverses the SS. Our material did not study efferents from the thalamus, and so this conclusion is necessarily tentative.

Within the SS there is segregation of the corticofugal and corticopetal fibers. This understanding dates back to Flechsig (1896), based on his myelination studies in human, supported by the work of Probst (1901b) in the cat and Biemond (1930) in rabbits and monkeys. Fibers afferent to the cortex from the lateral geniculate nucleus are relayed in the external layer of the SS, whereas those efferent from the cortex to the LGN are in the internal layer of the SS. This observation that the connections between the LGN and the primary visual cortex run in separate tracts in the white matter in the SS has been examined recently in the rat using the isotope technique (Woodward and Coull, 1984) and confirmed electrophysiologically (Woodward et al., 1990).

The SS may thus be considered the equivalent of the "internal capsule" of the posterior part of the hemispheres. It is the major corticosubcortical afferent and efferent system that links the cerebral cortex with the thalamus and pons, as well as with other diencephalic and brainstem structures. It contains fibers, such as those from the posterior parietal cortex, that often lead directly from the SS into the internal capsule to reach the subcortical destination. It contains a specialized corticosubcortical system, the optic radiation, but the SS and the optic radiation are not synonymous—except in the caudal regions of the occipital lobe, where only visual fibers are to be found.

The functional implications of these observations are also analogous to those of the internal capsule. Lesions of the geniculocalcarine pathway within the SS produce visual loss, just as lesions of the posterior limb of the internal capsule produce motor or sensory impairment, depending on the location of the lesion and the cortical-subcortical system that is interrupted. Damage to the rostral-ventral sector, SS-1 in this work, or the Flechsig-Meyer loop, produces a "pie-in-the-sky" hemianopsia, a slice of visual loss from the upper outer quadrant of the contralateral visual field in both eyes. More extensive lesions of the visual radiation produce varying degrees of hemianopsia, or loss of vision in the contralateral visual field, which is somewhat clumsily termed "incongruent" when the visual field deficit is not identical across the hemispheres.

In addition to the visual loss from the SS lesions that involve the optic radiation, the anatomical observations suggest that damage to selected regions of the SS may result in impairments and distortion of visual information at a higher level. Lesions of the middle and dorsal aspects of sector SS-3 are likely to disrupt posterior parietal and visual association cortex projections to and from thalamic nuclei such as pulvinar, lateral posterior, and lateral dorsal nucleus (Jones, 1985; Schmahmann and Pandya, 1990; Yeterian and Pandya, 1985). Similarly, they may damage the parieto-occipital links with the cerebellum through the dorsolateral pontine nuclei in particular (Brodal, 1978; Glickstein et al., 1985; Schmahmann and Pandya, 1989), limiting the cerebellar modulation of high-level visual information as required for the visual control of reaching (Stein and Glickstein, 1992), as well as more abstract spatial cognition (Schmahmann and Sherman, 1998), and other functions subserved by posterior parietal and temporal regions.

Thus, the term "optic radiation" for SS is not accurate, and the SS is not exclusively a tract of the striate cortex; rather, it subserves more complex visual and higher-order sensory processing. Lesions of the SS may thus be analogous to lesions of the anterior limb of the internal capsule that damage frontal-subcortical networks (corticothalamic and corticopontine) and produce deficits in high-level cognition but largely spare motor function. Similarly, like the lesions of the anterior limb of the internal capsule that largely spare motor function because the posterior limb of the capsule is preserved, lesions of the dorsal part of the sagittal stratum spare the visual fields because the ventral part of the SS, namely the optic radiation, is preserved.

Now that imaging can detect the different components of the SS *in vivo* in humans (Hosoya et al., 1998), it should be possible in the future to develop more precise structure–function correlations between the SS and visual-spatial analysis.

Thalamic Peduncles

Corticosubcortical fibers enter the thalamus in specific locations determined by their site of origin. The afferent and efferent fibers are arrayed around the thalamus and are collectively termed the thalamic peduncles. Charles Judson Herrick (1868–1960) observed fibers passing between the thalamus and cortex to be grouped into somesthetic radiations from the lateral and ventral thalamic nuclei to the cerebral cortex; auditory radiations from the medial geniculate body to the superior temporal gyrus; optic radiations from the pulvinar and lateral geniculate nucleus to the cuneus in the occipital lobe; other temporothalamic fibers; and frontal thalamic tracts between the medial nucleus of thalamus and the frontal lobe (Herrick, 1915, pp. 165–171). According to our observations, there are five principal thalamic peduncles: the superior, lateral, inferior, and anterior thalamic peduncles and the ventral subcortical bundle. These peduncles represent staging areas of the fibers from the cerebral cortex before they pass through the reticular nucleus to enter the respective thalamic nuclei.

Superior Thalamic Peduncle

The superior thalamic peduncle is bounded laterally by the internal capsule and is situated between the caudate nucleus superiorly and the thalamus below. It joins the internal medullary lamina and extends medially to the midline of the thalamus. It contains fibers from the caudal inferior parietal lobule, caudal cingulate gyrus, parahippocampal gyrus, and dorsolateral prefrontal cortex.

Lateral Thalamic Peduncle

The lateral thalamic peduncle is located between the thalamus proper and the reticular nucleus, adjacent to the posterior limb of the internal capsule. For purposes of description, its dorsal-ventral extent is divided into dorsal, middle, and ventral sectors. This peduncle conveys fibers from the superior and inferior parietal lobules, superior temporal gyrus and sulcus, cingulate gyrus, and motor cortices, with topographical ordering as described below.

Anterior Thalamic Peduncle

The anterior thalamic peduncle emerges from the anterior limb of the internal capsule and enters the most rostral part of the thalamus. It conveys fibers from all regions of the prefrontal cortex, as well as from the supplementary motor area.

Inferior Thalamic Peduncle

The inferior thalamic peduncle (ITP) emerges from the orbital frontal cortex and courses to the thalamus. It has a ventral and a dorsal sector. The ventral component lies beneath the globus pallidus and curves upward around its medial border. Here the ventral component of the ITP merges with the dorsal component that lies medial to the globus pallidus rostrally and that penetrates the rostral thalamus at its medial and ventral aspects. Within the thalamus the ITP courses caudally, situated between the midline thalamic nuclei and the ventral anterior thalamic nucleus. It conveys fibers to the thalamus from the caudal orbital cortex, and has been reported to convey fibers to the thalamus from the anterior and medial temporal lobe and from the amygdala (Whitlock and Nauta, 1956; see Klingler and Gloor, 1960, for further discussion). Klingler designated this, the extracapsular thalamic peduncle, "pedunculus thalami extracapsularis" (Klingler and Gloor, 1960; Ludwig and Klingler, 1956).

Ventral Subcortical Bundle

We have used the term "ventral subcortical bundle" (VSB) to denote an aggregation of fibers that occupies a unique position lateral to the thalamus. This appears to correspond in part to what Stephen Walter Ranson (1921) referred to as the temporothalamic fasciculus of Arnold (1851), and what Klingler and Gloor (1960) termed the temporopulvinar fasciculus.[1] In Ranson's description, the Arnold bundle appears to merge with what Carl Wernicke in his *Atlas des Gehirns* (1897, 1900, 1903) depicted as the "corona radiata temporalis" in the temporal stem and that Dejerine (1895) named Wernicke's bundle. Using the gross dissection methodology, Ranson (1921, p. 367) reported that the fasciculus of Arnold "emerges from the ventrolateral part of the posterior extremity of the thalamus under cover of the external geniculate body. The fibers form a large strand directed forward in the inferior of the two layers of the sublenticular segment of the internal capsule along the roof of the inferior horn of the lateral ventricle. Here a few at a time they curve outward and then somewhat backward into the white matter of the temporal lobe. Thus as they spread out toward their distribution, the fibers describe broad curves with the convexity forward. The most medial of these fibers extend farthest forward reaching the anterior extremity of the roof of the inferior horn before they curve outward and backward toward their distribution."

As evident in our material, before reaching the various thalamic peduncles the corticothalamic fibers from frontal, parietal, occipital, and superior temporal regions are conveyed along with fibers destined for other brainstem or diencephalic sites, traveling within subcortical bundles that run in the internal capsule or the sagittal stratum. We considered it useful to maintain this convention of a subcortical bundle emanating from the rostral and inferior temporal regions, lying within the temporal stem. It appears to correspond to the Wernicke bundle (his "corona radiata temporalis"), it differs from the subcortical bundles in the capsule and sagittal stratum in that it conveys thalamic fibers exclusively, and it is continuous with the VSB.

According to our observations, fibers in the ventral subcortical bundle arise from the rostral parts of the superior temporal gyrus, superior temporal sulcus, and inferotemporal area, as well as from the parahippocampal gyrus. They course from the temporal lobe medially over the tail of the caudate nucleus and the stria terminalis. The fibers then move posteriorly, occupying a position above and medial to the stria terminalis, lateral to the lateral geniculate nucleus (rostrally) and the pulvinar inferior (caudally). The ventral subcortical bundle thus lies wedged between these thalamic nuclei and the stria terminalis. From there, fibers enter the caudal part of the thalamus, destined primarily for the medial pulvinar.

Cortical Origins of Thalamic Peduncles in the Present Analysis

Parietal Lobe

Fibers from the parietal lobe are present mostly in the lateral thalamic peduncle. Fibers from the medial convexity of the superior parietal lobule aggregate in its most dorsal sector. Those from the caudal parts of the inferior and superior parietal lobules occupy its midportion. The rostral part of the inferior parietal lobule, in contrast, occupies the most ventral sector. The fibers from the caudal Sylvian opercular area are situated in the lateral thalamic peduncle, below those from the superior and caudal inferior parietal lobule and above those from the rostral inferior parietal lobule. Fibers from the inferior parietal lobule also travel via the superior thalamic peduncle.

Superior Temporal Region

The fibers from the caudal part of the superior temporal gyrus travel via the midsector of the lateral thalamic peduncle caudally, situated above those from the midportion of the STS and STG, which are more ventrally located. Fibers from the STS also ascend in the lateral thalamic peduncle to reach the superior thalamic peduncle before entering and terminating in the thalamus. Fibers from the rostral part of the STG enter the thalamus after traveling in the ventral subcortical bundle.

Inferotemporal Area

Most of the fibers from the inferotemporal region enter the thalamus by way of the ventral subcortical bundle. This includes the posterior, middle, and rostral parts of the inferotemporal region, the parahippocampal gyrus, and the rostral part of the ventral bank of the STS.

Occipital Lobe

Fibers from the medial preoccipital region enter the thalamus via the dorsal sector of the lateral thalamic peduncle. Those from the dorsal preoccipital area course through its middle sector. The remainder of the preoccipital area sends fibers predominantly via the ventral two thirds of this peduncle.

Cingulate Gyrus

The caudal cingulate region sends fibers to the thalamus via the dorsal sector of the lateral thalamic peduncle caudally. A contingent of fibers also travels in the superior thalamic peduncle throughout its caudal to rostral extent. The rostral cingulate fibers are present in the rostral part of the lateral thalamic peduncle throughout its dorsal-ventral extent.

Motor Cortices

Fibers from the opercular region of the precentral gyrus enter the rostral part of the thalamus via the ventral sectors of the lateral thalamic peduncle. Fibers from the face representation are in this peduncle in its middle and ventral sectors, those from the hand representation are in its middle region, and trunk and leg fibers are in its dorsal and middle sectors. Fibers from the supplementary motor area enter the thalamus via the anterior thalamic peduncle.

Prefrontal Cortex

All regions of the prefrontal cortex send fibers to the thalamus via the anterior limb of the internal capsule, and from there the fibers enter the thalamus through the anterior thalamic peduncle. Fibers from the dorsolateral prefrontal cortex also enter the thalamus via the superior thalamic peduncle and the dorsal sector of the lateral thalamic peduncle. Some fibers from the orbital cortex descend from the anterior limb of the internal capsule into the inferior thalamic peduncle, from where they course toward the amygdala and hypothalamus.

Thus, it seems that thalamic fibers arising from most of the occipital lobe visual areas, the caudal parietal lobe, the cingulate gyrus, the motor cortices, and the caudal superior temporal gyrus penetrate the thalamus via the lateral thalamic peduncle. Fibers from rostral parts of the superior and inferior temporal regions and the parahippocampal gyrus enter the thalamus via the ventral subcortical bundle. Most of the prefrontal lobe fibers enter the thalamus via the anterior thalamic peduncle. Fibers from the parahippocampal gyrus, caudal cingulate area, caudal inferior parietal lobule, and dorsolateral prefrontal area course via the superior thalamic peduncle. Fibers in the inferior thalamic peduncle emerge mostly from the caudal orbital region.

Functional Notions

The functions of the thalamic peduncles may be inferred from the properties of the cortical areas from which the fibers are conveyed and from the considerable clinical information and evolving experimental evidence pointing to the different proposed roles of the various thalamic nuclei (see, e.g., Bogousslavsky et al., 1988; Graff-Radford et al., 1990; Jones, 1985; Schmahmann, 2003). Based on the available information, however, an attempt at a more precise delineation of the putative functional properties of the thalamic peduncles themselves is not currently warranted. We hope that the anatomical data presented in this work will facilitate such future investigations.

Composite Summary of Cerebral White Matter Fiber Systems in the Rhesus Monkey

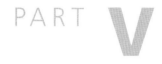

PART V

Composite Summary of Cerebral White Matter Fiber Pathways in the Rhesus Monkey

In this chapter a series of diagrams of rostral to caudal coronal sections of the brain of a rhesus monkey illustrates in a composite manner the association, commissural, projection, and striatal fiber bundles (figure 27-1). The fiber bundles are outlined on the coronal sections, and the fibers traveling within the bundles are color-coded according to the lobe in which they originate. Sections 69 and 78 are omitted in this series, as they were used to depict motor cases only, as seen in chapter 11.

27

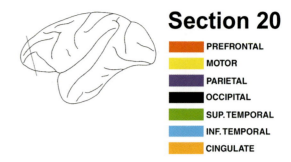

- PREFRONTAL
- MOTOR
- PARIETAL
- OCCIPITAL
- SUP. TEMPORAL
- INF. TEMPORAL
- CINGULATE

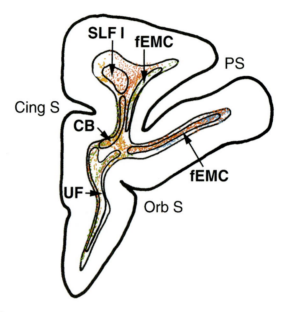

Figure 27-1

Composite summary diagrams of rostral-caudal coronal sections of the template brain (Scs. 20–165) showing the locations of the association, commissural, striatal, and subcortical fiber tracts. Fiber pathways are labeled in bold; sulci and other anatomical structures are labeled in regular font. Fibers within the different fasciculi are color-coded according to the schematic at the top right: prefrontal (red), motor (yellow), parietal (purple), occipital (black), superior temporal region (green), inferior temporal region (blue), and cingulate gyrus (orange). The schematic of the hemispheric diagrams above shows the level at which each coronal section is taken. The striatal bundle (StB) linking the subcallosal fasciculus of Muratoff (MB) and the external capsule (EC) is traversed by subcortical fibers destined for the internal capsule and traveling almost perpendicular to the striatal fibers. Similarly, the superior longitudinal fasciculus II (SLF II) in particular and the fronto-occipital fasciculus (FOF) appear to contain fibers from motor regions (labeled in yellow), but these are subcortical bundle fibers (SB) from the motor cortex descending through these association fiber pathways en route to the internal capsule (see, for example, Scs. 73, 81, 85, and 89). See list of abbreviations, p. 617.

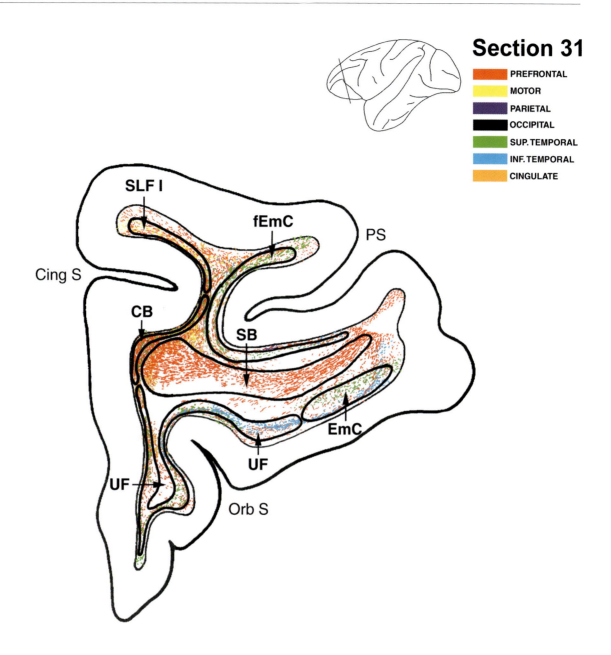

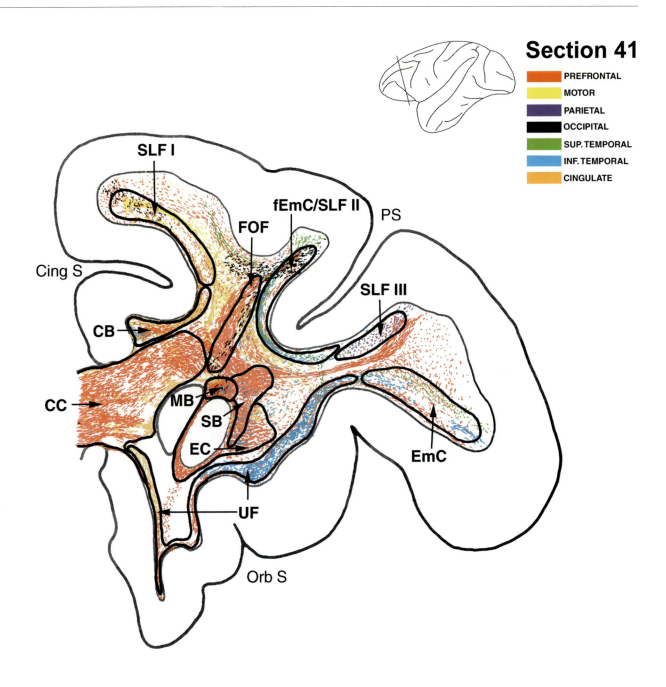

PREFRONTAL
MOTOR
PARIETAL
OCCIPITAL
SUP. TEMPORAL
INF. TEMPORAL
CINGULATE

SLF I

fEmC/SLF II

FOF

PS

Cing S

SLF III

CB

CC

MB

SB

EC

EmC

UF

Orb S

Figure 27-1 (continued)

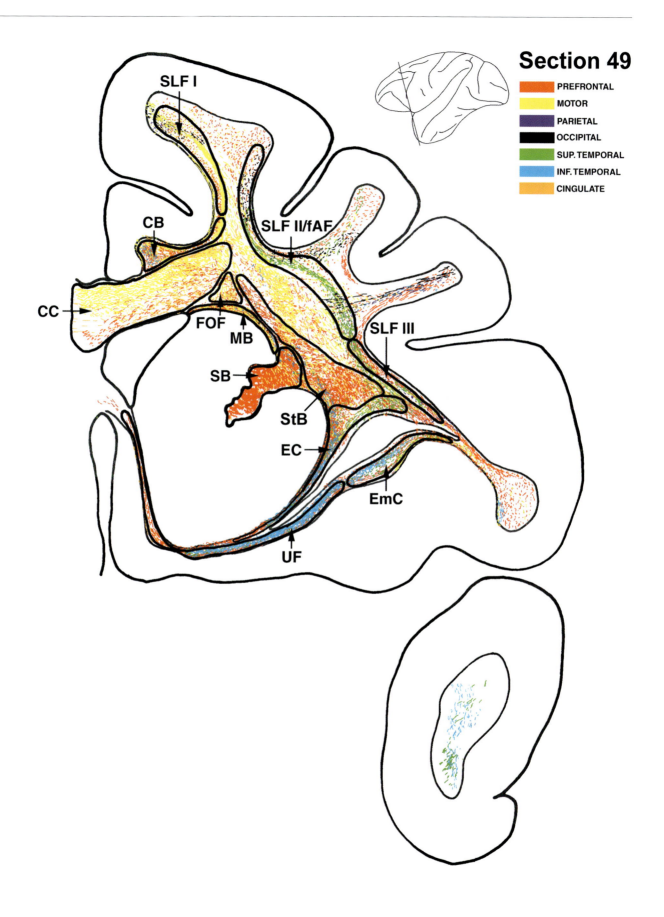

Section 49

PREFRONTAL
MOTOR
PARIETAL
OCCIPITAL
SUP. TEMPORAL
INF. TEMPORAL
CINGULATE

SLF I

CB

SLF II/fAF

CC

FOF

MB

SB

StB

SLF III

EC

EmC

UF

537

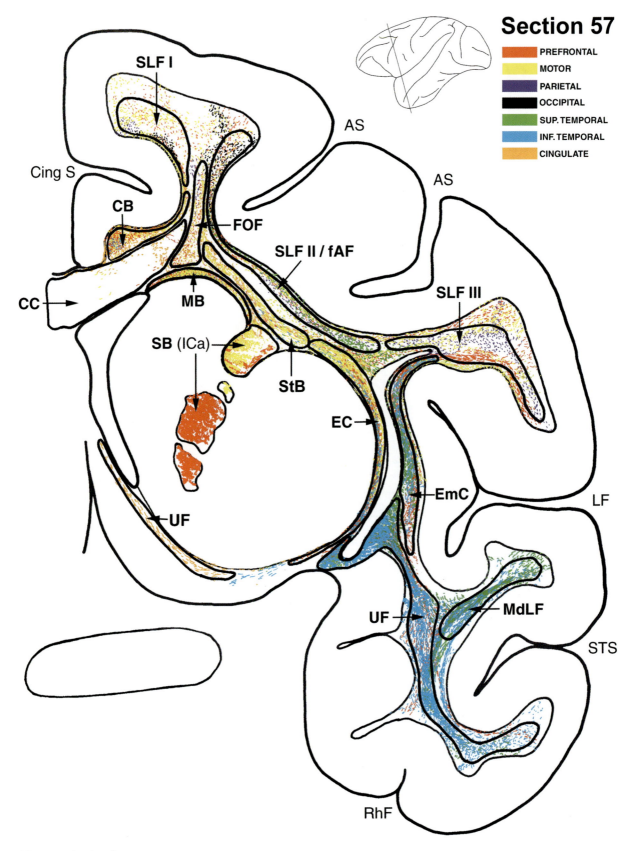

Figure 27-1 (continued)

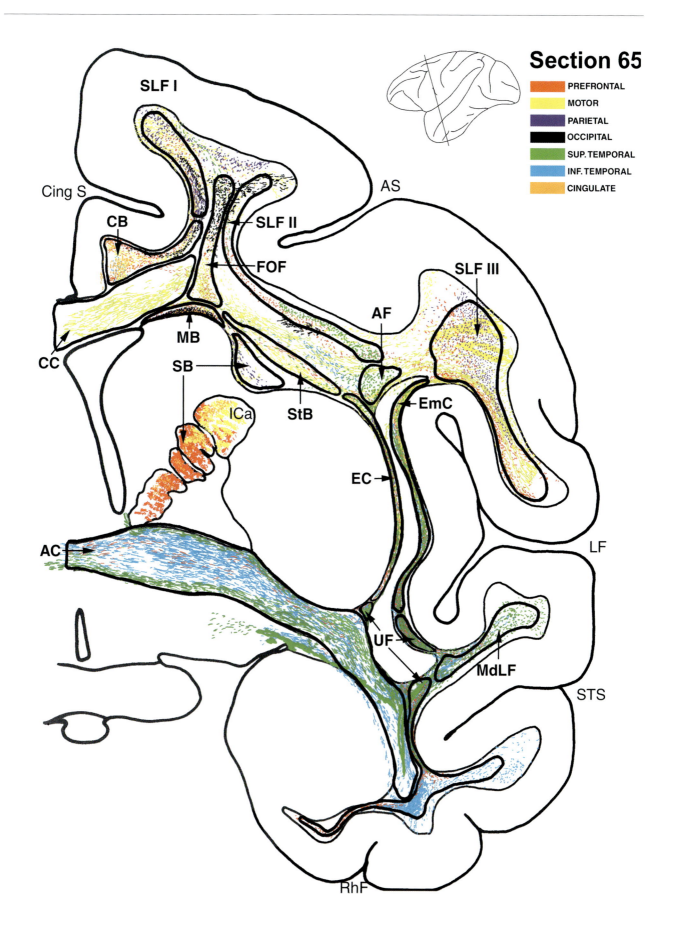

SLF I

Cing S

CB

SLF II

FOF

AS

SLF III

AF

MB

CC

SB

StB

ICa

EmC

EC

AC

UF

MdLF

LF

STS

RhF

Section 65

	PREFRONTAL
	MOTOR
	PARIETAL
	OCCIPITAL
	SUP. TEMPORAL
	INF. TEMPORAL
	CINGULATE

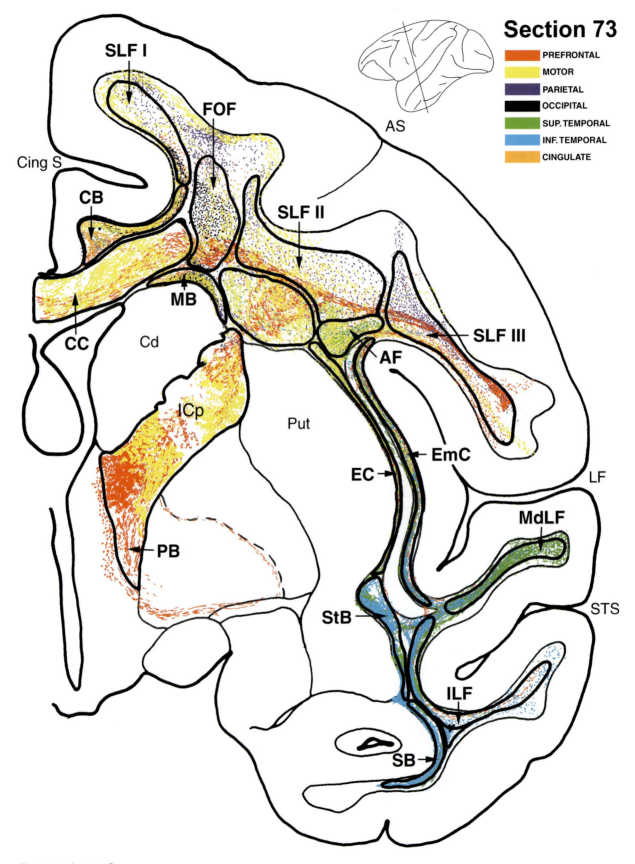

PREFRONTAL
MOTOR
PARIETAL
OCCIPITAL
SUP. TEMPORAL
INF. TEMPORAL
CINGULATE

SLF I

FOF

AS

Cing S

CB

SLF II

MB

SLF III

CC

Cd

AF

ICp

Put

EmC

EC

LF

MdLF

PB

STS

StB

ILF

SB

Figure 27-1 (continued)

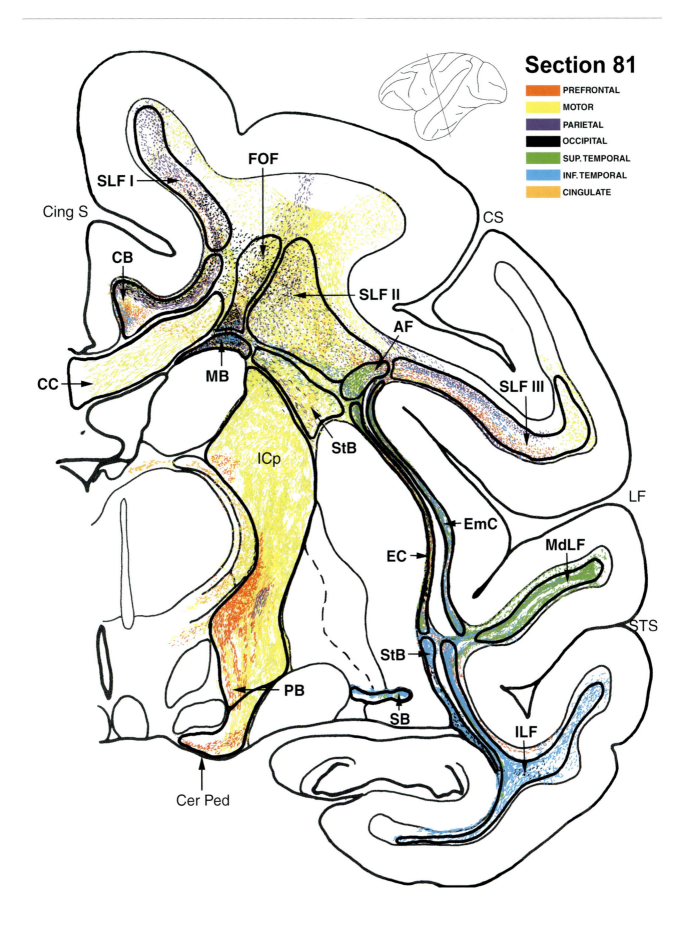

Section 81

PREFRONTAL
MOTOR
PARIETAL
OCCIPITAL
SUP. TEMPORAL
INF. TEMPORAL
CINGULATE

SLF I
FOF
Cing S
CS
CB
SLF II
AF
CC
MB
SLF III
ICp
StB
EmC
EC
MdLF
LF
StB
PB
SB
ILF
STS
Cer Ped

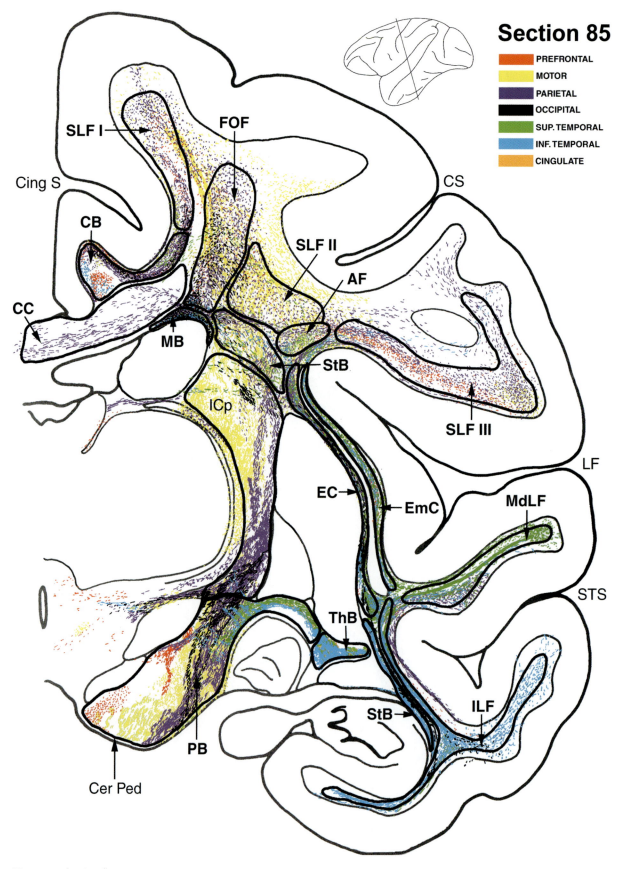

PREFRONTAL
MOTOR
PARIETAL
OCCIPITAL
SUP. TEMPORAL
INF. TEMPORAL
CINGULATE

SLF I

FOF

Cing S

CB

SLF II

AF

CC

MB

StB

ICp

SLF III

CS

LF

EC

EmC

MdLF

ThB

STS

StB

ILF

PB

Cer Ped

Figure 27-1 (continued)

542

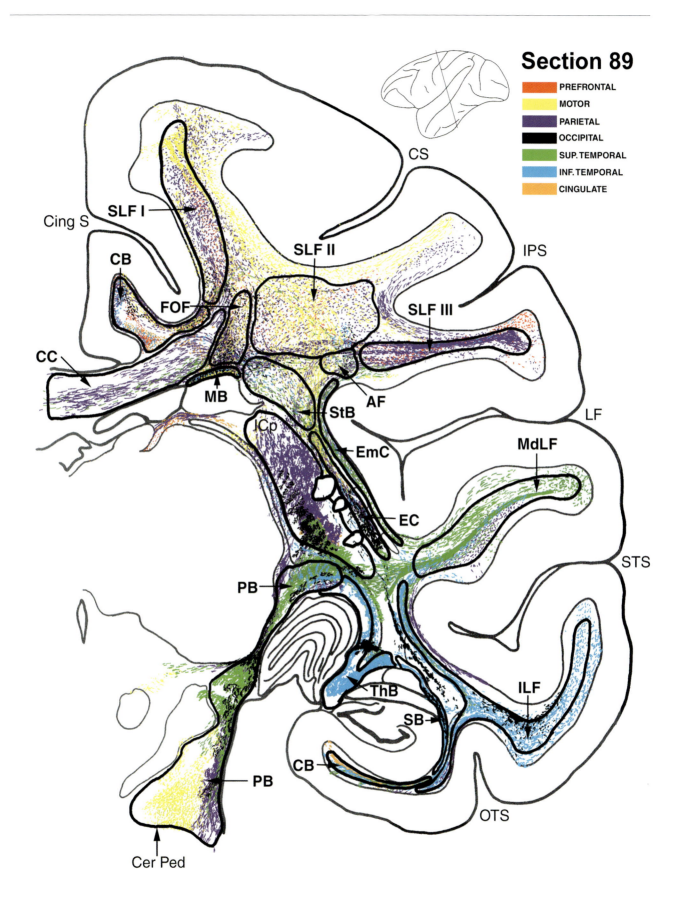

Section 89

PREFRONTAL
MOTOR
PARIETAL
OCCIPITAL
SUP. TEMPORAL
INF. TEMPORAL
CINGULATE

CS

IPS

LF

STS

Cing S

SLF I

SLF II

SLF III

CB

FOF

AF

CC

MB

StB

ICp

EmC

MdLF

EC

PB

ThB

SB

ILF

CB

PB

Cer Ped

OTS

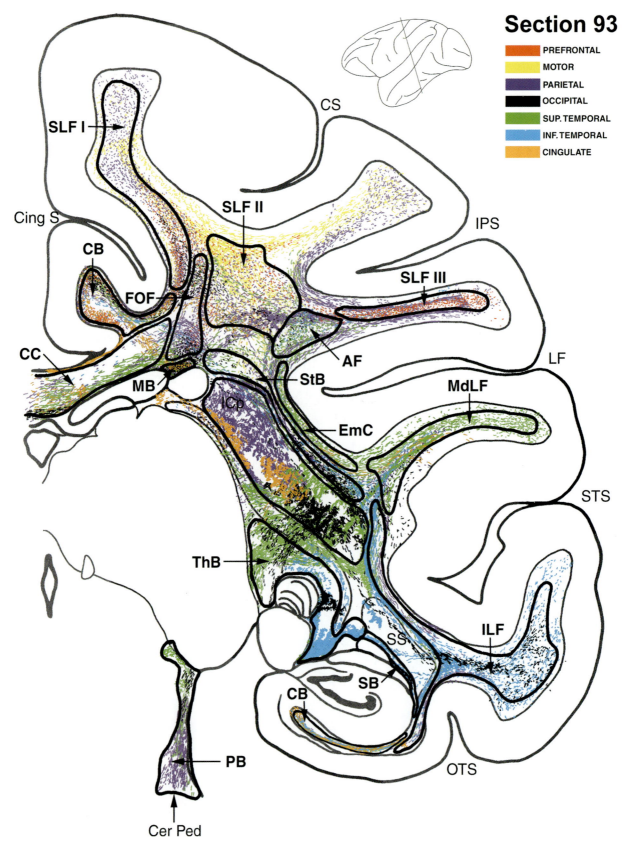

PREFRONTAL
MOTOR
PARIETAL
OCCIPITAL
SUP. TEMPORAL
INF. TEMPORAL
CINGULATE

SLF I

CS

SLF II

Cing S

CB

FOF

SLF III

IPS

AF

CC

StB

LF

MB

ICp

MdLF

EmC

STS

ThB

SS

ILF

SB

CB

PB

OTS

Cer Ped

Figure 27-1 (continued)

544

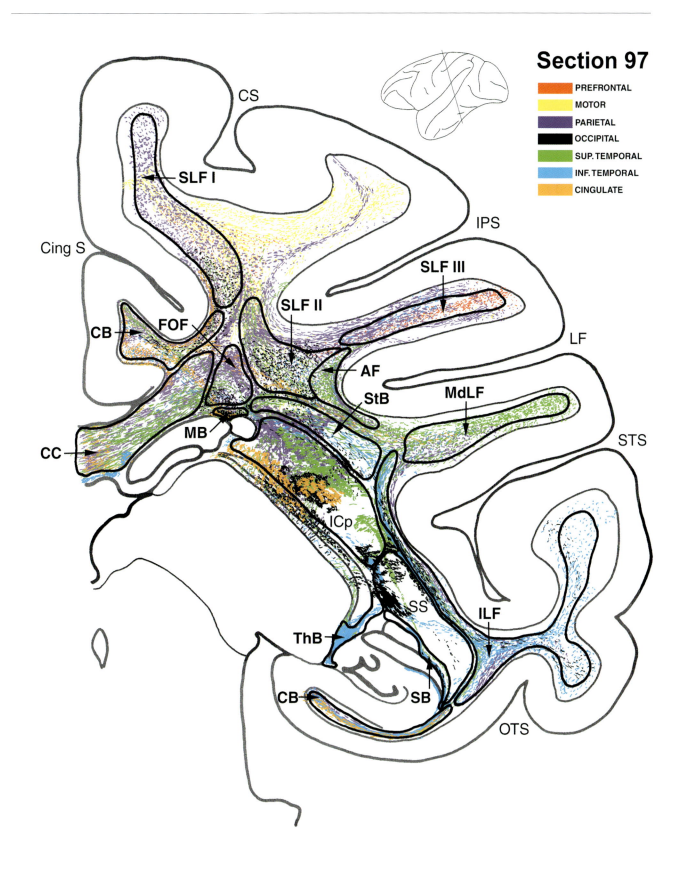

Section 97

PREFRONTAL
MOTOR
PARIETAL
OCCIPITAL
SUP. TEMPORAL
INF. TEMPORAL
CINGULATE

CS

Cing S

SLF I

IPS

SLF III

SLF II

FOF

CB

AF

StB

MdLF

LF

MB

CC

ICp

STS

SS

ILF

ThB

CB

SB

OTS

545

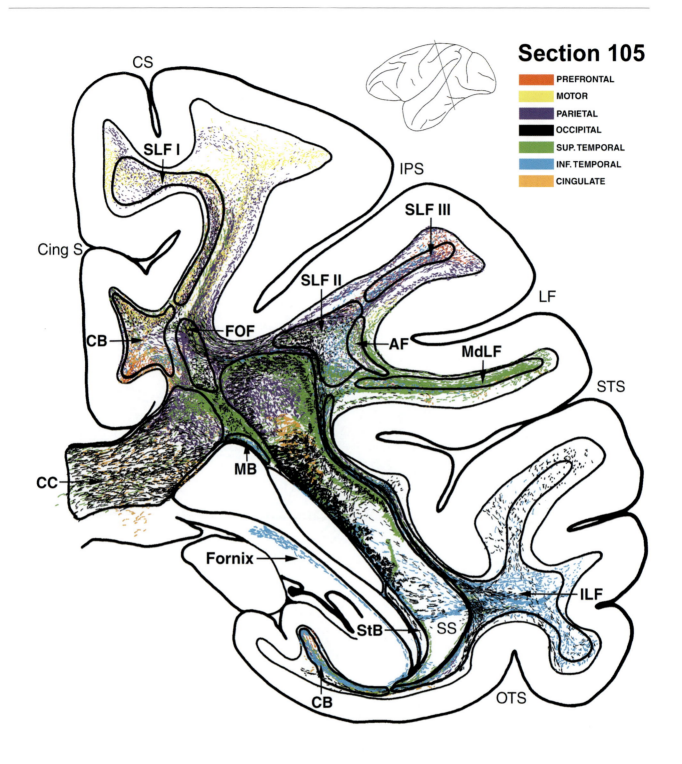

Figure 27-1 (continued)

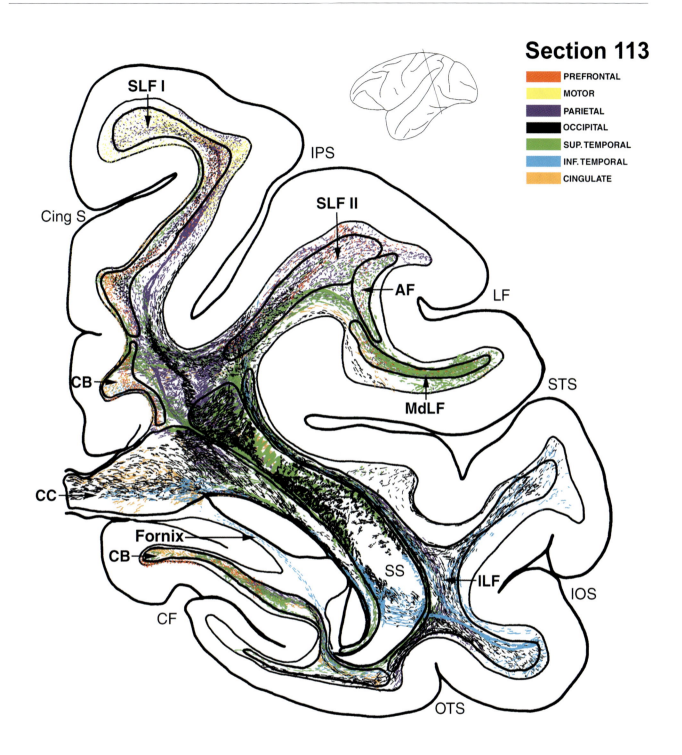

PREFRONTAL
MOTOR
PARIETAL
OCCIPITAL
SUP. TEMPORAL
INF. TEMPORAL
CINGULATE

SLF I

IPS

Cing S

SLF II

AF

LF

CB

STS

MdLF

CC

Fornix

CB

SS

ILF

IOS

CF

OTS

547

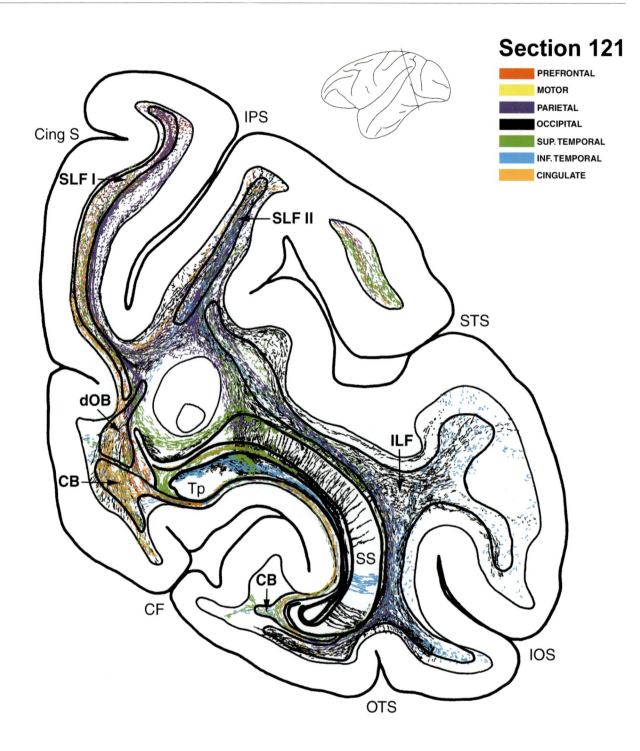

PREFRONTAL
MOTOR
PARIETAL
OCCIPITAL
SUP. TEMPORAL
INF. TEMPORAL
CINGULATE

Cing S

IPS

SLF I

SLF II

STS

dOB

ILF

CB

Tp

SS

CF

CB

IOS

OTS

Figure 27-1 (continued)

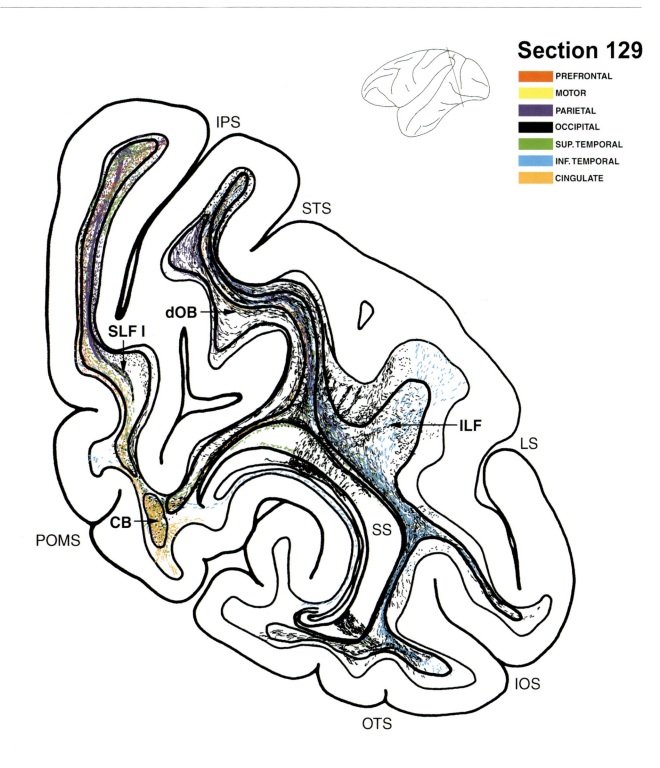

Section 129

PREFRONTAL
MOTOR
PARIETAL
OCCIPITAL
SUP. TEMPORAL
INF. TEMPORAL
CINGULATE

IPS

STS

dOB

SLF I

ILF

LS

POMS

CB

SS

IOS

OTS

549

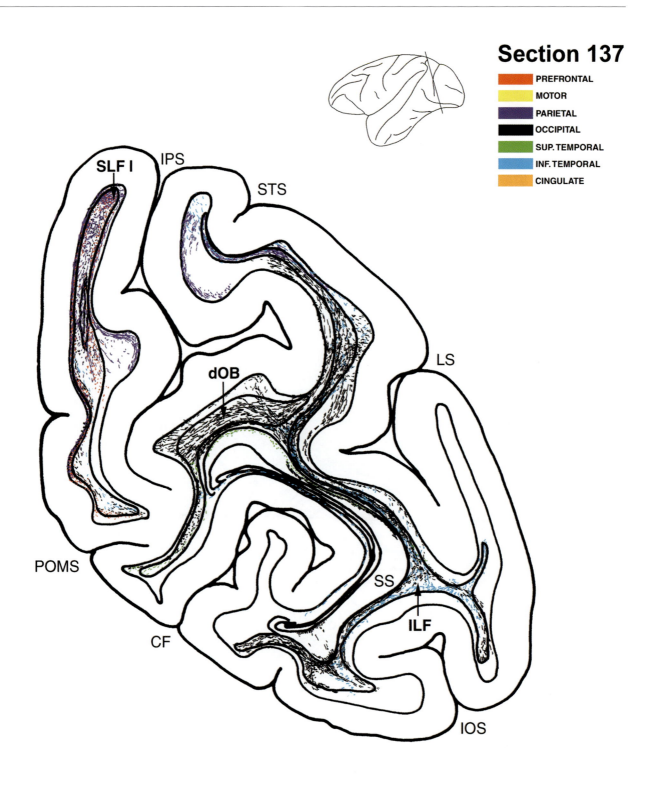

Figure 27-1 (continued)

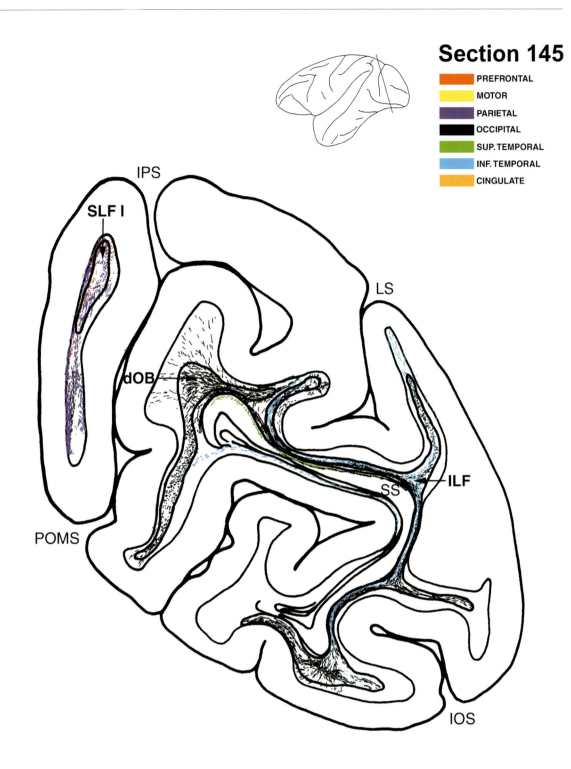

PREFRONTAL
MOTOR
PARIETAL
OCCIPITAL
SUP. TEMPORAL
INF. TEMPORAL
CINGULATE

IPS

SLF I

LS

dOB

ILF

SS

POMS

IOS

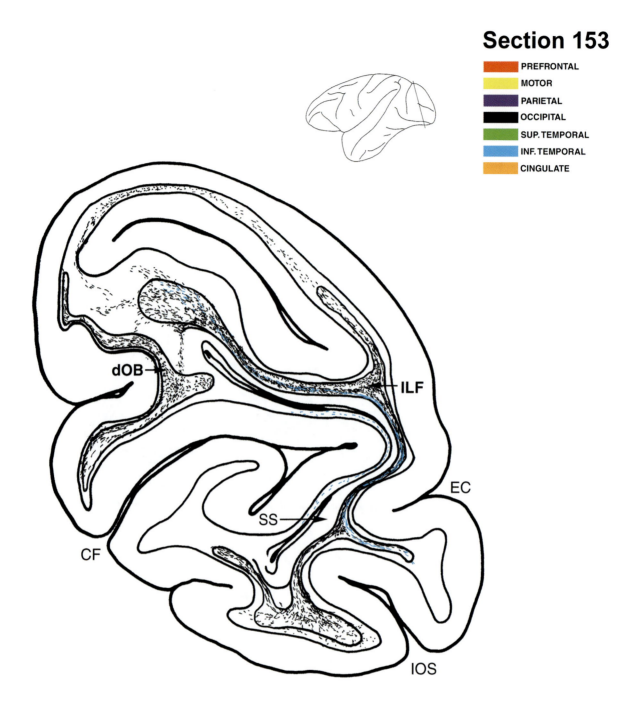

PREFRONTAL
MOTOR
PARIETAL
OCCIPITAL
SUP. TEMPORAL
INF. TEMPORAL
CINGULATE

dOB

ILF

EC

SS

CF

IOS

Figure 27-1 (continued)

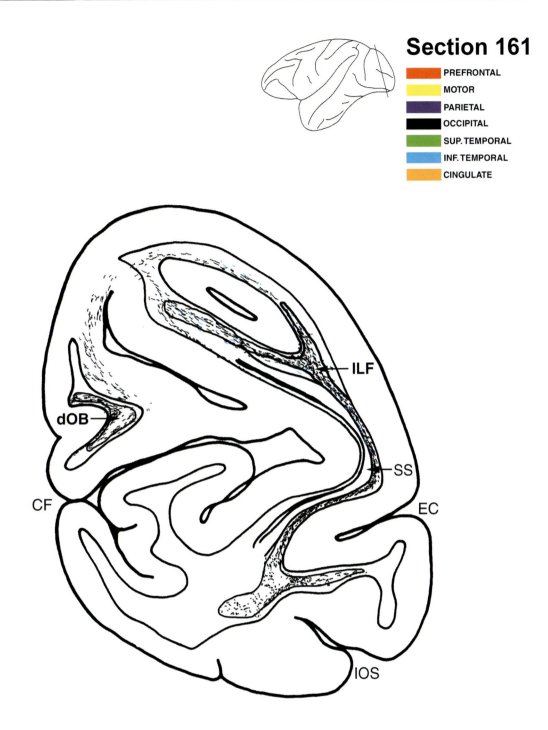

PREFRONTAL
MOTOR
PARIETAL
OCCIPITAL
SUP. TEMPORAL
INF. TEMPORAL
CINGULATE

ILF

dOB

CF

SS

EC

IOS

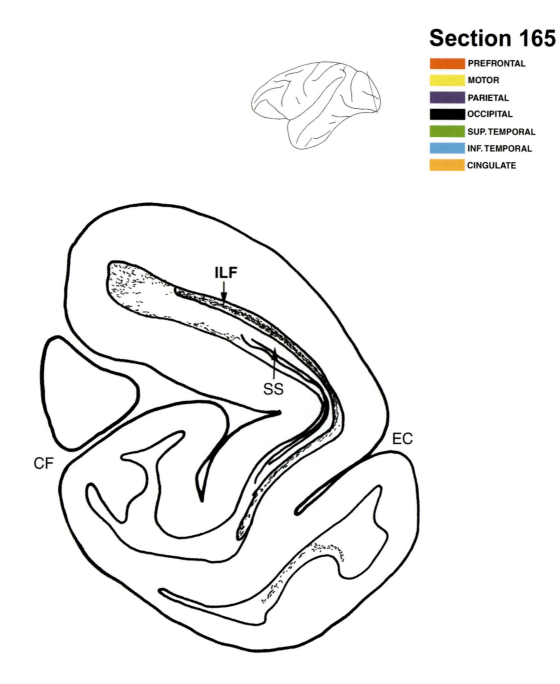

PREFRONTAL
MOTOR
PARIETAL
OCCIPITAL
SUP. TEMPORAL
INF. TEMPORAL
CINGULATE

ILF

SS

CF

EC

Figure 27-1 (continued)

Functional Considerations

 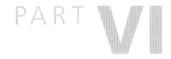

Clinical Significance

In two of his seminal papers, Geschwind (1965a,b) discussed the clinical disconnection syndromes resulting from lesions of cerebral association areas and from damage to some of the specific white matter tracts that link them. This approach highlighted the observations of earlier investigators such as Liepmann and Dejerine, and it also reflected the time-honored neurological approach of deriving deeper understanding of brain function by paying close attention to the details of cortical organization and connectivity. Written during the waning days of what may be regarded as the first era of psychosurgery, characterized by the introduction of prefrontal leucotomy for psychiatric indications (see Ballantine et al., 1967; Freeman and Watts, 1942; Fulton, 1949; Moniz, 1937; Pressman, 1988), Geschwind's ideas presaged further fundamental advances in both the understanding of cerebral organization and the range of clinical manifestations of white matter lesions.

Since the 1960s it has become increasingly apparent that there is an intricate organization of the fiber tracts linking the different cortical areas with each other and with subcortical areas, as can be gathered from the present work. These fiber bundles are likely to be critical elements in the anatomical underpinning of the distributed neural systems that subserve cognition and emotion.

Further, the clinical consequences of white matter lesions appear to extend considerably beyond the scope of the original disconnection syndromes. There is a growing recognition that high-level cognitive impairments and even dementia may result from lesions confined to the white matter (Filley, 2001; Rao, 1996). This underscores the practical relevance of these fiber pathways for the understanding of neuropsychiatry and behavioral neurology, and for helping advance diagnosis and management.

Throughout this monograph, we have emphasized the possible functional significance in humans of the fiber bundles that we have observed in the monkey. In the relevant chapters we have also mentioned neurosurgical approaches to the white matter for relief of neurological and psychiatric disorders. These include prefrontal leucotomy, the utility of more precise cingulotomy for obsessive-compulsive disorder and management of intractable pain (see chapter 17), corpus callosum section for epilepsy (see chapter 22), the recent introduction of deep brain stimulation of the anterior limb of the internal capsule for obsessive-compulsive disorder (see chapter 24), and the possible consequences on behavior of disruption of the uncinate fasciculus (see chapter 16).

In this chapter we draw upon the cases of selected individual patients, mostly from our personal clinical experience, to focus on the apparent wider clinical relevance of white matter anatomy and disorders. We discuss diseases of the white matter that cause dementia, selected examples of focal white matter lesions that produce cognitive and sensorimotor manifestations, and the phenomena of white matter attrition and pruning. Finally, we touch on the question of the effect of lesion location on recovery from neurological deficit.

Diseases of the White Matter Causing Dementia

Cognitive deficits occur in a number of disorders that predominantly or exclusively affect the white matter (table 28-1). This disease-oriented approach considers the conditions that have a major impact on the myelinated axons of the central nervous system and is a clinically important step in the process of reaching a diagnosis so that the pathophysiology can be better appreciated and appropriate management may be instituted. The onset and evolution of symptoms and signs in a particular patient (the history) and the results of the clinical examination and specifically targeted laboratory investigations will usually lead to the correct diagnosis.

The following are examples of some white matter diseases that are associated with dementia, depicted through neuroimaging abnormalities and synopses of the major features of the clinical presentations. A wider and more detailed discussion is beyond the scope of this work (see Filley, 2001). A clinical feature common to most of these presentations is the prominent "frontal lobe" component of the disorders, present in the early stages and notable throughout (see, e.g., Dimitrov et al., 1996; Fisher, 1983; Grafman et al., 1990; Koechlin et al., 1999; Luria, 1966; Mesulam, 2000; and Stuss and Benson, 1986, for accounts of the behavioral syndromes of the frontal lobe). This complex neurobehavioral constellation in the setting of white matter disorders is likely a reflection of the interruption of the transmission of information through the association fiber bundles between the frontal lobe and other cortical association areas, as well as between association areas and subcortical regions.

White matter abnormalities on neuroimaging do not often provide obvious clues to the nature of the underlying pathology. Studies of these white matter lesions suggest that risk factors such as hypertension, diabetes, and aging produce changes in the blood-brain barrier, hyalinization of arterioles, and obliteration of the lumen of the vessel, leading to microinfarcts. Astrocytic gliosis is a common pathological feature identified at the site of the white matter lesion (Baloh et al., 1995; Baloh and Vinters, 1995; Leifer et al., 1990; Marshall et al., 1988). These findings are thus often commented upon in clinical reports as representing "gliosis, demyelination, or ischemia," and there is continuing interest in the degree to which FLAIR (fluid attenuated inversion recovery) and T2 hyperintensities on MRI in later adulthood are incidental or clinically relevant (e.g., Almkvist et al., 1992; Bradley et al., 1991; Christiansen et al., 1994; Coffey et al., 1989; Gunning-Dixon and Raz, 2000; Schmidt et al., 2002; Tupler et al., 1992; Whitman et al., 2001).

The following clinical cases help highlight the relevance for human disease of the neuroanatomical observations in the monkey. The underlying pathology in some of these cases may be consistent with astrocytic gliosis, and many of the patients discussed here have diseases known to produce pathologic change in the white matter, as confirmed in some by brain biopsy or at autopsy.

Table 28-1
Diseases Primarily Affecting Cerebral White Matter

Hereditary congenital diseases

    Mitochondrial encephalopathy with lactic acidosis and stroke-like episodes (MELAS)

    Metachromatic leukodystrophy (arylsulfatase A deficiency)

    Krabbe's globoid cell leukodystrophy (galactocerebrosidase deficiency)

    Adrenoleukodystrophy (very long chain fatty acid excess), adrenomyeloneuropathy

    Alexander's disease

    Leukoencephalopathy with vanishing white matter

    Leukodystrophy with axonal spheroids

    Callosal agenesis

Trauma

    Diffuse axonal injury

    Focal lesions of white matter tracts (e.g., fornix transection)

Infectious/postinfectious

    Human immunodeficiency virus (HIV)

    Progressive multifocal leukoencephalopathy (PML)

    Leukoencephalitis from varicella, rubella, cytomegalovirus

    Lyme disease

    Subacute sclerosing panencephalitis (SSPE)

Inflammatory

    Vasculitis (systemic lupus erythematosus, Sjögren's, temporal arteritis, polyarteritis
        nodosa, Wegener's granulomatosis, isolated angiitis of the central nervous system)

    Sarcoidosis

    Behçet's disease

Tumors

    Gliomatosis cerebri

    Primary cerebral lymphoma

Metabolic

    Vitamin B_{12} deficiency

    High-altitude cerebral edema

Vascular

    Binswanger's subcortical ischemic leukoencephalopathy

    Cerebral autosomal dominant arteriopathy with strokes and ischemic
        leukoencephalopathy (CADASIL)

    Amyloid angiopathy

    Posterior reversible encephalopathy syndrome

    Intravascular lymphomatosis

Demyelinating

    Multiple sclerosis and variants (Balo, Schilder, Marburg)

    Acute disseminated encephalomyelopathy (ADEM)

Toxins

    Postradiation demyelination

    Chemotherapy (methotrexate, BCNU)

    Solvents (toluene)

    Alcohol (Marchiafava–Bignami disease)

    Carbon monoxide intoxication

Hydrocephalus

    Normal pressure hydrocephalus

Degenerative

    White matter component of Alzheimer's disease

    Changes concomitant with "normal aging"

Leukodystrophy with Axonal Spheroids

A 37-year-old woman developed progressive cognitive failure leading to death in 5 years. Initial symptoms included impaired spatial cognition and forgetfulness. Within 2 years she became increasingly paranoid, agitated, and suicidal. She developed incontinence, profound abulia, fidgeting, and restlessness. She had normal vision, hearing, strength, and gait. In contrast, examination revealed hyperreflexia, Babinski signs, and "frontal release signs." Elementary sensation was normal. She was disoriented and had severely impaired declarative memory, semantic fluency, and reverse digit span test. Language was sparse, with occasional paraphasic errors and impaired naming, but comprehension was preserved for simple instructions and short written sentences, and repetition was preserved. All forms of praxis and complex logical reasoning were markedly deficient. The neuroimaging is shown in figure 28-1. Preterminally, she became mute and showed neglect of left hemispace progressing to cortical blindness. A diagnosis of mitochondrial cytopathy was suspected based on elevated urinary excretion of organic acids, and muscle biopsy showing enlarged mitochondria with complex cristae and disturbed biochemistry. Genetic analysis for mitochondrial mutations was negative. She did not improve with treatment by a number of different agents, including immune suppression.

At autopsy the brain revealed normal cerebral cortex but a severe leukoencephalopathy. The white matter was discolored and spongy in the frontal, temporal, and parietal lobes, relatively spared in the occipital lobe, and grossly normal beneath primary motor and sensory cortices. The corpus callosum was atrophied and discolored except in the region corresponding to the location of sensorimotor fibers. There was focal cavitation in the anterior limb of the internal capsule, but the posterior limb, external capsule, and extreme capsule were relatively spared. The medial aspect of the crus cerebri containing prefrontopontine fibers was discolored and atrophied, as were the thalamus, subthalamic nucleus, and hypothalamus. The U-fibers were largely spared. More recent areas of involvement were in the optic radiation, the corpus callosum, and the white matter of the somatosensory and visual cortices (figure 28-2). Histological examination confirmed the leukoencephalopathy, with loss of axons and myelin sheaths to a similar extent, preservation of U-fibers, reactive astrocytes and macrophages, and numerous axon retraction balls (neuroaxonal spheroids) highlighted by neurofilament stain. These features are consistent with the diagnosis of leukodystrophy with neuroaxonal spheroids (e.g., Marotti et al., 2004; Terada et al., 2004).

This case delineates the phenomenon of white matter dementia. It portrays the Jacksonian picture of dissolution of the nervous system (James Hughling Jackson [1835–1911]; Jackson, 1931–1932) commencing with cognitive and emotional failure, leading eventually to loss of vision. Early deficits were loss of the ability to plan and sequence information and engage in problem solving (functions subserved by the prefrontal cortex), and problems with visual-spatial analysis, under the control of posterior parietal regions. The dementia resulted from a rare form of a leukodystrophy affecting principally the white matter association pathways, with involvement late in the course of the visual projection system producing cortical blindness. The preservation of the ability to repeat a sentence quite late into the illness despite the many language deficits is consistent, perhaps, with the relative sparing of the extreme capsule, as discussed in chapter 4. Preservation of elementary sensorimotor function was matched by the rela-

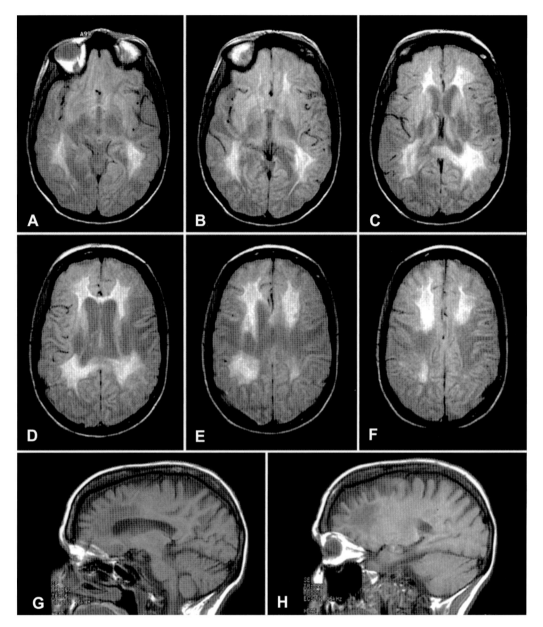

Figure 28-1

FLAIR MRI images in the horizontal plane (A–F) of a patient with leukodystrophy with axonal spheroids shown pathologically to be confined to the white matter and sparing cerebral cortex. The hyperintense signal abnormality tends to spare the white matter beneath the pericentral cortices. The parasagittal T1-weighted MRI scans in G and H show the hypointense signal abnormality located maximally within the white matter of the prefrontal region.

Figure 28-2

Photographs of the formalin-fixed right hemisphere of the brain of the patient whose MRI is seen in figure 28-1. A, Coronal section through the frontal lobe and temporal pole, with arrow pointing to the discoloration and atrophy of the association fiber tracts and corona radiata. B, Coronal section through the parieto-occipital region, with arrow pointing to the lesion involving the association pathways of the posterior hemisphere. Arrowheads point to the anterior limb of the internal capsule in A and the ventral component of the sagittal stratum containing the optic radiation in B. The midsagittal view in C shows the changes in the corpus callosum. The left arrow denotes the atrophy and discoloration of the rostrum, genu, and anterior part of the body, and the arrow on the right points to the lesion of the splenium. In contrast, the arrowhead points to a relatively preserved part of the corpus callosum, which corresponds in the monkey to the callosal sector linking the sensorimotor cortices across the hemispheres. (Figures courtesy of Dr. E.T. Hedley-Whyte, department of neuropathology, Massachusetts General Hospital).

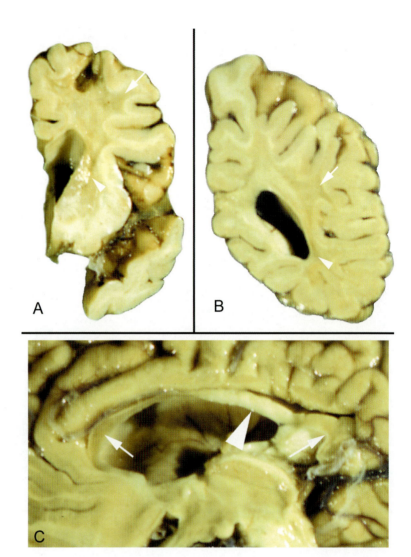

tively normal anatomy of the white matter of the sensorimotor projection pathways, including the posterior limb of the internal capsule and relative sparing of sector 3 of the corpus callosum, which transmits peri-Rolandic fibers between the hemispheres.

Mitochondrial Encephalopathy with Lactic Acidosis and Stroke-like Episodes (MELAS)

A 45-year-old landscape architect presented with a fluctuating but progressive course over a 6-year period of cognitive decline with perseveration, poor insight, lack of motivation, and abulia. He was evaluated in psychiatric institutions and noted to have transient impairments on visual field testing, a history of headache, and white matter abnormalities in occipital and frontal lobe regions on MRI. Clinical suspicion of a mitochondrial disease at the time of his presentation to our unit with catatonia led to a muscle biopsy showing characteristic ragged red fibers, and genetic testing confirmed the A3243G MELAS mutation in the mitochondrial DNA, establishing the diagnosis. Subsequent clinical exacerbations were associated with elevated lactate peaks in affected

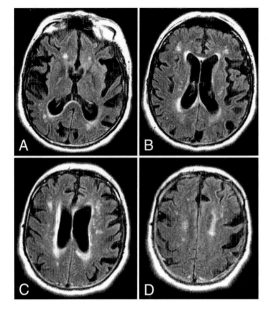

Figure 28-3

FLAIR MRI horizontal images of the brain from inferior (A) to superior (D) taken from a patient with A3243G mutation of mitochondrial encephalopathy with lactic acidosis and stroke-like episodes (MELAS). The periventricular and subcortical white matter location of the multiple hyperintensities is evident, as is the presence of mild generalized atrophy.

brain regions on magnetic resonance spectroscopy. Some clinical improvement was noted with oral antioxidants and avoidance of cigarette smoking. Representative sections from the MRI are shown in figure 28-3. (See discussion of this case in Kim et al., 1999.)

Cerebral Autosomal Dominant Arteriopathy with Strokes and Ischemic Leukoencephalopathy (CADASIL)

A highly educated 48-year-old man developed changes in personality and intellect with problems making decisions and dealing with complex abstractions, loss of eloquence, and difficulty with mathematics. He became withdrawn, appeared depressed, had deficient short-term memory, became lost while driving, and exhibited poor judgment. He experienced discrete clinical episodes of subcortical stroke and became incontinent, and progressive gait failure led to wheelchair dependency and admission to a long-term care facility in year 7 of the illness. Sequential examinations showed progressive deterioration in motor and mental performance, with restricted vocabulary, circumlocution, and semantic paraphasic errors. Conversation was vacuous and simplified, replete with stock phrases. He was inaccurate about current events and displayed perseverative intrusions, but was able to repeat complex phrases. He was severely apraxic in all domains. He demonstrated the major elements of the Gerstmann syndrome as reiterated by Geschwind, namely agraphia, acalculia, right–left disorientation, and finger or body part agnosia (Benson and Geschwind, 1970; Gerstmann, 1924, 1927, 1930; Strub and Geschwind, 1974). Complex reasoning was impossible. He had a right hemiparesis, diffuse hyperreflexia, bilateral Babinski signs, and palmar grasps. Elementary sensation was normal.

MRI scans of the brain 6 years into the illness show severe and diffuse T2 and FLAIR bright signal abnormality (figure 28-4) and T1 dark signal throughout the cerebral white matter. Multiple cavitated lacunar infarctions are noted throughout

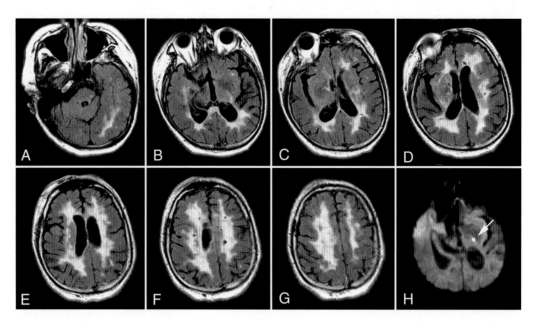

Figure 28-4

MRI images of the brain of a patient with cerebral autosomal dominant arteriopathy with strokes and ischemic leukoencephalopathy (CADASIL). A–G, Horizontal sections from inferior to superior showing the FLAIR signal hyperintensity within the cerebral white matter, including the splenium more than the genu of the corpus callosum. Areas of lacunar infarction are seen as punctate dark signal within the corona radiata, as well as in the body of the caudate nucleus (seen optimally in sections D and G). H, Diffusion-weighted image (DWI) taken at the time of presentation with acute right-arm weakness shows the restricted diffusion (bright signal, shown by arrow) indicating acute infarction in the posterior limb of the left internal capsule.

the deep white matter and involve the anterior limb of the internal capsule, pons, and basal ganglia. Notch 3 gene analysis confirmed the diagnosis of CADASIL. (For further insights into this disorder, see, e.g., Chabriat et al., 1995; Joutel et al., 1997; Mas et al., 1993; Sabbadini et al., 1995; Taillia et al., 1998).

Progressive Subcortical Ischemic Leukoencephalopathy (Presumptive Diagnosis)

A 79-year-old man with hypertension and hypercholesterolemia exemplifies the white matter dementia that is difficult to diagnose in the absence of biopsy. Genetic testing for CADASIL revealed a DNA sequence alteration presently regarded as benign and a nonpathogenic polymorphism. He experienced loss of initiative, memory, insight, and ability to care for himself, and after 5 years he became disoriented, perseverative, and unaware of the degree of his incapacity, and his memory was severely impaired. Naming, verbal fluency, and reverse digit span were poor. He had hyperreflexia and extensor plantar responses, and gait was slow, magnetic (stuck to the floor and difficulty initiating), and threatened by retropulsion. Speech was slow but not aphasic. Vision was intact.

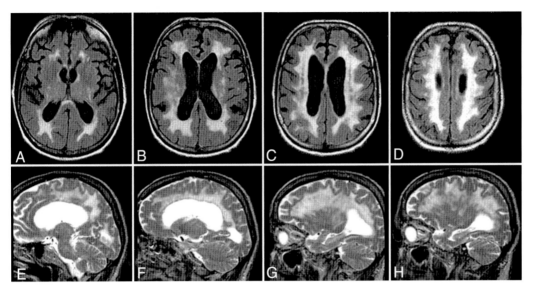

Figure 28-5

Horizontal FLAIR MRI sequences from inferior to superior (A–D) in a patient with dementia and presumed ischemic leukoencephalopathy. T2-weighted MRI sequences in the parasagittal plane (E–H) show the cerebral white matter involvement with sparing of the cerebral cortex.

The MRI (figure 28-5) reveals the white matter lesions involving predominantly cerebral association areas, with the internal capsule relatively preserved.

Progressive Multifocal Leukoencephalopathy (PML)

This 25-year-old man developed changes in personality including social withdrawal, apathy, and disinterest. Over 2 months, verbal output declined, leading to mutism. Examination revealed right hemiparesis with hyperreflexia and extensor plantar response and homonymous hemianopsia on the left. His neuroimaging is shown in figure 28-6.

A 66-year-old immunocompromised man with chronic lymphatic leukemia and recent chemotherapy developed progressive confusion, forgetfulness, and abulia over a period of 3 months. Previously energetic and talkative, he became forgetful, apathetic, and withdrawn. He was disoriented, had a flattened affect, and was slow to answer questions, but language was fluent. Comments to house staff and students were overfamiliar. Recall of newly learned information was impaired but could be prompted with clues. He had a left inferior quadrantanopsia and a neglect of the left superior visual field with double simultaneous stimulation. He moved the left arm only minimally spontaneously, but strength on the left was full when formally tested. He had a left hyperreflexia and extensor plantar response. MRI (figure 28-7A,B,C) reveals bilateral frontal lobe white matter lesions spreading across the rostrum and genu of the corpus callosum, with lesions also in the right parieto-occipital white matter. These lesions do not enhance with contrast, and in this clinical setting are indicative of PML. Figure 28-7D reveals the loss of axonal integrity in the corpus callosum, as shown by decreased diffusivity across the callosum on diffusion-weighted imaging. Also, the parasagittal images in figure 28-7E,F reveal that the pathology tracks between the two frontal lobes in

Figure 28-6

Neuroimages showing features characteristic of progressive multifocal leukoencephalopathy. A, CT scan showing hypodensity in the left frontal lobe and involving the genu of the corpus callosum. B, T2-weighted MRI of the frontal lobe lesion. Note additional small areas of signal abnormality in the white matter of the left posterior parietal region and right frontal lobe, consistent with the multifocal nature of this disorder. C, White matter signal hyperintensity in the right occipital lobe, accounting for the clinical finding of left homonymous hemianopsia.

Figure 28-7

The FLAIR MRI images in this patient with lymphoma are strongly indicative of the diagnosis of progressive multifocal leukoencephalopathy. A through C, from inferior to superior in the horizontal plane, show the white matter lesion in the right anterior and ventral prefrontal region tracking into the anterior limb of the internal capsule (A) and across the rostrum and genu of the callosum into the prefrontal white matter of the left hemisphere (B, C). D, Diffusion tensor image with arrows indicating the bright signal in the normal white matter of the splenium of the corpus callosum posteriorly, but absence of corresponding signal in the affected genu of the callosum anteriorly. E and F, Parasagittal T1-weighted MRI scans of the right hemisphere and midline showing the hypointense signal abnormality indicating the site of the lesion in the orbitofrontal and ventral prefrontal regions. The abnormal signal tracking across the corpus callosum and linking these frontal lobe regions is within the rostrum and genu(G, H). This topography within the callosum of the abnormal fibers may be expected from the tract tracing observations in the monkey.

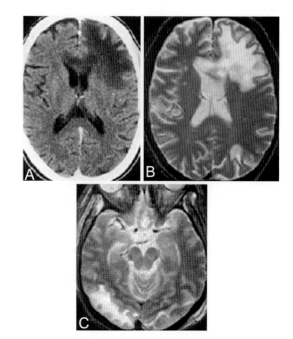

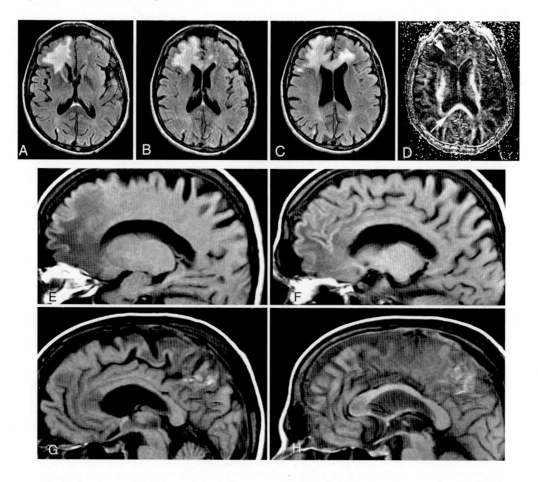

the rostrum and genu of the corpus callosum, a very similar location in the callosum to that assumed by the orbital and ventral prefrontal fibers in the monkey (see chapters 12 and 22).

Amyloid Angiopathy with Vasculitis

A 65-year-old man died after a 7-year illness with amyloid angiopathy and associated vasculitis that manifested as a change in personality and decline in intellect. His symptoms initially suggested depression, as he became withdrawn, apathetic, and lethargic, with substantial weight loss. He was unable to manage complex spatial concepts and was increasingly irritable, unmotivated, and quiet in company, and his affectionate nature vanished. Memory was intact initially (scoring 30 on the Mini-Mental State test, Folstein et al., 1975) but later declined. There was lack of insight and restricted semantic fluency, verbal working memory, and mental flexibility. He demonstrated perceptual fragmentation on tests of visual organization, copy, and recall. Decreased awareness of right hemispace was accompanied by levitation of the right arm when his attention was directed elsewhere, a phenomenon thought to be influenced by the parietal lobe (see Critchley, 1953; Denny-Brown et al., 1952; Richer et al., 1993). He became mute and prominently abulic. There was a dramatic improvement in function for over a year on a combination of methylphenidate, azathioprine, and donepezil, but the course inexorably progressed. He remained ambulatory throughout with preserved strength and sensation, although tone was increased with a cogwheeling component.

Figure 28-8
MRI images of the brain in the horizontal plane in a patient with dementia from amyloid angiopathy and associated cerebral vasculitis. A through D, FLAIR images from inferior to superior, showing high-signal-intensity abnormality principally affecting white matter regions containing association pathways and sparing the internal capsule. E through H, Gradient echo (susceptibility) images from inferior to superior showing multiple minute areas of hemorrhage at the cortical–white matter junction throughout the hemispheres and involving the thalamus and basal ganglia.

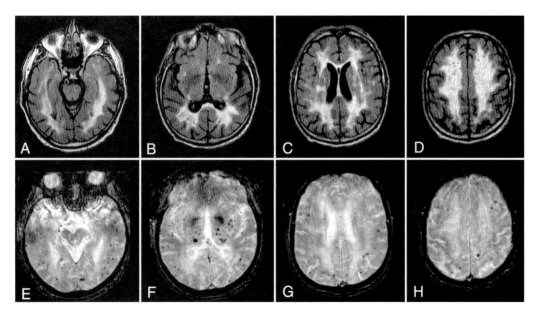

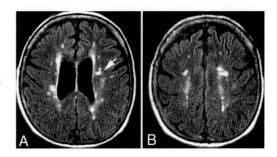

Figure 28-9
Scattered white matter hyperintensities seen in horizontal FLAIR MRI images of a patient with MS. These include the characteristic Dawson's fingers aligned perpendicular to the long axis of the ventricles, highlighted by the arrow in A.

The MRI shows diffuse cerebral white matter hyperintensities with evidence of hemorrhage on gradient echo sequences in basal ganglia and thalamus (figure 28-8). Brain biopsy indicated a component of vasculitis (see Greenberg et al., 1993, and Vonsattel et al., 1991, for further discussion of this entity).

Multiple Sclerosis (MS)

A 63-year-old woman with a history of MS developed progressive cognitive failure manifesting predominantly as impairment of executive function, including verbal working memory, set shifting, and poverty of spontaneity. Visual spatial skills were also affected. Selected images from her MRI are in figure 28-9.

There is a growing recognition from imaging and neuropathological studies that in MS, the disease is not confined to the myelin, but that axonal transection is an important component of the illness and may be the pathological correlate of the irreversible neurological impairment of this disease (Davie et al., 1995; Narayan et al., 1997; Trapp et al., 1998).

Human Immunodeficiency Virus (HIV)

One of the great successes of contemporary management for HIV-AIDS is the response to therapy of HIV dementia and the prevention of this devastating complication by protease inhibitors. In its full-blown form, the hallmark pathology of microglial nodules and multinucleated giant cells has a predilection for the white matter. The presentation is typically characterized by poverty of initiation, motivation, and speech, slowing of mental operations, forgetfulness progressing to memory loss, impaired new learning, and apathy.

A 48-year-old man had a background of bipolar affective disorder, drug and alcohol abuse, and a two-decade history of HIV infection. His MRI shows white matter changes, particularly in the frontal lobe, and generalized atrophy with ventriculomegaly and thinning of the corpus callosum (figure 28-10).[1] He reported headache, poor short-term memory, and clouding of mentation. He demonstrated difficulty with concentration and sustained attention, visual-spatial construction, and graphomotor set shifting. Although he scored 29/30 on a Mini-Mental State exam, neuropsychological testing revealed weaknesses in a number of cognitive domains, including attention/executive functioning, perseveration, impairment of verbal reasoning, and set-shifting. The poor

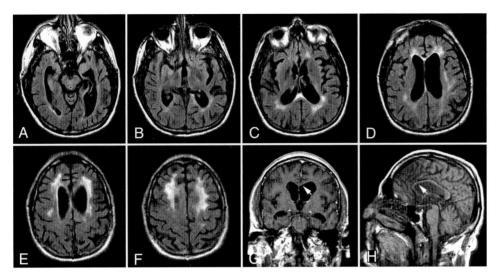

Figure 28-10

FLAIR MRI images of the brain of a patient with HIV dementia. A through F, Horizontal images from inferior to superior showing the signal hyperintensity most prominently in the prefrontal white matter and in the posterior periventricular area, including the splenium of the corpus callosum. The generalized atrophy is seen in these images, as well as in the coronal T1-weighted image in G showing ventricular dilatation. Thinning of the corpus callosum is highlighted by the arrow in G and the sagittal T1-weighted image in H.

executive ability to organize information interfered with memory, and visuospatial skills and motor dexterity were also weak. He acknowledged many symptoms of depression.

HIV dementia remains a scourge of this worldwide pandemic in the many regions where appropriate therapy is not widely available.

Methotrexate-Induced White Matter Changes with Cognitive Impairment

A 51-year-old physician received methotrexate for prevention of CNS lymphoma in the setting of vitreous lymphoma. Over a period of 3 months he reported difficulty expressing his thoughts and visual-spatial disorientation so severe that he was becoming lost in familiar places. Cognitive testing revealed a 20-point decline in his IQ compared to baseline testing, and there was relative weakness in measures of verbal comprehension, confrontation naming, verbal fluency, executive functioning, processing speed, perceptual organization, and most measures of memory.

The MRI shows marked changes in the white matter (figure 28-11)[2] that had not been present before institution of the methotrexate chemotherapy.

Postradiation Demyelination

A young woman who had received whole brain radiation for intracranial lymphoma 15 years earlier developed progressive dementia, abulia, and mutism that required placement in a long-term care facility. Her MRI was dominated by massive white matter de-

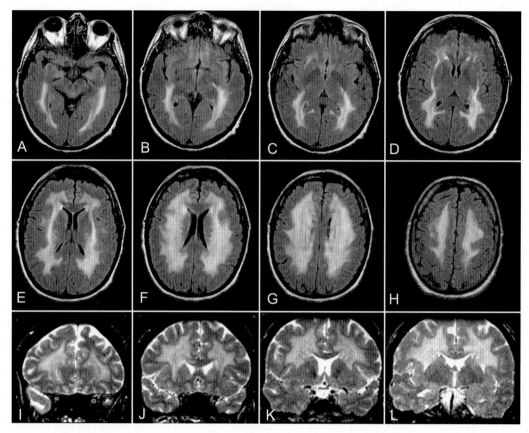

Figure 28-11

Representative sections of a FLAIR MRI of the brain in a patient with cognitive changes following chemotherapy with methotrexate. A through H, Horizontal images from inferior to superior show the abnormality diffusely involving the cerebral white matter with relative sparing of the internal capsule. Similar findings are noted on the selected coronal images from I, rostral, to L, caudal.

myelination in both cerebral hemispheres, similar to that of the methotrexate patient above, but with substantial atrophy evident as well.

Binswanger's Subcortical Ischemic Leukoencephalopathy: Vascular Dementia

The precise nomenclature, pathogenesis, and natural history of Binswanger's disease remain a matter of ongoing investigation and discussion (see, e.g., Babikian and Ropper, 1987; Hachinski, 1990; Korczyn, 2002; Loeb, 2000; Loeb and Meyer, 1996; Roman, 1999; Roman et al., 2002). It was originally described as a disease of the subcortical white matter with multiple focal ischemic infarctions in subcortical nuclei and associated ventriculomegaly, with impairment of gait, cognitive failure, and urinary incontinence. Some classifications of the etiology of dementia maintain this nomenclature, whereas others consider Binswanger's disease within the larger framework of vascular dementia. Mixed dementia (vascular dementia plus Alzheimer's disease) is the most common disorder affecting cognition. The complexity of this constellation is exempli-

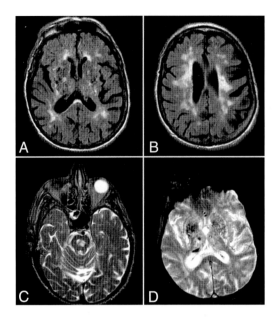

Figure 28-12

MRI images of the brain in the horizontal plane in a patient with the Binswanger form of vascular dementia in addition to amyloid angiopathy. A and B, FLAIR sequences reveal multiple lacunes in the thalami and basal ganglia bilaterally (dark signal) and hyperintensity (bright signal) scattered throughout the periventricular and subcortical white matter, including the splenium of the corpus callosum. Sulcal prominence indicates generalized cerebral atrophy. C, T2-weighted image showing the location of infarction involving the central part of the basis pontis. D, Gradient echo sequence showing the presence of small hemorrhages within the thalamus and basal ganglia bilaterally (right more than left) and scattered small areas of hemorrhage at the cortical–white matter junction posteriorly.

fied by the case of an 81-year-old man with progressive motor and cognitive disability over a period of at least 10 years, accompanied by an accumulating burden of subcortical lacunar infarction, evolving and extensive white matter devastation, and evidence of amyloid angiopathy (figure 28-12). In the absence of pathologic confirmation, a diagnosis of Alzheimer's disease as an additional component cannot be determined, but his age and the dense memory loss that has become superimposed upon his overall state in the past 2 years makes that a distinct possibility. In this patient, as described also in the literature (e.g., Cummings, 1988), early manifestations included a slowing of mentation and apathy that suggested depression. The course evolved in a stepwise fashion with upper motor neuron signs first unilaterally then bilaterally, motor slowing, gait failure, urinary incontinence, and then more recently severe impairment of memory. The white matter abnormalities are a major component of this man's neuroanatomical and neuropathological condition, but the extent to which the neuropsychiatric manifestations are a result specifically of the white matter involvement must of necessity be inferred from other conditions in which the white matter is affected in isolation.

Endovascular Lymphoma

Progressive dementia in this 78-year-old man was thought to be a manifestation of Binswanger's disease, but his course was too rapid, and brain biopsy for suspected isolated angiitis of the CNS led to the correct diagnosis of intravascular lymphoma. The course was characterized by progressive subcortical strokes. The initial presentation was transient loss of vision in the right eye and right-hand clumsiness resulting from a stroke in the left internal capsule and posterior temporal lobe. Further infarcts 5 months later in the left internal capsule and corona radiata and the right centrum semiovale manifested as right arm clumsiness and dysarthria, and repeat neuroimaging 1 year into the course revealed new infarcts in the white matter of the left occipital lobe and in the deep white matter in the watershed vascular territories between the left middle cerebral artery and the posterior and anterior cerebral arteries. White matter infarcts were also seen in the

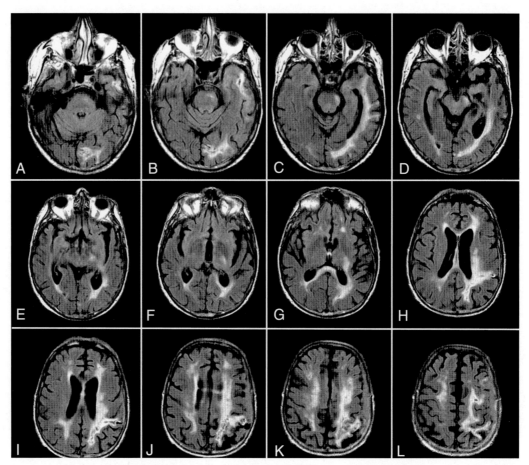

Figure 28-13

FLAIR MRI images from inferior (A) to superior (L) of a patient with predominantly white matter ischemia resulting from intravascular lymphoma. Note the Wallerian degeneration tracking from the left parietal lobe (H) into the internal capsule (G, F, E), crus cerebri (D), lateral part of the basis pontis (C), and the corticofugal fibers within the lateral and ventral regions of the basis pontis (B, A); the abnormal signal tracking from the parietal lesion across the splenium of the corpus callosum to the right hemisphere (H, G); and the involvement of the region in the occipitotemporal area containing the horizontal limb of the inferior longitudinal fasciculus (D, C), and involvement of the optic radiation in the occipital white matter (C, B, A).

cerebellum. Immediately before the diagnostic brain biopsy, the patient presented with deteriorating right-sided weakness and expressive aphasia. He was oriented only to place, and verbal communication was limited by transcortical motor aphasia: he had poor verbal output, frequent paraphasic errors, anomia, alexia, and agraphia. In contrast, he was able to repeat sentences well, and his comprehension was relatively preserved. He displayed prominent perseveration. He was barely able to ambulate with two assistants, had a right hemiparesis, and had hyperreflexia and extensor plantar responses bilaterally.

MRI shows new lesions on the diffusion-weighted images scattered throughout the white matter of the left cerebral hemisphere, as well as in the right precentral and posterior parietal regions. FLAIR hyperintensity in the splenium of the corpus callosum appears to correspond to Wallerian degeneration across the corpus callosum, a finding seen more prominently in a scan taken a year after definitive treatment was instituted. The same scan also traces fiber tracts from the left parieto-occipital lobe through the internal capsule to the lateral part of the cerebral peduncle and the traversing corticofugal fibers in the center of the basis pontis (see MRI in figure 28-13). The subcortical location of the infarcts in this uncommon case of intravascular lymphoma is likely related to the caliber of vessels involved, and the intellectual, language, and motor manifestations appear to be a result of damage localized predominantly, if not exclusively, in association and projection fiber bundles in the cerebral white matter.

Subacute Sclerosing Panencephalitis (SSPE)

This late complication of measles is usually insidiously progressive over 1 to 3 years but is occasionally more fulminant, evolving over a matter of weeks. The white matter is often abnormal on neuroimaging studies, and the pathology includes demyelination, gliosis, and inflammatory infiltrates, as well as neuronal loss, degeneration of dendrites, and neurofibrillary tangles. Patients usually have behavioral changes, myoclonus, dementia, visual disturbances, and pyramidal and extrapyramidal signs. The diagnosis is based upon the clinical manifestations, the presence of characteristic periodic EEG discharges, and demonstration of raised antibody titers against measles in the plasma and cerebrospinal fluid (see, e.g., Garg, 2002).

In the early stages, lesions on MRI are usually asymmetric and involve parieto-occipital corticosubcortical regions (Ozturk et al., 2002). Symmetric periventricular white matter changes become more prominent with time, but there appears to be no definite correlation between the clinical stage and either the duration from the onset or the MRI findings.

These observations are reflected in the MRI of this pregnant woman age 24 who was raised in Haiti. Her case was brought to neurological attention when she was unable to read or sign the hospital admission forms prior to her labor and delivery, and the MRI (figure 28-14) revealed the abnormalities in the occipital lobes bilaterally. The

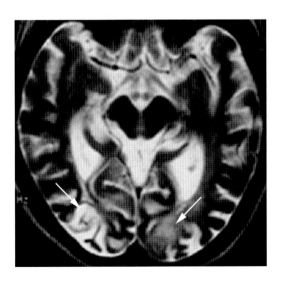

Figure 28-14
Occipital lobe abnormalities bilaterally on this representative T2-weighted MRI image in a young woman with subacute sclerosing panencephalitis and cortical blindness.

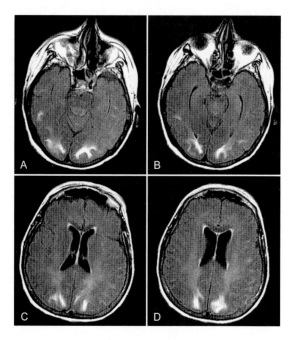

Figure 28-15
The T2-weighted MRI images in the horizontal plane in this patient with hypertension-induced posterior reversible encephalopathy syndrome (PRES) show the signal abnormality in the white matter in posterior brain regions from the occipital lobe (A, B) into the superior aspects of the posterior parietal region (C, D).

progression of findings on the MRI, lack of contrast enhancement of the lesion, and EEG findings with characteristic sharp wave complexes led to spinal fluid analysis for measles virus antibody, confirming the diagnosis, which at present is still incurable.

Posterior Reversible Encephalopathy Syndrome (PRES)

A syndrome of headaches, vomiting, confusion, seizures, motor signs, and cortical blindness and other visual abnormalities occurs in the setting of abrupt increases in blood pressure and with the use of immunosuppressive agents such as cyclosporine (Hinchey et al., 1996). MRI findings indicate a predominantly posterior leukoencephalopathy, as seen in figure 28-15 in a 65-year-old woman with recent onset of hypertension. Endothelial cell damage appears to be the central pathophysiological mechanism of this syndrome, with vasogenic edema resulting from dysfunction of cerebral vascular autoregulation. The involvement of the posterior hemisphere regions is thought to reflect a relative predisposition of the blood–brain barrier in these areas to extravasation of fluid into the extracellular space. The clinical manifestations are thought to reflect distortion of occipital lobe projection and association pathways. This syndrome is usually confined to the cerebral white matter and is not always reversible. Therapy needs to be instituted appropriately (see, e.g., Antunes et al., 1999; Kinoshita et al., 2003).

Traumatic Brain Injury

Diffuse axonal injury (DAI) is a major complication of severe closed head trauma. It results in debilitating clinical deficits, including the persistent vegetative state and is associated with diffuse degeneration of cerebral white matter (Gennarelli et al., 1982; Strich, 1956). The pathophysiology in the experimental rat model includes increased permeability of the blood–brain barrier with vasogenic cerebral edema followed by cytotoxic edema and then diffuse axonal damage (Cernak et al., 2004). Histopathological changes include axonal disruption in cerebral white matter as well as in the corpus callosum, brainstem, and cerebellar peduncles and white matter, with more severe cases associated with additional multifocal lesions (Adams et al., 1989). Conventional MRI (Paterakis et al., 2000) and diffusion-weighted (Schaefer et al., 2004) and diffusion tensor MRI (Huisman et al., 2004) rely on the extent and location of lesions in cerebral white matter for diagnosis and prognosis of these patients. Such strategies have implications for management, including secondary prevention of the neurobiological processes initiated by the trauma that are now known to evolve over subsequent hours and days (Reilly, 2001). The sensitivity of axons to mechanical injury (Gentleman et al., 1995; Medana and Esiri, 2003) and the consequences of closed head trauma on cognition further emphasize the importance of the cerebral white matter.

Normal Pressure Hydrocephalus

This is a disease of the white matter "by proxy." The primary event is not in the white matter itself, but the pathophysiology appears to reflect disruption of conductance within cerebral white matter pathways as a consequence of cerebrospinal fluid extravasation from the ventricles and/or pressure effects on the periventricular axons.

This 89-year-old man made a dramatic recovery of gait, bladder function, and intellect following ventriculoperitoneal shunting (figure 28-16; case described in detail in Schwartzschild et al., 1997).

Structure–Function Correlations in Focal Lesions of the White Matter

A second conceptual approach to elucidating the clinical relevance of the cerebral white matter pathways is to take advantage of "nature's experiment" by studying the clinical consequences of restricted white matter lesions. There is a dictum in clinical

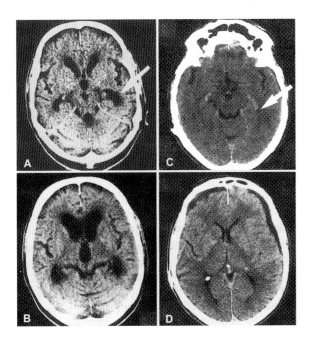

Figure 28-16

Axial CT scans of the brain of a patient with normal pressure hydrocephalus before (A, B) and 3 weeks after (C, D) ventriculoperitoneal shunting. A and C are images taken at the level of the interpeduncular fossa. B and D are images taken at the level of the frontal horns of the lateral ventricles. The ventricular spans between the caudate nuclei at the level of the frontal horns measured 34 mm before shunting and 9 mm after shunting. The marked improvement in the size of the temporal horns of the lateral ventricles is highlighted by the arrows in A (before shunt) and C (after shunt). Small subdural collections are seen in the post-shunt scan (D), but these were not of clinical significance. Lower images not shown here demonstrated dilation of the fourth, third, and lateral ventricles on the initial CT, with diminution after shunting. (Reproduced from Schwartzschild et al., 1997.)

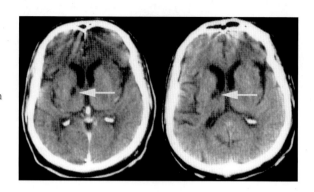

Figure 28-17
Horizontal images from the CT scan of a patient with lacunar infarction involving the genu of the right internal capsule (arrows). The image on the left is ventral to that on the right.

neurology that defining the location of a lesion is the key to understanding its effects on nervous system function. The deeper appreciation of the organization of the fiber bundles in the cerebral white matter has the potential to expand this approach to structure–function correlations of lesions of specific fiber tracts and to bring greater clarity and precision to the understanding of the clinical consequences of damage to the white matter. The following representative cases help illustrate these principles.

Focal Lesions with Cognitive Change ("Strategic Location Dementia") or Sensorimotor Deficits

Infarct in Genu of Internal Capsule

This 63-year-old truck driver had a stroke in the genu of the right internal capsule (figure 28-17), and the major finding on examination, in addition to mild and transient hemiparesis, was contralateral neglect and visual spatial disorganization (Schmahmann, 1984). He neglected the left side with double simultaneous visual and tactile stimulation, and he neglected left hemispace when bisecting lines, searching for stimuli on a page, and in his drawings. He could not locate major cities of the northeastern United States on a map, even though this had been his truck route, and he could not adequately draw the floor plan of his house or a reasonable outline of a generic "house" (figure 28-18).

Subsequent descriptions of the capsular genu syndrome report disturbances in language with left genu and anterior capsule lesions, spatial awareness deficits with lesions on the right, and deficits of emotion with lesions on either side (e.g., Chukwudelunzu et al., 2001; Tatemichi et al., 1992). These behavioral changes may result from disconnection of thalamic nuclei from cortical areas involved in these cognitive domains, and the role of the corticopontocerebellar fibers passing through the genu may be pertinent here as well.

Marchiafava-Bignami Disease of Corpus Callosum

The pathophysiology of this complication of alcohol abuse is still mysterious, although its clinical manifestations have long been recognized. In an early description, Leventhal et al. (1965) reported prominent frontal lobe pathological features, including personality change and abulia, together with memory impairment in the setting of the lesion affecting the anterior and midsections of the callosum.

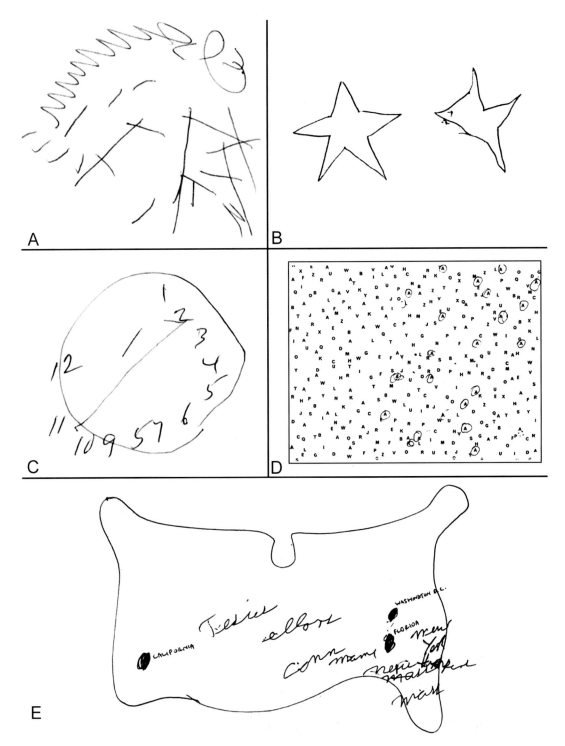

Figure 28-18

The performance of the patient with right capsular genu syndrome on selected tasks of spatial awareness and constructional praxis. A, Fragmented drawing of a person. B, The five-pointed star drawn for the patient on the left is copied with a missing portion at bottom left. C, The numbers on the left half of the clock are poorly placed. D, The instruction to circle all the "A's" on the page results in neglect of the left side. E, Placement of major cities and states on a rudimentary map of the United States is markedly impaired, particularly given that this patient was a truck driver whose route was in the northeastern United States.

Fornix Transection

Reports of lesions of the fornix in monkeys (Gaffan et al., 2001; Owen and Butler, 1981) and humans (D'Esposito et al., 1995; Gaffan et al., 1991; Heilman and Sypert, 1977; Sweet et al., 1959) describe amnesia as a major consequence. These cases emphasize the role of the fornix in memory. They also illustrate an important principle of white matter connectivity, as the posterior fornix conveys hippocampal input into the mamillary bodies and the dorsomedial nucleus of the thalamus.

Alexia Without Agraphia: The Classic Anatomy

This is the scenario well described by Dejerine (1892) and subsequent authors. Geschwind (1965a,b) reprised the original observations, traced the evolution of case reports and hypotheses about this phenomenon, and further analyzed it within the context of the association areas and the pathophysiology of the disconnection syndromes. Dejerine followed his patient for more than 4 years, and as related by Geschwind (1974, pp. 151–152): "This patient suffered from the acute loss of the ability to read letters, words or musical notation in association with a right hemianopia . . . he could write correctly (in script) either spontaneously or to dictation but could not read what he had written a short time previously . . . At post-mortem the brain showed an infarct of the left occipital lobe and of the splenium of the corpus callosum." The left occipital lobe lesion destroys the striate cortex and renders it impossible for visual information from that hemisphere to reach the left posterior temporal (Wernicke) language area. The visual word form information that would lead from the intact right occipital lobe across the splenium of the corpus callosum to the left hemisphere for decoding by the Wernicke language area is now interrupted by the additional lesion in the splenium, and hence the alexia. The ability to write is preserved, however, because the language-related cortices in the left hemisphere are not damaged—hence alexia without agraphia.

Alexia Without Agraphia from a Single Subcortical Lesion

A single lesion strategically placed in the white matter deep to Wernicke's area in the posterior left temporal lobe may also result in alexia without agraphia. The pathophysiology is similar to the dual lesion case, as in this instance the white matter lesion blocks input to the posterior language area from visual cortices of both the left and right hemispheres, but the language cortex itself is spared. There may be a partial right homonymous hemianopsia, as the white matter lesion may also interrupt some of the visual radiations.

Parietal Pseudothalamic Pain

The thalamic pain syndrome described by Dejerine and Roussy (1906) from lesions of the inferolateral thalamic artery (Caplan et al., 1988; Nasreddine and Saver, 1997; Schmahmann, 2003) is characterized by a deep, burning, uncomfortable pain with dysesthesia and perversion of sensation. A similar clinical presentation results from white matter lesions deep to the second somatosensory cortex in the inferior postcentral gyrus and the parietal operculum (figure 28-19), postulated to interrupt the interac-

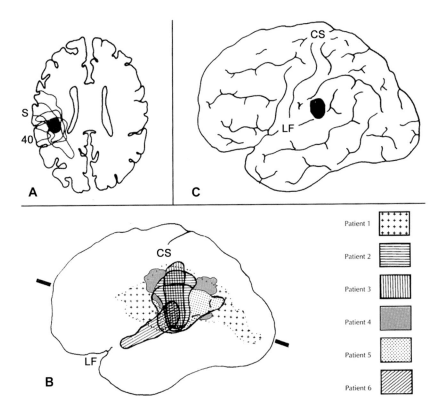

Figure 28-19
Sites of the lesions in six patients with upper extremity pain following focal infarction in the contralateral cerebral hemisphere. A, Section through the brain taken at the angle shown by the markers in B. An outline of the extent of the lesion in each case was mapped onto this section, and the site of involvement common to all the lesions is shown by the blackened area. Area 40 in the inferior parietal lobule and the primary somatosensory cortex (S) are indicated. B, The extent of the lesions when projected laterally onto the hemisphere. The individual patients are identified by the accompanying legend. The lesion common to all cases is shown by the blackened area in figure C. This area was situated deep to both the caudal insula and to the opercular part of the rostral inferior parietal lobule. Abbreviations: CS, central sulcus; LF, lateral (Sylvian fissure). (Figure from Schmahmann and Leifer, 1992.)

tion between the SII cortex and pain-mediating regions of the thalamus (Schmahmann and Leifer, 1992).

Anterior Aphasia from a Posterior Subcortical Lesion

This 23-year-old man developed inability to use his right arm despite full strength, and in addition had reduced verbal output and word-finding difficulty but preservation of comprehension. His white matter lesion seen on neuroimaging (figure 28-20) was shown by cerebral biopsy and response to treatment to be tumefactive sclerosis, a fulminant focal form of MS (Schmahmann et al., 2003).

Volitional Facial Paresis, Impaired Dexterity, and Stuttering from a Motor-Premotor Subcortical Lesion

A 28-year-old woman reported an episode of being "tongue-tied" with stuttering and difficulty finding words to say in conversation. This recurred 2 weeks later, associated with right facial weakness, and impairment of hand movements with attempts at writing, brushing her hair, applying make-up, or using a razor. Examination revealed right volitional facial paresis (facial weakness with forced grimace, but normal facial movements with spontaneous smile). There was a slight decrease in dexterity of the right hand and dystonic posturing of that hand with stress-gait. Hand dexterity improved with a course of intravenous steroids instituted after the MRI revealed a large demyelinating plaque deep to the left motor and premotor cortices, with smaller demyelinating lesions scattered in the left more than right hemispheres (figure 28-21). The dichotomy

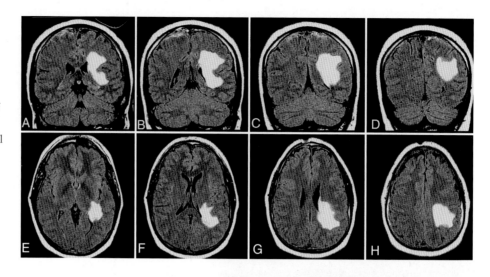

Figure 28-20

FLAIR MRI images of the brain of a patient with biopsy-proven tume-factive MS. A through D are coronal sequences from rostral to caudal showing the lesion restricted to the white matter of the posterior temporal and parietal regions. The lesion is seen in the horizontal plane from inferior to superior in E through H.

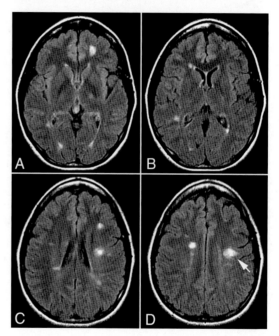

Figure 28-21

FLAIR MRI images in the horizontal plane from inferior to superior (A–D) in a patient with MS. The lesion highlighted by the arrow in D was the first to appear, and the subsequent lesions developed over the ensuing 4 years.

in facial paresis likely reflects involvement of the face motor fibers emanating from the precentral and premotor cortices but sparing of face fibers from the SMA and the cingulate motor cortices (Morecraft et al., 2001).

Visual Loss: Optic Radiation

Visual loss from lesions of the optic radiation are a classic in neurologic diagnosis, as shown in a 25-year-old man with a contralateral hemianopsia from PML affecting the white matter of the right occipital lobe (see figure 28-6C). Similarly, in a 65-year-old woman with eclampsia, loss of vision accompanied by confusion was associated with the posterior reversible encephalopathy syndrome, or posterior hypertensive encephalopathy (neuroimaging in this case was similar to that shown in figure 28-15).

Focal Deficits From Lesions of the Posterior Limb of the Internal Capsule

Lacunes in the posterior limb of the internal capsule produce sensorimotor deficits. More anterior lesions tend to cause weakness of the contralateral face and upper limb with impaired dexterity, whereas lesions further caudally situated in the capsule generally cause greater deficit in the lower extremity. The pattern of motor deficit following lacunes in different regions of the posterior limb of the internal capsule requires closer scrutiny.

Topography of the Corpus Callosum in Humans

The arrangement of fibers in the midsagittal plane of the corpus callosum of the monkey appears to be quite precise, as shown in the experimental cases in this series and in previous investigations (see chapter 22). Two clinical cases in the present chapter are consistent with the notion that the human corpus callosum is similarly arranged.

The lesion on MRI in figure 28-7G,H is evident in the rostrum and genu of the corpus callosum, in the setting of PML affecting predominantly the orbitofrontal and the ventral prefrontal cortices bilaterally. It is these cortical areas that send efferents through the rostrum and genu of the corpus callosum in the monkey.

Further, in the patient whose pathology is shown in figure 28-2C, the corpus callosum is discolored and atrophied in all areas except the region in closest anatomical proximity to the peri-Rolandic cortices. This patient's clinical scenario was marked by overwhelming cognitive failure with demyelination on MRI and at postmortem examination, but there was relative sparing radiographically and clinically of elementary sensorimotor function, and the white matter deep to the pericentral cortices was also relatively preserved at autopsy. The spared callosal segment in this case corresponds approximately to sector CC3 of the corpus callosum of the monkey, which transmits pre- and postcentral fibers between the hemispheres.

Diffuse White Matter Attrition

Aging

It has become apparent through studies in monkeys that an important concomitant of the aging process is loss of white matter within the cerebral cortex, as well as in the subcortical regions (Peters, 2002; Peters et al., 1994, 1996). These studies have shown that in the aging monkey there is a breakdown in the integrity of myelin around axons, an overall reduction in the volume of white matter in the cerebral hemispheres, thinning of layer I in area 46 of prefrontal cortex, and decrease in the cell density in cortically projecting brainstem nuclei. Further, old monkeys display memory impairment on tasks of spatial and visual recognition that correlate with the extent of degeneration of myelinated fibers in the cortex and white matter. White matter changes occur with advancing age in humans, and the effects of these changes on cognition and speed of information processing is under active investigation (e.g., Head et al., 2004; Fellgiebel et al., 2005; Longstreth et al., 2005; Salat et al., 2005; Schmidt et al., 2005; Sullivan et al., 2005; Tuch et al., 2005).

Alzheimer's Disease

The pathology of this devastating disorder is not thought to be primarily in white matter, but the cerebral atrophy and loss of white matter that is so marked in the later stages of Alzheimer's disease (e.g., Brinkman et al, 1981; Hubbard and Anderson, 1981) places the white matter pathways squarely within the discussion of the pathophysiology of this illness. Patients with dementia, including Alzheimer's disease, were found to have lesions with the appearance of incomplete infarction of the white matter (Brun and Englund, 1986; Englund and Brun, 1990). The lesions were characterized by partial loss of myelin, axons, and oligodendroglial cells, mild reactive astrocytic gliosis, and sparsely distributed macrophages. In addition, these authors noted stenosis resulting from hyaline fibrosis of arterioles and smaller vessels, and they thought the observed changes were due to hypoperfusion of the white matter, as many of the patients had signs of cardiovascular disease, usually with hypertension. White matter dementia, the clinical entity that results from large-scale disconnection of cerebral association areas from interrelated cortical and subcortical regions, may thus be an additional burden, if not the primary pathophysiology, in Alzheimer's disease and mixed dementia (e.g., Scheltens et al., 1992; Capizzano et al., 2004; de Leeuw et. al., 2005).

The significance of diffuse white matter atrophy for other disorders affecting cognition is also becoming apparent, as in the case of the white matter atrophy seen in patients with cognitive decline in the setting of chronic alcohol abuse (Mochizuki et al., 2005), and disordered fractional anisotropy in the white matter of recovering alcoholics (Pfefferbaum et al., 2005).

Excess White Matter

Disruption of the natural phenomenon of pruning of excess axons in the developing brain (Innocenti, 1995; Lamantia and Rakic, 1990a) appears to be relevant in some clinical disorders. The volume of cerebral white matter is greater in boys with autism than in age-matched controls (Herbert et al., 2003), and this enlargement is noted in the outer "radiate" white matter containing association fiber systems but not in the "inner zone containing sagittal and bridging system compartments" (Herbert et al., 2004). In addition, diffusion tensor imaging in autism reveals disruption of white matter (as determined by reduced fractional anisotropy) between regions implicated in social functioning. These areas included the ventromedial prefrontal cortex, anterior cingulate gyrus, and temporoparietal junction and in clusters in the superior temporal sulcus, temporal lobes approaching the amygdala, occipitotemporal tract, and corpus callosum (Barnea-Goraly et al., 2004). The pruning of axonal connections during development appears to be necessary for optimal sculpting of neural circuits, and thus persistence into adulthood of excess and perhaps chaotically organized fiber systems may be as detrimental to healthy cognition as the loss of the required axonal connections in the mature brain.

Effect of Location of the White Matter Lesion on Recovery from Deficit

In some conditions, the size of the lesion alone is the major determinant of prognosis. This applies particularly to intracranial hemorrhage, including intraparenchymal, intraventricular, and subarachnoid locations (e.g., Caplan and Stein, 1986). In general, large bleeds have a graver prognosis, both in terms of the quality of function and the preservation of life itself. A similar approach has sometimes been adopted in the analysis of neurological deficits from ischemic infarction. One study found good correlation between infarct size and weakness severity in patients with infarction in the territory of the middle cerebral artery, but there was poor correlation between lesion location and specific syndromes of focal weakness. No two cases shared the same lesion for the same syndrome, and several cases with different patterns of weakness shared the same location of the lesion (Mohr et al., 1993).

Other studies of ischemic infarction, however, have determined that outcome depends more on the particular structures damaged rather than the size of the lesion. A proof of principle of this statement may be derived from consideration of the degree of recovery from hemiplegia and from aphasia. Clinical experience indicates that hemiparesis is more profound and more persistent as the lesion location moves from the anterior limb of the internal capsule to the posterior limb. This pattern is thought to reflect the observation that supplementary motor and M3 fibers are in the anterior limb, but fibers from the primary motor cortices are in the posterior limb (Morecraft et al., 2002; the present work). The size of the lesion may be equivalent, but the effect on motor function is quite different.

Patients with aphasia recover more slowly when the lesion involves the area between the corpus callosum medially, the corona radiata laterally, and the caudate nucleus ventrally (Naeser et al., 1989). This is the territory of the Muratoff bundle immediately above the head and body of the caudate nucleus that transmits fibers from dorsal cortical areas to the caudate nucleus (see chapter 20), and of the fronto-occipital fasciculus (see chapter 19) that links the dorsal and medial prestriate and posterior parietal cortices with the dorsolateral prefrontal cortex. This finding provides support for the notion that the location of the lesion (i.e., which specific white matter tracts are damaged) is crucial in recovery from aphasia. It also emphasizes the importance of intact communication between the cortical and subcortical nodes in the distributed neural circuits that support language processing.

Finally, the combination of a more precise understanding of the organization of the white matter pathways in the monkey and the increasingly sophisticated techniques available to study these tracts in the human *in vivo* has the potential to further elucidate the clinical consequences of focal white matter lesions (e.g., Makris et al., 1997; Molko et al., 2002a,b; Schmahmann et al., 2003).

Conclusions

29

In this work we set out to study the intricacies of the white matter pathways emanating from the cerebral cortex of the monkey to better understand the organization of the distributed systems that subserve neural functions, and in an attempt to provide new insights into the clinical manifestations of focal white matter lesions in patients.

By examining the evolution of ideas concerning the fiber tracts, we were able to clarify a number of persistent uncertainties regarding anatomy and nomenclature that have confounded the understanding of the organization of these fiber pathways. Application of the autoradiographic technique to the study of the fiber trajectories in the experimental animal made it possible to delineate more precisely the entire trajectory of these pathways arising from different cortical areas. Information about the fiber fascicles that constitute the white matter was analyzed in different cases and synthesized on a single template brain.

We were struck by the exquisitely precise arrangement of the fiber bundles as they emanate from each cortical area and course through the cerebral white matter to their destinations in cortical and subcortical sites. Further, it appears that there is a common principle of organization of the efferent fibers that applies to all cortical areas.

The association fibers comprise local, neighborhood, and long association fibers, and they are immediately distinguishable from the commissural and projection fibers that emerge from the cortex in the form of a compact cord. This cord of fibers then divides into its two major components, the commissural fibers, which head toward the opposite hemisphere, and the projection or subcortical fibers, which travel in the major subcortical fiber tracts, including the internal capsule and sagittal stratum. The subcortical fibers themselves separate further into two major components, one destined for the basis pontis, other brainstem regions, and the spinal cord, and the other group destined for the thalamus. The thalamic fibers are relayed to different thalamic nuclei via the superior, lateral, ventral, and anterior thalamic peduncles. These thalamic peduncle fibers encase the periphery of the thalamus proper. The striatal fibers are distinct from both the association and the subcortical fibers and are conveyed by two distinct fasciculi. Those coming from the medial occipital, posterior parietal, cingulate, and frontal lobes mainly course via the subcallosal fasciculus of Muratoff. The fibers from the temporal lobe, ventral occipital, and ventral prefrontal cortices travel predominantly via the external capsule.

Fibers are topographically arranged in the corpus callosum and anterior commissure according to their origin in the cerebral cortex. Similarly, fibers in the sagittal stratum and the anterior and posterior limbs of the internal capsule are topographically arranged according to the site of origin in the cerebral cortex.

All the fiber pathways are precisely arranged into bundles that link specific brain regions, and in many instances there is topographical organization within the bundles themselves, determined by the site of origin of the fibers in the cerebral cortex. The association, commissural, and corticothalamic fibers convey information in a bidirectional manner.

Dichotomy of Cerebral Function and Association Pathways

It has been suggested that cerebral cortical architecture and function conform to a fundamental dichotomy in the visual, somatosensory, and auditory domains, as well as in limbic and multimodal dimensions (Pandya and Yeterian, 1985). The overall pattern of organization of the association fiber pathways may be viewed within the context of this dual organizing principle.

In the visual system two distinct association fiber tracts can be discerned in the occipital lobe: the fronto-occipital fasciculus and the inferior longitudinal fasciculus. The fronto-occipital fasciculus links the dorsal and medial parts of the occipital lobe with the caudal dorsolateral prefrontal cortex and is thought to subserve the peripheral visual field and visual-spatial information. In contrast, the inferior longitudinal fasciculus, which links the ventrolateral and ventromedial parts of the occipital lobe with the inferotemporal cortex and parahippocampal gyrus, is postulated to be involved with the central visual field, and hence with object discrimination and object memory.

In the auditory domain, the two long association pathways leading to the prefrontal cortex are the arcuate and the uncinate fascicles. The arcuate fascicle links the caudal superior temporal gyrus with dorsal area 8 and may subserve sound localization and audiospatial analysis. By contrast, part of the uncinate fascicle links the rostral superior temporal gyrus with the orbital and medial prefrontal cortex and may have a role in sound recognition and memory.

Long association fibers emanating from the somatosensory cortex are also organized in a dual manner. Thus, the dorsal component of the superior longitudinal fasciculus, SLF I, links the superior and medial parietal cortices predominantly with the dorsal premotor and supplementary motor areas and may have a role in initiation and the intentional aspect of somatomotor control. The role of SLF III, which links the rostral part of the inferior parietal lobule with the ventral premotor and prefrontal area, is likely related to the articulatory aspects of language and gestural communication.

The long association fiber tracts emerging from the post-Rolandic multimodal areas appear to respect this duality as well. The SLF II fibers link the caudal inferior parietal lobule with the dorsolateral prefrontal cortex, and by its involvement with visual spatial and oculomotor function, this fiber bundle is likely to contribute to spatial awareness. The extreme capsule, on the other hand, that links the temporal multimodal area with the ventral prefrontal region, including area 45, homologous with the pars triangularis, is thought to contribute to the nonarticulatory aspects of language.

Finally, the pathways from the limbic areas are also organized into two major components. The cingulum bundle links the caudal cingulate area with the mid-dorsolateral prefrontal region and is thought to play a role in the processes of self-monitoring, working memory, and motivation. The uncinate fasciculus, by contrast, links the parahippocampal gyrus with the orbitofrontal cortex and may play a role in emotional and self-regulatory aspects of behavior.

Future Directions

The observations presented here have a great deal of contemporary relevance. They show how fibers are relayed in a precise manner between cortical areas, indicating that they are critical elements in the distributed neural circuits that subserve all forms of behavior. This applies not only to the corticocortical association pathways but also to the corticosubcortical projections and to the topographically arranged fibers within the commissures.

Increasingly sophisticated neuroimaging techniques delineate trajectories of these pathways in the human brain *in vivo*, and these observations may now be interpreted in the light of correspondingly detailed anatomical knowledge derived from the experimental animal. The detail of the origins, trajectories, and patterns of termination of the fibers tracts as determined in the monkey will be particularly relevant in maximizing the ability of these techniques to help develop a finer understanding of similar pathways in imaging studies of the human brain, in which the cortical origins and termination patterns of fiber tracts cannot yet be identified.

This work has direct clinical relevance because diseases of the white matter produce a plethora of manifestations, from sensorimotor impairment to disturbances of the highest levels of intellectual capability. Variations in lesion size and location may have profoundly different clinical consequences, and the present work emphasizes that this reflects the fact that fibers in adjacent regions of the white matter may have markedly different origins, destinations, and functional significance.

Thus, one potentially important clinical outcome of this work is the realization that a lesion of the cortex destroys more than just the cortical area involved: it also affects the afferent and efferent cortical fibers and thereby disrupts the interaction of that cortical region with multiple other ipsilateral and contralateral cortical areas, as well as with thalamic, striatal, and pontocerebellar regions. Similarly, a lesion localized to the white matter disrupts the communication between cortical areas, and it also interrupts the cortical links with these subcortical nodes, which are essential to the normal function of the distributed neural circuit.

The wider importance of this work is that by judicious extrapolation and application to the human, we are now in a position to understand the pathways in terms of their normal anatomy and function, as well as in pathological situations. This anatomical exploration may help to elucidate the functions of the nodes within the distributed neural systems that are linked by the fiber pathways, and thus promote the discovery of fundamental ideas regarding the interactions between the human brain and human behavior.

Notes

1. According to Garrison/McHenry (1969), Galen defined the scientific method by pointing out that to obtain knowledge concerning the function of the nervous system and the diseases that afflict it, clinical observation must be combined with careful anatomical and experimental investigation. He showed in experimental studies on spinal cord that hemisection leads to paralysis below the lesion on the ipsilateral side, that transection of the cord between cervical levels 1 and 2 produces instant death and between cervical levels 3 and 4 stops respiration, damage below the sixth vertebra produces paralysis of thoracic muscles with respiration continued by the diaphragm, and lesions lower in the spinal cord produce paralysis confined to the lower limbs and bladder. He distinguished between sensory and motor nerves in experimental studies and in clinical observations. Voluntary power and sensation were derived from the brain. Total abolition of these functions, such as in apoplexy, indicated brain lesions. A local effect, as in the arm or leg of one side, or portions of the extremities, pointed to a spinal cord lesion. When the face is involved, the disease must be in the brain. Galen's anatomical and clinical observations led him to the view that the brain is "an organ where all sensations arrive, and where all mental images, and all intelligent ideas arise, a place of imagination, memory, and comprehension" (quoted in Polyak, 1957, p. 80).

2. In addition to assigning memory to the gyri, Willis placed imagination in the corpus callosum, perception in the corpora striata, and instinct in the midbrain. He developed the notion that the cerebellum was the essential anatomic substrate needed to support life, and that it was the controller of such involuntary mechanisms as heartbeat, respiration, and gastrointestinal motility. The cerebellum does indeed play a role in autonomic function (see Schmahmann, 1997), but Willis' conclusion that vital functions are destroyed by cerebellar extirpation was based on primitive experimental technique that probably damaged the brainstem. In Neuburger's view, this notion, one of the first attempts at localization of physiological function (i.e., the cerebellum is vital for life), generated the field of hypothesis-driven scientific investigation introduced by Nicolaus Steno (Niels Stensen, 1638–1686), who decried what he regarded as poorly substantiated claims, and performed experiments to test, and ultimately disprove, Willis' assertion.

3. Lancisi was convinced of the location of the soul in the corpus callosum by the fact that during great mental exertion an unpleasant sensation could be clearly felt in just that region. Sensory perceptions ended in it, and in keeping with its delicate texture, imagination and judgment, the products of the mingling of sensation, originated there. Unlike René du Perron Descartes (1596–1650), who considered the soul to be in the pineal body, Lancisi regarded the pineal body as having a reinforcing effect, giving propulsive force to the animal spirits streaming out of the corpus callosum.

4. This *sensorium commune* was that point in the brain "that is the meeting point for all the sensation and excitation of the whole organism, and from where they, in their turn, act as from a *motorium commune*, or the common point for movement" (Georgius [Jiří] Procháska [1749–1820], 1800, quoted in Neuburger/Clarke, 1897/1981, p. 240), and it was the only site for the conversion of sensory stimuli into motion, forming a reflex center under the influence of the soul. According to Steven Polyak, a number of "even the most emancipated" scientific thinkers in the 150 to 200 years after Vesalius, the "Vesalian Epigoni," including such writers as Willis, Descartes, and Vieussens, were still "under the complete domination of the idea of a mysterious animal spirit supposed to fill the brain ventricles" (Polyak, 1957, p. 96). Doubts about the presence of a "spirit" in the brain were raised by some "lucid intellectuals" in the late 17th and early 18th centuries, however, including Steno, and Johann Jakob Wepfer (1620–1695), whose work in apoplexy helped initiate the discipline of cerebrovascular neurology. Richard Lower (1631–1691) in *De Catarrhis* (1655) ascertained that catarrh was nothing more than nasal secretions, dispelling Galen's concept that catarrh drained vital juices from the brain. After the discovery by Luigi Galvani (1737–1798) of the electrical properties of excised tissue in 1786, the hypothesis of the nervous system's activation by the soul, by animal spirits, or by nerve fluid finally had to be discarded. It also meant that the concept of soul had to be disentangled from the notion of a life force. As the soul now became identified exclusively with the mind, it became necessary to differentiate between the origins of voluntary actions and involuntary, or reflex, actions.

5. The experimental conditions under which Reil was working were less than ideal. He portrayed these difficult circumstances in his writing on the anterior commissure (Reil, 1812a, Volume XI. Erstes Heft, p. 91): "I could not examine whether its [the anterior commissure] fibers dissolve into even more delicate fibrils by dissection

using dilute hydrochloric acid as is the case with nerves, because a certain Mr. Langermann, who himself is in danger of dissolving in his own mud, placed a court order against me to forbid me from dissection at this location where entire streams of blood from the slaughterhouses foul the public roads."

6. Burdach also described the cuneate fasciculus of the spinal cord that bears his name. (The gracile fasciculus of F. Goll [1829–1903] was described in 1860.) Burdach's notion of thalamus and thalamocortical interactions mediated through the fiber systems has contemporary relevance: "Of all the ganglia, [the thalami] have the greatest influence upon the incipient expression of mental spontaneity, upon the capacity for unifying sensory impressions into a whole, and thus they allow their owner to realize that he is thinking . . . they are the root of consciousness, which develops in the corona radiata and is perfected in the 'Belungsorganen' [covering organs—the cerebral cortex and white matter, including the corpus callosum and fornix]" (translated and presented in Neuburger/Clarke, 1897/1981, p. 280).

7. Todd, for example, while noting that "layers of the brain will separate most readily when torn in the direction of their fibres" (Todd, 1845, p. 133) observed that the method of Reil, Gall and Spurzheim, and others "consisted in tracing the course of the fibres chiefly from below upwards" (that is, from the inferior aspect of the brain, used in order to trace the destinations of the major brainstem fiber systems). In his text for students, however, Todd favored dissection from the superior aspect of the hemisphere, and his comment epitomized the prevailing debate concerning methodology in the following manner:

> Such is the mode of dissection from above downwards, against which it has been greatly the fashion of late years to declaim with much vehemence. But, however the advocates of a particular theory may object, there can be no doubt that this method is by far the most useful for all practical purposes . . . It is plain, therefore, that all who are desirous of becoming acquainted with the anatomy of this organ should begin by making dissections in this way (ibid., p. 131).

The recurring and sometimes heated debate in the early and middle part of the 1800s between those who would dissect the brain from the top versus those who would do so from the lower end, is strangely reminiscent of the "most obstinate war" between the Big-Endians of Blefuscu (those who break their eggs at the larger end) and the Small-Endians of Lilliput (who break their eggs from the smaller end), described by Jonathan Swift (1667–1745) in *Gulliver's Travels* fully a century earlier (1726).

8. The compound microscope had been invented a few years previously, and its advantages were explained by George Adams (1798, pp. 14–15):

> A compound microscope, as it consists of two, three, or more glasses, is much more easily varied, and is susceptible

of greater changes in its construction, than the single microscope. The number of the lenses, of which it is formed, may be increased or diminished, their respective positions may be varied, and the form in which they are mounted be altered almost *ad infinitum*. But among these varieties, some will be found more deserving of attention than others.

9. From *Mikroskopische Untersuchungen über die Übereinstimmung in der Struktur und dem Wachstum der Thiere und Pflanzen*, Berlin, 1839, translated and quoted in Clarke and O'Malley, p. 57.

10. Meynert presented a major synopsis of his understanding of the anatomical organization of the nervous system of mammals, included in Stricker's text that was translated by Henry Power in 1872. (See figure N-1, A for the figures of the bat brain to which Meynert refers in the following passages, and figures N-1, B–D, for his gross dissections and diagrammatic representations of fiber tracts in the human and monkey brain.) Pp. 372–374:

> The form of the cerebral cortex, which resembles a cap covering the outer surface of the hemispheres, appears specially fitted for this comprehension of the conductive tracts (figs. 230, 231, and 232, F, O, Tp, R, H). This form results from the grouping of the innumerable sensory elements occupying the cortex, namely the *nerve cells*. The sensory nerves constitute their feelers, the motor their arms. Since this convoluted mass of fibres must in great part pass through the occipital foramen in order to reach the several organs, there is a *convergence* of them from all sides, both in the peduncles of the brain and in the spinal cord, towards the grey matter of the central cavities. After however they have traversed this central grey substance, they *diverge*, as the peripheral nervous system, to all parts of the body. Since now this organization effects the contact of the sensory shell of the cortex of the cerebrum with the various forms of sensory impressions derived from the external world, the image of which is coincidentally projected upon the cortex, the name of *projection system* is very appropriate to this great segment of the nervous system, and in this comparison the cortex of the cerebrum is to be regarded as the surface on which the projection is received, while the external world stands for the projected object ($P_1 P_2 P_3$).
>
> In fig. 230, $P_1 P_2 P_3$ represent the successive links of the projection system, which last is interrupted several times by masses of grey matter. The first and uppermost link (*P1 P1'* and *Br*) is a medullary system springing for the most part in a radial manner from the cortex, and extending peripherically into the second principal mass of grey substance, the ganglia at the base of the hemispheres (corpus striatum and optic thalamus) (figs. 230, 231, 232, *Cs, Th, Qu*). From the interrupting network of the *ganglionic masses* springs the second link of the projection system, the *system of the crus cerebri* (P2), the peripheric extremity of which is found in the grey substance of the third category, i.e., the grey substance around the central cavi-

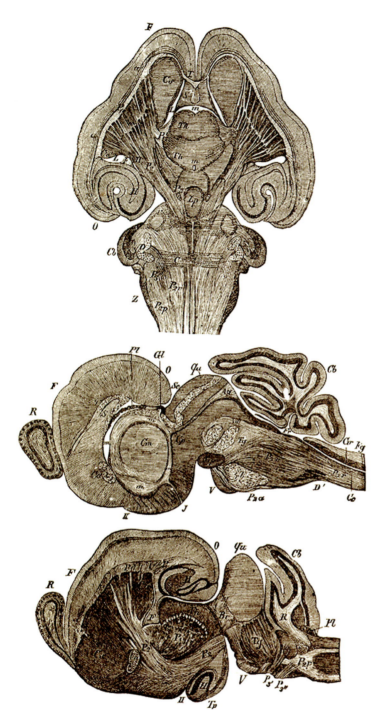

Figure N-1, A

Reproduction of Theodore Meynert's figures 230 (top), 231 (middle) and 232 (lower) illustrating the brain of the bat. (From his chapter in Stricker, 1872, translation by Power, p. 370). The legend reads: "One horizontal and two perpendicular longitudinal sections from the brain of *Vespertilio pipistrella*, intended to expose the principal features of the cerebral structure."

ties. The third link of the projection system is formed by the nerves which arise from the above-named grey substance of the central cavities, extending from the origin of the third pair of cerebral nerves in the grey matter around the aquaeductus Sylvii to the nucleus or origin of the lowermost coccygeal nerves of the spinal cord. These, perhaps without exception, end peripherically in definite microscopic terminal organs that have already been described in several chapters of this work.

The region through which the *first link of the projection system* pursues its course is that formed by the cerebral hemispheres, within which it is apparently accompanied by two medullary formations, *the trabecular fibres (fibres of the corpus callosum)* and the *arcuate* system. While the projection system forms the medium of communication for the cells of the cortex with the outer world, the communication of the cortical cells of the cerebral hemispheres amongst themselves is

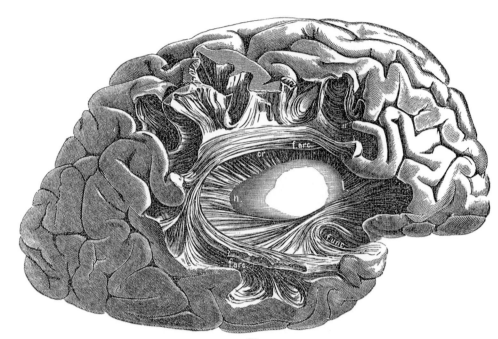

Fig. 19.

Dissection of Cortex and Medullary Substance of the Convexity of the Brain.

n. l. Lenticular nucleus. f.unc. Fasciculus uncinatus. f.arc. Fasciculus arcuatus. cr. Corona radiata, projection-system.

Figure N-1, B

Figure 19 from Meynert (1885, p. 43) illustrating fibers in a gross dissection of the lateral convexity of the human brain. Abbreviations as noted in his legend.

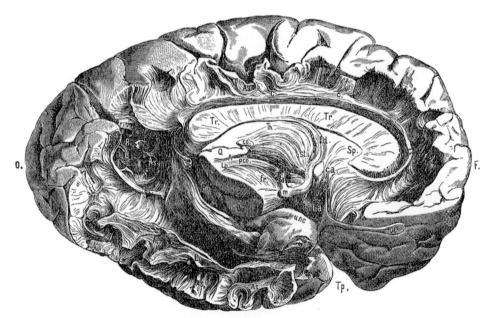

Fig. 18.

Dissection of the Cortex and the Medullary Substance of the Median Surface of the Brain.

Fr., Tp., Occ. Frontal, temp., and occip. region. Tr. Corp. callosum (trabs cerebri). c. c. Cingulum. As. Fibræ propriæ (association fibres). R. Cortex. bi. Fasciculus basalis internus (Burdach). Li. Fasciculus longitudinalis inferior. Olf. Olfactory lobe. La. Lamina perforata anterior. ca. Anterior commissure. unc. Uncus. Sp. Septum pellucidum. Th. Optic thalamus. fd. Descending fornix. m. Corpus mammillare. fa. Ascending fornix. Q. Corp. quadrigemina. A. Aquæductus Sylvii. Pv. Pulvinar thalami. Gi. Internal geniculate body. T. Tegmentum. Pd. Pes pedunculi cerebri. St.i. Stilus intern. thalami optici. Lp. Posterior longitudinal fasciculus. Above pco., descent of post. commissure. co. Conarium.

Figure N-1, C

Figure 18 from Meynert (1885, p. 40) illustrating fibers in a gross dissection of the medial surface of the human brain. Abbreviations as noted in his legend.

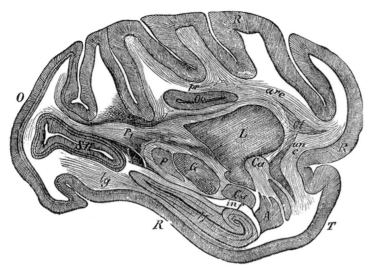

Fig. 256. *Profile section, from the brain of Circocebus cinomolgus (somewhat enlarged)*. *F*, frontal extremity. *O*, occipital extremity. *T*, temporal extremity. *R*, cortex cerebri. *Op*, cortex of the inner side of the operculum (Klappdeckel, part of 1st primitive convolution* overhanging the island of Reil) which forms one boundary of Burdach's superior fissure, the other being formed by the cortical substance of the island. *H*, the ammon's horn. *SH*, sulcus hypocampi. *L*, the third member of the nucleus lenticularis. *Cl*, claustrum (sometimes nucleus tæniæformis, Vormauer). *A*, nucleus amygdalæ. *Cs*, tail of the nucleus caudatus†. *P*, tuberculum posterius thalami optici (Polster d. Sehhügels). *G*, corpus geniculatum externum. *pr*, fibræ propriæ uniting two convolutions. *arc*, fasciculus arcuatus. *unc*, fasciculus uncinatus. *lg*, fasciculus longitudinalis inferior. *Ca*, anterior commissure. *inf*, inferior horn of the lateral ventricle. *P₁*, upper member of the projection-system.

Figure N-1, D
Meynert's illustration of a schematic view of fibers in the sagittal orientation in the brain of a fascicularis monkey. Figure 256, p. 659 in Meynert's chapter in the original German version of Stricker; reproduced as figure 233 on p. 380 in Henry Power's translation of Stricker, 1872. Abbreviations as noted in his legend.

accomplished in a threefold manner, so that that portion of the protoplasm of the primordial cells from which the innumerable cells of the cortex are developed, again unites to form a morphological unity; a process that can only be regarded as an instance of reunion. This view is most obviously based on the union of the transverse commissural fibres in the middle line during foetal life, after which they have perforated the median wall of the vesicles of the hemispheres. The commissural trabeculae (callosal fibres, figs. 230 and 231, T) unite *the corresponding and identical regions* of the cortex of the two opposite halves of the *cerebral hemispheres*.

The different regions of the cortex of the *same* hemisphere are, on the other hand, continuously connected together by the grey fibre plexus formed by the anastomoses of the cell processes. It forms, however, the most satisfactory proof of the law of isolated conduction, which is even here in operation, that in addition the regions of the cortex are also connected together by medullated fibres (figs. 230 and 232, *aa*), the fasciculi of the fibrae propriae, fibrae arcuatae, which form a continuous layer, lining the inner surface of the cortex, composed of fasciculi of variable length. As the connection of the several territories of the cortex must correspond to a functional connection of their states of excitation, through the agency of this medu-

rally system, its fasciculi may be termed a connecting system (*Associations system*).

A fourth collection of medullary fasciculi belonging to the cerebral hemispheres consists of those forming a connection between the cortex of the cerebrum and the cortex of the cerebellum, which are collected in the superior peduncle of the cerebellum as a distinct band, situated superficially in the back of the pons; but from the intermediate nature of the course of these fibres between the two cortical substances as well as from their long and close connection with the projection system of the cerebrum, it is impossible in such a general description as the present to give a clear notion of them, or to disentangle their relations.

Pp. 420–421:

Thus, upon the whole, there are four territories of origin for the crusta of the cerebral peduncle: 1. The *cortex* of the occipital and temporal lobes of the cerebrum; 2. The *nucleus caudatus* (corpus striatum internum); 3. The *nucleus lenticularis* (corpus striatum externum); and 4. The *substantia nigra*. The parts taking origin from these centers are distributed over the transverse section of the crusta that the most external area proceeds from the cortex of the cerebrum, and the innermost from the lenticular nucleus, whilst the intermediately placed and widest tract is common to the caudate and lenticular nuclei.

11. The validity of Haeckel's hypothesis has subsequently been roundly criticized as a "disastrous union of embryology and evolutionary biology" (Gilbert, 2003, http://www.devbio.com), and its uncritical acceptance has been blamed for introducing untenable notions of race and gender into philosophy, theology, and politics. (See discussions in Gilbert 2003; Gould, 1977).

12. Flechsig's projection systems relate to five primordial regions, or sensory areas of the cerebral hemisphere corresponding to the terminal areas of the principal afferent fiber tracts, and to the motor system. The projection systems are the somatosensory and somatomotor regions of the pre- and postcentral gyri, the primary auditory area in the transverse temporal convolution (Heschl's gyrus), the visual sphere (transmitted in the optic radiations of Gratiolet) around the calcarine fissure, the olfactory sphere in the uncus of the hippocampus, and a gustatory area in the hippocampal formation. The sensory areas are not contiguous and do not spread over the whole hemisphere but rather are relatively small patches separated by considerable distances, and together represent less than one third of the entire cortex. Further, the corticofugal or efferent descending tracts originate either in the sensory sphere or in their immediate vicinity, thus providing each sensory sphere with both afferent and efferent connections: Flechsig's "conjugate tracts" (From Polyak, 1957).

13. Lewellys Franklin Barker summarized Flechsig's conclusions regarding association areas in the first American neuroscience textbook in 1899 (Barker, 1899, pp. 1070–1078):

[T]he areas of the cortex in which projection neurons play a part in the architecture are much more limited in extent than we have been accustomed to suppose. When all the sense areas and motor areas have become medullated, only about one third of the surface of the cerebrum has been involved. . . . [A]ll or very nearly all of the projection fibers of the cerebrum are accounted for when the corticofugal and corticopetal paths of the different sensory-motor areas . . . are summed up. What is the significance of the nearly two-thirds of the cortex that remain unaccounted for? [Flechsig's] anatomical investigations indicate that these hitherto "silent areas" ("silent, not because they do not speak, but because we are too dull of understanding to hear what they say"—Thomas and Keen 1896, [reference quoted in Barker's footnote]) possess functions of the greatest importance and interest . . . [and] are concerned in the higher manifestations of the intellect, in the process of memory, recognition, judgment and reflection.

In Flechsig's view, the extensive areas of cortex that lie interposed between the sensory areas consist of the belt areas that adjoin the sensory spheres (the "marginal zones") and four "terminal zones" that myelinate one month after birth. These "association centers" or "association areas" are located in most of the frontal lobe, the insula of Reil, the greater part of the temporal lobe, and a large part of the parietal and occipital lobes. Flechsig considered them to be a substratum of psychic functions and postulated that because of their relatively large size in the human brain, they were likely to be a specific human acquisition and the material foundation of man's mastery over other creatures. The association cortices serve as the repository of past impressions arising through the afferent channels via the sensory spheres and serve as the essential substratum of memory in integration or building of complex processes. (This concept has been carried forward into the contemporary debate, as reflected in Mesulam, 1998.) The posterior association area, representing a large portion of the parietal, occipital, and temporal lobes, would be concerned with the integration of visual, somesthetic, and auditory impulses. Its task would be to retain visual, auditory, and somesthetic experiences, integrate them, and perform complex acts such as reading, visual understanding, written language, understanding spoken word, and auditory language. The functions of the largest association area, representing most of the frontal lobe, would be uppermost in the hierarchy of cerebral mantle functions and faculties: consciousness of one's own personality or ego, conscious and purposeful planning and acting, willpower, "character," logical thinking, and judgment. The frontal lobes would be the anatomical substratum of a "unified person conscious of itself, and capable of free and independent action" (Modifed from Polyak, 1957, p. 176). (These notions predated the work of Aleksandr Romanovich Luria [1902–1977, e.g., Luria, 1966] and were postulated in the aftermath of the famous account of Phineas Gage in the *Proceedings of the Massachusetts Medical Society* in 1868 by John Martyn Harlow [1819–1907].)

14. Cajal, 1933 (translated in Clarke and O'Malley, p. 445):

There is a ramification in the gray matter, of the sensory nerve fibers that originate from other regions of the nervous system and perhaps from the sensory nerves. Monakow suggested that all cerebral regions give rise to association fibers. These fibers are ordinarily the biggest among those that cross the gray matter of the cerebral cortex. Their thickness considerably surpasses that of the axis cylinders of the giant pyramidal cell. Further they are differentiated from the latter because their course is sometimes oblique, sometimes horizontal and zigzag. These fibers come from the white matter across which we have followed them for some distance. They bend to right or obtuse angles in order to enter the cortex, and after a variable course, but which is almost always oblique, they divide into two or three large divergent branches. These branches go off obliquely, and proceed over a large area. They then branch many times and finally their finest rootlets end in diffuse free varicose arborization, usually close to small or medium sized pyramidal cells. All these fibers, and their main branches, possess a very thick myelin sheath. Because of the great thickness of myelin and above all, because of their irregular course, now horizontal, now oblique, they can be distinguished from the axis cylinder of the pyramids whose course, as may be said, is nearly straight and descending (radiating bundle of medullary fibers).

15. Baillarger's date of birth is 1815 according to http://www .whonamedit.com, but 1806 according to Clarke and O'Malley.

16. Baillarger found the cortex to be composed of six parallel layers, alternating white and gray and differing in structure, although in some places there were only two layers. He determined that the white cortical strata are made up partly of fibers penetrating from the white subcortical substance, and partly from the fibers within the cortex. The fibers that entered the cortex from the subjacent white matter were most numerous in the summit of the gyrus, less prominent on the wall of the sulci, and least evident around the sulcal floor, where they were arranged obliquely. In different locations the fibers terminated in the lowermost layer of the cortex or in layers closer to the cortical surface. Baillager's naked-eye determination of the bands of white matter in the cortex were subsequently verified with the use of the myelin stain and became an important tool in myeloarchitecture.

Chapter 3
Materials Analyzed

1. The procedures for non-human primate care and experimentation were followed according to NIH guidelines for the experimental use of nonhuman primates, as published in the "NIH Guide for the Care and Use of Laboratory Animals." The anterograde tract-tracing method using the autoradiographic technique was employed (Cowan et al., 1972) because this allows excellent visualization of the fiber pathways, as well as their sites of termination. In all cases, animals were anesthetized with ketamine hydrochloride (10 mg/kg) and sodium pentobarbital (30 mg/kg), and the cerebral cortex was exposed by craniotomy and reflection of the dura. Regions of interest in the cerebral cortex were identified by inspection of the sulcal pattern. Two closely adjacent injections of 0.5 μL tritiated leucine and proline (volume range 0.4–1.2 μL, specific activity range 40–80 μCu, aqueous solution) were made in defined cortical areas under direct visual guidance with a 1-μL Hamilton syringe and a microdrive attachment. Injection sites were confirmed by microscopic analysis of architectonic features. Cortical injections were made at a depth of 2 mm, sulcal injections at a depth of 4 to 6 mm. After a survival period of 7 to 10 days the animals were deeply anesthetized with Nembutal and perfused transcardially with saline and then 10% formalin, and the brains were removed. The brainstem was separated from the cerebral hemispheres rostral to the level of the inferior colliculus at 90 degrees to the long axis of the pons. The cerebral hemispheres were blocked in the coronal plane to facilitate sectioning with the microtome. The brains were then embedded in paraffin, cut in the coronal plane at a

thickness of 10 μm, and mounted on glass slides. The slides were immersed in Kodak NTB-2 nuclear track emulsion in a humidified darkroom, allowed to dry, wrapped in silver foil to prevent light contamination, and exposed for 4 to 6 months. Slides were then developed in Kodak D-19 and fixed in Kodak Rapid-Fix. Counterstaining for Nissl substance was performed using thionin in most cases and cresyl violet in some before the slides were coverslipped and stored (Cowan et al., 1972).

2. The brain was postfixed in 10% formalin for 10 days and dehydrated in a series of 80%, 95%, and 100% ethanol and ethanol/ether. It was then placed in 3% celloidin for 1 week, followed by 12% celloidin for 3 days to harden. The celloidin block was trimmed, placed on a sliding microtome, and cut coronally at 36 μm. Every fifth section was mounted on glass slides, stained for Nissl substance with cresyl violet, and coverslipped using Permount.

Chapter 13
Superior Longitudinal Fasciculus and Arcuate Fasciculus

1. Burdach writes that the fibers "bildet," or form, the gyri. The descriptions of Reil and Burdach predated the clear understanding that axons are the extensions in the white matter of the neurons situated within the cerebral cortex. See the discussion concerning Neuron Theory, in Chapter 2.

2. The term "Stammlappen" is maintained in our text, as it refers to an earlier concept of brain anatomy that does not translate into contemporary terminology. It seems to correspond to a "hilum" of the brain, at the intersection of the mesodiencephalic structures and the telencephalon. To the best of our understanding from Burdach's description quoted below, it includes gray and white matter structures in the basal forebrain region and extends laterally underneath the lentiform nucleus and the external capsule to include the insula. Burdach, 1822, p. 169:

> The medial portion of the lower surface of the "Stammlappen" is situated below the lower surface of the lentiform nucleus and the striatum. Anteriorly it forms the lower cribriform plate through which the arteries ascend to the lentiform nucleus. It consists of fibers that run like an arc from medial to posterolateral. Most medially and posteriorly in this fiber system the optic tract is situated. Superiorly and more laterally it is the belt layer and the stem of the septum ("Scheidewand"). More laterally it is the tapetum and the anterior commissure and then the longitudinal tract and the corona radiata.

Burdach, 1822, paragraph 205, p. 165:

> The brainstem is situated freely with its superior and medial surfaces in the cisterns and the posterior portion of its lower surface lying exposed above the basal layer of the skull. Along with its lateral surfaces and the anterior portions of

its lower surface it assumes a similarity with the cortical mantle so that here it earns its designation "Stammlappen (lobus caudicis)." On its lateral surfaces it is covered with gyri like the cerebral cortex ("Mantel"), and it is connected with it by "Belegungsmasse." ["Belegungsmasse" refers to the white matter fiber systems, literally—allocation substance, associated ("gehörige") with the cortex ("Mantel") of the brain [that] contains, in addition to the shorter fibers, four large pairs of bundles that run longitudinally. (Burdach, 1822, Paragraph 194, p. 148).] In the anterior portion of the lower surface of the "Stammlappen," the crura cerebri with their longitudinal fibers are covered by oblique fibers that are connected with the gyri and "Belegungsmasse." The lateral surfaces of the "Stammlappen" or the superior part of the brainstem that are gyrated and face away from each other constitute the insula.

Chapter 14
Extreme Capsule

1. Dejerine, 1895 (pp. 808–809):

The fibers of the external capsule . . . contribute a contingent of the fibers in the extreme capsule. The extreme capsule, in addition, contains large numbers of short association fibers connecting neighboring convolutions, or convolutions that are separated from the insula by variable distances. The fibers of the external and extreme capsules . . . are frequently surrounded by hemorrhagic centers that accumulate at the external aspect of the putamen. . . . [I]n these instances, as we have been able to observe more than once, the degeneration of these various fibers, with the exception of the fibers of the anterior commissure and the uncinate fasciculus, cannot be followed beyond the immediate vicinity of the primary locus. This feature demonstrates that a large number of fibers in the external capsule and in particular the extreme capsule, belong to a system of short associative fibers.

Chapter 17
Cingulum Bundle

1. Burdach, 1822 (p. 370, annotation to paragraph 194):

(Reil) designates them (the cingulum bundles) at times as covered stripes, at times longitudinal stripes, despite the fact that they are not covered in all places, nor are they stripe like. According to him ([Reil, 1809a] Archiv IX, page 144) they are situated lateral to the midline in the two gyri, above the corpus callosum that supports the hemispheres. They encircle the brain so that the entrance into the oblique fissure and cribri-

form plate is situated between its two ends. They thus have the same orientation as the fornix. Anteriorly they run with the genu backwards to the cribriform plate and the anterior commissure, then bend forward and form the medial wall of the fissure of the olfactory stripe, or end in the angle that is formed by the termination of the rostrum of the corpus callosum with the "Leistchen"—[little bar, likely the precommissural septum] (Archiv IX, p. 352). Posteriorly they attach to the gyrus and cover the medial wall of the lower horn up to the pes hippocampi (Archiv IX, p. 173 and p. 193). Together with the crura of the fornix they connect to the pes hippocampi and form its gray substance. They give off a radiation below that which comes from the gyrus, and form the most medial layer of the lower walls of the posterior and lower horns [of the lateral ventricle] and continue in the lower horn.

2. Burdach, 1822 (p. 148, paragraph 194):

Zwingen (Cingulum). The "Belegungsmasse" [white matter fiber systems, literally—allocation substance] that is associated only with the cortex of the brain contains, in addition to the shorter fibers, four large pairs of bundles that run longitudinally. Three of these, the cingulum, the arcuate fasciculus, and the unciform fasciculus, form a posteriorly convex and anteriorly open arc, whereas the inferior longitudinal fascicle runs in one plane. We will begin with the cingulum because it represents the transition point from the 'Belegungsorgan' [the cerebral cortex and white matter, including the corpus callosum and fornix, according to Neuburger/Clarke, 1897/1981, p. 280, note 62] to the "Belegungsmasse" and because it belongs not only to the cortex, but also to the core of the brain.

3. Burdach, 1822 (p. 148, paragraph 194):

If one scrapes out the medial surface of one hemisphere either above or within the surroundings of the corpus callosum until one reaches the horizontal fibers, one exposes the cingulum and recognizes it because it is closely adjacent to the corpus callosum, although its fibers run in the opposite direction, and form a self-contained peculiar structure. Only after peeling it away does one reach the radiations that come from the superior layer of the body of the corpus callosum. Similarly, one can convince oneself of its independence by cutting off the lower portion of the brain, and then from the inferior aspect peeling off the body of the corpus callosum with all of its radiations. The cingulum bundles then remain as peculiar constructions preserved in mint condition.

4. Burdach further described his conception of the cingulum bundle as follows (ibid., p. 148, paragraph 194):

The anterior origin of the cingulum is situated at the basal surface of the "Stammlappen" below the striatum at the cribriform plate between the optic tract that lies medially, and the anterior commissure that lies laterally. From there, it runs along the lateral surface of the optic tract anteriorly and medially, then along the lateral surface of the gray lamina terminalis anteriorly and superiorly, and then anteriorly and inferiorly along the lateral surface of the taenia of the corpus callosum and the handle of the septum. It forms an arc that is convex superiorly alongside the floor of the septum. At times it appears as if it is connected with the handle of the septum, or as if it receives descending fibers from it. Also, it appears occasionally that the origin of the cingulum is joined by fibers that come from the temporal lobe, namely from its apex, or from the lateral wall of the temporal horn. Here the cingulum reaches the frontal lobe, runs along the lower surface of the genu of the corpus callosum anteriorly, and ascends in an arc-like fashion along its anterior surface towards the superior surface of the body of the corpus callosum. It thereby forms the gyri of the inner surface of the frontal lobe by running around the anterior portion of the body of the corpus callosum, but it also reaches into the most medial gyri of the lower and anterior surface, that is, towards those that extend to the medial portion of the olfactory tract.

5. As noted by Gustav Huguenin (1840–1920; 1879, translated and quoted in Beevor, 1891, p. 142), the contemporary view of the cingulum bundle was that:

numerous other fibres from the neighbouring parts of the cortex join it and then leave it again after a longer or shorter course; this small system of arciform fibres is united to the fibres which go the whole length of the cingulum . . . [T]he cingulum receives at its anterior part fibres from the medulla of the olfactory lobe . . . [L]ongitudinal fibres of the cingulum are crossed by transverse fibres from the medullary center of the hemispheres; these terminate in the cortex of the gyrus fornicatus, and are the fibres of the corpus callosum . . . [T]he fibres of the cingulum itself are distributed to the cortex of all the parts situated above it . . . We have called the bundle of fibres lying beneath the gyrus fornicatus a system of association fibres . . . And as the different parts which they unite have such marked physiological differences we are quite justified in considering these fibres as systems connecting the various functional regions of the brain.

6. Dejerine, 1895 (p. 751):

According to Meynert, Schwalbe, Obersteiner, etc. the most inferior and internal fibers of the cingulum are not covered by gray cortex, but form the superior aspect of the corpus callosum, the fibers of Lancisi, the taenia tecta at the level of the hippocampal convolution, and the reticular substance of Arnold. However, these structures [fibers of Lancini, Taenia tecta, and the reticular substance] are quite distinct from the cingulum, because as we have seen earlier they represent tangential fibers of cortical origin. . . . The origin and termination of cingulum fibers is very controversial. According to Foville the two ends of the cingulum terminate in the anterior perforated substance. According to Broca, they connect the internal olfactory root to the external olfactory root. Broca compared this system of the cingulum to a [tennis] racket with the olfactory peduncle being the handle. According to Meynert, Huguenin, etc., the anterior-inferior extremity of the cingulum is connected to the amygdala. . . . The functions of the cingulum are very unclear; Horsley sectioned the cingulum rostral to the precuneus in the ouistiti monkey (*Hapale jactans*) and did not notice any paralytic or anesthetic effect. The animal was sacrificed two months later and upon examination of the brain, Beevor noticed degeneration of the fibers occupying the posterior part of the horizontal fascicle. Not all the fibers in this region were degenerated, and this can be explained by the widely accepted notion that the cingulum contains fibers of different lengths that belong to these fascicles for only a small part of their trajectory."

Cajal had shown in 1890 (La Cellule, Vol. VII, referenced in Cajal 1901, translated by Kraft, 1955) using the Golgi technique in the rat that axons within the cingulate gyrus originate in the interhemispheric gray matter and follow an anteroposterior course. He later observed (1899–1904, translated into English 1999 by Pasik and Pasik; 1901, translated into English 1955 by Kraft, pp. 110–111; 1901, translated into English by DeFelipe and Jones, 1988; 1909–1910, translated into English by Swanson and Swanson, 1995, pp. 665–666) that in the rabbit and mouse, the supracallosal white matter contained two distinct bundles, one medial and the other lateral. He regarded the medially situated fibers as the "cingulum or longitudinal fascicle of the cingulate cortex" (Cajal, 1995 translation, p. 666), whereas he regarded the fibers situated more dorsally and laterally as the "arcuate or superior longitudinal fascicle of the hemispheres" (ibid.) and equated them in part with the bundle described by Forel and Onufrowicz (see chapters 13, 17, and 19 for discussion of these fiber systems).

7. Yakovlev and Locke, 1961b (p. 389):

Not all of the fibers in the medullary core of the cingulate gyrus belong to the cingulum proper. The cingulum proper constitutes less than half of the medullary core and occupies a characteristic position. It is immediately adjacent to the subarea LA$_3$ [nomenclature of von Economo and Koskinas, 1925]. Most of its fibers arise from this subarea, few are contributed from subarea LA$_2$ in the inferior part of the crown of the gyrus, and none from subarea LA$_1$ in the bank of the cingulate sulcus [figure N-2]. The relationships are thus inverse to those obtaining with regard to the commissural callosal fibers. On emerging from Lamina VI of subarea LA$_3$, the fibers of the cingulum run anteriorly and posteriorly in

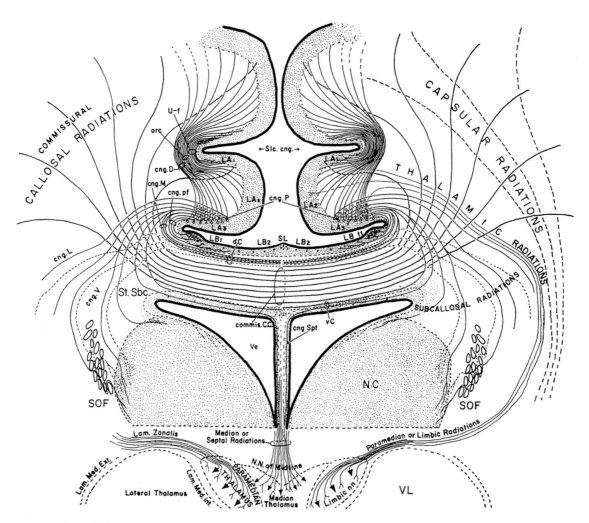

Figure N-2

Reproduction of figure 6A from Yakovlev and Locke (1961b, p. 374) showing their conception of relations of the cingulate gyrus. The legend to their figure with abbreviations reads: "[T]he efferent and thalamic afferent connections of the cingulate gyrus in coronal plane. Arc–arcuate fibers of Arnold, commisCC–corticocortical commissural fibers in the core of the corpus callosum, cngD–dorsal (arcuate) radiations of the cingulum to the supralimbic cortex, cngL–lateral (subcallosal) radiations of the cingulum to the ipsilateral striatum and limbic thalamus, cngM–medial subcallosal radiations of the cingulum to the contralateral striatum and limbic thalamus via dorsal (dC) and ventral (vC) laminae of the corpus callosum, cngP–ground bundle of the cingulum (cingulum proper), cng pf–corticoperforant radiations of the cingulum to the hippocampua (indusium), cng S pt–fibers from the ventral radiation of the cingulum to septum, cngV–ventral subcallosal radiations of the cingulum to the ipsilateral striatum and limbic thalamus, dC–dorsal lamina of corpus callosum, NC–caudate nucleus, Slc cng–cingulate sulcus, StSbc–stratum subcallosum, tt–taenia tecta, U-f–U-fibers of Meynert, vC–ventral lamina of corpus callosum, Ve–lateral ventricle, VL–ventral lateral nucleus of the thalamus."

the parasagittal plane. They constitute the ground bundle, or the cingulum proper. At the subrostral level, this ground bundle is thin and flattened in the parasagittal plane; in the supracallosal sector it is roughly triangular in cross section; however in the posterior supracallosal and retrosplenial sectors, as the cingulate gyrus becomes broader and the agranular limbic cortex in the bank of the callosal sulcus approaches the area entorhinalis TH in the bank of the hippocampal sulcus, the cingulum spreads vertically in the parasagittal plane.

8. Yakovlev and Locke, 1961b (p. 390):

There are several distinctive and significant features peculiar to the organization of the efferent connections of the cingulate gyrus. As has been clearly shown by Cajal and will presently be developed further, the significant feature of the majority of the pyramids of the limbic cortex in rodents is their bifurcation into anteriorly and posteriorly running branches. However, in monkey . . . there occurs an enrichment of branching also in the transverse, i.e., mediolateral, plane. This was evident in the "Indian war bonnet" disposition of the fibers radiating from the cingulum proper dorsally, laterally, and ventrally, as seen in coronal plane" (see figure N-2).

Page 391:

Another characteristic feature of the pyramids of the limbic cortex is the extraordinarily wide distribution of the axonal terminals of apparently each single cell to the supralimbic cortex, to the hippocampus, to the striatum, to the thalamus, and to the nuclei of the tegmentum of the brainstem. This feature was shown by Cajal "with ultimate evidence" with regard to the cells with bifurcated axonal fibers, the posteriorly running branches terminating in the cerebral cortex—Cajal's "associational fibers"—and the anteriorly running branches—Cajal's "projectional fibers"—descending to the striatum and the "inferior regions" of the brain. Such a widespread distribution of the fibers radiating from the cingulum was described by Showers in Marchi preparation and was evident also in our material.

Chapter 18
Inferior Longitudinal Fasciculus

1. This passage was also translated by Davis (1921, pp. 370–371). In Davis' translation: "Its inner part forms the inner margin of this groove and unites with the tapetum and cingulum. Its outer part unites with the ground bundles that ascend in the lateral border of the temporal lobe." The original text reads: "Sein innrer Theil, der den innern Rand dieses Gleises bildet, hängt mit der Tapete und der Zwinge, sein äußsrer Theil mit dem in die seitlichen Randwülste des Unterlappens heraufsteigenden Bogenbündel, zusammen" (Burdach, 1822, paragraph 196, p. 152).

2. Davis translates "Stammlappen" as "insular cortex of Reil," but see footnote 2 of chapter 13 for our working definition of this term.

3. Burdach described his internal basal bundle as follows:

Finally, fiber bundles which we would like to designate as an internal basal bundle ("innre Grundbündel [fasciculi baseos interni]") originate from the apex of the medial part of the lower surface of the occipital lobe, running anteriorly along with the gyri, initially below the cuneus, then below the cingulum in the temporal lobe, through the continuation of the medial parieto-occipital sulcus but distinct from it, finally passing through it and merging with the cingulum. Thus the cingulum contains the fiber bundles from the occipital lobe as it runs anteriorly along the internal rim of the lower surface of the temporal lobe where it forms the inner part of the floor of the temporal horn of the lateral ventricle [literally, lower horn], situated below Ammon's horn, and then forms the uncus. It reaches the end of the temporal horn of the lateral ventricle and appears to ascend anterior to the amygdala and to enter its lower portion.

The legend to his Tafel IX, figure 2, states: "the cingulum and internal basal bundle merge below the uncus" (Burdach, 1822, paragraph 194, p. 151).

4. Dejerine (1895) discussed the inferior longitudinal fasciculus as follows (pp. 765–775):

Inferior Longitudinal Fasciculus of Burdach—Sagittal layers of the occipital lobe (Wernicke). The external sagittal stratum (Sachs). Sensory fascicle (Charcot, Ballet). The inferior longitudinal fasciculus of Burdach is a fascicle that has an anterior-posterior orientation. It is situated at the edge of the inferior and external temporo-occipital lobe and extends from the occipital to the temporal lobe. The inferior longitudinal fasciculus forms the external layer of the sagittal fibers from the occipito-temporal lobe and it is extremely easy to dissect on hardened brains, because the direction of the fibers is perpendicular to those that cover them. Considered as a whole, this fascicle forms a kind of gutter that is tightly bent with the opening oriented superiorly and medially. In the concavity we see the projection fibers of the occipito-temporal lobe. It has an external wall, an inferior wall, and a very sharp, thick angle, which corresponds to the inferior and external edge of the hemisphere, particularly at the base of the third temporal convolution and third occipital convolution. The external wall corresponds to the first and second temporal convolutions.

The inferior longitudinal fasciculus exhibits this particular shape only in the temporal lobe. In the occipital lobe, the inferior wall of the gutter moves dorsally and medially and covers the stratum calcarinum. At the base of the cuneus, the two edges of the gutter are so close that they are joined and transform this fascicle into a kind of oval cone, the summit of which is located about 2.5 centimeters from the occipital pole. Because of this particular organization, when we look at coronal sections the inferior longitudinal fasciculus takes the shape of a ring that is more or less irregular and angular, and within the temporal lobe it takes the shape of a gutter that is sharply curved. The inferior longitudinal fasciculus therefore forms a clearly delineated fasciculus. Some authors incorrectly thought that this fasciculus includes commissural fibers as well as projection and association fibers that cover the floor of the occipital and temporal horns, and that are located between the ventricular ependyma and the most superficial part of the collateral sulcus. . . . Like all long association fascicles, the inferior longitudinal fasciculus contains a complex system of fibers of variable length. Secondary degeneration studies following cortical lesions restricted to the occipital lobe have shown that these fascicles contain a large number of long fibers with degenerating fibers that can be followed within the white matter of the temporal lobe.

The fibers of the inferior longitudinal fasciculus originate in the superficial part of the pole of the occipital lobe. Laterally they cross the projection and commissural fibers and the white matter of the occipital lobe, they then group together behind the occipital horn and form a thin angular fascicle that is easily visualized on sections processed with the Weigert stain. This fascicle receives a large number of fibers from the cuneate, lingual lobule, fusiform lobule, and the three convolutions of the convex aspect of the occipital lobe. These fibers are not all oriented in the same direction. Fibers that originate from the inferior half and external part of the occipital lobe travel from the back to the front and along the inferior and external edge of the occipital and sphenoidal horns. The fibers that originate from the superior and external part of the occipital lobe travel obliquely from the ventral to the rostral direction, along the external wall of the atrium. The fibers that originate from the most superficial regions become oblique. The fibers that originate from the cortex of the cuneus are also obliquely oriented and travel along the internal wall of the occipital horn outside the stratum calcarinum and then over the floor of the occipital horn. All these fibers are close to the compact fascicle of sagittal fibers that cover the inferior and external edge of the atrium, which in the temporal lobe takes the shape of a gutter.

In the temporal lobe, the inferior longitudinal fasciculus gives off many fibers. The fibers from the inferior layers go to the hippocampal convolution, the fusiform lobule, and the third temporal convolution. Even larger numbers project in the first temporal convolution, and reach the temporal lobe, where they cross the fibers of the arcuate fasciculus or the so-called superior longitudinal fasciculus of Burdach, as well as the fibers of the uncinate fasciculus. A small number of fibers enter the external capsule where they contribute to the formation of the inferior layers. These fibers barely pass the posterior third of the external capsule and intermingle with the fibers of the anterior commissure and of the uncinate fasciculus, but they can be distinguished from them by their larger caliber and intense staining. Finally, other fibers radiate into the cortex of the hook or U convolution in the temporal cortex that limits the anterior perforated substance,

and into the adjacent cortex of the first temporal convolution. The rostral termination of the inferior longitudinal fasciculus and its intermingling with the uncinate fasciculus are easily visualized on serial horizontal sections.

Near the first temporal convolution, the inferior longitudinal fasciculus exhibits a quite special feature on horizontal microscopic sections. It is traversed by a large number of undulated fascicles strongly stained with hematoxylin that curve rostrally and medially across the thalamic radiations and enter into the body of the retro-lenticular segment of the internal capsule. They then radiate into the pulvinar, into the external and internal geniculate bodies, and within the external and internal nucleus of the thalamus. The most anterior of these undulating fascicles arrives in the subthalamic region, the posterior segment of the internal capsule, and descends with the fibers of the posterior segment into the base of the cerebral peduncle where it contributes to the formation of its external fifth.

Do all these fibers that cross the thalamic radiation and the retro-lenticular segment of the internal capsule belong to the inferior longitudinal fasciculus, a part of which enters the corona radiata? Or rather, are they projection fibers from the temporal lobe that cross the inferior longitudinal fasciculus to reach their final destination? This question is very important because it involves the functional role of this inferior longitudinal fasciculus. In the latter case, the fascicle would exclusively be an associative fascicle; in the former case, it would contain both associative and projection fibers. For authors who consider this fascicle to be the same as that made of projection fibers from the occipital lobe and who describe these fibers under the names of optic radiations (Gratiolet), lame des faisceaux optiques (Meynert), substance sagittale du lobe occipital (Wernicke), or fasceau sensitif (Charcot, Balet, Brisaud), the inferior longitudinal fasciculus would be formed of projection fibers.

According to Sachs, the fibers that this author calls stratum sagittale externum would be mainly made of associative fibers, but would in addition contain a small number of projection fibers.

It is obvious that in the inferior longitudinal fasciculus, the origin of projection and associative fibers can not be determined with normal anatomy. The intermingling of these fibers is too extensive, and therefore we have to use secondary degeneration techniques to address the issue of their origin. We consider that the inferior part of the inferior longitudinal fasciculus is exclusively an associative fascicle, and that its superior part is intimately united to the retro-lenticular segment of the internal capsule, and contains projection fibers that are destined for subcortical centers (such as the thalamus, lentiform nucleus, globus pallidus, etc.)

We insisted in previous paragraphs on the fact that the inferior longitudinal fasciculus is traversed in all of its occipital parts by fibers which travel from the occipital cortex to the tapetum and to the thalamic radiations. At the same time we believe that most fibers in the temporal division of this fascicle originate from the sagittal layer of the occipito-temporal lobe, and radiate in the pulvinar, the internal and external geniculate body, the external thalamic nucleus, the suboptic region, the posterior segment of the internal capsule, etc., etc. As we said, [we believe] that these fibers do not belong to the inferior longitudinal fasciculus, but rather they merely traverse the inferior longitudinal fasciculus, and they belong either to the corona radiata of the occipital lobe or to the corona radiata of the temporal lobe.

5. Flechsig (1896, p. 2) regarded the constituents of the inferior longitudinal fasciculus in the following manner:

The inferior longitudinalis fasciculus of Burdach has previously been described as an association system, connecting the occipital lobe with the temporal lobe, in particular with its anterior portions. I have stated previously that this assumption is incorrect. This inferiorly situated long bundle is one of the earliest myelinated bundles of the brain and one can, as a consequence, see this in a one-week-old newborn, completely and in detail. The fascicles in question end posteriorly in the occipital lobe, particularly in the visual area, but anteriorly they do not connect with the cortex, but rather with the optic thalamus. They assume a considerably longer course by running medially into the temporal lobe, up to the area lateral and posterior to the lenticular body where they curve sharply upwards and reach around the lower horn from anterior. [This is the loop of visual fibers within the temporal lobe that later came to bear the name of Meyer]. In the thalamus, they connect in part to the basal part of the lateral nucleus, in the structure that has the form of a bowl. Other parts ascend on the posterior surface of the pulvinar in the stratum zonale and reach the main nucleus (Flechsig—von Tschisch). Here they intertwine. A strong fiber bundle goes from the superior surface of the lateral geniculate through the pulvinar to the posterior stratum zonale, and the fibers of both bundles are probably partly connected. The inferior longitudinal fasciculus is therefore nothing more than a part of the optic radiation of Gratiolet. It is accompanied on its way from the thalamus to the lateral side of the lower horn by corona radiata bundles of the thalamus that run to the olfactory area and the Ammon's horn and which curve anteriorly, lateral to the amygdaloid nucleus.

6. Flechsig, 1896 (p. 3):

These facts are particularly critical in opposing the position of Sachs that was based on the view that the inferior longitudinal fasciculus, identical to the external sagittal stratum,

comprises the most important association system between the visual cortex and the cortical areas of the temporal lobe that are involved with language, especially the first temporal gyrus. The external sagittal stratum is entirely unrelated to association processes, and therefore also has nothing to do with the association of facial and auditory impressions [that subserve] visual memory—it is a bundle of the corona radiata.

Chapter 19
Fronto-Occipital Fasciculus

1. Onufrowicz obtained the brain of a patient with callosal agenesis (Onufrowicz, 1887, p. 305) "through the courtesy of my previous employer, Dr. Moore, who was the previous director of the mental institution in Rheinau (Kanton Zürich), where this brain was stored." Onufrowicz stated that he was (p. 305):

indebted to Professor Dr. Forel for letting me use his library, and for his willingness to guide me through this work and for teaching me how to interpret the brain and its parts, and for making the illustrations in this article. . . . Although many cases of agenesis of the corpus callosum have been described in the human brain, we are in a position to make a small contribution to the knowledge of the anatomy of this condition with this case. Further, we are able to make a contribution to brain anatomy in general that should be valuable, because, to our knowledge, cross sections were performed only in the most recently described case of Anton. In that case of a fetal brain, myelinated fiber systems were not yet developed. That previously described case did not produce any further insights into the internal structural changes of the brain because no cross sections were taken. In the current case we performed coronal sections of the left half of the brain, and stored the other half in the collection of the Burghölzli institution.

2. Page 313:

Description of our case. Gottlieb Hoffman von Seen (Kanton Zürich). Born in 1842, died in Rheinau Feb. 22, 1879 from pneumonia. Thanks to the priest Meister in Seen I received the following valuable remarks about Hoffman. "One could see even in the cradle, he was completely stupid and without all sense. As a young boy, he walked around the house with pitiful screaming. He was even unable to learn how to eat. He either tried to stuff a whole slice of bread into his mouth or he made little pieces and crumbled them on the floor. His father was a farmer and weaver, and Hoffman used the basket cane to vandalize mirrors and the glass in windows. The only sign of intelligence was that he would return to his parents' house in response to a particular whistle. The behavior of Hoffman during his stay in Rheinau is as follows. He sat in a chair that was specially constructed for him. He would walk close to walls. He was filthy and had to be fed since he put food all over himself and as described above, he tried to stuff food in big pieces in his mouth. From time to time he made inarticulate noises. His sensory organs were unfortunately not examined, but he was able to see, he was able to feel, and it appears he was able to hear. Furthermore, he had deformed hands and feet. This was the reason he could not walk." A detailed history of his illness is unfortunately not available, and the very poorly performed autopsy is as follows. He had scoliosis of the spine, severe stiffness [after death], he had stains in dependent areas and he was very cachectic. He had a small round and pointed skull, slightly asymmetric, somewhat thickened in the midline, and tethered to the pia, which was injected. The gyri were very flattened because of compression, and the sulci were flat due to poor preservation. The olfactory nerves were absent and the pia was difficult to detach from the skull. (Autopsy on Feb 24th 1879.)

3. Page 313:

When the brain was taken out it immediately fell apart in 2 pieces and it became apparent at once that the corpus callosum and the olfactory bulb were missing. The brain in our descriptions is depicted as normal size, was put in a solution of potassium bichromate, but unfortunately became foul. It was subsequently immersed in cognac, and as a consequence of this treatment, the surface of the brain became very fragile. The gyri at the base, in particular, were compressed, so that no clear interpretation of those could be done.

4. Dejerine, 1895 (pp. 760–761):

This fascicle that we call in our serial sections, occipital frontal fascicle, is in fact the fascicle that was described by Meynert under the name of corona radiata of the caudate nucleus, and by Wernicke under the name of fascicle of the corpus callosum traveling to the internal capsule. According to Meynert the corona radiata of the caudate nucleus is formed by numerous fibers that originate in the caudate nucleus, merge along the angle of the superior and external aspect of the caudate nucleus and radiate within the convolutions of the superior aspect of the hemisphere. Wernicke has shown that these fibers have no connection with the caudate nucleus, and when we examine serial sections we do not see any fiber terminating in the caudate nucleus.

According to Wernicke these fibers form a fascicle of callosal fibers reaching the internal capsule. They originate

from the anterior wall of the frontal horn, that is, from the genu of the corpus callosum and from the white matter of the frontal lobe. They then unite in one compact fascicle 1.5 centimeters thick, and run along the superior and external edge of the caudate nucleus. The fibers enter the internal capsule between the caudate nucleus and the superior edge of the putamen at the level of the middle part of the thalamus. This fascicle is not part of the anterior segment of the internal capsule.

From the examination of serial sections, whether coronal sections or horizontal or sagittal sections, we have been able to reach the conclusion that none of these fibers make contact with the caudate nucleus.

5. Dejerine, 1895 (p. 761):

Because we have no anatomical-pathological or experimental data supporting the previous idea of Gratiolet and of Foville, an idea that has been supported by Wernicke regarding the existence of callosal fibers traveling within the internal capsule, we believe we can identify this fascicle as the occipital-frontal fascicle described by Forel and Onufrowicz when they discuss agenesis of the corpus callosum.

Page 765:

These observations made in the human are consistent with the lessons learned from experimental pathology. Experimental work by Muratoff that is being performed in the dog indicates that the occipito-frontal fascicle of Forel and Onufrowicz (subcallosal fasciculus of Muratoff), partially degenerates following ablation of the motor sphere, or the destruction of frontal or occipital convolutions.

6. Dejerine, 1895 (p. 758):

Forel and Onufrowicz demonstrated, and this has been confirmed by Kaufmann and Hochhaus, that in the case of complete agenesis of the corpus callosum the arrest of development concerns mainly the corpus callosum, the forceps and the commissural system of the cerebral trigone (David's Lyre). The tapetum, in contrast, which corresponds to the layer of fibers that cover the external wall of the temporal and occipital horns, develops normally and continues rostrally with a fascicle that is directed sagittally, located medial to the corona radiata and lateral to the body of the trigone with which it is intimately united. These facts demonstrate that the tapetum does not belong to the corpus callosum, but belongs to the intra-hemispheric association fascicle that Forel and Onufrowicz termed the occipital-frontal fascicle . . . In the temporo-occipital lobe, after it forms the tapetum, the occipito-frontal fascicle radiates in the convolutions of the external aspect and the inferior external aspect of the lobe.

7. Schröder, 1901 (pp. 94–95):

The assumption of Onufrowicz . . . was no doubt a conclusion *per exclusionem*. The corpus callosum, i.e., the horizontal connecting bridge between both hemispheres, was missing, the bundle could not easily be regarded as belonging to the corona radiata and therefore the only remaining option was the interpretation that it is an association system. The first and only one who doubted this interpretation was H. Sachs. Sachs said that in the described cases of callosal agenesis the callosal fibers were not missing, but present, and that the trunk of the corpus callosum did not connect both hemispheres but the poles of the same hemisphere. What Onufrowicz thought to be the fronto-occipital bundle was this trunk portion of the corpus callosum. This attempt at an explanation has not been very popular. Vogt called it untenable and not viable. Dejerine likewise had his doubts. On first inspection this explanation does indeed appear surprising.

Onufrowicz saw that the corpus callosum was missing and concluded without any reasoning that the entire callosal fiber system was missing completely (agenesis). He did not even try to search for possible remnants of the corpus callosum. He found an exceptional fiber tract but did not consider the possibility that it could possibly have something to do with the corpus callosum.

Sachs now postulates that the normally developed callosal fibers have grown from the cortex until they reach their gathering place in proximity to the lateral ventricle. Here they are prevented by an unknown circumstance from crossing the midline, they have therefore curved posteriorly and anteriorly and made connections to cortical areas of the same, instead of the contralateral, hemispheres (heterotopia of the corpus callosum).

Sachs' assumption is just a hypothesis, but a hypothesis that facilitates the understanding of certain teratological cases much more than the forced interpretation by Onufrowicz. One thing has to be mentioned: according to Sachs the controversial fiber tract also represents an association bundle in cases lacking the corpus callosum, i.e., a system that connects cortical areas of the same hemisphere with each other and since it can be traced from the frontal lobe to the occipital pole, one could not argue with its name "fronto-occipital bundle." But, and this is the core message, this fronto-occipital bundle does not have an analogue in the normal brain, such as the superior longitudinal fascicle or another of the known fiber tracts. It has formed in an abnormal manner from the corpus callosum that was prevented from crossing the midline. The finding of such a fiber tract in the normal brain is therefore excluded from the outset since this bundle only forms under certain pathological conditions and forms a replacement for the missing corpus callosum. It contains fibers that were meant to connect with cortical areas of the contralateral hemisphere, but

since they were prevented from doing so, have made a connection with the corresponding cortical areas of the same hemisphere. If they did not find the connection to adequate cortical territories they would have perished, as we know from experience.

How the axis cylindrical processes of callosal cells form such unusual connections is impossible to explain. But according to the current status of our knowledge on the embryological mechanisms in the brain it is equally difficult to explain how each cell finds its partner in the other hemisphere under normal circumstances.

If one familiarizes oneself with the thought that a heterotopia in the sense of Sachs is possible, the illustrations by Kaufmann and Onufrowicz are in fact evidence of such heterotopia. What is designated as fronto-occipital bundle assumes the position of the trunk of the normal corpus callosum, but the connecting bridge between both hemispheres is missing. In the anterior horn, the fiber layer lies like the normal corpus callosum medial to the ventricle and not at its lateral edge where the authors are searching for the fronto-occipital bundle. Posteriorly it moves gradually laterally like the normal corpus callosum, and finally sends the main portion of its fibers on the lateral side of the posterior horn as the tapetum in the occipital direction. (At the time of Onufrowicz's work everyone considered that the tapetum contained only callosal fibers. If he had concluded more correctly: my bundle continues posteriorly directly into the tapetum which we know represents callosal fibers, consequently my bundle has to do with the corpus callosum, if he had concluded this, the currently favored but entirely unfruitful tapetum question would not have arisen).

8. Schröder, 1901 (pp. 84–86):

On coronal section through the area of the central gyri (Taf II, Fig. 1-The image is from the same preparation as in Wernicke's Atlas des Gehirns, Part 1) we see the lateral angle of the lateral ventricle surrounded by a brighter fiber-mass (fnc), which sits broadly on the caudate nucleus and reaches the corpus callosum superiorly. Its medial lower rim continues in a thin fiber layer that covers the caudate nucleus on its free surface, its medial superior rim reaches below the corpus callosum towards the midline. This bundle is remarkable because of the abundance of coarse vessels. A clearly defined direction of fibers cannot be recognized. Even under the microscope one sees only within the lateral part, a predominance of sagittal fibers by means of its slightly darker coloration. Sachs has called this bundle, fasciculus nuclei caudati ("Schwanzkernbündel"). We agree with his nomenclature.

In the frontal lobe, where the fasciculus nuclei caudati is best developed, it descends in front of the head of the caudate close to the base of the brain and one finds it therefore on coronal sections that lie in front of the tip of the anterior horn (see Wernicke Atlas I, Taf. 2), where it lies encircled by the corpus callosum. In the most anterior portion of the anterior horn it forms a thick layer at its lateral wall; the head of the caudate, which pushes the bundle gradually into the superior and lateral corner of the ventricle, appears on adjacent cuts. Here, one can track it posteriorly up to the area of the pulvinar.

Laterally, a sharply demarcated area of thick, dark and convoluted fiber bundles borders the fasciculus nuclei caudati (r). The formation of this bundle is subject to individual variability. In more anterior planes, the space it takes up is larger and its formation is therefore different, as it has a characteristic net-like appearance, i.e., dark fiber bundles form a meshwork in which the mesh is filled by bright oblique bundles (compare Wernicke Atlas I, Taf. 7-12). H. Sachs has introduced these bundles as corona radiata bundles that ascend from the internal capsule initially for a stretch along the caudate before they run towards the cortex. He called this the net-like or reticulated corona radiata area ("reticulirtes Stabkranzfeld"), we simply refer to as "area r." It descends like the fasciculus nuclei caudati in front of the caudate towards the base and it runs posteriorly. The further one gets posteriorly, the more the bright, gap-filling fiber mass diminishes and the closer the darker bundles move together. One constantly finds here, however, a thin layer of bright fibers on the lateral side of the area. From the description of area r it becomes immediately apparent that it is not a bundle in the strong anatomical sense, but that it is formed by fibers that run in only a portion of it; this also explains its changing characteristics in different brains and in different parts of the same brain. The position of area r is always lateral to the fasciculus nuclei caudati within the area of the corona radiata radiations (cr), i.e., close to their exit from the internal capsule, i.e., close above a line that connects the superior edge of the caudate and the putamen.

Area r consists superiorly only of a few crowded bundles. It moves superiorly between the caudate bundle and the corpus callosum and sits with its base on the remaining corona radiata fibers. In the lower horn, we find it in corresponding formation: the basis is directed superiorly at the corona radiata, the tip wedged between the fasciculus nuclei caudati and the tapetum. On fortuitous coronal sections one can see the descending part of this bundle in considerable length. We see therefore that the formation of the area r is not limited to the area of the parietal and frontal lobe as Sachs stated, but can also be clearly recognized in the temporal lobe. Neither area r nor the caudate bundle continues into the occipital lobe.

9. Schröder, 1901 (pp. 91–93):

Dejerine addresses the fronto-occipital bundle in detail in his great work. At the outset it should be mentioned that

Dejerine calls what Sachs designated fasciculus nuclei caudati "substance grise sous-ependymaire"; we will not elaborate upon whether this name is justified. Sachs has already pointed out that nerve cells can not be found in it, so that one can not talk of a 'gray [area]'. . . . Dejerine begins also with the cases of callosal agenesis (Onufrowicz, Kaufmann, Hochhaus). He is convinced that the fronto-occipital bundle of these authors cannot be identified with the superior longitudinal fascicle of Burdach. He then describes a fiber tract in great detail that he considers to be the analogue of Onufrowicz's bundle in the normal brain. He describes it as a fiber tract that on anterior cross section is shaped like a pyramid and about 0.5 cm thick, separated from the ventricle by the gris sous-ependymaire, lateral to the corona radiata, superior to the corpus callosum, inferiorly abutting the caudate nucleus. This is nothing other than Sachs' reticulated corona radiata area ("reticulirtes Stabkranzfeld") our area r (see above). Further posteriorly the bundle is said to curve inferiorly and anteriorly and to form the tapetum together with the callosal fibers from the forceps major. This precise [feature] cannot be seen on Dejerine's images.

Dejerine's figures (figs 281-287 and 301-302) do not show an indication of the border between the fiber-complex he designates as a fronto-occipital bundle and the base of the corona radiata; the naïve viewer could rather see evidence for an affiliation of this bundle with the corona radiata in these illustrations. Further, Dejerine discusses in detail fiber tracts that he believes run from the frontal portion of the bundle to the cortex. He distinguishes on the horizontal cut (page 570, fig 295) three groups of such fibers. The first runs from the main bundle anteriorly and is embedded into the lateral part of the substance grise sous-ependymaire, crosses the corpus callosum and radiates into the frontal gyri. According to my preparations, this fiber tract appears to me to be an artificial construct. It was previously mentioned above that the lateral portion of the fasciculus nuclei caudati (Dejerine's substance grise sous-ependymaire) contains darker fibers than the medial portion. There is no relationship of these fibers to the formation that Dejerine designates as fronto-occipital bundle (our area r). Furthermore, like the fasciculus nuclei caudati, this dark bundle generally has its border on the posterior edge of the corpus callosum. What not infrequently impresses one as its anterior-bound continuation through the corpus callosum, is a bundle of rectangular callosal fibers, described above, that frequently come off here. It should not be denied that a part of the delicate fibers of the fasciculus nuclei caudati is also interspersed with the corpus callosum. However, I have never seen a compact fiber tract such as Dejerine has illustrated. On the contrary, I almost always saw a callosal bundle that comes off right in this location (compare Wernicke Atlas II (4B) Text p. 13 and Taf. 9).

As a second group of fibers, Dejerine describes those that run medially from the corona radiata together with the corona radiata fibers to the medial surface of the hemisphere. These fibers can easily be identified and construed (see Taf. II, Fig 2, r2), if one recognizes that Dejerine's fronto-occipital bundle is a corona radiata region: those fibers are corona radiata fibers from this region that join the remaining corona radiata fibers.

As a third grand group of fibers, Dejerine finally mentions fibers that run from his fronto-occipital bundle laterally and inferiorly through the base of the corona radiata to the external capsule. Those are obviously the same fibers that Sachs considers to be fibers moving into the fasciculus nuclei caudati, and they are also mentioned by other authors. According to my preparations, these are largely callosal radiations; it is very probable that the fasciculus nuclei caudati also sends fibers to the cortex here, but these are not the easily recognizable, markedly firm, straight-running fibers that remain visible even when the preparations are so far differentiated that the caudate nucleus bundle that easily decolorizes has lost its colored fibers. One will understand the relationship of these fibers with the corpus callosum if one considers what was said about the callosal radiation above. (Footnote—Much more noticeable is a tract of fine fibers that leaves the fasciculus nuclei caudati posteriorly, as can be seen on horizontal cuts, and which can be tracked to the base of the corona radiata and the internal capsule, but not through them [see Wernicke Atlas II, Taf.6-8]).

The cited literature lets us sufficiently recognize a fact that will need to be emphasized next: What different authors describe as a fronto-occipital bundle in the normal brain, is by no means a uniform structure. All consider the tapetum to be its occipital portion, either as a whole or in part. For the frontal portion however, at least two different tracts come into consideration, the fasciculus nuclei caudati and the area r, according to our description above. von Monakow is probably the only one who still adheres, together with Onufrowicz, to the identification of the fronto-occipital bundle as the superior longitudinal fasciculus. It appears therefore obvious that it is unacceptable to talk of a "fronto-occipital bundle" in pathologic-anatomical descriptions.

As concerns the area r, in which Dejerine in particular sees a fronto-occipital association system, as mentioned above one can recognize most easily on sagittal cuts that it belongs to the corona radiata.

10. Obersteiner and Redlich (1902, p. 301) found it "completely inadmissible to draw conclusions regarding normal anatomy from findings in brains with hereditary agenesis of the corpus callosum" and they (pp. 302–306):

agree with those authors (Sachs, Marchand, Roemer, Probst, Bischoff and others) who assume that the so-called

fronto-occipital fascicle in the brain with corpus callosum agenesis consists of callosal fibers. . . . First of all we would like to emphasize that a bundle characterized by the location and size of the so-called fronto-occipital fasciculus [seen] in the brain without a corpus callosum does not exist in the normal human brain. If we admit the assumption, that due to the missing callosal fibers the fasciculus fronto-occipitalis could have changed its location and emerged more visibly, by all means we would have to find evidence for such a bundle in the normal brain. But that is not the case. If we follow, for example, Dejerine's description and illustrations, which we can compare especially well in frontal and basal cuts of brains of young children, we have to admit that a fiber system exists in the area of the caudate nucleus that is set apart moderately well in certain areas of the brain. However, it is located lateral to the caudate nucleus, as Schröder has already mentioned, and not medially as is the case with the fronto-occipital fasciculus of Onufrowicz.

If we try to clarify the course of this bundle on frontal and basal cuts, we have to state that it appears in front of the caudate nucleus in the form of a few bundles of coarse fibers that appear to emerge from the posterior layer of the corpus callosum ("rückläufigen Balkenschichte," Sachs). Those fibers then form an arc that runs dorsally and remains lateral to the caudate nucleus. New fibers from the frontal and dorsal areas of the brain enter the tract, because on frontal cuts of the white matter we see a few of those fibers appearing, arranged in thin bundles, breaking into the callosal fibers and running to the lateral part of the caudate nucleus and—as we learn from horizontal sections—they turn dorsally. This is the reason that the fiber bundle becomes more bulky dorsally. The bulkiest portion is in the plane in which the caudate nucleus has just been capped ("gekappt"). But even here (Fig. 4) the bundle is not impressive and by no means comparable to the massive bundles described in brains without a corpus callosum. Furthermore it cannot be traced much further in the caudal direction, even along the entire dimensions of the caudate nucleus. Its rostral and dorsal aspect that has a fuzzy (indistinct) border with the corona radiata becomes progressively more washed-out and it essentially dissolves in it. If anything, this bundle can be separated best [from the corona radiata] in young children due to the slightly different caliber and color of its fibers. One can almost always easily separate this bundle from the callosal fibers (due to the bigger caliber of the fibers). Again, a combination of frontal and basal cuts teaches us that a very small tract of this bundle can be traced backwards where it runs apparently along the tail of the caudate nucleus to the lower horn in a dorsally-convex arc (Fig. 5), slightly lateral to the stratum subcallosum. But it is necessary to re-emphasize the fact that these bundles are minute and can only be seen in certain cuts.

Another detail has to be added. The thick fibers that belong to this bundle are, as more rostrally-made frontal cuts illustrate, arranged in small bundles that become interwoven and dissolve towards the caudate nucleus. The coarse fibers that constitute the bundles are braided around the fibers that build a thick meshwork (also in Schröder and Fig. 1). Further back, the fine braided fibers disappear again, and only bundles of coarse fibers remain. The fine fibers become myelinated later than the coarse ones.

In the animal we find very different circumstances. A sharply delineated fiber system that would correspond to the one that we have just described in the human cannot be found. At most, we see a few bundles that maintain the same direction as the bundles just discussed in the monkey and in martens, which cannot be separated from the corona radiata in any way.

We believe that these few remarks justify the claim that the normal bundle cannot be identified as the fronto-occipital bundle of Onufrowicz. We can exclude the possibility that the former contains association fibers based on what we have said (see also Probst). Therefore the assumptions of certain authors who previously ascribed certain physiological roles to the system are invalid (for example Kirchhoff). Its origin in the frontal brain seems to be certain, but we cannot trace it to the occipital lobe. The assumption by Sachs, who agrees with Schröder, that this system contains corona radiata fibers, seems quite plausible. Also Flechsig, Romer and Probst ascribe the fasciculus fronto-occipitalis of Dejerine to the projection fibers. The latter designates this fiber area in the second volume of his Anatomie des Centres nerveux as OF+P, "faisceau complexe contenant a la fois des fibres du faisceau occipito-frontal et des fibres de projections." The designation by Sachs "reticulated corona radiata field" ("reticulirtes Stabkranzfeld") is quite correct. In considering the intimate spatial relationship of this bundle to the caudate nucleus—we refer among other things to the part following the tail of the caudate—it appears quite likely that this bundle, that stands out from the remaining projection fibers to a certain degree, contains fibers that run directly from the cortex to the caudate nucleus, so that we would suggest the designation reticulated cortico-caudal bundle. It would not be impossible that the fibers that constitute the coarse bundle dissolve into the fine braided fibers and from here transition into their terminal station, the caudate nucleus. A definite conclusion will only be possible after examining circumscribed fresh cortical foci that have been prepared according to the method of Marchi. An experimental-anatomical examination is excluded since the bundle cannot be separated sufficiently in the animal.

11. As Muratoff wrote in 1893 (1893a, p. 724): "The tapetum, the posterior end of the subcallosal fasciculus, is . . . not affected by a transection of the corpus callosum." Page 725:

In experiment 24, during the transection of the corpus callosum, I injured the subcallosal fasciculus and this resulted in degeneration of large numbers of its fibers. The degeneration was much more severe than following destruction of various parts of the cortex. I could not follow the degenerated fibers throughout the entire course of the system. After a long course in the sagittal direction they curve upwards and disappear in the cortex after the curvature around the corpus callosum. Therefore the subcallosal fasciculus and the tapetum of the corpus callosum represent one and the same fiber system. Both are long tracts that connect different areas in the cortex of one hemisphere with each other, and therefore they are association fibers in the sense of Meynert. This is a complicated system. All its fibers have the same physiological characteristics but their terminations in the cortex are different. Based on the results of my experiments, one can assume that all fibers of the system originate and terminate in the cortex.

12. In Schröder (1901, p. 90), von Monakow (1892) is quoted as follows: "The fibers of the so-called tapetum of the corpus callosum ('Balkentapete') . . . I consider as association fibers that connect the occipital lobe partly with the parietal and partly with the frontal lobe (fasciculus longitudinalis superior). In normal brains one sees that these fiber bundles cease to be a cohesive fiber tract in the area of the posterior central gyrus and start to scatter from here." In a later work, von Monakow (1899) argues in a similar manner, except that he modifies his opinion concerning the tapetum, which he regards as consisting largely of callosal fibers, and then he says: "The parts of the tapetum that enter the superior longitudinalis fasciculus curve initially in an upward direction and disperse with numerous fascicles through the . . . splenium-portions of the callosum, and only gather again in the area of the posterior thalamus, in fact in a portion that lies between the internal capsule, the tail of the striate and the hemispheric myelin substance."

13. Obersteiner and Redlich, 1902 (p. 286):

Schröder can take credit for pointing out the confusion and its causes surrounding the "Tapetum-question" in two recently published essays. While on the one hand, the tapetum is considered a part of the corpus callosum, on the other hand—especially based on findings on brains lacking the corpus callosum—the callosal nature of the tapetum has been denied, and [instead] it has been allocated to a long association bundle (fasciculus fronto-occipitalis), which itself has been identified respectively as the fasciculus nuclei caudati (Sachs) and the fasciculus subcallosus (Muratoff). Schröder has correctly pointed out that things were brought in parallel here whose relationship cannot be proven. Schröder now argues that this fasciculus subcallosus does not represent the tapetum in a strict sense; he also doubts, that it contains exclusively association fibers. Herewith, Schröder returns with Sachs to the original assumption, that the tapetum exclusively contains callosal fibers. We have previously mentioned that on the one hand people adhere to the callosal nature of the tapetum, while on the other hand it has been assigned to the fasciculus fronto-occipitalis either in whole or in part (for example by Dejerine, Edinger, Monakow, Gianelli, Zingerle). From the fronto-occipital fasciculus we could only track a very small and thin bundle to the lower horn, otherwise it is not in consideration here. The statement by Bianchi, that after ablating the frontal lobe in the monkey, a degeneration of the fronto-occipital association-system according to Marchi cannot be traced to the tapetum may be mentioned here.

14. Muratoff, 1893b (p. 98):

Through faradic excitation, I determined the center of this or that extremity, of the facial muscles and the center of the entire motor area. Afterwards, I removed the corresponding area with a sharp spoon. . . . The operated animals were kept alive for two weeks up to one month . . . The anatomical examination was identical in all cases. I used a new method that was introduced by Marchi.

In his experiment 5 he removed the entire motor area:

The defect in the left hemisphere covers almost the entire area of the motor cortex. The superior border of the defect reaches almost the medial edge of the hemisphere. . . . The lesion is exclusively bordered by cortical substance and only the most superficial layer of the corona radiata fibers is here and there affected. The lesion produced motor weakness of both extremities, inversion of the right-sided paws when walking, and all modalities of sensation were affected on the right side.

15. Muratoff, 1893b (p. 98):

In our material, only its broadened angulated mid-portion is degenerated, [comprising] in fact, the majority of fibers. The medial and inferior portions, which face the corpus callosum and the caudate, are normal. (Fig I and Fig II) . . . [T]he degeneration within this system is always localized to a certain portion, i.e., an expanded protrusion situated above the body of the caudate. On sagittal section one can recognize long degenerated fibers within this bundle; the number of the degenerated fibers depends again on the size of the lesion. On some cuts one can see how the fibers from the cortex run into the subcallosal fascicle. Its degeneration is always on the same side as the lesion. Within this system, the fibers have the following order: from the lesioned area

of the cortex they descend downwards, run around the corpus callosum and enter the subcallosal fascicle. Here they run a longer or shorter distance sagittally, and terminate in the cortex of the frontal or occipital lobe. These are the long bow-like fibers that run below the corpus callosum. The fact that the degeneration is always limited to the expanded mid-portion of the bundle is noteworthy.

16. Muratoff provided further detail in his description of the subcallosal fasciculus (1893a, pp. 721–722):

On sagittal cuts this fiber system is longitudinally oriented. As a consequence of the increase in caliber of the descending part, the thickness of this bundle is different on the various cuts—some taken from the medial border of the hemisphere and others from the lateral. On sections from the medial border of the hemisphere, it looks like a small fiber bundle in the form of a flat arc, corresponding to the curvature of the corpus callosum. On sections taken 0.5 cm further laterally, the subcallosal bundle is much thicker, equal in size to approximately half of the corpus callosum. One can follow the subcallosal fasciculus through the entire length of the corpus callosum. The lower surface is covered by ependyma. Posteriorly, below the splenium of the corpus callosum, this lower border becomes unclear, and merges together with the fornix in one structure. At high magnification, one can convince oneself that here, two leaves of ependyma touch each other. The superior leaf covers the surface of the subcallosal fasciculus, and the inferior leaf is on the upper surface of the fornix. Following the corpus callosum, the subcallosal fasciculus makes two flat curves—a posterior curve below the splenium of the corpus callosum, and an anterior curve below the genu of the corpus callosum. Here the fasciculus becomes much thicker, and without sharp delimitation it becomes a layer of fibers that covers the caudate body. These two fiber categories form, so to speak, an anatomically indivisible bundle at the anterior end of the genu. Further back, one again sees two layers of ependyma that cover the subcallosal fasciculus and the caudate body.

Therefore the parts in the above-mentioned areas have the following relation to one another. 1: corpus callosum; 2: subcallosal fasciculus; 3: superior ependymal layer; 4: the anterior end of the caudate body and the posterior end of the fornix. We provide this detailed topographical and anatomical description of the system because in textbooks it is mostly not described. On reviewing the literature in this regard we find multiple previous reports of this system. As far as I can ascertain, it was described first by Onufrowitz . . . [and subsequently] . . . Kauffman described this in more detail in a brain with agenesis of the corpus callosum. . . . If we imagine that in our cases the corpus callosum was missing, the anatomical position of our subcallosal fasciculus would be the same as the fronto-occipital bundle described by Onufrowitz and Kauffmann. . . . Both authors equate their system with Burdach's arcuate fasciculus. "The genius Burdach recognized this fiber tract, or probably guessed it" (Onufrowicz, p. 322). Reading the original text, one can have doubts about this assumption. Burdach certainly described a bundle that connects the frontal and occipital lobes, but he localized it lateral to the corona radiata at the level of the corpus callosum. Sachs emphasizes this inconsistency. Indeed, our system is positioned as a compact bundle medial to the corona radiata and below the corpus callosum. Without denying the priority of the discovery of the system by Onufrowicz and Kaufmann, I would like to insist on the term "subcallosal fasciculus." As we will see further below, this bundle does not exclusively represent a frontal occipital association tract. In his recent book, Sachs described this system as the fasciculus of the caudate nucleus. Miraculously, Schnopfhagen did not recognize the neuronal nature of this structure, and concluded instead that it was an ependymal layer.

17. Muratoff, 1893 (p. 724):

The subcallosal fasciculus degenerates with destruction of the frontal or occipital gyri. In the latter case, degeneration is not limited to the descending part, but is more diffuse and involves the entire system. From a number of frontal cuts, one can convince oneself that the degenerated fibers do not traverse the entire system. In other words, the subcallosal fasciculus does not carry direct frontal occipital communication tracts. (von Monakow had the same opinion regarding the probable structure of the frontal occipital bundle when he referred to pathological anatomical examinations.) Fibers from the anterior sigmoid gyrus travel a short distance within this bundle anteriorly and posteriorly and then enter the cortex of more distant parts of the hemisphere. This seminal picture is evident from examination of sagittal cuts, regardless of whether the lesion is in the frontal or the occipital lobes.

18. Sachs (1893, pp. 78–79) chose the designation "fasciculus nuclei caudati" because of the:

intimate relationship of the so-called fiber layer to the caudate nucleus. . . . [T]he bundle, which connects the striatum ("Streifenhuegel") with the cortex, in particular with the cortex of the frontal and parietal lobe as well as the insula, and therefore contains association fibers of both parts of the brain, accompanies the caudate nucleus along its entire course lateral to the lateral ventricle. The cross section of this bundle becomes smaller posteriorly in relationship to the decrease in size of the caudate nucleus, so that only the outline of this bundle is present in the descending part of the caudate nucleus. With a thin tapering layer, like a capsule, this bundle covers also the free, ventricular surface of

the nucleus. From this bundle, fibers continually enter the bulk of the caudate nucleus, to dissolve here in its fine fiber meshwork. Another contribution comes also from the external capsule.

19. Dejerine, 1895 (pp. 760 and 765):

This fascicle that we call in our serial sections, occipital frontal fascicle, is in fact the fascicle that was described by Meynert under the name of corona radiata of the caudate nucleus, and by Wernicke under the name of fascicle of the corpus callosum traveling to the internal capsule . . . Experimental work in the dog being performed by Muratoff indicates that the occipito-frontal fascicle of Forel and Onufrowicz (subcallosal fasciculus of Muratoff), is partially degenerated following ablation of the motor sphere, or destruction of the frontal or occipital convolutions.

20. Flechsig, 1896 (p. 3):

The "subcallosal fasciculus" (Muratoff) contains corona radiata bundles that exit from the internal capsule in the area that is situated in front of the mid-portion of the thalamus. Tracts of different lengths run adjacent to the caudate body, in part reach anteriorly to the genu of the corpus callosum, and join the corona radiata of the gyrus fornicatus and the anterior portion of my cortical sensory area ("Tastsphäre"). Some of these corona radiata bundles run almost through a third of the hemispheric length in sagittal direction. Callosal fibers join them and while some accompany them leading rostrally, others curve posteriorly leading to the parietal and occipital lobes. There are only very few bundles that join from the stratum zonale of the caudate nucleus.

21. According to Schröder (1901, p. 89), Oskar Vogt (1895) recognized that Muratoff had described a subcallosal fasciculus, but Vogt:

distinguished the subcallosal fascicle from a very narrow, darkly tinged fiber layer that covers the caudate nucleus on its dorsal and medial surface, [that he regarded as] an association system of the caudate nucleus. Vogt considered the subcallosal fascicle to be an association system of the cortex that has nothing to do with the caudate nucleus. In contrast to Muratoff, he assumed the predominance of long fibers, based only on the experience that association fibers within the brain are always longer when they lie more closely adjacent to the ventricle. He saw especially prominent dispersion of fibers to the cortex frontally and laterally through the external capsule towards the insula.

22. Schröder, 1901 (p. 93):

Experiments by Muratoff and O. Vogt who saw degenerations within this bundle after removal of cortical parts are evidence that it has relationships to the cortex. Two facts however speak against considering this bundle as a pure association system of the cortex, i.e., to assume that its fibers come from the cortex and return to the cortex after a longer or shorter course. At first, the intimate positioning of this bundle to the caudate nucleus is remarkable, it accompanies it as we saw on its entire course and—this is also important—its cross section diameter is always proportional to that of the caudate. In the anterior horn at the head of the caudate nucleus, a massive fiber layer; along the tail of the caudate nucleus in the lower horn, a small and thin fiber layer underneath the ependyma. This seems to suggest with high probability that the caudate bundle and caudate nucleus have a close anatomical and physiological relationship to each other. The second point is the unusual position for a cortical association system in the deepest depth of the hemisphere, directly adjacent to the ventricular wall. It is inconceivable that association fibers from the cortex run so deep only to run back the same far distance, especially since these fibers, as Muratoff's degeneration experiments revealed, are not long ones that connect distant cortical areas, but only run a very short distance in the sagittal direction within the bundle. That must be the reason why O. Vogt disagreed with the findings of Muratoff and made the *a priori* assumption of the predominance of long fibers within the bundle, because of the empirical evidence that association fibers within the brain seem to be longer the further away they are from the cortex. The formation of the fasciculus nuclei caudati, however, argues against the predominance of long sagittal fibers within it. Fibers that run for long stretches in the same direction tend to form compact bundles, whereas the fasciculus nuclei caudati has more the appearance of a meshwork.

23. Obersteiner and Redlich, 1902 (pp. 290–301):

One of us (Redlich, 1897) has seen degeneration of the subcallosal fasciculus after an extensive lesion of the frontal brain that was not limited to the cortex alone, but it was insignificant and could only be seen in short stretches. There is therefore no evidence that the above-mentioned bundle contains fibers directly from the frontal lobe to the occipital lobe. In those cases the lesion extended beyond the cortex, so that a direct relationship between cortex and the fasciculus cannot be alleged, although we can confirm Muratoff's statement that the degeneration of this bundle is restricted to the same side. . . . [A]fter unilateral lesions of posterior parts of the brain, degeneration of the corpus callosum was seen above the lower horn on the other side, but medial to it, immediately adjacent to the ventricular ependyma, one can find a non-degenerated area. In contrast, the statement by Muratoff, that the subcallosal fascicle forms an anatomically indivisible bundle with the fiber layer that covers the caudate nucleus—he obviously means the stratum zonale of the caudate nucleus—is wrong. Moreover it is obvious that both fiber categories only have a spatial relationship—and this to only limited degree—but they are otherwise to be differentiated.

On frontal cuts of adult humans and also in most animals, the basal aspect of the subcallosal fascicle abuts the caudate nucleus and reaches along the medial plane of the caudate nucleus inferiorly, so that it appears that it merges with the thin layer of nerve fibers that wrap around the caudate nucleus on its dorsal and medial surface (Stratum zonale, nuclei caudati of Obersteiner). On closer view, the two layers can be separated from each other; whereas the fibers of the subcallosal fascicle have thin caliber, the fibers of the stratum zonale are a little thicker and represent an even thicker meshwork than the subcallosal fascicle. . . . Both fiber layers can also be separated by reference to their historical development. As Bechterew has described elsewhere, the fibers of the subcallosal fascicle myelinate relatively late; even in a child of several months (Fig. 1) we find the subcallosal fascicle unmyelinated, whereas the stratum zonale is fully developed and covers the caudate nucleus as a narrow and compact nerve fiber layer on its dorsal surface, reaching medially and downwards, separated from the ventricular surface by a thin and bright layer, the ependyma. Carmine preparations or other techniques that stain the cells permit the separation of the subcallosal fascicle from the stratum zonale by yet another means (here one can also convince himself of the correct statement by Sachs that the fasciculus nuclei caudati does not contain ganglia). On such preparations in humans one can easily convince oneself that nests of relatively large cells, which resemble ependymal cells, can be found between the caudate nucleus and the subcallosal fascicle. Here, the glia frequently tend to show a slight aggregation, corresponding to Weigert's striped keel ("Kielstreifen"). These cells can also be found along the medial plane of the caudate nucleus between the ependyma and the stratum zonale, as well as on the outer plane of the caudate nucleus. They can also be seen on the dorsal surface of the subcallosal fascicle that trails dorsally along the corpus callosum, above the former. Not uncommonly one finds crosscut vessels or large lymphatic areas that create border zones. The aggregation of such cells is even more substantial between the subcallosal fascicle and the caudate nucleus in animals such as cats, dogs, horses, calves etc., where one can distinguish the subcallosal fascicle macroscopically. Our findings permit almost no other interpretation than that both formations are differentiated historically through development. The cells described must therefore be considered as remnants of further divisions that existed previously.

Whereas the subcallosal fascicle maintains an intimate spatial relationship to the caudate nucleus in humans so that Sachs suggested the term fascicle nuclei caudati, the situation is profoundly different in animals. Here, the spatial relationship between the caudate nucleus and the subcallosal fascicle is only regional, i.e., it exists only in certain portions of this bundle, if we may be permitted to say it like that. Concerning this matter, however, many differences exist in various animals. . . .

In the most anterior portion as well as posteriorly where it covers the lateral wall of the lower horn of the ventricle the fibers [of the subcallosal fasciculus] have a more parallel direction—at least in a few places—but here they follow a mostly dorso-ventral direction, not a fronto-occipital one, so that in the frontal cut the fibers are cut longitudinally and not transversely. This is in contrast to the assumption of Muratoff and Vogt that the subcallosal fascicle represents a fronto-occipital association system. Rather, the designation fasciculus subcallosus, as chosen by Muratoff, is more correct than the term fasciculus nuclei caudati (Sachs), particularly when considering the situation in animals. Whereas in the human the latter term may be right in that the aforementioned fiber system has a spatial relation to the caudate nucleus, this is not the case in animals as we have seen. But even in humans it is not entirely correct that the caudate nucleus and the subcallosal fascicle are proportional in size to each other. How much less this is true in animals—especially in those animals that have a well-developed bundle—we have previously described in detail. Here, we see a spatial relationship to the caudate nucleus only in certain stretches, but there is always very close attachment to the corpus callosum, which is why it is called subcallosus. It does not, however, represent a fascicle in the ordinary sense in which one understands it to contain fibers oriented in the same direction. Rather, it contains thickly woven fibers that have a great variety of directions. Therefore it seems that the term stratum subcallosum is possibly the best fitting one.

It appears quite difficult to comment on the significance of this fiber system, its origin and its terminations. I can state that the fibers contained in the stratum subcallosum do not originate within it, because, as mentioned earlier, the stratum subcallosum does not contain ganglion cells. Many authors count the subcallosal fascicle among the projection systems . . . Sachs also believes that his fasciculus nuclei caudati provides a connection between cortex and caudate nucleus . . .

An exclusive relation of the subcallosal fascicle to the caudate nucleus cannot be defended for we find the subcallosal fascicle particularly prominent in animals in which the caudate nucleus does not exist. However, a relation to the cortex does not appear to be implausible. On basal cuts in human one sees on extremely ventrally placed cuts, where the subcallosal fascicle is relatively poorly myelinated, more or less distinct bundles of fine fibers that run through its area and cross each other, apparently coming from the frontal cortex, according to what Dejerine designated as

"bundle of the fronto-occipital fascicle to the third frontal gyrus." Considering the small caliber of the fibers that are contained in the subcallosal fascicle it appears quite unlikely that those are long fibers, such as [one sees in] a long association system. We found no evidence for connections to the external capsule as has been assumed by several authors.

24. Riley (1960, p. 568) dismissed the existence of a "[f]asciculus cortico-caudalis reticulatus (Obersteiner-Redlich). This fasciculus is erroneously named and does not connect the cortex and caudate nucleus except for perhaps a few fibers. It is applied to the caudate nucleus laterally. Its fibers probably enter the internal capsule or the thalamic nuclei."

Chapter 20
Muratoff Bundle (Subcallosal Fasciculus) and the External Capsule

1. Burdach, 1822 (p. 130, paragraph 180):

The fibers of the external capsule do not come from the lentiform nucleus and do not have any relationship with it. They also do not come from the crus cerebri or the internal capsule because those lie too far medially. If one peels off the crus cerebri and the lentiform nucleus the external capsule remains preserved in its entirety. However, it is also not a pure "Belegungsmasse" [see FOOTNOTE 2 of chapter 13] which would originate from a focal point or any other place of the lateral surface, but rather it arises inferiorly and medially from the brainstem. To see this one has to remove the unciform fasciculus and the inferior longitudinal fasciculus ("Längenbündel") that are positioned below it. There then appears a horizontal myelinated bundle that runs from medial to lateral, above the uncinate fascicle and the temporal lobe that forms the base of the lentiform nucleus, or under its basal plane, and then curves around the lateral aspect of the basal plane and ascends vertically. The true continuity of this horizontal leaf with the vertical external capsule one can easily recognize on a vertical cross-section in the anterior part of the thalamus by peeling it off. But one can discern it even without peeling it off from the direction of the claustrum, which with its lower part also curves medially.

On the same cut one can now recognize that a layer from the superior part of the thalamus descends at its anterior end along the medial surface to the floor of the third ventricle and then continues laterally in the horizontal leaf, runs laterally and posteriorly in an oblique fashion below the lentiform nucleus and then forms the resting place of the "Markkügelchen" [this designation is unclear], the roots and pillars of the fornix, as well as the anterior commissure and the cribriform plate, and then transitions into the posterior part of the external capsule. But even without such a transection one can find the same relationship when peeling off the fibers of the basal plane of the "Stammlappen" [see FOOTNOTE 2 of chapter 13], and it is therefore certain that the external capsule originates from the fiber system of the tegmentum ("Haube"), and is also one part of the stratum zonale of the thalamus and represents its lower portion. Since the stratum zonale predominantly or exclusively seems to originate from the olivary bundle we are leaning towards assuming that the latter represents the origin of the external capsule. But even disregarding this situation, we sometimes succeeded in tracking the fibers from the olivary nucleus below the blue substance of the rhomboid cavity, through the black semicircle, through the thalamus and along its medial surface and downwards, and through the horizontal myelin leaf below the lentiform nucleus up to the external capsule. We therefore believe that the external capsule, the pale lump of the lentiform nucleus [globus pallidus] and its cover are all initially continuations of the thalamus.

2. Dejerine, 1895 (pp. 807–808):

The external capsule contains a large number of commissural and associative fibers . . . Nevertheless, the external capsule is not devoid of projection fibers, and it provides the main contingent of fibers that are found in the inferomedial thalamic peduncle. The external capsule is covered by the convolutions of the insula, the extreme capsule and the claustrum. It is located on the external aspect of the putamen, and is united with the putamen by a few myelinated fibers. Indeed, there is no separation between these two structures, although many blood vessels are present (lenticulo-caudate and lenticulo-striate arteries) that often are the site of cerebral hemorrhage. In a brain hardened by alcohol or bichromate, following the removal of the insula, extreme capsule and claustrum, the external capsule has the appearance of a half-opened fan, the base of which is traversed by the fibers of the arcuate or superior longitudinal fasciculus. The base exhibits a smooth curve that corresponds to the superior border of the putamen, and the foot of the corona radiata. The top of the fan corresponds to the anterior commissure. The fibers of the medial part of the external capsule are vertically oriented towards the top, those of the posterior and anterior aspects are oriented obliquely in the superior, lateral and anterior directions, or superiorly, laterally and posteriorly, and the most inferior fibers tend to be more horizontally oriented.

The fibers of the external capsule have a very complex origin. Fibers in the medial aspect probably originate from the occipitofrontal fascicle and the medial aspect of the corpus callosum. They reach the external capsule after crossing perpendicular to the fibers in the foot of the corona radiata. In cases of agenesis of the corpus callosum, the external

capsule appears to have developed normally, and thus the callosal contingent of the external capsule does not appear to be very prominent.

The anterior fibers of the external capsule originate from the uncinate fasciculus, and, according to Schnopf-hagen, from the genu and the rostrum of the corpus callosum. These latter fibers travel beneath the rostral end of the corpus striatum and therefore do not intermingle with the foot of the corona radiata. The posterior fibers are provided by the inferior longitudinal fasciculus, the anterior commissure, and the temporal fibers of the uncinate fasciculus. This latter fascicle occupies the entire region of the external capsule that is located beneath the pole of the insula and divides up ("morcelle") the horizontal aspect of the claustrum.

A certain number of obliquely oriented fibers of the external capsule probably belong to a projection system, particularly the inferomedial thalamic peduncle.

Throughout its extent, very small fascicles originate from the external capsule and traverse the claustrum creating small indentations in the claustrum, and terminate in the crest of the convolutions of the insula. Other fibers course towards the gray matter belonging to the vertical or fenestrated portion of the claustrum.

3. The corticostriate projections have received considerable attention in recent years, and some of the salient and representative observations are presented here for reference.

Nauta and Domesick (1984) determined from their studies in the rat that that the striatum is subdivided into a ventromedial, limbic system-afferented region and a dorsolateral, "non-limbic" region largely corresponding to the main distribution of corticostriatal fibers from the motor cortex, and they suggested that the limbic-afferented striatal sector is an interface between the motivational and the more strictly motor aspects of movement. Alexander et al. (1986) viewed the anatomically segregated circuits within the multisynaptic cortico-striatal-thalamic-cortical loops as forming skeletomotor, oculomotor, prefrontal and limbic circuits.

Primary sensorimotor projections to putamen were identified by Kemp and Powell (1970). Jones et al. (1977) observed that sensory projections to striatum overlap projections from the motor cortex, with each cortical area resulting in striatal terminations within interrupted clusters, strips or bands.

The pattern of associative projections to striatum were studied by a number of investigators, including Saint-Cyr et al. (1990), Cavada and Goldman-Rakic (1991), and Yeterian and Pandya (1991, 1993, 1995, 1998) that are summarized below.

Prefrontal projections: Medial and dorsal prefrontal areas project predominantly to the dorsal and central portion of the head and body of the caudate nucleus. Orbital and inferior prefrontal areas are related mainly to the ventral and central portion. There is a medial-lateral topography in the caudate nucleus projections, such that medial and orbital prefrontal areas project medially, and dorsal and ventral arcuate regions project laterally. Prefrontal regions adjacent to the principal sulcus project mainly to the intermediate sector of the head and body. There is some degree of overlap of corticostriatal projections from the different prefrontal sectors, and minor projections are directed to the tail of the caudate nucleus and to the putamen (Yeterian and Pandya, 1991).

Posterior parietal projections: According to Cavada and Goldman-Rakic (1991) all regions of the parietal lobe project to the striatum, but the zones of densest projections vary according to each parietal subdivision. Further, all parietal lobe regions project to a rather extended anteroposterior area in the contralateral striatum, less extensively than the ipsilateral side, but with a similar topographical distribution. The details of the termination patterns from the parietal lobe were similar to those identified by Yeterian and Pandya (1993) as follows. The supplementary sensory area in the caudal portion of the cingulate gyrus projects to the dorsal part of the putamen; the second somatosensory area in the rostral parietal opercular region projects to the ventral part of the putamen, thus resembling the pattern seen from the primary somatosensory cortex. As one progresses from rostral to caudal within both the superior and the inferior parietal regions, projections shift from the putamen to the caudate nucleus. The rostral part of the superior parietal lobule projects predominantly to the dorsal portion of the putamen, whereas caudal superior parietal lobule and the cortex of the upper bank of the intraparietal sulcus have connections with the caudate nucleus as well as the dorsal portion of the putamen. The medial parietal convexity cortex projects strongly to the caudate nucleus, with less extensive projections to the putamen. The rostral portion of the inferior parietal lobule projects mainly to the ventral sector of the putamen and has only minor connections with the caudate nucleus. The middle portion of the inferior parietal lobule has sizable projections to both the putamen and the caudate nucleus. The caudal portion of the inferior parietal lobule and the lower bank of the intraparietal sulcus project predominantly to the caudate nucleus, with relatively minor connections with the putamen.

Superior temporal region projections: The primary auditory cortex has limited projections to the caudoventral putamen and to the tail of the caudate nucleus. The second auditory area within the circular sulcus has connections to the rostral and caudal putamen and to the body and tail of the caudate nucleus. Association areas in the rostral part of the superior temporal gyrus project to rostroventral and caudoventral portions of the putamen, and to ventral portions of the head and body of the caudate nucleus and to the tail. The midportion of the gyrus projects to similar striatal regions, but the connections to the head of the caudate nucleus are less extensive. The caudal portion of the superior temporal gyrus projects more dorsally within the caudal putamen and the head and the body of the caudate nucleus (Yeterian and Pandya, 1998).

Visual projections: Using retrograde and anterograde tracing techniques, Saint-Cyr et al. (1990) determined that temporal, occipital, and parietal visual cortical areas project into the caudate nucleus largely according to proximity, although certain multimodal cortical

areas seem to have a much wider projection. The rostral tail of the caudate nucleus receives cortical afferents from area TE, adjacent portions of areas TF, TH, TG, and occasionally area 35. The posterior tail and ventral genu inputs are from areas TE and TF, TEO, and the ventral parts of prestriate areas V4, V3, and (sparsely) V2. Cortical afferents to the dorsal part of the genu of the caudate nucleus are from prestriate areas MT and PO, parietal area PG, the ventral and lateral intraparietal sulcal areas, and area PE and adjacent area 23. The cortex around the principal sulcus/frontal eye field region, the anterior cingulate cortex, and the superior temporal polysensory area project to each of these caudate nucleus regions. These findings were substantiated by Yeterian and Pandya (1995), who showed that medial and dorsolateral extrastriate regions project to dorsal and lateral parts of the head and body of the caudate nucleus, and to the caudal and dorsal sector of the putamen. The rostral portion of the annectant gyrus has connections to the caudal sector of the body and to the genu of the caudate nucleus, whereas projections from the caudal portion of the lower bank of the superior temporal sulcus are directed to dorsal and central sectors of the caudate head and body as well as the genu and tail, and to the caudal putamen. The ventromedial extrastriate cortex projections resemble those of the medial and dorsolateral regions. Those from the ventrolateral extrastriate region are related mainly to the ventral sector of the body of the caudate nucleus, as well as to the genu and tail, and the caudal putamen. The caudal inferotemporal cortex is related strongly to the tail of the caudate nucleus and to the ventral putamen.

Chapter 21
Anterior Commissure

1. According to Burdach (1822, annotations to paragraph 188), the anterior commissure had been identified by Eustach, Willis, Albin, Haller, Schönlein, Meckel, Lieutaud, Santorini, Malacarne, Rolando, Carus, Tiedemann, Chaussier, and Gordon.

2. Reil, 1812a; Volume XI. Erstes Heft (pp. 91–92):

> One can divide the anterior commissure into a body and two extremities. The body is cylindrical and at least double the caliber of the optic nerve . . . The commissure has entirely the construction of a nerve fiber tract. Indeed, it is a peculiar formation situated in the middle of the brain and running straight through it as distinct nerve fiber tract, which must have a very particular role. The commissure consists of bundles, and the bundles consist of such delicate fibers that they are almost invisible. It separates immediately into these fibers if one cuts into the sheath and divides the delicate cell tissue by which it is contained. . . . The commissure runs from one temporal lobe ("Mittellappen") to the other through the brain. Its mid-portion that separates it into two completely identical halves is situated freely between the two hemispheres of the brain. Above it

the arcs of the fornix ("Zwillingsbinde") curve downwards and reach behind the fornix to the little buttons ("Knöpfchen") [mamillary bodies] behind it. The septum [pellucidum] attaches to the anterior and convex rims of these arcs. In front of the septum, the little bar ("Leistchen") [likely the precommissural septum] ascends from the cribriform plate, runs close to it, and enters the septum above the beak [rostrum] of the corpus callosum. Both little bars are connected by a delicate membrane, are situated in front of the commissure, and join the optic nerves at the superior surface of the commissure. Between these little bars and the crura of the fornix, the commissure enters through an oval hole into the corpus striatum. It runs at the anterior extremity of the thalamus between the thalamus and the posterior edge of the corpus striatum, i.e., into the neck between the two of them, into which the taenia descend. The middle and free portion of the commissure is situated a little higher and posteriorly and sinks to both sides into the gray matter of the corpus striatum, and runs below the first radiation of the corona radiata which it touches and which lies lateral to it. But at times one or two radiations lie medially and surround it like a forceps ("Zange"). More medially, towards the lateral wall of the capsule of the large brain ganglion in which the commissure enters through the oval hole, the corpus striatum and large brain ganglion merge into each other. In this way the anterior commissure enters the large brain ganglion that is situated and expands below the corona radiata, continues through it at a distance of 2 to 3 Lines above the cribriform plate, and curves during this course with a flat horizontal arc, encompasses the crura cerebri concentrically with the optic nerves, curves again towards the temporal lobe and downwards, then runs strongly backwards below the posterior part of the unciform bundle in the entrance to the Sylvian fissure, where its extremities expand like radiations. It therefore follows in its course a superiorly and inferiorly, and anteriorly and posteriorly continuous serpentine line in the horizontal plane. In this way the body of the commissure runs towards the mid-portion of the medial surface of the unciform fascicle and appears on the base of the large brain ganglion from its canal that has its opening facing obliquely and backwards. Behind the bundle it curves backwards in a round, almost, rectangular shape, loses its cylindrical form, and expands in fan-like radiating extremities. These radiations attach to the medial surface of the unciform fascicle and run with it backwards towards the round end of the descending horn and its superior wall. They lie between the external capsule of the large brain ganglion in the Sylvian fissure and the internal capsule that comes from the crus cerebri, and amalgamate with these radiations to form one radiation. This continues in the superior wall of the descending and posterior horn above the tapetum and crosses the radiation

of the superior extremity of the thalamus that runs anteriorly in the lateral horn.

3. Burdach, 1822 (paragraph 188, p. 139):

The anterior commissure is a tract that originates in radiations from the occipital and temporal lobes. It is situated below the corona radiata, running anteriorly along the lentiform nucleus, curves medially, and crosses the midline to the other hemisphere in an oblique fashion. It therefore represents a connection of the occipital lobe, temporal lobe, and Stammlappen [see FOOTNOTE 2 of chapter 13] of both hemispheres . . . [It] remains a compact bundle that forms an uninterrupted single structure with the bundle from the other hemisphere.

Chapter 22
Corpus Callosum

1. Burdach, 1822 (p. 141, paragraph 189):

The corpus callosum ("Balken") is the largest and most evolved ("highest") of all the structures of the brain, and of the "Belegungsorgan" [see Footnote 2, chapter 17] which in its radiation neighbors and equals the radiations of the brainstem, but in its body at the center of the brain opposes its stem and is separated from it by a cave the ceiling of which it forms, and the floor of which is formed by the brainstem. As the corpus callosum arches over the brainstem it lies initially over the entire striatum, but it belongs to all the lobes with the exception of the "Stammlappen" [see Footnote 2, chapter 13]. The breadth is predominant and freely developed.

2. Lamantia and Rakic (1990a) estimate that in the human, the callosum contains axons derived from 2% to 3% of the neurons of the cerebral cortex. Myelinated fibers are present mostly in regions of the callosum linking primary sensory cortices. The smallest myelinated axons and the largest proportion of the unmyelinated axons (30%) are present in callosal areas carrying projections from association cortices. These authors (Lamantia and Rakic, 1990b) further determined that the number of axons in the callosum of the newborn rhesus monkey exceeds that of the adult animal by at least 3.5 times, with the progressive increase in callosal axons occurring from midgestation through birth. The elimination of supernumerary axons that takes place in two phases over approximately 4 months of postnatal life is thought to occur during a process that results in the local proliferation of synapses from a subset of initial interhemispheric projections. Innocenti (1995) views this pruning of callosal axons as playing a role in the evolution of the cerebral cortex by enabling adjustments of cortical connectivity to changes in the number, size, internal organization, and cellular composition of cortical areas.

3. Beevor (1891, p. 165) referred to the work of Quain (1882, volume 2, p. 344) and translated Quain's text as follows:

> From the posterior end, or splenium, of the corpus callosum they (the fibres) arch round the posterior and inferior cornua of the lateral ventricle, forming the upper and outer wall of those parts of the cavity, into the temporo-sphenoidal and the lower part of the occipital lobes. Lastly, from the under part of the splenium fibres pass with a bold sweep (forceps major) into the posterior and superior parts of the occipital lobes.

Beevor also referenced and translated Schwalbe (1881, p. 494), who stated that the hinder part of the body of the corpus callosum and its splenium are destined for the temporal and occipital convolutions:

> The fibres from the posterior part of the body run laterally and inferiorly in an arch, convex outwards, and course in the upper lateral wall of the posterior and inferior horns of the lateral ventricle as a thin layer of white matter, being only covered over by the ependyma, and called the tapetum. This structure contains the callosal fibres for the temporal and the inferior part of the occipital convolutions. The swelling formed on the under surface of the callosal body by the rolling under of the fibres—the splenium proper—sends it fibres to the posterior and upper part of the occipital convolutions in such a way that the latter are supplied by the callosal fibres coming from the angle formed by the splenium with the body, while the posterior part of the occipital convolutions gets its callosal fibres from the splenium itself . . . The arrangement on each side of these concavely-shaped tracts from the splenium forms what is known as the forceps major posterior. It will be seen that, as the splenium is attached directly to the corpus callosum, so the forceps major is in immediate contact with the tapetum, and represents the portion of the tapetum which is rolled up towards the middle line.

4. In de Lacoste et al. (1985), sector I of the human corpus callosum represented 25% of the total anteroposterior distance of the callosum in order to include the rostrum and the genu. The remaining sectors II through V each subtended 18.75% of the total anteroposterior distance of the callosum. The subdivisions of the corpus callosum according to these authors is reproduced here in figure N-3.

5. Witelson (1989) divided the human corpus callosum into seven rostrocaudal divisions. These seven segments are not of equal extent. Her figure 1 on page 805 and the legend to that figure are reproduced here as figure N-4.

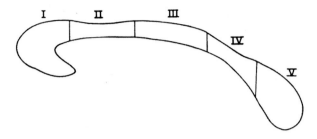

Figure N-3

Diagrammatic representation of the human corpus callosum, subdivided according to deLacoste et al. (1985), figure 30.1.

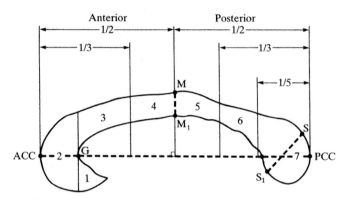

Figure N-4

Diagrammatic representation of the human corpus callosum and its subdivisions according to Witelson, 1989 (p. 805, figure 1). The legend to that figure is as follows: "Diagram of the midsagittal view of the corpus callosum of the human adult, showing the seven regional subdivisions used for area measurement, numbered 1–7. The dashed lines represent the three linear measurements. ACC and PCC indicate the anteriormost and posteriormost points of the callosum, with ACC-PCC defined as the length of the callosum; M and M1, superior and inferior points, respectively, of the callosum at its midpoint, with MM1 defined as the width of the midcallosum; S and S1, superior and inferior points on the posterior bulbous region which is the splenium, chosen such that SS1 is the length of the maximal perpendicular between two parallel lines drawn as tangents to the superior and inferior surfaces of the splenium; G, the anteriormost point on the inner convexity of the anterior callosum. ACC-PCC was used as the linear axis to subdivide the callosum into anterior and posterior halves; anterior, middle and posterior thirds; and the posterior one-fifth region (region 7), which is roughly congruent with the splenium. The line perpendicular to the axis at point G was used to define the anteriormost division of the callosum, roughly congruent with the genu (region 2), and the rostrum (region 1). Region 3 [rostral body] was defined as the anterior one-third minus regions 1 and 2. Region 4 [anterior body] was defined as the anterior one-half minus the anterior one-third. Region 5 [posterior body] was defined as the posterior one-half minus the posterior one-third. Region 6, the isthmus, was defined as the posterior one-third minus the posterior one-fifth. Regions 3, 4, 5 and 6 constitute the body of the callosum."

6. Burdach's views on the corpus callosum were addressed in the monograph of Neuburger/Clarke, 1897/1981 (p. 280, footnote 62). These historians stated that in Burdach's view, "The corpus callosum . . . was associated with mental activity, and by way of its anatomical situation, it constituted the organ of the unifying psyche (i.e., the psyche unified all impressions in a sense of 'I who hear also feel')." In their footnote, Neuburger/Clarke translated Burdach, 1826 (volume 3, p. 484, paragraph 1011): "By means of the corpus callosum both hemispheres can act together in perceiving sensation. The activity aroused by impression on corresponding points in the two hemispheres will therefore be able to produce one and the perceptive image." Further (ibid., paragraph 1012, pp. 484–485): "its [corpus callosum] higher function will be to separate the spatial aspect from sensory perceptions and, by the (abstract) cognition of the phenomena, to proceed to the essence (i.e., the faculty of generalization, as against the perception of individual objects only). It must thus be the organ of reason and, consequently, also of the higher mental functions."

Chapter 24
Internal Capsule

1. Early studies of the internal capsule were conducted in a variety of species, including guinea pig, rabbit, cat, dog, and monkey, as well as in degeneration studies in man. These investigations were performed by such luminaries as Türck, von Monakow, von Gudden, Flechsig, Ferrier, Charcot, Brissaud, Meynert, Dejerine, Obersteiner, Vulpian, Wernicke, Beevor, Horsely, Ferrier, Yeo, and Schäfer, as well as Burdon-Sanderson, Carville and Duret, Franck, Pitres, Nothnagel, Probst, and Veysièrre. This early literature is summarized and referenced in Beevor and Horsely (1890a), as well as in Mellus (1899), Simpson and Jolly (1907), Holmes and May (1909), Levin (1936), Lassek (1954), Bucy (1957), Hanaway and Young (1977), Ross (1980), Davidoff (1990), Fries et al. (1993), and Morecraft et al. (2002).

Chapter 25
Sagittal Stratum

1. Sachs thought the tapetum was the most medial part of the sagittal stratum, hence three strata.

2. Polyak, 1957 (p. 407):

The fibers of the visual radiation are a part of the sagittal fiber system of the brain with which they are continuous. The "inferior" and "superior longitudinal bundles" of the parieto-temporo-occipital lobes of the older anatomists as they appear in macroscopically dissected specimens are a single, solid fiber lamina, precisely as it appears in microscopic sections stained for fibers. There are no visible features by which parts of this lamina belonging to the visual system may be distinguished from those serving other functions. The only criterion for such differentiation is the origin of a particular segment of this lamina in a subcortical nucleus with a known function, e.g., the lateral geniculate nucleus, and its termination in a cortical area whose functional significance is ascertained, e.g., the striate cortex.

Chapter 26
Thalamic Peduncles

1. Klingler held (Klingler and Gloor, 1960, p. 347; Ludwig and Klingler, 1956) that the temporopulvinar bundle of Arnold, the thalamic bundle that we refer to as the ventral subcortical bundle, should be termed the inferior thalamic peduncle, analogous to the "anterior, superior and posterior thalamic peduncles which all pass through different segments of the internal capsule." The bundle that remains named the inferior thalamic peduncle received the designation "extracapsular thalamic peduncle" by Klingler, although this term has not been adopted by other anatomists.

Chapter 28.
Clinical Significance

1. This case was kindly provided to us by Dr. Nagagopal Venna, Massachusetts General Hospital.

2. This case was kindly provided to us by Dr. Fred H. Hochberg, Massachusetts General Hospital.

Abbreviations

II	optic tract		Hy	hypothalamus
AC	anterior commissure		Ia	agranular insular
AD	anterodorsal thalamic nucleus		ICa	internal capsule, anterior limb
AF	arcuate fasciculus		ICp	internal capsule, posterior limb
Am/AMG	amygdala		Idg	dysgranular insula
AM	anteromedian thalamic nucleus		Ig	granular insula
AS	arcuate sulcus		ILF	inferior longitudinal fasciculus
ASi	arcuate sulcus inferior ramus		IOS	inferior occipital sulcus
ASs	superior limb of arcuate sulcus		IPCD	inferior precentral dimple
AV	anteroventral thalamic nucleus		IPro	proisocortex of the insula
BF	basal forebrain		IPS	intraparietal sulcus
CB	cingulum bundle		LF	lateral fissure
CC	corpus callosum		LGN	lateral geniculate nucleus
Cd/CN	caudate nucleus		LP	lateral posterior thalamic nucleus
Cer Ped	cerebral peduncle		LS	lunate sulcus
CF	calcarine fissure		MI	primary motor cortex
CFe	ectocalcarine fissure		MB	Muratoff bundle
Cing S	cingulate sulcus		MDdc	medial dorsal thalamic nucleus, densocellular part
Cl	claustrum		MdLF	middle longitudinal fasciculus
CL	central lateral thalamic nucleus		MDmc	medial dorsal thalamic nucleus, magnocellular part
CM	centromedian thalamic nucleus		MDpc	medial dorsal thalamic nucleus, parvicellular part
CMA	cingulate motor area		MG/MGN	medial geniculate nucleus
CoS	collateral sulcus		NBM	nucleus basalis of Meynert
CS	central sulcus		NRTP	nucleus reticularis tegmenti pontis
Csl	superior central lateral thalamic nucleus		OlfS	olfactory sulcus
DB	diagonal band of Broca		Orb S	orbital sulcus
DHC	dorsal hippocampal commissure		Orb S l	lateral orbital sulcus
dOB	dorsal occipital bundle		Orb S m	medial orbital sulcus
EC	external capsule		OT	olfactory tract
EmC	extreme capsule		OTS	occipitotemporal sulcus
ENTO	entorhinal cortex		pAll	periallocortex
fAF	fibers of the arcuate fasciculus		parahippo	parahippocampal gyrus
fBF	fibers to the basal forebrain		Parasub	parasubiculum
fEMC	fibers of the extreme capsule		PB	pontine bundle
fFOF	fibers of the fronto-occipital fasciculus		Pcn	paracentralis thalamic nucleus
fHy	fibers to the hypothalamus		PeriAm	periamygdaloid area
fSMA	fibers to the supplementary motor area		Perirh	perirhinal area
fZI	fibers to the zona incerta		Pf	parafascicular thalamic nucleus
FOF	fronto-occipital fasciculus		PM	medial pulvinar thalamic nucleus
For	fornix		POMS	parieto-occipital medial sulcus
G	gustatory area		Presub	presubiculum
GP	globus pallidus		Pro	proisocortex
HIPPO	hippocampal formation		ProM	motor proisocortex

Prostr	prostriata	SS	sagittal stratum
PS	principal sulcus	StB	striatal bundle
Put	putamen	STS	superior temporal sulcus
R	reticular nucleus	Th	thalamus
RhF	rhinal fissure	ThB	thalamic bundle
RN	red nucleus	Tma	anterior middle temporal sulcus
RS	rostral sulcus	Tmp	posterior middle temporal sulcus
SB	subcortical bundle	Tp	tapetum
Sc.	section	UB	uncinate bundle
Scs.	sections	UF	uncinate fasciculus
SI	substantia innominata	V	ventricle
SII	second somatosensory area	VHC	ventral hippocampal commissure
SLF I	superior longitudinal fasciculus subcomponent I	VL	ventral lateral thalamic nucleus
SLF II	superior longitudinal fasciculus subcomponent II	VLc	ventral lateral thalamic nucleus, caudal part
SLF III	superior longitudinal fasciculus subcomponent III	VLm	ventral lateral thalamic nucleus, medial part
SMA	supplementary motor area	VSB	ventral subcortical bundle
SN	substantia nigra	X	thalamic nucleus X
SPCD	superior precentral dimple	ZI	zona incerta
SpS	suprasplenial sulcus		

References

Abe O, Masutani Y, Aoki S, et al. (2004). Topography of the human corpus callosum using diffusion tensor tractography. J Comput Assist Tomogr 28:533–539.

Adams G. (1798). Essays on the Microscope; Containing a Practical Description of the Most Improved Microscopes; A General History of Insects, Their Transformation, Peculiar Habits, and Economy Etc. Second edition with considerable additions and improvements by Frederick Kanmacher. London: Dillon and Keating. Dedication to the King, pp. v–viii.

Adams JH, Doyle D, Ford I, Gennarelli TA, Graham DI, McLellan DR. (1989). Diffuse axonal injury in head injury: definition, diagnosis and grading. Histopathology 15:49–59.

Adey WR. (1951). An experimental study of the hippocampal connexions of the cingulate cortex in the rabbit. Brain 74:233–247.

Adey WR, Meyer M. (1952). An experimental study of hippocampal afferent pathways from prefrontal and cingulate areas in the monkey. J Anat 86:58–74.

Aicardi J, Chevrie JJ. (1994). The Aicardi syndrome. In: Lassonde M, Jeeves MA, eds. Callosal Agenesis, pp. 7–17. New York: Plenum Press.

Akelaitis AJ. (1941a). Studies on the corpus callosum: (II) The higher visual functions in each homonymous field following complete section of the corpus callosum. Arch Neurol Psychiat 45:788–796.

Akelaitis AJ. (1941b). Studies on the corpus callosum: (VIII) The effects of partial and complete seciont of the corpus callosum on psychopathic epileptics. Am J Psych 98:409–414.

Akelaitis AJ. (1942). Studies on the corpus callosum: (VI) Orientation (temporal-spatial gnosis) following section of the corpus callosum. Arch Neurol Psychiat 48:914–937.

Akelaitis AJ, Smith KR. (1942). Studies on the corpus callosum: (I) Laterality in behavior and bilateral motor organization in man before and after section of the corpus callosum. Arch Neurol Psychiat 47:519–543.

Albert ML, Feldman RG, Willis AL. (1974). The "subcortical dementia" of progressive supranuclear palsy. J Neurol Neurosurg Psychiatry 37:121–130.

Alexander GE, Crutcher MD, DeLong MR. (1990). Basal ganglia-thalamocortical circuits: parallel substrates for motor, oculomotor, "prefrontal" and "limbic" functions. Prog Brain Res 85:119–146.

Alexander GE, DeLong MR, Strick PL. (1986). Parallel organization of functionally segregated circuits linking basal ganglia and cortex. Annu Rev Neurosci 9:357–381.

Alexander MP, Baker E, Naeser MA, Kaplan E, Palumbo C. (1992). Neuropsychological and neuroanatomical dimensions of ideomotor apraxia. Brain 115:87–107.

Alivisatos B, Milner B. (1989). Effects of frontal or temporal lobectomy on the use of advance information in a choice reaction time task. Neuropsychologia 27:495–503.

Almkvist O, Wahlund LO, Andersson-Lundman G, Basun H, Backman L. (1992). White-matter hyperintensity and neuropsychological functions in dementia and healthy aging. Arch Neurol 49:626–632.

Amaral DG, Behniea H, Kelly JL. (2003). Topographic organization of projections from the amygdala to the visual cortex in the macaque monkey. Neuroscience 118:1099–1120.

Amaral DG, Insausti R, Cowan WM. (1983). Evidence for a direct projection from the superior temporal gyrus to the entorhinal cortex in the monkey. Brain Res 275:263–277.

Amaral DG, Price JL. (1984). Amygdalo-cortical projections in the monkey (Macaca fascicularis). J Comp Neurol 230:465–496.

Amunts K, Weiss PH, Mohlberg H, et al. (2004). Analysis of neural mechanisms underlying verbal fluency in cytoarchitectonically defined stereotaxic space: the roles of Brodmann areas 44 and 45. Neuroimage 22:42–56.

Amunts K, Zilles K. (2001). Advances in cytoarchitectonic mapping of the human cerebral cortex. Neuroimaging Clin North Am 11:151–169.

Andermann F, Andermann E. (1994). The Andermann syndrome: agenesis of the corpus callosum and sensorimotor neuropathy. In: Lassonde M, Jeeves MA, eds. Callosal Agenesis, pp. 19–26. New York: Plenum Press.

Andersen RA, Asanuma C, Essick G, Siegel RM. (1990). Corticocortical connections of anatomically and physiologically defined subdivisions within the inferior parietal lobule. J Comp Neurol 296:65–113.

Anderson D, Ahmed A. (2003). Treatment of patients with intractable obsessive-compulsive disorder with anterior capsular stimulation. Case report. J Neurosurg 98:1104–1108.

Angrilli A, Palombo D, Cantagallo A, Maietti A, Stegagno L. (1999). Emotional impairment after right orbitofrontal lesion in a patient without cognitive deficits. NeuroReport 10:1741–1746.

Anton G, Zingerle H. (1902). Bau, Leistung und Erkrankung des menschlichen Stirnhirnes. Graz: Leuschner & Lubensky.

Antunes NL, Small TN, George D, Boulad F, Lis E. (1999). Posterior leukoencephalopathy syndrome may not be reversible. Pediatr Neurol 20:241–243.

Aouizerate B, Cuny E, Martin-Guehl C, et al. (2004). Deep brain stimulation of the ventral caudate nucleus in the treatment of obsessive-compulsive disorder and major depression. Case report. J Neurosurg 101:682–686.

Archambault LS. (1905). Le faisceau longitudinal inferieur et le faisceau optique central. Revue Neurol 13:1053–1066.

Archambault LS. (1909). The inferior longitudinal bundle and the geniculocalcarine fasciculus. A contribution to the anatomy of the tract-systems of the cerebral hemisphere. Albany Med Ann 30:118–143.

Ariëns-Kappers CU, Huber GC, Crosby EC. (1936). The Comparative Anatomy of the Nervous System of Vertebrates, Including Man. New York: Macmillan.

Arnold F. (1838a). Tabulae Anatomicae. Fasciculus I. Continens Icones cerebri et medullae spinalis. Turici, Impensis Orelii, Fuesslini et sociorum.

Arnold F. (1838b). Untersuchungen im Gebiete der Anatomie und Physiologie mit besonderer Hinsicht auf seine anatomischen Tafeln. Bemerkungen über den Bau des Hirns und Rückensmarks nebst Beiträgen zur Physiologie des zehnten und eilften Hirnnerven, mehrern kritischen Mitteilungen so wie verschiedenen pathologischen und anatomischen Beobachtung. Zürich: Verlage von S. Höhr.

Arnold F. (1851). Handbuch der Anatomie des Menschen mit besondere Rücksicht auf Physiologie und praktische Medicin, Volume 2. Freiburg im Breslau: Herder'sche Verlagshandlung.

Asanuma C, Andersen RA, Cowan WM. (1985). The thalamic relations of the caudal inferior parietal lobule and the lateral prefrontal cortex in monkeys: divergent cortical projections from cell clusters in the medial pulvinar nucleus. J Comp Neurol 241: 357–381.

Asanuma C, Thach WR, Jones EG. (1983). Anatomical evidence for segregated focal groupings of efferent cells and their terminal ramifications in the cerebellothalamic pathway of the monkey. Brain Res 286:267–297.

Avicenna (Abu 'Ali al-Husayn ibn 'Abd Allah ibn Sina). Canon medicinae (Kitab al-Qanun fi al-tibb). Venice: Simon Bevilaqua, 1500. http://www.nlm.nih.gov/hmd/arabic/E8.html.

Azuma M, Suzuki H. (1984). Properties and distribution of auditory neurons in the dorsolateral prefrontal cortex of the alert monkey. Brain Res 298:343–346.

Babikian V, Ropper AH. (1987). Binswanger's disease: a review. Stroke 18:2–12.

Bachevalier J, Mishkin M. (1986). Visual recognition impairment follows ventromedial but not dorsolateral prefrontal lesions in monkeys. Behav Brain Res 20:249–261.

Bagchi AK. (1979). The evolution and chronology of ancient Indian medical sciences. Bull Indian Inst Hist Med Hyderabad. 9:21–26.

Bailey P, Bonin G von, Davis EW, Garol H, McCulloch WS, Roseman E, Silveira A. (1944). Functional organization of the medial aspect of the primate cortex. J Neurophysiol 7:51–55.

Bailey P, Bonin G von, Garol HW, McCulloch WS. (1941). Cortical origin and distribution of corpus callosum and anterior commissure in chimpanzee (Pan satyrus). J Neurophysiol 4:564–571.

Bailey P, Bonin G von, Garol HW, McCulloch WS. (1943a). Functional organization of temporal lobe of monkey (Macaca mulatta) and chimpanzee (Pan satyrus). J Neurophysiol 6:121–128.

Bailey P, Bonin G von, Garol HW, McCulloch WS. (1943b). Long association fibers in cerebral hemispheres of monkey and chimpanzee. J Neurophysiol 6:129–134.

Baleydier C, Mauguiere F. (1980). The duality of the cingulate gyrus in monkey. Neuroanatomical study and functional hypothesis. Brain 103:525–554.

Ballantine HT, Bouckoms AJ, Thomas EK, Gitiunas IE. (1987). Treatment of psychiatric illness by stereotactic cingulotomy. Biol Psychiatry 22:807–819.

Ballantine HT, Cassidy WL, Flanagan NB, Marino R Jr. (1967). Stereotaxic anterior cingulotomy for neuropsychiatric illness and intractable pain. J Neurosurg 26:488–495.

Ballowitz E, Ehrlich P, Mosse M, Krause R, Rosin H, Weigert C. (1903). Encyklopädie der mikroskopischen Technik, mit besonderer Berücksichtigung der Färbelehre. Berlin: Urban & Schwarzenberg.

Baloh RW, Vinters HV. (1995). White matter lesions and disequilibrium in older people. II. Clinicopathologic correlation. Arch Neurol 52:975–981.

Baloh RW, Yue Q, Socotch TM, Jacobson KM. (1995). White matter lesions and disequilibrium in older people. I. Case-control comparison. Arch Neurol 52:970–974.

Bammer R, Acar B, Moseley ME. (2003). In vivo MR tractography using diffusion imaging. Eur J Radiol 45:223–234.

Barbas H. (1988). Anatomic organization of basoventral and mediodorsal visual recipient prefrontal regions in the rhesus monkey. J Comp Neurol 276:313–342.

Barbas H, De Olmos J. (1990). Projections from the amygdala to basoventral and mediodorsal prefrontal regions in the rhesus monkey. J Comp Neurol 300:549–571.

Barbas H, Mesulam M-M. (1981). Organization of afferent input to subdivisions of area 8 in the rhesus monkey. J Comp Neurol 200:407–431.

Barbas H, Pandya DN. (1984). Topography of commissural fibers of the prefrontal cortex in the rhesus monkey. Exp Brain Res 55:187–191.

Barbas H, Pandya DN. (1987). Architecture and frontal cortical connections of the premotor cortex (area 6) in the rhesus monkey. J Comp Neurol 256:211–228.

Barbas H, Pandya DN. (1989). Architecture and intrinsic connections of the prefrontal cortex in the rhesus monkey. J Comp Neurol 286:353–375.

Barbieri C, De Renzi E. (1988). The executive and ideational components of apraxia. Cortex 24:535–543.

Barker LF. (1899). The Nervous System and Its Constituent Neurones. New York: D. Appleton and Co.

Barnea-Goraly N, Kwon H, Menon V, Eliez S, Lotspeich L, Reiss

AL. (2004). White matter structure in autism: preliminary evidence from diffusion tensor imaging. Biol Psychiatry 55:323–326.

Barnes CL, Pandya DN. (1992). Efferent cortical connections of multimodal cortex of the superior temporal sulcus in the rhesus monkey. J Comp Neurol 318:222–244.

Basser PJ, Mattiello J, LeBihan D. (1994). MR diffusion tensor spectroscopy and imaging. Biophys J 66:259–267.

Basser PJ, Pajevic S, Pierpaoli C, Duda J, Aldroubi A. (2000). In vivo fiber tractography using DT-MRI data. Magnetic Resonance Imaging in Medicine 44:625–632.

Bassetti C, Bogousslavsky J, Barth A, Regli F. (1996). Isolated infarcts of the pons. Neurology 46:165–175.

Bayard S, Gosselin N, Robert M, Lassonde M. (2004). Inter- and intra-hemispheric processing of visual event-related potentials in the absence of the corpus callosum. J Cogn Neurosci 16:401–414.

Bechara A, Damasio AR, Damasio H, Anderson SW. (1994) Insensitivity to future consequences following damage to human prefrontal cortex. Cognition 50:7–15.

Bechterew W von. (1899). Die Leitungsbahnen im Gehirn und Rückenmark: ein Handbuch für das Studium des Aufbaues und der innerne Verbindungen des Nervensystemes. Second edition. Deutsch von Richard Weinberg. Leipzig: A. Georgi. Translated into French as Bechterew W. (1900). Les voies de conduction de cerveau et de la möelle. Lyon: A. Storck & Cie.

Beck PD, Kaas JH. (1998). Thalamic connections of the dorsomedial visual area in primates. J Comp Neurol 396:381–398.

Beevor CE. (1886). On Professor Hamilton's theory concerning the corpus callosum. Brain 8:377–379.

Beevor CE. (1891). On the course of the fibres of the cingulum and the posterior parts of the corpus callosum and fornix in the marmoset monkey. Phil Trans Roy Soc London B 182:135–199.

Beevor CE. (1898). Diseases of the Nervous System: A Handbook for Students and Practitioners. Philadelphia: P. Blackiston, Son & Co.

Beevor CE, Horsley V. (1887). A minute analysis (experimental) of the various movements produced by stimulating in the monkey different regions of the cortical centre for the upper limb, as defined by Professor Ferrier. Phil Trans Roy Soc Lond B 178:153–167.

Beevor CE, Horsley V. (1888). A further minute analysis by electrical stimulation of the so-called motor region of the cortex cerebri in the monkey (Macacus sinicus). Phil Trans Roy Soc Lond B 179:205–256.

Beevor CE, Horsley V. (1890a). An experimental investigation into the arrangement of the excitable fibres of the internal capsule of the bonnet monkey (Macacus sinicus). Phil Trans Roy Soc Lond B 181:49–88.

Beevor CE, Horsley V. (1890b). A record of the results obtained by electrical excitation of the so-called motor cortex and internal capsule in an orang-outang (Simia satyrus). Phil Trans Roy Soc Lond B 181:129–158.

Beevor CE, Horsley V. (1894). A further minute analysis by electrical stimulation of the so-called motor region (facial area) of the cortex cerebri in the monkey (Macacus sinicus). Phil Trans Roy Soc Lond B 185:39–81.

Benson DA, Hienz RD, Goldstein MH Jr. (1981). Single-unit activity in the auditory cortex of monkeys actively localizing sound sources: spatial tuning and behavioral dependency. Brain Res 219:249–267.

Benson DF, Geschwind N. (1970). Developmental Gerstmann syndrome. Neurology 20:293–298.

Benson DF, Sheramata WA, Bouchard R, Segarra JM, Price D, Geschwind N. (1973). Conduction aphasia: a clinicopathological study. Arch Neurol 28:339–346.

Berke JJ. (1960). The claustrum, the external capsule and the extreme capsule of Macaca mulatta. J Comp Neurol 115:297–321.

Bianchi L, D'Abundo G. (1886). Le degenerazioni discendenti sperimentali nel cervello e nel midollo spinale a contributo della dotrina della localizzazioni cerebrali. La Psichiatria 4:249–268.

Biber MP, Kneisley LW, LaVail JH. (1978). Cortical neurons projecting to the cervical and lumbar enlargements of the spinal cord in young and adult rhesus monkeys. Exp Neurol 59:492–508.

Bielschowsky M. (1902). Die Silberimprägnation der Achsencylinder. Neurologisches Zentralblatt 21:579–84.

Biemond A. (1930). Experimentell-anatomische Untersuchungen über die corticofugalen optischen Verbindungen bei Kaninchen und Affen. Zeitschrift für die gesamte Neurologie und Psychiatrie 129:65–127.

Black P, Myers RE. (1965). A neurological investigation of eye-hand control in the chimpanzee. In: Ettlinger EG, ed. Functions of the Corpus Callosum, pp. 47–59. Ciba Foundation Study Group No. 20, in honour of Lord Adrian. Boston: Little, Brown and Company.

Blatt GJ, Andersen RA, Stoner GR. (1990). Visual receptive field organization and cortico-cortical connections of the lateral intraparietal area (area LIP) in the macaque. J Comp Neurol 299:421–445.

Blatt GJ, Pandya DN, Rosene DL. (2003). Parcellation of cortical afferents to three distinct sectors in the parahippocampal gyrus of the rhesus monkey: an anatomical and neurophysiological study. J Comp Neurol 466:161–179.

Blum F. (1893). Der Formaldehyd als Härtungsmittel. Ztschr f Wissensch Mikr 10:314–315.

Bogen JE, Bogen GM. (1988). Creativity and the corpus callosum. Psychiatr Clin North Am 11:293–301.

Bogousslavsky J, Regli F, Uske A. (1988). Thalamic infarcts: clinical syndromes, etiology, and prognosis. Neurology 38:837–848.

Bonin G von. (1960). Some Papers on the Cerebral Cortex. Translated from the French and German. Springfield, Ill: Thomas.

Bonin G von, Bailey P. (1947). The Neocortex of Macaca mulatta. Urbana, IL: University of Illinois Press.

Boussaoud D, Desimone R, Ungerleider LG. (1991). Visual topography of area TEO in the macaque. J Comp Neurol 306:554–575.

Braak H. (1978). The pigment architecture of the human temporal lobe. Anat Embryol 154:213–240.

Bradley WG Jr, Whittemore AR, Watanabe AS, Davis SJ, Teresi LM, Homyak M. (1991). Association of deep white matter infarction with chronic communicating hydrocephalus: implications regarding the possible origin of normal-pressure hydrocephalus. AJNR Am J Neuroradiol 12:31–39.

Brinkman SD, Sarwar M, Levin HS, Morris HH 3rd. (1981). Quantitative indexes of computed tomography in dementia and normal aging. Radiology 138:89–92.

Broca P. (1878). Anatomie comparée des circonvolutions cérébrales. Le grand lobe limbique. Revue d'Anthropologie, 1:385–498.

Brodal A. (1948). The origin of the fibres of the anterior commissure in the rat. Experimental studies. J Comp Neurol 88:157–205.

Brodal A. (1981). Neurological Anatomy in Relation to Clinical Medicine, 3rd ed. New York: Oxford University Press.

Brodal P. (1978). The corticopontine projection in the rhesus monkey. Origin and principles of organization. Brain 101:251–283.

Brodmann K. (1905). Beitraege zur histologischen Lokalisation der Grosshirnrinde. III Mitteilung. Die Rindenfelder der niederen Affen. J Psychol Neurol 4:177–226.

Brodmann K. (1908). Beiträge zur histologischen Lokalisation der Grosshirnrinde. J Psychol Neurol 10:231–246.

Brodmann K. (1909). Vergleichende Lokalisationslehre der Grosshirnrinde in ihren Principien, dargestellt auf grund des Zellenbaues. Leipzig:Johann Ambrosius Barth Verlag. Translated into English by Laurence J. Garey as Localisation in the Cerebral Cortex. (London: Smith-Gordon, 1994; new impression, London: Imperial College Press, 1999).

Brown JW, ed. (1988). Agnosia and Apraxia: Selected Papers of Liepmann, Lange, and Pötzl. Translations by George Dean, Ellen Perecman, Emil Franzen, Joachim Luwisch. Hillside, NJ: Lawrence Erlbaum Associates.

Bruce A. (1887–1888). On a case of absence of the corpus callosum in the human brain. Proc R Soc Edinb 15:320–341.

Bruce A. (1889). On the absence of the corpus callosum in the human brain, with the description of a new case. Brain 12:171–190.

Brun A, Englund E. (1986). A white matter disorder in dementia of the Alzheimer type: a pathoanatomical study. Ann Neurol 19:253–262.

Buccino G, Binkofski F, Fink GR, et al. (2001). Action observation activates premotor and parietal areas in a somatotopic manner: an fMRI study. Eur J Neurosci 13:400–404.

Bucy P, Klüver H. (1940). Anatomic changes secondary to temporal lobectomy. Arch Neurol Psychiatry 44:1142–1146.

Bucy PC. (1957). Is there a pyramidal tract? Brain 80:376–392.

Bullier J, Schall JD, Morel A. (1996). Functional streams in occipito-frontal connections in the monkey. Behav Brain Res 76:89–97.

Burdach KF (CF). (1822–1826). Vom Baue und Leben des Gehirns. Leipzig: Zweyter Band, 1822; Dritter band,1826. In der Dyk'schen Buchhandlung.

Butter CM, Snyder DR, McDonald JA. (1970). Effects of orbital frontal lesions on aversive and aggressive behaviors in rhesus monkeys. J Comp Physiol Psychol 72:132–144.

Cajal S Ramón y. (1894). La fine structure des centres nerveux (Croonian Lecture). Proc R Soc Lond 55:444–468.

Cajal S Ramón y. (1899–1904). Textura del sistema nervioso del hombre y de los vertebrados. Estudios sobre el plan estructural y composición histológica de los centros nerviosos adicionados de consideraciones fisiológicas fundadas en los nuevos descubrimientos. Nicolás Moya; Madrid. Translated into English by P. Pasik and T. Pasik as Texture of the Nervous System of Man and the Vertebrates: Studies on the Structural Plan and Histologic Composition of the Neural Centers with Physiologic Considerations based on New Discoveries (two volumes; an annotated and edited translation of the original Spanish text with the additions of the French version. Wien, New York:Springer, 1999.)

Cajal S Ramón y. (1901). Estudios sobre la corteza cerebral humana IV: Estructura de la corteza cerebral olfativa del hombre y mamíferos. Trabajos del Laboratorio de Investigaciones Biológicas de la Universidad de Madrid. 1:1–140. Translated into English by J. DeFelipe and E.G. Jones as Studies on the human cerebral cortex IV. Structure of the olfactory cerebral cortex of man and mammals. In: Cajal on the Cerebral Cortex. An Annotated Translation of the Completed Writings, pp. 289–362 (New York: Oxford University Press, 1988).

Cajal S Ramón y. (1901–1902). Trabajos del Laboratorio de Investigaciones Biológicas de la Universidad de Madrid, Tomo I. Translated by L. M. Kraft as Studies on the Cerebral Cortex (Limbic Structures). Chicago: Year Book, 1955.

Cajal S Ramón y. (1909–1910). Histologie du système nerveux de l'homme et des vertébrés. Translated into French by L. Azoulay. Paris: Maloine. Translated into English by N. Swanson N and L. W. Swanson as Histology of the Nervous System of Man and Vertebrates. New York: Oxford University Press, 1995.

Cajal S Ramón y. (1933). Neuronismo o reticularismo? Las pruebas objetivas de la unidad anatómica de las células nerviosas. Archivos Neurobiol 13:570–646.

Campbell AW. (1905). Histological Studies on the Localisation of Cerebral Function. Cambridge: CambridgeUniversity Press.

Capizzano AA, Acion L, Bekinschtein T, et al. (2004). White matter hyperintensities are significantly asssociated with cortical atrophy in Alzheimer's disease. J Neurol Neurosurg Psychiatry 75:822–827.

Caplan LR, DeWitt LD, Pessin MS, Gorelick PB, Adelman LS. (1988). Lateral thalamic infarcts. Arch Neurol 45:959–964.

Caplan LR, Schmahmann JD, Kase CS, et al. (1990). Caudate infarcts. Arch Neurol 47:133–143.

Caplan LR, Stein RW. (1986). Stroke: A Clinical Approach. Boston: Butterworths.

Carpenter MB. (1976). Human Neuroanatomy, 7th ed. Baltimore: Williams & Wilkins.

Carville C, Duret H. (1875). Sur les functions des hemisphères cérébraux. Arch de Physiologie Normale et Pathologique 2:352–491.

Catani M, Howard RJ, Pajevic S, Jones DK. (2002). Virtual in vivo interactive dissection of white matter fasciculi in the human brain. Neuroimage 17:77–94.

Catani M, Jones DK, Donato R, Ffytche DH. (2003). Occipito-temporal connections in the human brain. Brain 126:2093–2107.

Cavada C, Goldman-Rakic PS. (1989). Posterior parietal cortex in rhesus monkey: II. Evidence for segregated corticocortical networks linking sensory and limbic areas with the frontal lobe. J Comp Neurol 287:422–445.

Cavada C, Goldman-Rakic PS. (1991). Topographic segregation of corticostriatal projections from posterior parietal subdivisions in the macaque monkey. Neuroscience 42:683–696.

Cellerini M, Konze A, Caracchini G, Santoni M, Dal Pozzo G. (1997). Magnetic resonance imaging of cerebral associative white matter bundles employing fast-scan techniques. Acta Anat (Basel) 158:215–221.

Cernak I, Vink R, Zapple DN, et al. (2004). The pathobiology of moderate diffuse traumatic brain injury as identified using a new experimental model of injury in rats. Neurobiol Dis 17:29–43.

Chabriat H, Tournier-Lasserve E, Vahedi K, et al. (1995). Autosomal dominant migraine with MRI white-matter abnormalities mapping to the CADASIL locus. Neurology 45:1086–1091.

Charcot JM. (1878). Lectures on localization in diseases of the brain, delivered at the Faculté de Médicine, Paris in 1875. Bourneville DM, ed. Translated by Edward P. Fowler. New York: William Wood.

Charcot JM. (1883). Leçons sur les localisations dans les maladies du cerveau et de la moëlle épinière. Lectures on the Localisation of Cerebral and Spinal Diseases: delivered at the Faculty of Medicine of Paris, translated and edited by Walter Baugh Hadden. London: New Sydenham Society.

Chavis DA, Pandya DN. (1976). Further observations on cortico-frontal connections in the rhesus monkey. Brain Res 117:369–386.

Christakou A, Robbins TW, Everitt BJ. (2004). Prefrontal cortical-ventral striatal interactions involved in affective modulation of attentional performance: implications for corticostriatal circuit function. J Neurosci 24:773–780.

Christiaens JL, Blond S. (1998). Acquired lesions of the corpus callosum. Neurochirurgie 44(Suppl 1):116–124.

Christiansen P, Larsson HB, Thomsen C, Wieslander SB, Henriksen O. (1994). Age-dependent white matter lesions and brain volume changes in healthy volunteers. Acta Radiol 35:117–122.

Chrysikopoulos H, Andreou J, Roussakis A, Pappas J. (1997). Infarction of the corpus callosum: computed tomography and magnetic resonance imaging. Eur J Radiol 25:2–8.

Chukwudelunzu FE, Meschia JF, Graff-Radford NR, Lucas JA. (2001). Extensive metabolic and neuropsychological abnormalities associated with discrete infarction of the genu of the internal capsule. J Neurol Neurosurg Psychiatry 71:658–662.

Chung CS, Caplan LR, Yamamoto Y, et al. (2000). Striatocapsular haemorrhage. Brain 123:1850–1862.

Ciccarelli O, Parker GJ, Toosy AT, et al. (2003). From diffusion tractography to quantitative white matter tract measures: a reproducibility study. Neuroimage 18:348–359.

Cipolloni PB, Pandya DN. (1985). Topography and trajectories of commissural fibers of the superior temporal region in the rhesus monkey. Exp Brain Res 57:381–389.

Clarke E, O'Malley CD. (1996). The Human Brain and Spinal Cord. A Historical Study Illustrated by Writings from Antiquity to the Twentieth Century, 2nd ed. San Francisco: Norman Publishing.

Clarke S, Bellmann Thiran A, Maeder P, et al. (2002). What and where in human audition: selective deficits following focal hemispheric lesions. Exp Brain Res 147:8–15.

Clarke S, Lindemann A, Maeder P, Borruat FX, Assal G. (1997). Face recognition and postero-inferior hemispheric lesions. Neuropsychologia 35:1555–1563.

Clarke S, Thiran AB. (2004). Auditory neglect: what and where in auditory space. Cortex 40:291–300.

Coffey CE, Figiel GS, Djang WT, Saunders WB, Weiner RD. (1989). White matter hyperintensity on magnetic resonance imaging: clinical and neuroanatomic correlates in the depressed elderly. J Neuropsychiatry Clin Neurosci 1:135–144.

Colby CL, Gattass R, Olson CR, Gross CG. (1988). Topographical organization of cortical afferents to extrastriate visual area PO in the macaque: A dual tracer study. J Comp Neurol 269:392–413.

Colombo M, Rodman HR, Gross CG. (1996). The effects of superior temporal cortex lesions on the processing and retention of auditory information in monkeys (Cebus apella). J Neurosci 16:4501–4517.

Combs CM. (1949). Fiber and cell degeneration in the albino rat brain after hemidecortication. J Comp Neurol 90:373–401.

Cooper IS, Upton AR, Amin I. (1980). Reversibility of chronic neurologic deficits. Some effects of electrical stimulation of the thalamus and internal capsule in man. Appl Neurophysiol 43:244–258.

Cooper IS, Upton AR, Amin I. (1982). Chronic cerebellar stimulation (CCS) and deep brain stimulation (DBS) in involuntary movement disorders. Appl Neurophysiol 45:209–217.

Corti A. (1851). Recherches sur l'organe de l'ouïe des mammifères. Ztschr f Wissensch Zool 3:109–169. Referenced in Walker EA (1938).

Cosgrove GR, Rauch SL. (2003). Stereotactic cingulotomy. Neurosurg Clin North Am 14:225–235.

Courtney SM, Petit L, Haxby JV, Ungerleider LG. (1988). The role of prefrontal cortex in working memory: examining the contents of consciousness. Philos Trans R Soc Lond B 353:1819–1828.

Cowan WM, Gottlieb DI, Hendrickson AE, Price JL, Woolsey TA. (1972). The autoradiographic demonstration of axonal connections in the central nervous system. Brain Res 37:21–51.

Crick F, Jones E. (1993). Backwardness of human neuroanatomy. Nature 361:109–110.

Critchley M. (1953). The Parietal Lobes. London: E. Arnold.

Critchley M. (1979). The Divine Banqet of the Brain, and Other Essays. New York: Raven Press.

Crosby EC, Humphrey T, Lauer EW. (1962). Correlative Anatomy of the Nervous System. New York: Macmillan.

Crosby EC, Schnitzlein HN. (1982). Comparative Correlative Neuroanatomy of the Vertebrate Telencephalon. New York: Macmillan.

Crosson B. (1985). Subcortical aphasia: a working model. Brain and Language 25:257–292.

Crosson B. (1999). Subcortical mechanisms in language: lexical-semantic mechanisms and the thalamus. Brain Cogn 40:414–438.

Cummings JL. (1988). Depression in vascular dementia. Hillside J Clin Psychiatry 10:209–231.

Cumming WJ. (1970). An anatomical review of the corpus callosum. Cortex 6:1–18.

Curran EJ. (1909). A new association fiber tract in the cerebrum with remarks on the fiber tract dissection method of studying the brain. J Comp Neurol Psychiat 19:645–656.

Damasio AR, Damasio H, Van Hoesen GW. (1982). Prosopagnosia: anatomic basis and behavioral mechanisms. Neurology 32:331–341.

Damasio H, Damasio AR. (1980). The anatomical basis of conduction aphasia. Brain 103:337–350.

Danek A, Bauer M, Fries W. (1990). Tracing of neuronal connections in the human brain by magnetic resonance imaging in vivo. Eur J Neurosci 2:112–115.

Davidoff RA. (1990). The pyramidal tract. Neurology 40:332–339.

Davie CA, Barker GJ, Webb S, et al. (1995). Persistent functional deficit in multiple sclerosis and autosomal dominant cerebellar ataxia is associated with axon loss. Brain 118:1583–1592.

Davis LE. (1921). An anatomic study of the inferior longitudinal fasciculus. Arch Neurol Psychiat 5:370–381.

Deacon TW. (1992). Cortical connections of the inferior arcuate sulcus cortex in the macaque brain. Brain Res 573:8–26.

Deecke L. (1987). Bereitschaftspotential as an indicator of movement preparation in supplementary motor area and motor cortex. Ciba Found Symp 132:231–250.

Degos JD, Gray F, Louarn F, Ansquer JC, Poirier J, Barbizet J. (1987). Posterior callosal infarction. Clinicopathological correlations. Brain 110:1155–1171.

Dejerine JJ. (1892). Contribution à l'étude anatomo-patholoqique et clinique des différentes variétés de cécité verbale. Mém Soc Biol 4:61–90.

Dejerine JJ. (1895). Anatomie des centres nerveux. Paris: Rueff et Cie.

Dejerine J, Dejerine Mme J. (1897). Sur les dégénérescences secondaires consécutives aux lésions de la circonvolution de l'hippocampe, de la corne d'Ammon, de la circonvolution godronné et du pli rétrolimbique (trigone cerebral, commissure antérieure, faisceau inférieur du forceps calleux, tapetum et faisceau occipito-frontal. Compt Rend Soc Biol 49:587–590.

Dejerine J, Roussy G. (1906). Le syndrome thalamique. Rev Neurol 14:521–532.

de Lacoste MC, Kirkpatrick JB, Ross ED. (1985). Topography of the human corpus callosum. J Neuropath Exp Neurol 44:578–591.

de Leeuw FE, Barkhof F, Scheltens P. (2005). Progression of cerebral white matter lesions in Alzheimer's disease: a new window for therapy? J Neurol Neurosurg Psychiatry 76:1286–1288.

Demeter S, Rosene DL, Van Hoesen GW. (1985). Interhemispheric pathways of the hippocampal formation, presubiculum, and entorhinal and posterior parahippocampal cortices in the rhesus monkey: the structure and organization of the hippocampal commissures. J Comp Neurol 233:30–47.

Demeter S, Rosene DL, Van Hoesen GW. (1990). Fields of origin and pathways of the interhemispheric commissures in the temporal lobe of macaques. J Comp Neurol 302:29–53.

Denny-Brown D (1962). The Basal Ganglia and Their Relation to Disorders of Movement. London: Oxford University Press.

Denny-Brown D, Meyer JS, Horenstein S. (1952). The significance of perceptual rivalry resulting from parietal lesion. Brain 75:433–471.

D'Esposito M, Verfaellie M, Alexander MP, Katz DI. (1995). Amnesia following traumatic bilateral fornix transection. Neurology 45:1546–1550.

Devinsky O, Laff R. (2003). Callosal lesions and behavior: history and modern concepts. Epilepsy Behav 4:607–617.

Di Virgilio G, Clarke S, Pizzolato G, Schaffner T. (1999). Cortical regions contributing to the anterior commissure in man. Exp Brain Res 124:1–7.

Dimitrov M, Grafman J, Hollnagel C. (1996) The effects of frontal lobe damage on everyday problem solving. Cortex 32:357–366.

Divac I, Öberg RGE, eds. (1979). The Neostriatum: Proceedings of a WorkshopSponsored by the European Brain and Behaviour Society, Denmark, 17–19 April 1978. Oxford: Pergamon Press.

Donchin E, Otto D, Gerbrandt LK, Pribram KH. (1971). While a monkey waits: electrocortical events recorded during the foreperiod of a reaction time study. Electroencephalogr Clin Neurophysiol 31:115–127.

Doty RW. (1989). Schizophrenia: a disease of interhemispheric processes at forebrain and brainstem levels? Behav Brain Res 34:1–33.

Doty RW, Negrão N, Yamaga K. (1973). The unilateral engram. Acta Neurobiol Exp (Warsaw) 33:711–728.

Doyon J, Penhune V, Ungerleider LG. (2003). Distinct contribution of the cortico-striatal and cortico-cerebellar systems to motor skill learning. Neuropsychologia 41: 252–262.

Dubb A, Gur R, Avants B, Gee J. (2003). Characterization of sexual dimorphism in the human corpus callosum. Neuroimage 20:512–519.

Duffy FH, Burchfiel JL. (1971). Somatosensory system: organizational hierarchy from single units in monkey area 5. Science 172:273–275.

Dunnett SB, Iversen SD. (1981). Learning impairments following selective kainic acid-induced lesions within the neostriatum of rats. Behav Brain Res 2:189–209.

Dunsmore RH, Lennox MA. (1950). Stimulation and strychninization of supracallosal anterior cingulate gyrus. J Neurophysiol 13:207–214.

Dusser de Barenne JG. (1916). Experimental researches on sensory localizations in the cerebral cortex. Q J Exp Physiol 9:355–390.

Dusser de Barenne JG. (1924a). Experimental researches on sensory localization in the cerebral cortex of the monkey (*Macacus*). Proc R Soc London B. 96:272–291.

Dusser de Barenne JG. (1924b). Experimentelle Untersuchungen über die Lokalisation des sensiblen Rindengebietes im Grosshirn des Affen (*Macacus*). Deutsche Ztschrift für Nervenheilkunde 83:273–361.

Duval M. (1879). Technique de l'emploi du collodion humide our la pratique des coupes microscopiques. J de l'Anat et de la Physiol 15:185–188.

Ebeling U, von Cramon D. (1992). Topography of the uncinate fascicle and adjacent temporal fiber tracts. Acta Neurochir 115:143–148.

Eccles JC. (1982). The initiation of voluntary movements by the supplementary motor area. Arch Psychiatr Nervenkr 231:423–441.

Economo C von, Koskinas GM. (1925). Die Cytoarchitektonik der Hirnrinde des erwachsenen Menschen. Berlin: Springer.

Edinger L. (1904). Vorlesungen über den Bau der nervösen Zentralorgane des Menschen und der Tiere. Für Ärzte und Studierende. Leipzig: F.C.W. Vogel.

Eichler G. (1878). Ein Fall von Balkenmangel im menschlichen Gehirn. Archiv Psychiatrie 8:355–366.

Englund E, Brun A. (1990). White matter changes in dementia of Alzheimer's type: the difference in vulnerability between cell compartments. Histopathology 16:433–439.

Erickson TC. (1940). Spread of the epileptic discharge. An experimental study of the after-discharge induced by electrical stimulation of the cerebral cortex. Arch Neurol Psychiat 43:429–452.

Ettinger AB. (2004). Commentary on "Personality changes following temporal lobectomy for epilepsy." Epilepsy Behav 5:601–602.

Everitt BJ, Parkinson JA, Olmstead MC, Arroyo M, Robledo P, Robbins TW. (1999). Associative processes in addiction and reward. The role of amygdala-ventral striatal subsystems. Ann NY Acad Sci 877:412–438.

Fallon JH, Ziegler BTS. (1979). The crossed corticocaudate projection in the rhesus monkey. Neurosci Lett 15:29–32.

Felleman DJ, Van Essen DC. (1991). Distributed hierarchical processing in the primate cerebral cortex. Cereb Cortex 1:1–47.

Fellgiebel A, Muller MJ, Wille P et al. (2005). Color-coded diffusion-tensor imaging of posterior cingulate fiber tracts in mild cognitive impairment. Neurobiol Aging 26:1193–1198.

Fernandez-Ruiz J, Wang J, Aigner TG, Mishkin M. (2001). Visual habit formation in monkeys with neurotoxic lesions of the ventrocaudal neostriatum. Proc Natl Acad Sci USA 98:4196–4201.

Ferraina S, Bianchi L. (1994). Posterior parietal cortex: functional properties of neurons in area 5 during an instructed-delay reaching task within different parts of space. Exp Brain Res 99:175–178.

Ferrari PF, Gallese V, Rizzolatti G, Fogassi L. (2003). Mirror neurons responding to the observation of ingestive and communicative mouth actions in the monkey ventral premotor cortex. Eur J Neurosci 17:1703–1714.

Ferrier D, Yeo G. (1884). A record of experiments on the effects of lesions of different regions of the cerebral hemispheres. Phil Trans R Soc Lond B 175:479–564.

Filley CM. (2001). The Behavioral Neurology of White Matter. New York: Oxford.

Fink RP, Heimer L. (1967). Two methods for selective silver impregnation of degenerating axons and their synaptic endings in the central nervous system. Brain Res 4:369–374.

Fisher CM. (1967). A lacunar stroke: the dysarthria-clumsy hand syndrome. Neurology 17:614–617.

Fisher CM. (1978). Ataxic hemiparesis. Arch Neurol 35:126–128.

Fisher CM. (1983). Honored guest presentation: abulia minor vs. agitated behavior. Clin Neurosurg 31:9–31.

Fisher CM, Cole M. (1965). Homolateral ataxia and crural paresis: a vascular syndrome. J Neurol Neurosurg Psychiatry 28:48–55.

Fisher CM, Curry HB. (1965). Pure motor hemiplegia of vascular origin. Arch Neurol 13:30–44.

FitzPatrick KA, Imig TJ. (1978). Projections of auditory cortex upon the thalamus and midbrain in the owl monkey. J Comp Neurol 177:573–555.

Flaherty AW, Graybiel AM. (1991). Corticostriatal transformations in the primate somatosensory system. Projections from physiologically mapped body-part representations. J Neurophysiol 66:1249–1263.

Flaherty AW, Graybiel AM. (1993). Two input systems for body representations in the primate striatal matrix: experimental evidence in the squirrel monkey. J Neurosci 13:1120–1137.

Flechsig P. (1896). Weitere Mitteilungen über den Stabkranz des menschlichen Grosshirns. Neurologishes Centralblatt 15:2–4.

Folstein MF, Folstein SE, McHugh PR. (1975). "Mini-mental state": a practical method for grading the cognitive state of patients for the clinician. J Psychiatr Res 12:189–198.

Foltz EL, White LE. (1962). Pain "relief" by frontal cingulumotomy. J Neurosurg 19:89–100.

Forel A. (1881). Fall von Mangel des Balkens in einem Idiotenhirn. Tageblatt d.54. Versammlung Deutscher Naturforscher und Aerzte, Salzburg. Tageblatt 54, S. 186.

Forel A. (1907). Balkendefecte. In: Gesammelte Hirnanatomische Abhandlungen: mit einem Aufsatz über die Aufgaben der Neurobiologie. München: Ernst Reinhardt, pp. 225–234.

Foville M. (1844). Traité complet de l'anatomie, de la physiologie et de la pathologie système nerveux cérébro-spinal. Premiere partie. Anatomie. Atlas par MM Émile Beau et F. Bion. Paris: Fortin, Masson et cie.

Fox CA, Fisher RR, Desalva SJ. (1948). The distribution of the anterior commissure in the monkey (*Macaca mulatta*). J Comp Neurol 89:245–278.

Fox CA, Schmitz JT. (1943). A Marchi study of the distribution of the anterior commissure in the cat. J Comp Neurol 79:297–314.

Freeman W. (1948). Transorbital leucotomy. Lancet 2:371–373.

Freeman W, Watts J. (1942). Psychosurgery: Intelligence, Emotion and Social Behavior Following Prefrontal Lobotomy for Mental Disorders. Springfield, Ill.: Charles C Thomas.

French JD, Sugar O, Chusid JG. (1948). Corticocortical connections of the superior bank of the sylvian fissure in the monkey (*Macaca mulatta*). J Neurophysiol 11:185–192.

Frey S, Kostopoulos P, Petrides M. (2000). Orbitofrontal involvement in the processing of unpleasant auditory information. Eur J Neurosci 12:3709–3712.

Fries W, Daneck A, Scheidtmann K, Hamburger C. (1993). Motor recovery following capsular stroke: role of descending pathways from multiple motor areas. Brain 116:369–382.

Fritsch GT, Hitzig E. (1870). Über die elektrische Erregbarkeit des Grosshirns. Arch Anat Physiol Wiss Med 37:300–332. Translated in Bonin G von, 1960, pp. 73–96.

Fulton JF. (1949). Functional Localization in Relation to Frontal Lobotomy. New York: Oxford University Press.

Funnell MG, Corballis PM, Gazzaniga MS. (2000). Insights into the functional specificity of the human corpus callosum. Brain 123:920–926.

Gaddi. (1871). Fisiol dei centri nervosi. Padova 1: 206.

Gaffan D, Parker A, Easton A. (2001). Dense amnesia in the monkey after transection of fornix, amygdala and anterior temporal stem. Neuropsychologia 39:51–70.

Gaffan EA, Gaffan D, Hodges JR. (1991). Amnesia following damage to the left fornix and to other sites. A comparative study. Brain 114:1297–1313.

Gage SH. (1892–1893). An aqueous solution of hematoxylin which does not really deteriorate. Proc Amer Microsc Soc 14:125–127.

Galaburda A, Sanides F. (1980). Cytoarchitectonic organization of the human auditory cortex. J Comp Neurol 190:597–610.

Galaburda AM, Pandya DN. (1983). The intrinsic architectonic and connectional organization of the superior temporal region of the rhesus monkey. J Comp Neurol 221:169–184.

Gall FJ, Spurzheim G. (1810). Anatomie et physiologie du systeme nerveux en general, et du cerveau en particulier. Atlas. Paris: Chez F. Schoell.

Gall FJ, Spurzheim G. (1813). Anatomie du cerveau. Dictionnaire des Sciences Medicales, volume 4. Reproduced in Gordon J (1817), pp. 185–207.

Garg RK. (2002). Subacute sclerosing panencephalitis. Postgrad Med J 78:63–70.

Garrison FH. (1969). History of Neurology. Revised and enlarged with a bibliography of classical, original, and standard works in neurology, by Lawrence C. McHenry, Jr. With a foreword by Derek E. Denny-Brown. Springfield, Ill.: Charles C Thomas.

Gattas R, Sousa AP, Mishkin M, Ungerleider LG. (1997). Cortical projections of area V2 in the macaque. Cereb Cortex 7:110–129.

Gattass R, Gross CG. (1981). Visual topography of striate projection zone (MT) in posterior superior temporal sulcus of the macaque. J Neurophysiol 46:21–38.

Gazzaniga MS. (1964). Cerebral mechanisms involved in ipsilateral eye-hand use in split-brain monkeys. Exp Neurol 10:148–155.

Gazzaniga MS. (1967). The human brain is actually two brains, each capable of advanced mental functions. When the cerebrum is divided surgically, it is as if the cranium contained two separate spheres of consciousness. Sci Am 217:24–29.

Gazzaniga MS. (2000). Cerebral specialization and interhemispheric communication: does the corpus callosum enable the human condition? Brain 123:1293–1326.

Gazzaniga MS, Kutas M, Van Petten C, Fendrich R. (1989). Human callosal function: MRI-verified neuropsychological functions. Neurology 39:942–946.

Gazzaniga MS, LeDoux JE, Wilson DH. (1977). Language, praxis, and the right hemisphere: clues to some mechanisms of consciousness. Neurology 27:1144–1147.

Gazzaniga MS, Risse GL, Springer SP, Clark DE, Wilson DH. (1975). Psychologic and neurologic consequences of partial and complete cerebral commissurotomy. Neurology 25:10–15.

Gazzaniga MS, Sperry RW. (1967). Language after section of the cerebral commissures. Brain 90:131–148.

Geesaman BJ, Born RT, Andersen RA, Tootell RB. (1997). Maps of complex motion selectivity in the superior temporal cortex of the alert macaque monkey: a double-label 2–deoxyglucose study. Cereb Cortex 7:749–757.

Gennarelli TA, Thibault LE, Adams JH, Graham DI, Thompson CJ, Marcincin RP. (1982). Diffuse axonal injury and traumatic coma in the primate. Ann Neurol 12:564–574.

Gentleman SM, Roberts GW, Gennarelli TA, et al. (1995). Axonal injury: a universal consequence of fatal closed head injury? Acta Neuropathol (Berl) 89:537–543.

Geoffroy G. (1994). Other syndromes frequently associated with callosal agenesis. In: Lassonde M, Jeeves MA, eds. Callosal Agenesis. New York: Plenum Press, pp. 55–62.

Gerdeman GL, Partridge JG, Lupica CR, Lovinger DM. (2003). It could be habit forming: drugs of abuse and striatal synaptic plasticity. Trends Neurosci 26:184–192.

Gerfen CR, Sawchenko PE. (1984). An anterograde neuroanatomical tracing method that shows the detailed morphology of neurons, their axons and terminals: immunohistochemical localization of an axonally transported plant lectin, Phaseolus vulgaris leucoagglutinin (PHA-L). Brain Res 290:219–238.

Gerlach J. (1858). Mikroskopische Studien aus dem Gebiete der menschlichen Morphologie, pp. vi, 72. Erlangen: F Enke.

Gerstmann J. (1924). Fingeragnosie. Eine umschriebene Störung der Orientierung am eigenen Körper. Wien Klin Wochenschr 40:1010–1012.

Gerstmann J. (1927). Fingeragnosie und isolierte Agraphie–ein neues Syndrom. Zeitschr Gesamte Neurologie Psychiatrie 108:152–177.

Gerstmann J. (1930). Zur Symptomatologie der Hirnläsionen im

Übergangsgebiet der unteren Parietal- und mittleren Occipital-windung. Der Nervenarzt 3:691–695.

Geschwind N. (1965a). Disconnexion syndromes in animals and man. I. Brain 88:237–294.

Geschwind N. (1965b). Disconnexion syndromes in animals and man. II. Brain 88:585–644.

Geschwind N. (1974). Selected papers on language and the brain. In: Cohen RS, Wartofsky MW, eds. Boston Studies in the Philosophy of Science, vol. 16. Boston: Reidel.

Geschwind N, Fusillo MG. (1964). Color-naming defects in association with alexia. Trans Am Neurol Assoc 89:172–176.

Geschwind N, Kaplan E. (1962). A human cerebral deconnection syndrome. A preliminary report. Neurology 12:675–685.

Ghashghaei HT, Barbas H. (2002). Pathways for emotion: interactions of prefrontal and anterior temporal pathways in the amygdala of the rhesus mokey. Neuroscience 115:1261–1279.

Giguere M, Goldman-Rakic PS. (1988). Mediodorsal nucleus: areal, laminar, and tangential distribution of afferents and efferents in the frontal lobe of rhesus monkeys. J Comp Neurol 277:195–213.

Gilbert SF. (2003). Developmental Biology, 7th ed. Sunderland, MA: Sinauer Associates.

Glaser GH. (1980). Treatment of intractable temporal lobe-limbic epilepsy (complex partial seizures) by temporal lobectomy. Ann Neurol 8:455–459.

Glees P. (1946). Terminal degeneration within the central nervous system as studied by a new silver method. J Neuropathol Exp Neurol 5:54–59.

Glees P, Cole J, Whitty CWM, Cairns HWB (1950). The effects of lesions in the cingular gyrus and adjacent areas in monkeys. J Neurol Neurosurg Psychiatr 13:178–190.

Gloor P, Salanova V, Olivier A, Quesney LF. (1993). The human dorsal hippocampal commissure. An anatomically identifiable and functional pathway. Brain 116:1249–1273.

Glickstein M, May JG, Mercier BE. (1985). Corticopontine projection in the macaque: the distribution of labelled cortical cells after large injections of horseradish peroxidase in the pontine nuclei. J Comp Neurol 235:343–359.

Gluhbegovic N, Williams TH. (1980). The Human Brain: A Photographic Guide. Hagerstown, MD: Harper & Row.

Gnadt JW, Andersen RA. (1988). Memory-related motor planning activity in posterior parietal cortex of macaque. Exp Brain Res 70:216–220.

Godschalk M, Lemon RN, Kuypers HG, Ronday HK. (1984). Cortical afferents and efferents of monkey postarcuate area: an anatomical and electrophysiological study. Exp Brain Res 56:410–424.

Goeppert HR, Cohn F. (1849). Ueber die Rotation des Zellinhaltes in Nitella flexilis. Bot Ztg 7:665–673, 681–691, 697–705, 713–719. Referenced in Walker EA (1938).

Goldberg G. (1987). From intent to action: evolution and function of the premotor systems of the frontal lobe. In: Perecman E, ed. The Frontal Lobes Revisited, pp. 273–306. New York: IRBN Press.

Goldberg ME, Bisley J, Powell KD, Gottlieb J, Kusunoki M. (2002). The role of the lateral intraparietal area of the monkey in the generation of saccades and visuospatial attention. Ann NY Acad Sci 956:5–15.

Goldberg ME, Segraves MA. (1987). Visuospatial and motor attention in the monkey. Neuropsychologia 25(1A):107–118.

Goldman PS, Nauta WJ. (1977). An intricately patterned prefronto-caudate projection in the rhesus monkey. J Comp Neurol 72:369–386.

Goldman-Rakic PS. (1988). Topography of cognition: parallel distributed networks in primate association cortex. Annu Rev Neurosci 11:137–156.

Goldman-Rakic PS. (1999). The "psychic" neuron of the cerebral cortex. Ann NY Acad Sci 868:13–26.

Goldman-Rakic PS, Selemon LD. (1990). New frontiers in basal ganglia research. Introduction. Trends Neurosci 13:241–244.

Goldman-Rakic PS, Selemon LD, Schwartz ML. (1984). Dual pathways connecting the dorsolateral prefrontal cortex with the hippocampal formation and parahippocampal cortex in the rhesus monkey. Neuroscience 12:719–743.

Golgi C. (1883). Recherches sur l'histologie des centers nerveux. Arch Ital de Biol 3:285–317.

Goodale MA, Milner AD. (1992). Separate visual pathways for perception and action. Trends Neurosci 15:20–25.

Gordinier HC. (1899). The Gross and Minute Anatomy of the Central Nervous System. Philadelphia: P. Blakiston's Son & Co.

Gordon J. (1817). Observations on the Structure of the Brain: Comprising an Estimate of the Claims of Drs. Gall and Spurzheim to Discovery in the Anatomy of That Organ. Edinburgh: William Blackwood.

Gould SJ. (1977). Ontogeny and Phylogeny. Cambridge, MA: Harvard University Press.

Graff-Radford NR, Tranel D, Van Hoesen GW, Brandt JP. (1990). Diencephalic amnesia. Brain 113(Pt 1):1–25.

Grafman J, Litvan I, Gomez C, Chase TN. (1990). Frontal lobe function in progressive supranuclear palsy. Arch Neurol 47:553–558.

Graham J, Lin CS, Kaas JH. (1979). Subcortical projections of six visual cortical areas in the owl monkey, Aotus trivirgatus. J Comp Neurol 187:557–580.

Gray's Anatomy, 38th ed. (1995). Williams PL (ed). New York: Churchill Livingstone.

Graybiel AM. (1998). The basal ganglia and chunking of action repertoires. Neurobiol Learn Mem 70:119–136.

Graybiel AM, Ragsdale CW Jr. (1978). Histochemically distinct compartments in the striatum of human, monkeys, and cat demonstrated by acetylthiocholinesterase staining. Proc Natl Acad Sci USA 75:5723–5726.

Greenberg SM, Vonsattel JP, Stakes JW, Gruber M, Finklestein SP. (1993). The clinical spectrum of cerebral amyloid angiopathy: presentations without lobar hemorrhage. Neurology 43:2073–2079.

Gross CG, Weiskrantz L. (1962). Evidence for dissociation of impairment on auditory discrimination and delayed response following lateral frontal lesions in monkeys. Exp Neurol 5:453–476.

Growdon JH, Corkin S. (1987). Cognitive impairments in Parkinson's disease. Adv Neurol 45:383–392.

Gudden B von. (1870). Experimentaluntersuchungen über das peripherische und centrale Nervensystem. Archiv Psychiatrie Nervenkrankheiten 2:693–723.

Gunning-Dixon FM, Raz N. (2000). The cognitive correlates of white matter abnormalities in normal aging: a quantitative review. Neuropsychology 14:224–232.

Hachinski VC. (1990). The decline and resurgence of vascular dementia. Can Med Assoc J 142:107–111.

Hackett TA, Preuss TM, Kaas JH. (2001). Architectonic identification of the core region in auditory cortex of macaques, chimpanzees, and humans. J Comp Neurol 441:197–222.

Hackett TA, Stepniewska I, Kaas JH. (1999). Prefrontal connections of the parabelt auditory cortex in macaque monkeys. Brain Res 817:45–58.

Haeckel E. (1879). Anthropogenie, 3rd ed. Leipzig: W. Engelmann.

Haeckel E. (1902). The Riddle of the Universe. New York: Harper and Brothers.

Halsband U, Passingham R. (1982). The role of premotor and parietal cortex in the direction of action. Brain Res 240:368–372.

Hamilton DJ. (1886). On the corpus callosum in the embryo. Brain 8:145–163.

Hanaway J, Young RR. (1977). Localization of the pyramidal tract in the internal capsule of man. J Neurol Sci 34:63–70.

Hannover A. (1840). Die Chromsäure, ein vorzügliches Mittel bei mikroskopischen Untersuchungen. Archiv für Anatomie, Physiologie und wissenschaftliche Medicin, pp. 549–558.

Harbaugh RE, Wilson DH, Reeves AG, Gazzaniga MS. (1983). Forebrain commissurotomy for epilepsy. Review of 20 consecutive cases. Acta Neurochir (Wien) 68:263–275.

Harper CG, Gonatas JO, Stieber A, Gonatas NK. (1980). In vivo uptake of wheat germ agglutinin-horseradish peroxidase conjugates into neuronal GERL and lysosomes. Brain Res 188:465–472.

Hartig T. (1854). Ueber das Verfahren bei Behandlung des Zellenkerns mit Farbstoffen. Bot Ztg 12:877–881. Referenced in Walker EA (1938).

Haxby JV, Gobbini MI, Furey ML, Ishai A, Schouten JL, Pietrini P. (2001). Distributed and overlapping representations of faces and objects in ventral temporal cortex. Science 293:2425–2430.

Haxby JV, Hoffman EA, Gobbini MI. (2000). The distributed human neural system for face perception. Trends Cogn Sci 4:223–233.

Haxby JV, Hoffman EA, Gobbini MI. (2002). Human neural systems for face recognition and social communication. Biol Psychiatry 51:59–67.

Head D, Buckner RL, Shimony JS, et al. (2004). Differential vulnerability of anterior white matter in nondemented aging with minimal acceleration in dementia of the Alzheimer type: evidence from diffusion tensor imaging. Cereb Cortex 14:410–423.

Heath CJ, Jones EG. (1971). Interhemispheric pathways in the absence of a corpus callosum. An experimental study of commissural connexions in the marsupial phalanger. J Anat 109:253–270.

Hedreen JC, Yin TC. (1981). Homotopic and heterotopic callosal afferents of caudal inferior parietal lobule in Macaca mulatta. J Comp Neurol 197:605–621.

Heilman K, Valenstein E. (2003). Clinical Neuropsychology. New York: Oxford University Press.

Heilman KM, Gilmore RL. (1998). Cortical influences in emotion. J Clin Neurophysiol 15:409–423.

Heilman KM, Pandya DN, Geschwind N. (1970). Trimodal inattention following parietal lobe ablations. Trans Am Neurol Assoc 95:259–261.

Heilman KM, Pandya DN, Karol EA, Geschwind N. (1971). Auditory inattention. Arch Neurol 24:323–325.

Heilman KM, Sypert GW. (1977). Korsakoff's syndrome resulting from bilateral fornix lesions. Neurology 27:490–493.

Heimer L. (1983). The Human Brain and Spinal Cord: Functional Neuronanatomy and Dissection Guide. New York: Springer-Verlag.

Heimer L. (1995). The Human Brain and Spinal Cord: Functional Neuronanatomy and Dissection Guide, 2nd ed. New York: Springer-Verlag.

Heimer L. (2003). The legacy of the silver methods and the new anatomy of the basal forebrain: implications for neuropsychiatry and drug abuse. Scand J Psychol 44:189–201.

Heinrich A, Runge U, Khaw AV. (2004). Clinicoradiologic subtypes of Marchiafava-Bignami disease. J Neurol 251:1050–1059.

Helgason C, Caplan LR, Goodwin J, Hedges T 3rd. (1986). Anterior choroidal artery-territory infarction. Report of cases and review. Arch Neurol 43:681–686.

Helmstaedter C, Kurthen M, Lux S, Reuber M, Elger CE. (2003). Chronic epilepsy and cognition: a longitudinal study in temporal lobe epilepsy. Ann Neurol 54:425–432.

Herbert MR, Ziegler DA, Deutsch CK, et al. (2003). Dissociations of cerebral cortex, subcortical and cerebral white matter volumes in autistic boys. Brain 126:1182–1192.

Herbert MR, Ziegler DA, Makris N, et al. (2004). Localization of white matter volume increase in autism and developmental language disorder. Ann Neurol 55:530–540.

Hermann F. (1894). Notiz über die Anwendung des Formalins (Formaldehyds) als Härtungs-und Conservirungsmittel. Anat Anz 9:112–115.

Herrick CJ. (1915). An Introduction to Neurology. Philadelphia: WB Saunders.

Highley JR, Walker MA, Esiri MM, Crow TK, Harrison PJ. (2002). Asymmetry of the uncinate fasciculus: a post-mortem study of normal subjects and patients with schizophrenia. Cerebral Cortex 12:1218–1224.

Hill D, Pond DA, Mitchell W, Falconer MA. (1957). Personality changes following temporal lobectomy for epilepsy. J Mental Sci 103:18–27. Reprinted as Classics in Epilepsy and Behavior: 1957, in Epilepsy Behav, 2004, 5:603–610.

628

Hinchey J, Chaves C, Appignani B, et al. (1996). A reversible posterior leukoencephalopathy syndrome. N Engl J Med 334:494–500.

His W. (1887). Zur Geschichte des menschlichen Rückenmarkes und der Nervenwurzeln. Abh. K. säch. Ges. Wiss., Math.-Phys. Classe 13:477–514.

Hitchcock E, Laitinen L, Vaernet K, eds. (1972). Psychosurgery: Proceedings of the Second International Conference on Psychosurgery, held in Copenhagen, Denmark. Springfield, Ill.: Charles C Thomas.

Hochhaus H. (1893). Ueber Balkenmangel im menschlichen Gehirn. Deutsche Zeitschrift für Nervenheilkunde (Leipzig) 4:79–93.

Hoeve HJH. (1909). A modern method of teaching the anatomy of the brain. Anat Rec 3:247–253.

Holmes G, May WP. (1909). On the exact origin of the pyramidal tracts in man and other mammals. Brain 32:1–43.

Holt DJ, Graybiel AM, Saper CB. (1997). Neurochemical architecture of the human striatum. J Comp Neurol 384:1–25.

Hopf A. (1954). Zur architektonischen Gliederung der menschlichen Hirnrinde. J Hirnforsch 1:442–496.

Hopper KD, Patel S, Cann TS, Wilcox T, Schaeffer JM. (1994). The relationship of age, gender, handedness, and sidedness to the size of the corpus callosum. Acad Radiol 1:243–248.

Horsely V, Schäfer EA. (1888). A record of experiments upon the functions of the cerebral cortex. Phil Trans R Soc Lond B 179:1–45.

Hosoya T, Adachi M, Yamaguchi K, Haku T. (1998). MRI anatomy of white matter layers around the trigone of the lateral ventricle. Neuroradiology 40:477–482.

Hubbard BM, Anderson JM. (1981). A quantitative study of cerebral atrophy in old age and senile dementia. J Neurol Sci 50:135–145.

Hughes Bennett A, Campbell CM. (1885). Case of brachial monoplegia due to a lesion of the internal capsule. Brain 8:78–84.

Huguenin G. (1879). Anatomie des centers nerveux. Traduit par Th. Keller; annoté par Mathias Duval. Paris: JB Baillière et fils.

Huisman TA, Schwamm LH, Schaefer PW, et al. (2004). Diffusion tensor imaging as potential biomarker of white matter injury in diffuse axonal injury. AJNR Am J Neuroradiol 25:370–376.

Huntley GW, Jones EG. (1991). The emergence of architectonic field structure and areal borders in developing monkey sensorimotor cortex. Neuroscience 44:287–310.

Hupperts RM, Lodder J, Heuts-van Raak EP, Kessels F. (1994). Infarcts in the anterior choroidal artery territory. Anatomical distribution, clinical syndromes, presumed pathogenesis and early outcome. Brain 117:825–834.

Hyman BT, Van Hoesen GW, Damasio AR. (1990). Memory-related neural systems in Alzheimer's disease: an anatomic study. Neurology 40:1721–1730.

Hyndman OR, Penfield W. (1937). Agenesis of the corpus callosum. Its recognition by ventriculography. Arch Neurol Psychiatry 37:1251–1270.

Ilinsky IA, Kultas-Ilinsky K. (1987). Sagittal cytoarchitectonic maps of the *Macaca mulatta* thalamus with a revised nomenclature of the motor-related nuclei validated by observations on their connectivity. J Comp Neurol 262:331–364.

Imig TJ, Ruggero MA, Kitzes LM, Javel E, Brugge JF. (1977). Organization of auditory cortex in the owl monkey (*Aotus trivirgatus*). J Comp Neurol 171:111–128.

Innocenti GM. (1995). Exuberant development of connections, and its possible permissive role in cortical evolution. Trends Neurosci 18:397–402.

Ishai A, Ungerleider LG, Martin A, Haxby JV. (2000). The representation of objects in the human occipital and temporal cortex. J Cogn Neurosci 12(Suppl 2):35–51.

Jackson JH. (1931–1932). Selected Writings of John Hughlings Jackson. Edited for the guarantors of Brain by James Taylor with the advice and assistance of Gordon Holmes and FMR Walshe. London: Hodder and Stoughton Ltd.

Jacobson S, Trojanowski JQ. (1974). The cells of origin of the corpus callosum in rat, cat, and rhesus monkey. Brain Res 74:149–155.

Jacobson S, Trojanowski JQ. (1977). Prefrontal granular cortex of the rhesus monkey. II. Interhemispheric cortical afferents. Brain Res 132:235–246.

James TW, Culham J, Humphrey GK, Milner AD, Goodale MA. (2003). Ventral occipital lesions impair object recognition but not object-directed grasping: an fMRI study. Brain 126:2463–2475.

Jamieson EB. (1908–1909). The means of displaying, by ordinary dissection, the larger tracts of white matter of the brain in their continuity. J Anat Physiol 43:225–234.

Jeeves MA. (1965). Psychological studies of three cases of congenital agenesis of the corpus callosum. In: Ettlinger EG, ed. Functions of the Corpus Callosum, Ciba Foundation Study Group, No. 20, pp. 73–94. Boston, Little, Brown & Co.

Jeeves MA. (1991). Stereo perception in callosal agenesis and partial callosotomy. Neuropsychologia 29:19–34.

Jenike MA, Baer L, Ballantine HT, et al. (1991). Cingulotomy for refractory obsessive-compulsive disorder. Arch Gen Psychiatry 48:548–555.

Johnson MD, Ojemann GA. (2000). The role of the human thalamus in language and memory: evidence from electrophysiological studies. Brain and Cognition 42:218–230.

Johnson PB, Ferraina S, Bianchi L, Caminiti R. (1996). Cortical networks for visual reaching: physiological and anatomical organization of frontal and parietal lobe arm regions. Cereb Cortex 6:102–119.

Johnston. (1908). A new method of brain dissection. Anat Rec 2:345–358.

Jones DK, Lythgoe D, Horsfield MA, Simmons A, Williams SC, Markus HS. (1999). Characterization of white matter damage in ischemic leukoaraiosis with diffusion tensor MRI. Stroke 30:393–397.

Jones EG. (1985). The Thalamus. New York: Plenum Press.

Jones EG. (2003). Chemically defined parallel pathways in the monkey auditory system. Ann NY Acad Sci 999:218–233.

Jones EG, Burton H. (1976). Areal differences in the laminar distribution of thalamic afferents in cortical fields of the insular, parietal and temporal regions of primates. J Comp Neurol 168:197–247.

Jones EG, Burton H, Porter R. (1975). Commissural and cortico-cortical "columns" in the somatic sensory cortex of primates. Science 190:572–574.

Jones EG, Coulter JD, Burton H, Porter R. (1977). Cells of origin and terminal distribution of corticostriatal fibers arising in the sensory-motor cortex of monkeys. J Comp Neurol 173:53–80.

Jones EG, Coulter JD, Hendry SH. (1978). Intracortical connectivity of architectonic fields in the somatic sensory, motor and parietal cortex of monkeys. J Comp Neurol 181: 291–347.

Jones EG, Coulter JD, Wise SP. (1979). Commissural columns in the sensory-motor cortex of monkeys. J Comp Neurol 188:113–136.

Jones EG, Powell TP. (1970). An anatomical study of converging sensory pathways within the cerebral cortex of the monkey. Brain 93:793–820.

Jouandet ML, Gazzaniga MS. (1979). Cortical field of origin of the anterior commissure of the rhesus monkey. Exp Neurol 66:381–397.

Joubert S, Felician O, Barbeau E, et al. (2003). Impaired configurational processing in a case of progressive prosopagnosia associated with predominant right temporal lobe atrophy. Brain 126:2537–2550.

Joutel A, Corpechot C, Ducros A, et al. (1997). Notch3 mutations in cerebral autosomal dominant arteriopathy with subcortical infarcts and leukoencephalopathy (CADASIL), a mendelian condition causing stroke and vascular dementia. Ann NY Acad Sci 826:213–217.

Kaada B, Pribram KH, Epstein J. (1949). Respiratory and vascular responses in monkeys from temporal pole, insula, orital surface and cingulate gyrus. J Neurophysiol 12:347–356.

Kaas J, Axelrod S, Diamon IT. (1967). An ablation study of the auditory cortex in the cat using binaural tonal patterns. J Neurophysiol 30:710–724.

Kareken DA, Unverzagt F, Caldemeyer K, Farlow MR, Hutchins GD. (1998). Functional brain imaging in apraxia. Arch Neurol 55:107–113.

Karol EA, Pandya DN. (1971). The distribution of the corpus callosum in the rhesus monkey. Brain 94:471–486.

Kaufmann E. (1887). Ueber Mangel des balkens im menschlichen Gehirn. Archiv Psychiatrie 18:769–781.

Kaufmann E. (1888). Ueber Mangel des Balkens im menschlichen Gehirn. Part B. Archiv Psychiatrie 19:229–243.

Keizer K, Kuypers HG, Huisman AM, Dann O. (1983). Diamidino yellow dihydrochloride (DY . 2HCl); a new fluorescent retrograde neuronal tracer, which migrates only very slowly out of the cell. Exp Brain Res 51:179–191.

Kemp JM, Powell TP. (1970). The cortico-striate projection in the monkey. Brain 93:525–546.

Kertesz A, Geschwind N. (1971). Patterns of pyramidal decussation and their relationship to handedness. Arch Neurol 24:326–332.

Kier EL, Staib LH, Davis LM, Bronen RA. (2004). MR imaging of the temporal stem: anatomic dissection tractography of the uncinate fasciculus, inferior occipitofrontal fasciculus, and Meyer's loop of the optic radiation. Am J Neuroradiol 25:677–691.

Kim HG, Schmahmann JD, Sims K, Falk W, Stern TA, Norris ER. (1999). A neuropsychiatric presentation of mitochondrial myopathy, encephalopathy, lactic acidosis and stroke-like episodes. Medicine Psychiatry 2:3–9.

Kim JS, Lee JH, Lee MC, Lee SD. (1994). Transient abnormal behavior after pontine infarction [Letter]. Stroke 25:2295–2296.

Kinoshita T, Moritani T, Shrier DA, et al. (2003). Diffusion-weighted MR imaging of posterior reversible leukoencephalopathy syndrome: a pictorial essay. Clin Imaging 27:307–315.

Klebs E. (1869). Die Einschmelzungs-Methode, ein Beitrag zur mikroskopischen Technik. Arch Micro Anat 5:164–166.

Kleist K. (1962). Sensory Aphasia and Amusia: The Myeloarchitectonic Basis. Translated by F. J. Fish and J. B. Stanton. Oxford, New York: Pergamon Press.

Klingler J, Gloor P. (1960). The connections of the amygdala and of the anterior temporal cortex in the human brain. J Comp Neurol 115:33–369.

Knowlton BJ, Mangels JA, Squire LR. (1996). A neostriatal habit learning system in humans. Science 273:1399–1402.

Knox DN. (1875). Glasgow Med J 7:227. Referenced in Bruce (1887–1888).

Koechlin E, Basso G, Pietrini P, Panzer S, Grafman J. (1999). The role of the anterior prefrontal cortex in human cognition. Nature 399:148–151.

Kolb B, Buhrmann K, McDonald R, Sutherland RJ. (1994). Dissociation of the medial prefrontal, posterior parietal, and posterior temporal cortex for spatial navigation and recognition memory in the rat. Cereb Cortex 4:664–680.

Koelliker A von. (1894). Ueber den Fornix longus von FOREL und die Riechstrahlungen im Gehirn des Kaninchens. Verhandlungen der Anatomischen Gesellscchaft 9:45–52.

Koelliker RA von. (1849). Berichte Königlichen zootomischen anstalt zu Würzburg. Leipzig:Wilhelm Engelmann.

Koob GF. (1999). The role of the striatopallidal and extended amygdala systems in drug addiction. Ann NY Acad Sci 877:445–460.

Korczyn AD. (2002). Mixed dementia: the most common cause of dementia. Ann NY Acad Sci 977:129–134.

Koski LM, Paus T, Petrides M. (1998). Directed attention after unilateral frontal excisions in humans. Neuropsychologia 36:1363–1371.

Kraft LM. (1955). Ramón y Cajal: Studies on the Cerebral Cortex (Limbic Structures). Chicago: Year Book.

Krieg WJ. (1954). Connections of the cerebral cortex. II. The macaque. E. The post-central gyrus. J Comp Neurol 101:101–165.

Krieg WJS. (1947). Connections of the cerebral cortex: I. The albino rat. J Comp Neurol 87:267–394.

Krieg WJS. (1975). Interpretive Atlas of the Monkey's Brain: 89 Cell- and Fiber-Stained Sections of the Brain of the Macaque, with an Illustrated Textbook. Evanston, Ill.: Brain Books.

Krubitzer LA, Kaas JH. (1990). Cortical connections of MT in four species of primates: areal, modular, and retinotopic patterns. Vis Neurosci 5:165–204.

Kubicki M, Westin C-F, Maier SE, et al. (2002). Uncinate fasciculus findings in schizophrenia: a magnetic resonance diffusion tensor imaging study. Am J Psychiatry 159:813–820.

Kuker W, Mayrhofer H, Mader I, Nagele T, Krageloh-Mann I. (2003). Malformations of the midline commissures: MRI findings in different forms of callosal dysgenesis. Eur Radiol 13:598–604.

Kumar K, Toth C, Nath RK. (1997). Deep brain stimulation for intractable pain: a 15-year experience. Neurosurgery 40:736–746.

Kunimatsu A, Aoki S, Masutani Y, Abe O, Mori H, Ohtomo K. (2003). Three-dimensional white matter tractography by diffusion tensor imaging in ischaemic stroke involving the corticospinal tract. Neuroradiology 45:532–535.

Künzle H. (1977). Projections from the primary somatosensory cortex to basal ganglia and thalamus in the monkey. Exp Brain Res 30:481–492.

Künzle H, Akert K. (1977). Efferent connections of cortical, area 8 (frontal eye field) in Macaca fascicularis. A reinvestigation using the autoradiographic technique. J Comp Neurol 173:147–164.

Kuypers HG, Bentivoglio M, Catsman-Berrevoets CE, Bharos AT. (1980). Double retrograde neuronal labeling through divergent axon collaterals, using two fluorescent tracers with the same excitation wavelength which label different features of the cell. Exp Brain Res 40:383–392.

Kuypers HG, Szwarcbart MK, Mishkin M, Rosvold HE. (1965). Occipitotemporal corticocortical connections in the rhesus monkey. Exp Neurol 11: 245–262.

Lamantia AS, Rakic P. (1990a). Cytological and quantitative characteristics of four cerebral commissures in the rhesus monkey. J Comp Neurol 291:520–537.

LaMantia AS, Rakic P. (1990b). Axon overproduction and elimination in the corpus callosum of the developing rhesus monkey. J Neurosci 10:2156–2175.

LaMantia AS, Rakic P. (1994). Axon overproduction and elimination in the anterior commissure of the developing rhesus monkey. J Comp Neurol 340:328–336.

Lassek AM. (1954). The Pyramidal Tract: Its Status in Medicine. Springfield, Ill.: Charles C Thomas.

LaVail JH, LaVail MM. (1972). Retrograde axonal transport in the central nervous system. Science 176:1416–1417.

Lawler KA, Cowey A. (1987). On the role of posterior parietal and prefrontal cortex in visuo-spatial perception and attention. Exp Brain Res 65:695–698.

Lazar M, Weinstein DM, Tsuruda JS, et al. (2003). White matter tractography using diffusion tensor deflection. Hum Brain Mapp 18:306–321.

LeBeau J. (1954). Anterior cingulectomy in man. J Neurosurg 11:268–276.

LeBihan D, Mangin JF, Poupon C, et al. (2001). Diffusion tensor imaging: concepts and applications. J Magn Reson Imaging 13:534–546.

Leichnetz GR. (2001). Connections of the medial posterior parietal cortex (area 7m) in the monkey. Anat Rec 263:215–236.

Leichnetz GR, Astruc J. (1975). Efferent connections of the orbitofrontal cortex in the marmoset (Saguinus oedipus). Brain Res 84:169–180.

Leifer D, Buonanno FS, Richardson EP Jr. (1990). Clinicopathologic correlations of cranial magnetic resonance imaging of periventricular white matter. Neurology 40:911–918.

Leinonen L, Hyvarinen J, Nyman G, Linnankoski I. (1979). I. Functional properties of neurons in lateral part of associative area 7 in awake monkeys. Exp Brain Res 34:299–320.

Leinonen L, Hyvarinen J, Sovijarvi AR. (1980). Functional properties of neurons in the temporo-parietal association cortex of awake monkey. Exp Brain Res 39:203–215.

Lennox MA, Dunsmore RH, Epstein JA, Pribram KH. (1950). Electrocorticographic effects of stimulation of posterior orbital, temporal and cingulate areas of Macaca mulatta. J Neurophysiol 13:383–388.

Lepage M, Ghaffar O, Nyberg L, Tulving E. (2000). Prefrontal cortex and episodic memory retrieval mode. Proc Natl Acad Sci USA 97:506–511.

Leuret F, Gratiolet P. (1839). Anatomir comparée du système nerveux. Considéré dans ses rapports avec l'intelligence. Atlas des 32 planches dess inées d'après nature et gravées. Paris: J-B Baillière et fils.

Leventhal CM, Baringer JR, Arnason BG, Fisher CM. (1965). A case of Marchiafava-Bignami disease with clinical recovery. Trans Am Neurol Assoc 90:87–91.

Levin PM. (1936). The efferent fibers of the frontal lobe of the monkey Macaca mulatta. J Comp Neurol 63:369–419.

Levine B, Black SE, Cabeza R, et al. (1998). Episodic memory and the self in a case of isolated retrograde amnesia. Brain 121:1951–1973.

Levine B, Katz DI, Dade L, Black SE. (2002). Novel approaches to the assessment of frontal damage and executive deficits in traumatic brain injury. In: Stuss DT, Knight RT, eds. Principles of Frontal Lobe Function, pp. 448–465. Oxford: Oxford University Press.

Levisohn L, Cronin-Golomb A, Schmahmann JD. (2000). Neuropsychological consequences of cerebellar tumor resection in children: cerebellar cognitive affective syndrome in a pediatric population. Brain 123:1041–1050.

Levy R, Friedman HR, Davachi L, Goldman-Rakic PS. (1997). Differential activation of the caudate nucleus in primates performing spatial and nonspatial working memory tasks. J Neurosci 17:3870–3882.

Levy R, Goldman-Rakic PS. (2000). Segregation of working memory functions within the dorsolateral prefrontal cortex. Exp Brain Res 133:23–32.

Lewine JD, Doty RW, Astur RS, Provencal SL. (1994). Role of the forebrain commissures in bihemispheric mnemonic integration in macaques. J Neurosci 14:2515–2530.

Leyton ASF, Sherrington CS. (1917). Observations on the excitable cortex of the chimpanzee, orangutan, and gorilla. Q J Exp Physiol 11:135–222.

Lichtheim L. (1885). On aphasia. Brain 7:433–484.

Liepmann H, Maas O. (1907). Fall von linksseitiger Agraphie und Apraxie bei rechtsseitiger Lähmung. J Psychol Neurol 10:214–227.

Lin CP, Wedeen VJ, Chen JH, Yao C, Tseng WY. (2003). Validation of diffusion spectrum magnetic resonance imaging with manganese-enhanced rat optic tracts and ex vivo phantoms. Neuroimage 19:482–495.

Locke S, Angevine JB Jr, Yakovlev PI. (1961). Limbic nuclei of thalamus and connections of limbic cortex. II. Thalamocortical projection of the lateral dorsal nucleus in man. Arch Neurol 4:355–364.

Locke S, Kruper DC, Yakovlev PI. (1964). Limbic nuclei of thalamus and connections of limbic cortex. 7. Transcallosal connections of cerebral hemisphere with striatum in monkey and man. Arch Neurol 11: 571–582.

Loeb C. (2000). Binswanger's disease is not a single entity. Neurol Sci 21: 343–348.

Loeb C, Meyer JS. (1996). Vascular dementia: still a debatable entity? J Neurol Sci 143:31–40.

Logothetis NK, Schall JD. (1989). Neuronal correlates of subjective visual perception. Science 245:761–763.

Longstreth WT Jr, Arnold AM, Beauchamp NJ Jr, et al. (2005). Incidence, manifestations, and predictors of worsening white matter on serial cranial magnetic resonance imaging in the elderly: the Cardioascular Health Study. Stroke 36:56–61.

López-Ibor Aliño JJ, Burzaco J. (1972). Stereotaxic anterior limb capsulotomy in selected psychiatric patients. In: Hitchcock E, Laitinen L, Vaernet K, eds. Psychosurgery: Proceedings of the Second International Conference on Psychosurgery held in Copenhagen, Denmark, pp. 391–399. Springfield, Ill: Charles C Thomas.

Ludwig E, Klingler J. (1956). Atlas Cerebri Humani. The Inner Structure of the Brain Demonstrated on the Basis of Macroscopical Preparations. Boston: Little Brown and Co.

Hackett TA, Preuss TM, Kaas JH. (2001). Architectonic identification of the core region in auditory cortex of macaques, chimpanzees, and humans. J Comp Neurol 441:197–222.

Luria AR. (1966). Higher Cortical Functions in Man. Preface to the English edition by Hans-Lukas Teuber and Karl H. Pribram. Authorized translation from the Russian by Basil Haigh. New York:Basic Books.

Lynch JC, Mountcastle VB, Talbot WH, Yin TC. (1977). Parietal lobe mechanisms for directed visual attention. J Neurophysiol 40:362–389.

Macchi G, Jones EG. (1997). Toward an agreement on terminology of nuclear and subnuclear divisions of the motor thalamus. J Neurosurg 86:670–685.

MacLean P, Pribram K. (1953). Neuronographic analysis of medial and basal cortex: II. Monkey. J Neurophysiol 16:323–340.

MacLean PD. (1949). Psychosomatic disease and the "visceral brain." Recent developments bearing on the Papez theory of emotion. Psychosom Med 11:338–353.

MacLean PD. (1952). Some psychiatric implications of physiological studies on the fronto-temporal portion of the limbic system (visceral brain). Electroenceph Clin Neurophysiol 4:407–418.

Maehara T, Shimizu H. (2001). Surgical outcome of corpus callosotomy in patients with drop attacks. Epilepsia 42:67–71.

Makris N, Kennedy DN, McInerney S, et al. (2005). Segmentation of subcomponents within the superior longitudinal fascicle in humans: a quantitative, in vivo, DT-MRI study. Cereb Cortex 15:854–869.

Makris N, Worth AJ, Sorensen AG, et al. (1997). Morphometry of in vivo human white matter association pathways with diffusion-weighted magnetic resonance imaging. Ann Neurol 42:951–962.

Malach R, Graybiel AM. (1986). Mosaic architecture of the somatic sensory-recipient sector of the cat's striatum. J Neurosci 6:3436–58.

Malkova L, Mishkin M. (2003). One-trial memory for object-place associations after separate lesions of hippocampus and posterior parahippocampal region in the monkey. J Neurosci 23:1956–1965.

Malpighi M (Marcelli Malpighii). (1669). De viscerum structura exercitatio anatomica. Elenchus exercitationum, de hepate, de cerebri cortice, de renibus, de liene, de polypo cordis. Typis T.R. Impensis Jo. Martyn, Londini. De cerebri cortice, pp. 50–71.

Mamelak AN, Barbaro NM, Walker JA, Laxer KD. (1993). Corpus callosotomy: a quantitative study of the extent of resection, seizure control, and neuropsychological outcome. J Neurosurg 79:688–695.

Marchi V, Algeri G. (1885). Sulle degenerazioni discendenti consecutive a lesioni della corteccia cerebrale. Riv sper d freniat 11: 492–494. Referenced in Walker EA (1938).

Marie P. (1901). Des foyers lacunaires de désintégration et de différents autres états cavitaires du cerveau. Rev Méd 21:281–298.

Marinkovic S, Gibo H, Milisavljevic M, Cetkovic M. (2001). Anatomic and clinical correlations of the lenticulostriate arteries. Clin Anat 14:190–195.

Marotti JD, Tobias S, Fratkin JD, Powers JM, Rhodes CH. (2004). Adult onset leukodystrophy with neuroaxonal spheroids and pigmented glia: report of a family, historical perspective, and review of the literature. Acta Neuropathol 107:481–8.

Marshall RS, Lazar RM, Mohr JP, Van Heertum RL, Mast H. (1996). "Semantic" conduction aphasia from a posterior insular cortex infarction. J Neuroimag 6:189–191.

Marshall VG, Bradley WG Jr, Marshall CE, Bhoopat T, Rhodes

RH. (1988). Deep white matter infarction: correlation of MR imaging and histopathologic findings. Radiology 167:517–522.

Marsland TA, Glees P, Erikson LB. (1954). Modification of the Glees silver impregnation for paraffin sections. J Neuropathol Exp Neurol 13:587–591.

Martinkauppi S, Rama P, Aronen HJ, Korvenoja A, Carlson S. (2000). Working memory of auditory localization. Cereb Cortex 10:889–898.

Mas JL, Cabanis EA, Baudrimont M, et al. (1993). Cerebral autosomal dominant arteriopathy with subcortical infarcts and leukoencephalopathy maps to chromosome 19q12. Nat Genet 3:256–259.

Mauritz KH, Wise SP. (1986). Premotor cortex of the rhesus monkey: neuronal activity in anticipation of predictable environmental events. Exp Brain Res 61: 229–244.

Mayo H. (1827). A Series of Engravings Intended to Illustrate the Structure of the Brain and Spinal Cord in Man. London: Burgess and Hill.

McCulloch WS. (1944). The functional organization of the cerebral cortex. Physiol Rev 24:390–407.

McCulloch WS, Garol HW. (1941). Cortical origin and distribution of corpus callosum and anterior commissure in the monkey (Macaca mulatta). J Neurophysiol 4:555–564.

McIntyre DC. (1975). Split-brain rat: transfer and interference of kindled amygdala convulsions. Can J Neurol Sci 2:429–437.

Medana IM, Esiri MM. (2003). Axonal damage: a key predictor of outcome in human CNS diseases. Brain 126:515 530.

Mellus EL. (1899). Motor paths in the brain and cord of the monkey. J Nerv Ment Dis 26:197–209.

Mellus EL. (1904). Bilateral relations of the cerebral cortex. Johns Hopkins Hosp Bull 12:108–112.

Merzenich M-M, Brugge JF. (1973). Representation of the cochlear partition of the superior temporal plane of the macaque monkey. Brain Res 50:275–296.

Mesulam M-M. (1976). The blue reaction product in horseradish peroxidase neurohistochemistry: incubation parameters and visibility. J Histochem Cytochem 24:1273–1280

Mesulam M-M. (1978). Tetramethyl benzidine for horseradish peroxidase neurohistochemistry: a non-carcinogenic blue reaction product with superior sensitivity for visualizing neural afferents and efferents. J Histochem Cytochem 26:106–117.

Mesulam M-M. (1981). A cortical network for directed attention and unilateral neglect. Ann Neurol 10:309–325.

Mesulam M-M. (1990). Large-scale neurocognitive networks and distributed processing for attention, language, and memory. Ann Neurol 28:597–613.

Mesulam M-M. (1998). From sensation to cognition. Brain 121:1013–1052.

Mesulam M-M. (2000). Principles of Behavioral and Cognitive Neurology, 2nd ed. New York: Oxford University Press.

Mettler R. (1935a). Corticofugal fiber connections of the cortex of Macaca mulatta. The occipital region. J Comp Neurol 61:221–256.

Mettler R. (1935b). Corticofugal fiber connections of the cortex of Macaca mulatta. The frontal region. J Comp Neurol 61:509–542.

Mettler R. (1935c). Corticofugal fiber connections of the cortex of Macaca mulatta. The temporal region. J Comp Neurol 63:25–47.

Mettler R. (1935d). Corticofugal fiber connections of the cortex of Macaca mulatta. The parietal region. J Comp Neurol 62:263–291.

Meyer A. (1907). The connections of the occipital lobes and the present status of the cerebral visual affections. Transactions of the Association of American Physicians. 22: 7–16.

Meyer A. (1971). Historical Aspects of Cerebral Anatomy. London: Oxford University Press.

Meyer G, MacElhaney M, Martin W, MacGraw CP. (1973). Stereotaxic cingulotomy with results of acute stimulation and serial psychological testing. In: Laitinen LV, Livingston KE, eds. Surgical Approaches in Psychiatry, pp. 38–58. Lancaster: Medical and Technical Publishing.

Meynert T. (1865). Anatomie der Hirnrinde als Träger des Vorstellungslebens und ihrer Verbindungsbahnen mit den empfindenden Oberflächen und den bewegenden Massen. In: Leidesdorf M, ed. Lehrbuch der psychichen Krankheiten, pp. 45–73. Erlangen: Verlag von Ferdinand Enke.

Meynert T. (1871–1872). Vom Gerhirne der Säugethiere. In: Stricker S, ed. Handbuch der Lehre von den Geweben des Menschen und der Thiere, volume 2, pp. 694–808. Leipzig: Englemann. Translated by Henry Power as The brain of mammals. In: Stricker S, ed. Manual of Human and Comparative Histology, volume 2, pp. 367–537 (London: New Sydenham Society).

Meynert T. (1885). Psychiatry. A Clinical Treatise on Diseases of the Forebrain Based Upon a Study of Its Structure, Functions and Nutrition. Part 1. The Anatomy, Physiology, and Chemistry of the Brain. Translated by B. Sachs. New York: GP Putnams' Sons.

Middleton FA, Strick PL. (1994). Anatomical evidence for cerebellar and basal ganglia involvement in higher cognitive function. Science 266:458–461.

Milch EC. (1932). Sensory cortical area: an experimental anatomic investigation. Arch Neurol Psychiat 28:871–872.

Milner B. (2003). Visual recognition and recall after right temporal-lobe excision in man. Epilepsy Behav 4:799–812.

Milner B. (2005). The medial temporal-lobe amnesic syndrome. Psychiatr Clin North Am 28:599–611.

Mingazzini G. (1922). Der Balken. Monographien aus dem. Gesamtgebiete der Neurologie und Psychiatrie. Berlin: Julius Springer, Heft 28.

Mishkin M. (1966). Visual mechanisms beyond the striate cortex. In: Russell RW, ed. Frontiers in Physiological Psychology. New York: Academic Press, pp. 93–119.

Mishkin M. (1982). A memory system in the monkey. Phil Trans R Soc Lond B. 298:85–95.

Mochizuki H, Masaki T, Matsushita S, et al. (2005). Cognitive impairment and diffuse white matter atrophy in alcoholics. Clin Neurophysiol 116:223–228.

Mohr JP, Foulkes MA, Polis AT, et al. (1993). Infarct topography and hemiparesis profiles with cerebral convexity infarction: the Stroke Data Bank. J Neurol Neurosurg Psychiatry 56:344–351.

Molko N, Cohen L, Mangin JF, et al. (2002a). Visualizing the neural bases of a disconnection syndrome with diffusion tensor imaging. J Cogn Neurosci 14:629–636.

Molko N, Pappata S, Mangin J-F, et al. (2002b). Monitoring disease progression in CADASIL with diffusion magnetic resonance imaging. A study with whole brain histogram analysis. Stroke 33:2902–2908.

Monakow C von. (1882a). Über einige durch Extirpation circumscripter Hirnrinden regionen bedingte Entwickelungshemmungen des Kanninchengehirns. Archiv Psychiatrie Nervenkranheiten 12:141–156.

Monakow C von. (1882b). Weitere Mittheilungen über durch Exstirpation circumscripter Hirnrindenregionen bedingte Entwickelungshemmungen des Kaninchengehirns. Archiv Psychiatrie Nervenkranheiten 12:535–549.

Monakow C von. (1885). Experimentelle und pathologisch-anatomische Untersuchungen über die Beziehungen der sogenannten Sehsphäre zu den infracorticalen Opticusentren und zum N. opticus. Archiv Psychiatrie Nervenkrankheiten 16:317–352.

Monakow C von. (1892). Experimentelle und pathologisch-anatomische Untersuchungen über die optischen Centren und Bahnen nebst klinischen Beiträgen zur corticalen Hemianopsie und Alexie. Archiv Psychiatrie Nervenkrankheiten 24:228–268.

Monakow C von. (1895). Experimentelle und pathologisch-anatomische Untersuchungen über die Haubenregion, den Sehhügel und die Regio subthalamica, nebst Beiträgen zur Kenntniss früh erworbener Gross- und Kleinhirndefecte. Archiv Psychiatrie Nervenkrankheiten 27:1–128.

Monakow C von. (1899). Zur Anatomie und Pathologie des unteren Scheitelläppchens. Archiv Psychiatrie Nervenkrankheiten 31:1–73.

Mondino dei Luzzi (Mundinus). (1478). Anathomia. Republished in 1926 as Anatomies de Mondino dei Luzzi et de Fguido de Vigevano, Paris, Droz.

Moniz E. (1937). Prefrontal leucotomy in the treatment of mental disorders. J Psychiatry 93:1379–1385.

Monro A Jr. (1813). Outlines of the Anatomy of the Human Body, in its Sound and Diseased State, volume 3. Edinburgh: Archibald Constable & Co.

Moody DM, Thore CR, Anstrom JA, Challa VR, Langefeld CD, Brown WR. (2004). Quantification of afferent vessels shows reduced brain vascular density in subjects with leukoariosis. Radiology 233:883–890.

Moran MA, Mufson EJ, Mesulam M-M. (1987). Neural inputs into the temporopolar cortex of the rhesus monkey. J Comp Neurol 256:88–103.

Morecraft RJ, Cipolloni PB, Stilwell-Morecraft KS, Gedney MT, Pandya DN. (2004). Cytoarchitecture and cortical connections of the posterior cingulate and adjacent somatosensory fields in the rhesus monkey. J Comp Neurol 469:37–69.

Morecraft RJ, Herrick JL, Stilwell-Morecraft KS, et al. (2002). Localization of arm representation in the corona radiata and internal capsule in the non-human primate. Brain 125:176–198.

Morecraft RJ, Louie JL, Herrick JL, Stilwell-Morecraft KS. (2001). Cortical innervation of the facial nucleus in the non-human primate: a new interpretation of the effects of stroke and related subtotal brain trauma on the muscles of facial expression. Brain 124:176–208.

Morecraft RJ, Hoesen GW van. (1993). Frontal granular cortex input to the cingulate (M3), supplementary (M2) and primary (M1) motor cortices in the rhesus monkey. J Comp Neurol 337:669–689.

Morecraft RJ, Hoesen GW van. (1998). Convergence of limbic input to the cingulate motor cortex in the rhesus monkey. Brain Res Bull 45:209–232.

Morel A, Garraghty PE, Kaas JH. (1993). Tonotopic organization, architectonic fields, and connections of auditory cortex in macaque monkeys. J Comp Neurol 335:437–459.

Morris R, Pandya DN, Petrides M. (1999a). Fiber system linking the mid-dorsolateral frontal cortex with the retrosplenial/presubicular region in the rhesus monkey. J Comp Neurol 407:183–192.

Morris R, Petrides M, Pandya DN. (1999b). Architecture and connections of retrosplenial area 30 in the rhesus monkey (Macaca mulatta). Eur J Neurosci 11:2506–2518.

Mott FW, Schaeffer EA. (1890). On movements resulting from faradic excitation of the corpus callosum in moneys. Brain 13: 174–177.

Motter BC, Steinmetz MA, Duffy CJ, Mountcastle VB. (1987). Functional properties of parietal visual neurons: mechanisms of directionality along a single axis. J Neurosci 7:154–176.

Mountcastle VB, Lynch JC, Georgopoulos A, Sakata H, Acuna C. (1975). Posterior parietal association cortex of the monkey: command functions for operations within extrapersonal space. J Neurophysiol 38:871–908.

Muakkassa KF, Strick PL. (1979). Frontal lobe inputs to primate motor cortex: evidence for four somatotopically organize "premotor" areas. Brain Res 177:176–182.

Mufson EJ, Pandya DN. (1984). Some observations on the course and composition of the cingulum bundle in the rhesus monkey. J Comp Neurol 225:31–43.

Muratoff W. (1893a). Secundäre Degenerationen nach Durchschneidung des Balkens. Neurologisches Centralblatt 12:714–729.

Muratoff W. (1893b). Sekundäre Degeneration nach Zerstörung der motorischen Sphäre des Gehirns in Verbindung mit der Frage von der Localisation der Hirnfunctionen. Archiv fur Anatomie und Entwicklungsgeschichte. Herausgegeben von Dr. Wilhelm His und Dr. Dubois-Reymond, Leipzig: Verlag von Veit & Comp, pp. 97–116.

Muratow W. (1893). Secundäre Degeneration nach Durchschneidung des Corpus callosum. Neurologisches Centralblatt 12:316.

Murray EA, Bussey TJ, Hampton RR, Saksida LM. (2000). The parahippocampal region and object identification. Ann NY Acad Sci 911: 166–174.

Murray EA, Coulter JD. (1981). Supplementary sensory area: the medial parietal cortex in the monkey. In: Woolsey CN, ed. Cortical Sensory Organization, Volume 1. Multiple Somatic Areas, pp. 167–196. Clifton, N.J.: Humana Press.

Myers RE. (1962). Commissural connections between occipital lobes of the monkey. J Comp Neurol 118:1–16.

Myers RE. (1965). The neocortical commissures and interhemispheric transmission of information. In: Ettlinger EG, ed. Functions of the Corpus Callosum, Ciba Foundation Study Group, No. 20, pp. 1–17. Boston: Little Brown & Co.

Myers RE, Sperry RW. (1953). Interocular transfer of a visual form discrimination habit in cats after section of the optic chiasma and the corpus callosum. Anat Rec 115:351–352.

Nadeau SE, Crosson B. (1997). Subcortical aphasia. Brain Lang 58:355–402; discussion 418–423.

Nadel L. (1991). The hippocampus and space revisited. Hippocampus 1:221–229.

Naeser MA, Palumbo CL, Helm-Estabrooks N, Stiassny-Eder D, Albert ML. (1989). Severe nonfluency in aphasia. Role of the medial subcallosal fasciculus and other white matter pathways in recovery of spontaneous speech. Brain 112:1–38.

Nakaji P, Meltzer HS, Singel SA, Alksne JF. (2003). Improvement of aggressive and antisocial behavior after resection of temporal lobe tumors. Pediatrics 112:e430.

Narayana A. (1995). Medical science in ancient Indian culture with special reference to Atharvaveda. Bull Indian Inst Hist Med Hyderabad 25:100–110.

Narayanan S, Fu L, Pioro E, et al. (1997). Imaging of axonal damage in multiple sclerosis: spatial distribution of magnetic resonance imaging lesions. Ann Neurol 41:385–391.

Nasreddine ZS, Saver JL. (1997). Pain after thalamic stroke: right diencephalic predominance and clinical features in 180 patients. Neurology 48:1196–99.

Nauta WJ. (1971). The problem of the frontal lobe: a reinterpretation. J Psychiatr Res 8:167–187.

Nauta WJ, Domesick VB. (1984). Afferent and efferent relationships of the basal ganglia. Ciba Foundation Symposium 107:3–29.

Nauta WJ, Gygax PA. (1951). Silver impregnation of degenerating axon terminals in the central nervous system: (1) Technic. (2) Chemical notes. Stain Technol 26:5–11.

Nauta WJ, Gygax PA. (1954). Silver impregnation of degenerating axons in the central nervous system: a modified technic. Stain Technol 29:91–93.

Nauta WJH. (1964). Some efferent connections of the prefrontal cortex in the monkey. In: Waren JM, Akert K, eds. The Frontal Granular Cortex and Behavior, pp. 397–409. New York: McGraw-Hill.

Neal JW, Pearson RC, Powell TP. (1990). The ipsilateral cortico- cortical connections of area 7 with the frontal lobe in the monkey. Brain Res 509:31–40.

Nemesius, Bishop of Emesa. (1512). Divini Gregori Nyssae [i.e. Nemesii emeseni] . . . Libri octo. i. De homine. ii. De anima. iii. De elementis. iiii. De viribus animae. v. De volutario et inuolutario. vi. De fato. vii. De libero arbitrio. viii. De prouidentia. Strassburg.

Neuburger M. (1897). Die historische Entwicklung der experimentellen Gehirn- und Rückenmarksphysiologie vor Flourens. Ferdinand Enke Verlag, Stuttgart. Translated and edited, with additional material, by Edwin Clarke, as The Historical Development of Experimental Brain and Spinal Cord Physiology Before Flourens. Baltimore/London: Johns Hopkins University Press, 1981.

Neuburger M, ed. (1910). Ludwig Türcks gesammelte neurologische Schriften, pp. 1–194. Leipzig und Wien: Franz Deuticke.

Niessl von Mayendorf. (1903). Vom fasciculus longitudinalis inferior. Arch Psychiat 37:537–563.

Niessl von Mayendorf. (1919). Die Assoziationssyteme des menschlichen Vorderhirns. Eine physiologische Studie. Archiv Anatomie Physiologie (Physiologische Abteilung) 283–390.

Nieuwenhuys R, Voogd J, van Hiujzen C. (1978). The Human Central Nervous System: A Synopsis and Atlas. Berlin: Springer-Verlag.

Nissl F. (1892). Ueber die Veranderungen der Ganglienzellen am Facaliskern des Kaninchens nach Ausreissung der Nerven. Allgemeine Zeitschrift Psychiatrie 48:197–198.

Nyby O, Jansen J. (1951). An experimental investigation of the corticopontine projection in macaca mulatta. Skrifter utgitt av det Norske Vedenskapsakademie: Oslo; 1. Mat Naturv Klasse 3:1–47.

Obersteiner H. (1896). Anleitung beim Studium des Baues der Nervösen Centralorgane im gesunden und kranken Zustande. Translated by Leonard Hill. Leipzig und Wien: Franz Deuticke.

Obersteiner H, Redlich E. (1902). Zur Kenntnis des Stratum (Fasciculus) subcallosum (Fasciculus nuclei caudati) und des Fasciculus fronto-occipitalis (reticulirtes cortico-caudales Bündel). Arbeiten aus dem Neurologischen Institut 8:286–307.

Ojemann GA. (1983). Brain organization for language from the perspective of electrical stimulation mapping. Behav Brain Sci 6:189–230.

Olszewski J. (1952). The Thalamus of the *Macaca mulatta*: An Atlas for Use with the Stereotaxic Instrument. Basel, New York: S. Karger.

Onufrowicz W. (1887). Das balkenlose Mikrocephalengehirn Hoffman. Ein Beitrag zur pathologischen und normalen Anatomie des menschlichen Gehirnes. Archiv Psychiatrie 18:305–328.

Oppenheim JS, Lee BC, Nass R, Gazzaniga MS. (1987). No sex-related differences in human corpus callosum based on magnetic resonance imagery. Ann Neurol 21:604–606.

Osborne SG. (1857). Vegetable cell-structure and its formation, as seen in the early stages of the growth of the wheat plant. Trans Micr Soc London 5:104–122.

Owen MJ, Butler SR. (1981). Amnesia after transection of the fornix in monkeys: long-term memory impaired, short-term memory intact. Behav Brain Res 3:115–123.

Ozturk A, Gurses C, Baykan B, Gokyigit A, Eraksoy M. (2002). Subacute sclerosing panencephalitis: clinical and magnetic resonance imaging evaluation of 36 patients. J Child Neurol 17:25–29.

Packard MG, Knowlton BJ. (2002). Learning and memory functions of the basal ganglia. Annu Rev Neurosci 25:563–593.

Pakkenberg B, Gundersen HJ. (1997). Neocortical neuron number in humans: effect of sex and age. J Comp Neurol 384:312–320.

Palmini AL, Gloor P, Jones-Gotman M. (1992). Pure amnestic seizures in temporal lobe epilepsy. Definition, clinical symptomatology and functional anatomical considerations. Brain 115:749–769.

Pandya DN. (1995). Anatomy of the auditory cortex. Rev Neurol (Paris) 151: 486–494.

Pandya DN, Barnes CL. (1987). Architecture and connections of the frontal lobe. In: Perecman E, ed. The Frontal Lobes Revisited, pp. 41–72. New York: IRBN Press.

Pandya DN, Hallett M, Mukherjee SK. (1969). Intra- and interhemispheric connections of the neocortical auditory system in the rhesus monkey. Brain Res 14:49–65.

Pandya DN, Karol EA, Heilbronn D. (1971). The topographical distribution of interhemispheric projections in the corpus callosum of the rhesus monkey. Brain Res 32:31–43.

Pandya DN, Karol EA, Lele PP. (1973a). The distribution of the anterior commissure in the squirrel monkey. Brain Res 49:177–180.

Pandya DN, Kuypers HG. (1969). Cortico-cortical connections in the rhesus monkey. Brain Res 13:13–36.

Pandya DN, Rosene DL. (1985). Some observations on trajectories and topography of commissural fibers. In: Reeves AG, ed. Epilepsy and the Corpus Callosum, pp. 21–39. New York: Plenum.

Pandya DN, Rosene DL, Doolittle AM. (1994). Corticothalamic connections of auditory-related areas of the temporal lobe in the rhesus monkey. J Comp Neurol 345:447–471.

Pandya DN, Sanides F. (1973). Architectonic parcellation of the temporal operculum in rhesus monkey and its projection pattern. Z Anat Entwicklungsgesch 139:127–161.

Pandya DN, Seltzer B. (1982). Intrinsic connections and architectonics of posterior parietal cortex in the rhesus monkey. J Comp Neurol 204:196–210.

Pandya DN, Seltzer B. (1986). The topography of commissural fibers. In: Leporé F, Ptito M, Jasper HH, eds. Two Hemispheres, One Brain: Functions of the Corpus Callosum, pp. 47–73. Proceedings of the Sixth International Symposium of the Centre de recherche en sciences neurologiques of the Université de Montréal, Québec, Canada, 1984. New York: Alan R. Liss, Inc.

Pandya DN, Van Hoesen GW, Domesick VB (1973b). A cingulo-amygdaloid projection in the rhesus monkey. Brain Res 61:369–373.

Pandya DN, Van Hoesen GW, Mesulam M-M. (1981). Efferent connections of the cingulate gyrus in the rhesus monkey. Exp Brain Res 42:319–330.

Pandya DN, Vignolo LA. (1968). Interhemispheric neocortical projections of somatosensory areas I and II in the rhesus monkey. Brain Res 7:300–303.

Pandya DN, Vignolo LA. (1969). Interhemispheric projections of the parietal lobe in the rhesus monkey. Brain Res 15:49–65.

Pandya DN, Yeterian EH. (1985). Architecture and connections of cortical association areas. In: Peters A, Jones EG, eds. Cerebral Cortex, Volume 4, pp. 3–61. New York: Plenum.

Pandya DN, Yeterian EH. (1990). Prefrontal cortex in relation to other cortical areas in rhesus monkey: architecture and connections. Prog Brain Res 85:63–94.

Pandya DN, Yeterian EH. (1996). Comparison of prefrontal architecture and connections. Philos Trans R Soc Lond B 351:1423–1432.

Pandya DN, Yeterian EH. (2003). Cerebral cortex: architecture and connections. In: Aminoff M, Daroff RB, eds. Encyclopedia of the Neurological Sciences, Volume 1, pp. 594–604. San Diego: Academic Press.

Papez JW. (1937). A proposed mechanism of emotion. Arch Neurol Psychiat 38:725–743.

Paterakis K, Karantanas AH, Komnos A, Volikas Z. (2000). Outcome of patients with diffuse axonal injury: the significance and prognostic value of MRI in the acute phase. J Trauma 49:1071–1075.

Paxinos G, Toga AW, Huan X-F. (1999). The Rhesus Monkey Brain in Stereotaxic Coordinates. San Diego: Academic Press.

Perkin WH. (1861). On colouring matters derived from coal tar. Quart J Chem Soc 14:230–255. Referenced in Walker EA (1938).

Perrett DI, Hietanen JK, Oram MW, Benson PJ. (1992). Organization and functions of cells responsive to faces in the temporal cortex. Philos Trans R Soc Lond B 335:23–30.

Peters A. (2002). The effects of normal aging on myelin and nerve fibers: a review. J Neurocytol 31:581–593.

Peters A, Leahu D, Moss MB, McNally KJ. (1994). The effects of aging on area 46 of the frontal cortex of the rhesus monkey. Cereb Cortex 4:621–635.

Peters A, Rosene DL, Moss MB, et al. (1996). Neurobiological bases of age-related cognitive decline in the rhesus monkey. J Neuropathol Exp Neurol 55:861–874.

Petr R, Holden LB, Jirout J. (1949). The efferent intercortical connections of the superficial cortex of the temporal lobe (*Macaca mulatta*). J Neuropathol Exp Neurol 8:100–103.

Petrides M. (1982). Motor conditional associative-learning after selective prefrontal lesions in the monkey. Behav Brain Res 5:407–413.

Petrides M. (1985). Deficits in non-spatial conditional associative learning after periarcuate lesions in the monkey. Behav Brain Res 16:95–101.

Petrides M. (1995). Impairments on nonspatial self-ordered and externally ordered working memory tasks after lesions of the mid-dorsal part of the lateral frontal cortex in the monkey. J Neurosci 15:359–375.

Petrides M. (1997). Visuo-motor conditional associative learning after frontal and temporal lesions in the human brain. Neuropsychologia 35:989–997.

Petrides M, Pandya DN. (1984). Projections to the frontal cortex from the posterior parietal region in the rhesus monkey. J Comp Neurol 228:105–116.

Petrides M, Pandya DN. (1988). Association fiber pathways to the frontal cortex from the superior temporal region in the rhesus monkey. J Comp Neurol 273:52–66.

Petrides M, Pandya DN. (1994). Comparative architectonic analysis of the human and the macaque frontal cortex. In: Boller F, Grafman J, eds. Handbook of Neuropyschology, Volume 9, pp. 17–58. Amsterdam: Elsevier.

Petrides M, Pandya DN. (1999). Dorsolateral prefrontal cortex: comparative cytoarchitectonic analysis in the human and the macaque brain and corticocortical connection patterns. Eur J Neurosci 11:1011–1036.

Petrides M, Pandya DN. (2002a). Association pathways of the prefrontal cortex and functional observations. In: Stuss DT, Knight RT, eds. Principles of Frontal Lobe Function. Oxford University Press.

Petrides M, Pandya DN. (2002b). Comparative cytoarchitectonic analysis of the human and the macaque ventrolateral prefrontal cortex and corticocortical connection patterns in the monkey. Eur J Neurosci 16:291–310.

Pfefferbaum A, Adalsteinsson E, Sullivan EV. (2005). Supratentorial profile of white matter microstructural integrity in recovering alcoholic men and women. Biol Psychiatry Aug 24 (Epub ahead of print).

Phillips AG, Carr GD. (1987). Cognition and the basal ganglia: a possible substrate for procedural knowledge. Can J Neurol Sci 14(3 Suppl):381–385.

Picard N, Strick PL. (1996). Motor areas of the medial wall: a review of their location and functional activation. Cereb Cortex 6:342–353.

Pierpaoli C, Jezzard P, Basser PJ, Barnett A, Di Chiro G. (1996). Diffusion tensor MR imaging of the human brain. Radiology 201:637–648.

Polyak S. (1957). The Vertebrate Visual System (Klüver H, ed). Chicago: University of Chicago Press.

Porrino LJ, Crane AM, Goldman-Rakic PS. (1981). Direct and indirect pathways from the amygdala to the frontal lobe in rhesus monkeys. J Comp Neurol 198:121–136.

Pressman JD. (1988). Sufficient promise: John F. Fulton and the origins of psychosurgery. Bull Hist Med 62:1–22.

Preuss TM, Goldman-Rakic PS. (1989). Connections of the ventral granular frontal cortex of macaques with perisylvian premotor and somatosensory areas: anatomical evidence for somatic representation in primate frontal association cortex. J Comp Neurol 282:293–316.

Preuss TM, Goldman-Rakic PS.(1991a). Myelo- and cytoarchitecture of the granular frontal cortex and surrounding regions in the strepsirhine primate Galago and the anthropoid primate Macaca. J Comp Neurol 310:429–474.

Preuss TM, Goldman-Rakic PS.(1991b). Architectonics of the parietal and temporal association cortex in the strepsirhine primate Galago compared to the anthropoid primate Macaca. J Comp Neurol 310:475–506.

Pribram KH, Fulton FJ. (1954). An experimental critique of the effects of anterior cingulate ablations in monkey. Brain 77:34–44.

Pribram KH, Lenox MA, Dunsmore RH. (1950). Some connections of the orbito-fronto-temporal, limbic and hippocampal areas of Macaca mulatta. J Neurophysiol 13:127–135.

Pribram KH, MacLean PD. (1953). Neuronographic analysis of medial and basal cerebral cortex. II. Monkey. J Neurophysiol 16: 324–340.

Price BH, Baral I, Cosgrove GR, et al. (2001). Improvement in severe self-mutilation following limbic leucotomy: a series of 5 consecutive cases. J Clin Psychiatry 62:925–932.

Probst FP. (1973). Congential defects of the corpus callosum. Morphology and encephalographic appearances. Acta Radiol (Suppl 331):1–152.

Probst M. (1901a). Ueber den Bau des vollständig balkenlosen Grosshirnes sowie über Mikrogyrie und Heterotopie der grauen Substanz. Archiv Psychiatrie Nervenkrankheiten 34:709–777.

Probst M. (1901b). Uber den Verlauf der centralen Sehfasern (Rinden-Sehhügelfasern) und deren Endigung im Zwischen- und Mittlehirne und über die Associations–und Commissuren-fasern der Sehsphäre. Archiv Psychiatrie Nervenkrankheiten 35:22–43.

Probst M. (1903). Ueber die Rinden-Sehhügelfasern des Riechfeldes, über das Gewölbe, die Zwinge, die Randbogenfasern, über die Schweifkernfaserung und über die Vertheilung der Pyramidenfasern im Pyramidenareal. Archiv Anatomie Entwickelungsgeschichte, pp. 138–152.

Proctor F. (1965). The spread of epileptic activity from one hemisphere to the other. In: Ettlinger EG, ed. Functions of the Corpus Callosum, Ciba Foundation Study Group, No. 20, pp. 121–127. Boston, Little, Brown & Co.

Purkinyĕ JE. (1837). Bericht die Versammlung deutscher Naturforscher und Ärzte in Prag im September. Prague. Pt. 3, sec. 5. Anatomisch-physiologische Verhandlungen. (Quoted in Clarke and O'Malley, 1996).

Quain J.(1882). Quain's Elements of Anatomy, 9th ed (Schafer EA, Thane GD, eds). New York:William Wood and Co.

Ragsdale CW Jr, Graybiel AM. (1981). The fronto-striatal projection in the cat and monkey and its relationship to inhomogeneities established by acetylcholinesterase histochemistry. Brain Res 208:259–266.

Rajkowska G, Goldman-Rakic PS. (1995a). Cytoarchitectonic definition of prefrontal areas in the normal human cortex: I. Remapping of areas 9 and 46 using quantitative criteria. Cereb Cortex 5:307–322.

Rajkowska G, Goldman-Rakic PS. (1995b). Cytoarchitectonic definition of prefrontal areas in the normal human cortex: II. Variability in locations of areas 9 and 46 and relationship to the Talairach Coordinate System. Cereb Cortex 5:323–337.

Ranson SW. (1921). A description of some dissections of the internal capsule, the corona radiata and the thalamic radiation to the temporal lobe. Arch Neurol Psychiatry 5:361–369.

Ranson WB. (1895). On tumors of the corpus callosum. Brain 18:531–550.

Rao SM. (1996). White matter disease and dementia. Brain Cogn 31:250–268.

Rasmussen T. (1980). Surgical aspects of temporal lobe epilepsy. Results and problems. Acta Neurochir Suppl (Wien) 30:13–24.

Rasmussen T, Milner B. (1975). Clinical and surgical studies of the cerebral speech areas in man. In: Zulch KJ, Creutzfeldt O, Galbraith GC, eds. Cerebral Localization: An Otfrid Foerster Symposium. New York: Springer-Verlag.

Rauch SL, Kim H, Makris N, et al. (2000). Volume reduction in the caudate nucleus following stereotactic placement of lesions in the anterior cingulate cortex in humans: a morphometric magnetic resonance imaging study. J Neurosurg 93:1019–1025.

Rauch SL, Savage CR. (1997). Neuroimaging and neuropsychology of the striatum. Bridging basic science and clinical practice. Psychiatr Clin North Am 20:741–768.

Rauch SL, Savage CR, Alpert NM, et al. (1997). Probing striatal function in obsessive-compulsive disorder: a PET study of implicit sequence learning. J Neuropsychiatry Clin Neurosci 9:568–573.

Rauschecker JP, Tian B. (2000). Mechanisms and streams for processing of what and where in auditory cortex. Proc Natl Acad Sci USA 97:11800–11806.

Rauschecker JP, Tian B, Hauser M. (1995). Processing of complex sounds in the macaque nonprimary auditory cortex. Science 268:111–114.

Ravel S. (2001). Reward unpredictability inside and outside of a task context as a determinant of the responses of tonically active neurons in the monkey striatum. J Neurosci 21:5730–5739.

Redlich E. (1897). Ueber die anatomischen Folgeerscheinungen ausgedehnter Exstirpationen der motorischen Rindencentren bei der Katze. Neurologisches Centralblatt 16:818–832.

Redlich E. (1905). Zur vergleichenden anatomie der Assoziationssysteme des Gehirns der Säugetiere. II. Der fasciculus longitudinalis inferior. Arbeiten aus dem Neurologischen Institute 12:109–206.

Reil JC. (1809a). Untersuchungen über den Bau des großen Gehirns im Menschen. Archiv fur die Physiologie. Halle, Curtschen Buchhandlung 9:136–146.

Reil JC. (1809b). Das Hirnschenkel–System oder die Hirnschenkel-Organisation im großen Gehirn. Archiv für die Physiologie. Halle, Curtschen Buchhandlung 9:147–171.

Reil JC. (1809c). Das Balken-System oder die Balken–Organisation im großen Gehirn. Archiv für die Physiologie. Halle, Curtschen Buchhandlung 9:172–195.

Reil JC. (1809d). Die Sylvische Grube oder das Thal, das gestreifte große Hirnganglium, dessen Kapsel und die Seitentheile des großen Gehirns. Archiv für die Physiologie. Halle, Curtschen Buchhandlung 9:195–208.

Reil JC. (1812a). Die vördere Commissur im großen Gehirn. Archiv für die Physiologie. Halle, Curtschen Buchhandlung 11:89–100.

Reil JC. (1812b). Mangel des mittleren und freyen Theils des Balkens im Menschengehirn. Archiv für die Physiologie. Halle, Curtschen Buchhandlung Physiol 11:341–344.

Reilly PL. (2001). Brain injury: the pathophysiology of the first hours. "Talk and Die revisited." J Clin Neurosci 8:398–403.

Reisch G. (1503). Margarita Philosophica. Freiburg im Breisgau.

Reutens DC, Bye AM, Hopkins IJ, et al. (1993). Corpus callosotomy for intractable epilepsy: seizure outcome and prognostic factors. Epilepsia 34:904–909.

Rhazes (Abu Bakr Mohammad Ibn Zakariya al-Razi, known in Latin as Rhazes and Rasis). Continens Liber or Kitab al-Hawi fi al-tibb. Translated into Latin in 1279 under the title Continens. Available at: http://www.nlm.nih.gov/hmd/arabic/bioR.html (accessed September 13, 2005).

Richer F, Martinez M, Robert M, Bouvier G, Saint-Hilaire JM. (1993). Stimulation of human somatosensory cortex: tactile and body displacement perceptions in medial regions. Exp Brain Res 93:173–176.

Riley HA. (1960). An Atlas of the Basal Ganglia, Brain Stem and Spinal Cord Based on Myelin-Stained Material. New York: Hafner.

Riolani, Ioannis. (1658). Petri Petiti Medici Parisiensis de Lacrymis, Libri tres. Enchiridii Anatomici et Pathologici. Libri IV, cap. 2, page 254.

Rizzolatti G, Camarda R, Fogassi L, Gentilucci M, Luppino G, Matelli M. (1988). Functional organization of inferior area 6 in the macaque monkey. II. Area F5 and the control of distal movements. Exp Brain Res 71:491–507.

Rizzolatti G, Fadiga L, Fogassi L, Gallese V. (1999). Resonance behaviors and mirror neurons. Arch Ital Biol 137:85–100.

Rizzolatti G, Fadiga L, Gallese V, Fogassi L. (1996). Premotor cortex and the recognition of motor actions. Brain Res Cogn Brain Res 3:131–141.

Rizzolatti G, Gentilucci M, Camarda RM, Gallese V, Luppino G, Matelli M, Fogassi L. (1990). Neurons related to reaching-grasping arm movements in the rostral part of area 6 (area 6a beta). Exp Brain Res 82:337–350.

Rizzolatti G, Matelli M. (2003). Two different streams form the dorsal visual system: anatomy and functions. Exp Brain Res 153:146–157.

Rizzolatti G, Matelli M, Pavesi G. (1983). Deficits in attention and movement following the removal of postarcuate (area 6) and prearcuate (area 8) cortex in macaque monkeys. Brain 106:655–673.

Robbins TW, Cador M, Taylor JR, Everitt BJ. (1989). Limbic-striatal interactions in reward-related processes. Neurosci Biobehav Rev 13:155–162.

Rockland KS, Pandya DN. (1979). Laminar origins and terminations of cortical connections of the occipital lobe in the rhesus monkey. Brain Res 179:3–20.

Rockland KS, Pandya DN. (1986). Topography of occipital lobe commissural connections in the rhesus monkey. Brain Res 365:174–178.

Roman GC. (1999). Vascular dementia today. Rev Neurol (Paris) 155(Suppl 4): S64–72.

Roman GC, Erkinjuntti T, Wallin A, Pantoni L, Chui HC. (2002). Subcortical ischaemic vascular dementia. Lancet Neurol 1:426–436.

Romanski LM, Bates JF, Goldman-Rakic PS. (1999a). Auditory belt and parabelt projections to the prefrontal cortex in the rhesus monkey. J Comp Neurol 403:141–157.

Romanski LM, Tian B, Fritz J, Mishkin M, Goldman-Rakic PS, Rauschecker JP. (1999b). Dual streams of auditory afferents target multiple domains in the primate prefrontal cortex. Nat Neurosci 2:131–136.

Rosene DL, Pandya DN. (1983). Architectonics and connections of the posterior parahippocampal gyrus in the rhesus monkey. Soc Neurosci Abstr 9:222.

Rosenow J, Das K, Rovit RL, Couldwell WT. (2002). Irving S. Cooper and his role in intracranial stimulation for movement disorders and epilepsy. Stereotact Funct Neurosurg 78:95–112.

Rosett J. (1933). The myth of the occipitofrontal association tract. Arch Neurol Psychiatry 30:1248–1258.

Ross ED. (1980). Localization of the pyramidal tract in the internal capsule by whole brain dissection. Neurology 30:59–64.

Rossion B, Caldara R, Seghier M, Schuller AM, Lazeyras F, Mayer E. (2003). A network of occipito-temporal face-sensitive areas besides the right middle fusiform gyrus is necessary for normal face processing. Brain 126:2381–2395.

Rudge P, Warrington EK. (1991). Selective impairment of memory and visual perception in splenial tumours. Brain 114:349–360.

Rundles RW, Papez JW. (1938). Fiber and cellular degeneration following temporal lobectomy in the monkey. J Comp Neurol 68:267–296.

Sabbadini G, Francia A, Calandriello L, et al. (1995). Cerebral autosomal dominant arteriopathy with subcortical infarcts and leucoencephalopathy (CADASIL). Clinical, neuroimaging, pathological and genetic study of a large Italian family. Brain 118:207–215.

Sachs H. (1892). Das Hemisphärenmark des menschlichen Grosshirns. 1. Der Hinterhauptlappen. Breslau. Universität. Pyschiatrische und Nervenklinik. Arbeiten. Leipzig: G. Thieme.

Sachs H. (1893). Vorträge über Bau und Thätigkeit des Grosshirns und die Lehre von der Aphasie und Seelenblindheit, für Aerzte und Studirende. Breslau: Verlag von Preuss & Junger.

Sachs H. (1897). Ueber Flechsig's Verstandescentren. Monatschrift für Psychiatrie und Neurologie 1:199–210 and 1:288–307.

Saint-Cyr JA. (2003). Frontal-striatal circuit functions: context, sequence, and consequence. J Int Neuropsychol Soc 9:103–127.

Saint-Cyr JA, Ungerleider LG, Desimone R. (1990). Organization of visual cortical inputs to the striatum and subsequent outputs to the pallido-nigral complex in the monkey. J Comp Neurol 298:129–156.

Sakata H, Takaoka Y, Kawarasaki A, Shibutani H. (1973). Somatosensory properties of neurons in the superior parietal cortex (area 5) of the rhesus monkey. Brain Res 64:85–102.

Salat DH, Tuch DS, Greve DN, et al. (2005). Age-related alterations in white matter microstructure measured by diffusion tensor imaging. Neurobiol Aging 26:1215–1227.

Sandell JH, Peters A. (2003). Disrupted myelin and axon loss in the anterior commissure of the aged rhesus monkey. J Comp Neurol 466:14–30.

Sanides F. (1968). The architecture of the cortical taste nerve areas in squirrel monkey (*Saimiri sciureus*) and their relationships to insular, sensorimotor and prefrontal regions. Brain Res 8:97–124.

Sarkisov SA. (1955). Atlas tsitoarkhitektoniki kory bol'shogo mozga cheloveka. Institut mozga (Akademiia meditsinskikh nauk SSSR).

Sauerwein HC, Lassonde M. (1994). Cognitive and sensori-motor functioning in the absence of the corpus callosum: neuropsychological studies in callosal agenesis and callosotomized patients. Behav Brain Res 64:229–240.

Savage CR. (1997). Neuropsychology of subcortical dementias. Psychiatr Clin North Am 20:911–931.

Schaefer PW, Huisman TA, Sorensen AG, Gonzalez RG, Schwamm LH. (2004). Diffusion-weighted MR imaging in closed head injury: high correlation with initial Glasgow Coma Scale score and score on modified Rankin scale at discharge. Radiology 233:58–66.

Schäfer EA. (1883). Report on the lesions, primary and secondary, in the brain and spinal cord of the Macaque monkey exhibited by Professors Ferrier and Yeo. J Physiol 4:316–326.

Scheltens P, Barkhof F, Valk J, et al. (1992). White matter lesions on magnetic resonance imaging in clinically diagnosed Alzheimer's disease. Evidence for heterogeneity. Brain 115:735–748.

Schlag J, Schlag-Rey M. (1987). Evidence for a supplementary eye field. J Neurophysiol 57:179–200.

Schleicher A, Amunts K, Geyer S, Morosan P, Zilles K. (1999). Observer-independent method for microstructural parcellation of cerebral cortex: a quantitative approach to cytoarchitectonics. Neuroimage 9:165–177.

Schmahmann JD. (1984). Hemi-inattention from right hemisphere subcortical infarction. Boston Society of Neurology and Psychiatry, Boston, MA, March 22.

Schmahmann JD. (1991). An emerging concept: the cerebellar contribution to higher function. Arch Neurol 48:1178–1187.

Schmahmann JD, ed. (1997). The Cerebellum and Cognition. International Review of Neurobiology, Volume 47. San Diego: Academic Press.

Schmahmann JD. (2003). Vascular syndromes of the thalamus. Stroke 34:2264–2278.

Schmahmann JD, Buchbinder B, Dickerson B, Makris N, Sherman J, Fischman A. (2003). Higher order deficits from a subcortical demyelinating white matter lesion: the mechanism, functional relevance, and significance of diaschisis. Massachusetts Hospital Clinical Research Day, Scientific Session.

Schmahmann JD, Leifer D. (1992). Parietal pseudothalamic pain syndrome. Clinical features and anatomical correlates. Arch Neurol 49:1032–1037.

Schmahmann JD, MacMore J, Ko R. (2004a). The human basis pontis. Clinical syndromes and topographic organization. Brain 127:1269–1291.

Schmahmann JD, Nitsch R, Pandya DN. (1992). The mysterious relocation of the bundle of Türck. Brain 115:1911–1924.

Schmahmann JD, Pandya DN. (1989). Anatomical investigation of projections to the basis pontis from posterior parietal association cortices in rhesus monkey. J Comp Neurol 289:53–73.

Schmahmann JD, Pandya DN. (1990). Anatomical investigation of projections from thalamus to the posterior parietal association cortices in rhesus monkey. J Comp Neurol 295:299–326.

Schmahmann JD, Pandya DN. (1991). Projections to the basis pontis from the superior temporal sulcus and superior temporal region in the rhesus monkey. J Comp Neurol 308:224–248.

Schmahmann JD, Pandya DN. (1992). Course of the fiber pathways to pons from parasensory association areas in the Rhesus monkey. J Comp Neurol 326:159–179.

Schmahmann JD, Pandya DN. (1993). Prelunate, occipitotemporal, and parahipppocampal projections to the basis pontis in rhesus monkey. J Comp Neurol 337:94–112.

Schmahmann JD, Pandya DN. (1994). Trajectories of the prefrontal, premotor, and precentral corticopontine fiber systems in the rhesus monkey. Soc Neurosci Abstr 20:985.

Schmahmann JD, Pandya DN. (1995). Prefrontal cortex projections to the basilar pons: implications for the cerebellar contribution to higher function. Neurosci Lett 199:175–178.

Schmahmann JD, Pandya DN. (1997a). Anatomic organization of the basilar pontine projections from prefrontal cortices in rhesus monkey. J Neurosci 17:438–458.

Schmahmann JD, Pandya DN. (1997b). The cerebrocerebellar system. In: Schmahmann JD, ed. The Cerebellum and Cognition. International Review of Neurobiology, Volume 41, pp. 31–60. San Diego: Academic Press.

Schmahmann JD, Rosene DL, Pandya DN. (2004b). The motor corticopontine projection in rhesus monkey. J Comp Neurol 478:248–268.

Schmahmann JD, Sherman JC. (1998). The cerebellar cognitive affective syndrome. Brain 121:561–579.

Schmidt R, Ropele S, Enzinger C, et al. (2005). White matter lesion progression, brain atrophy, and cognitive decline: the Austrian stroke prevention study. Ann Neurol 58:610–616.

Schmidt R, Schmidt H, Kapeller P, Lechner A, Fazekas F. (2002). Evolution of white matter lesions. Cerebrovasc Dis 13(Suppl 2):16–20.

Schnopfhagen F. (1909). In: Baur J. Aus den Gesellschaften. Versammlung Deutscher Natureforscher und Arzte in Salzburg vom 19 bis 25 September. Neurol Zentralblatt 32:1103–1114.

Schröder P. (1901). Das fronto-occipitale Associationsbündel. Ein kritischer Beitrag. Monatsschrift für Psychiatrie und Neurologie 9:81–99.

Schwalbe G. (1881). Lehrbuch der Neurologie, p. 494. Erlangen: Eduard Besold.

Schwann T. (1839). Mikroskopische Untersuchungen über die Übereinstimmung in der Struktur und dem Wachstum der Thiere und Pflanzen, Berlin. Translated and quoted in Clarke and O'Malley, p. 57.

Schwartzschild M, Rordorf G, Bekken K, Buonanno F, Schmahmann JD. (1997). Normal pressure hydrocephalus with misleading features of irreversible dementias. A case report. J Geri Psychiat Neurol 10:51–54. Reprinted in Dementia 1998;4:14–16.

Scoville WB, Milner B. (1957). Loss of recent memory after bilateral hippocampal lesions. J Neurol Neurosurg Psychiatry 20:11–21.

Selden NR, Gitelman DR, Salamon-Murayama N, Parrish TB, Mesulam M-M. (1998). Trajectories of cholinergic pathways within the cerebral hemispheres of the human brain. Brain 121:2249–2257.

Selemon LD, Goldman-Rakic PS. (1988). Common cortical and subcortical targets of the dorsolateral prefrontal and posterior parietal cortices in the rhesus monkey: evidence for a distributed neural network subserving spatially guided behavior. J Neurosci 8:4049–4068.

Seltzer B, Pandya DN. (1978). Afferent cortical connections and architectonics of the superior temporal sulcus and surrounding cortex in the rhesus monkey. Brain Res 149:1–24.

Seltzer B, Pandya DN. (1980). Converging visual and somatic sensory cortical input to the intraparietal sulcus of the rhesus monkey. Brain Res 192:339–351.

Seltzer B, Pandya DN. (1983). The distribution of posterior parietal fibers in the corpus callosum of the rhesus monkey. Exp Brain Res 49:147–150.

Seltzer B, Pandya DN. (1984). Further observations on parietotemporal connections in the rhesus monkey. Exp Brain Res 55:301–312.

Seltzer B, Pandya DN. (1989a). Frontal lobe connections of the superior temporal sulcus in the rhesus monkey. J Comp Neurol 281: 97–113.

Seltzer B, Pandya DN. (1989b). Intrinsic connections and architectonics of the superior temporal sulcus in the rhesus monkey. J Comp Neurol 290:451–471.

Semmes J, Mishkin M. (1965). A search for the cortical substrate of tactual memories. In: Ettlinger EG, ed. Functions of the Corpus Callosum, Ciba Foundation Study Group, No. 20, pp. 60–68. Boston, Little, Brown & Co.

Seymour SE, Reuter-Lorenz PA, Gazzaniga MS. (1994). The disconnection syndrome. Basic findings reaffirmed. Brain 117:105–115.

Shelton FN, Reding MJ. (2001). Effect of lesion location on upper limb motor recovery after stroke. Stroke 32:107–112.

Showers MJ. (1959). The cingulate gyrus: additional motor area and cortical autonomic regulator. J Comp Neurol 112:231–301.

Simpson S, Jolly WA. (1907). Degenerations following experimental lesions in the motor cortex of the monkey. Proc R Soc Edinb 27:281–301.

Sindou M, Guenot M. (2003). Surgical anatomy of the temporal lobe for epilepsy surgery. Adv Tech Stand Neurosurg 28:315–343.

Siwek DF, Pandya DN. (1991). Prefrontal projections to the mediodorsal nucleus of the thalamus in the rhesus monkey. J Comp Neurol 312:509–524.

Smith WK. (1944). The results of ablation of the cingular region of the cerebral cortex. Fed Proc 3:42–43.

Smith WK. (1945). The functional significance of the rostral cingular cortex as revealed by its responses to electrical excitation. J Neurophysiol 8:241–255.

Spangler WJ, Cosgrove GR, Ballantine HT, et al. (1996). Magnetic resonance image-guided stereotactic cingulotomy for intractable psychiatric disease. Neurosurgery 38:1071–1078.

Sperry R. (1982). Some effects of disconnecting the cerebral hemispheres. Science 217:1223–1226.

Sperry R. (1984). Consciousness, personal identity and the divided brain. Neuropsychologia 22:661–673.

Sperry RW. (1964). The great cerebral commissure. Sci Am 210:42–52.

Sperry RW. (1968). Hemisphere deconnection and unity in conscious awareness. Am Psychol 23:723–733.

Sperry RW, Vogel PJ, Bogen JE. (1970). Syndrome of hemisphere disconnection. In: Bailey P, Foil RE, eds. Proceedings of the Second Pan-American Congress of Neurology, Puerto Rico, pp. 195–200.

Squire LR. (1986). Mechanisms of memory. Science 232:1612–1619.

Squire LR. (1998). Memory systems. C R Acad Sci III 321: 153–156.

Squire LR, Zola-Morgan S. (1991). The medial temporal lobe memory system. Science 253:1380–1386.

Stamm JS, Sperry RW. (1957). Function of corpus callosum in contralateral transfer of somesthetic discrimination in cats. J Comp Physiol Psychol 50:138–143.

Stein DJ, Goodman WK, Rauch SL. (2000). The cognitive-affective neuroscience of obsessive-compulsive disorder. Curr Psychiatry Rep 2:341–346

Stein JF, Glickstein M. (1992). Role of the cerebellum in visual guidance of movement. Physiol Rev 72:967–1017.

Steno N. (1671). Dissertatio de cerebri anatome, spectatissimis viris dd Societatis apud dominum Thevenot collectae, dictata, atque è gallico exemplari. Parisiis edito 1669. Latinitate donata, opera & studio Guidonis Fanosii. Steno (Stensen) N. (1669).

Stilling B. (1842). Untersuchungen über die Funktionen des Rückenmarks und der Nerven. Mit specieller Beziehung auf die Abhandlungen. O Wigand, Leipzig, pp. xii, 316, plate 1. Referenced in Walker EA (1938).

Strich SJ. (1956). Diffuse degeneration of the cerebral white matter in severe dementia following head injury. J Neurochem 19:163–185.

Stricker S. (1870–1873). Handbuch der Lehre von den Geweben des Menschen und der Thiere. Leipzig: Englemann. Translated in three volumes by H. Power as Manual of Human and Comparative Histology (London: New Sydenham Society, 1870–1873; New York: William Wood & Co.).

Strub R, Geschwind N. (1974). Gerstmann syndrome without aphasia. Cortex 10:378–387.

Stuss DT, Benson DF. (1986). The Frontal Lobes. New York: Raven Press.

Sugar O, Amador LV, Griponissiotis B. (1950). Corticocortical connections of posterior wall of central sulcus in monkey (Macaca mulatta). J Neurophysiol 13:229–233.

Sugar O, French JD, Chusid JG. (1948). Corticocortical connections of the superior surface of the temporal operculum in the macaque (Macaca mulatta). J Neurophysiol 11:175–184.

Sullivan EV, Adalsteinsson E, Pfefferbaum A. (2005). Selective age-related degradation of anterior callosal fiber bundles quantified in vivo with fiber tracking. Cereb Cortex Oct 5 (Epub ahead of print).

Sullivan MV, Hamilton CR. (1973a). Memory establishment via the anterior commissure of monkeys. Physiol Behav 11:873–879.

Sullivan MV, Hamilton CR. (1973b). Interocular transfer of reversed and nonreversed discrimination via the anterior commissure in monkeys. Physiol Behav 10:355–359.

Sunderland S. (1940a). The projection of the cerebral cortex on the pons and cerebellum in the macaque monkey. J Anat 74:201–226.

Sunderland S. (1940b). The distribution of commissural fibers in the corpus callosum in macaque monkey. J Neurol Neurosurg Psychiatry 3:9–18.

Suzuki W, Zola-Morgan S, Squire LR, Amaral DG. (1993). Lesions of the perirhinal and parahippocampal cortices in the monkey produce long-lasting memory impairments in the visual and tactual modalities. J Neurosci 13:2430–2451.

Swedenborg E. (1882–1887). The Brain Considered Anatomically, Physiologically and Philosophically. Edited, translated, and annotated by R.L. Tafel. London: James Speirs.

Swedenborg E. (1938–1940). Three Transactions on the Cerebrum: A Posthumous Work by Emanuel Swedenborg (three volumes). Philadelphia: Swedenborg Scientific Association.

Sweet WH, Talland GA, Ervin FR. (1959). Loss of recent memory following section of fornix. Trans Am Neurol Assoc 84:76–82.

Taillia H, Chabriat H, Kurtz A, et al. (1998). Cognitive alterations in non-demented CADASIL patients. Cerebrovasc Dis 8:97–101.

Talairach J, Bancaud J, Geier S, et al. (1973). The cingulate gyrus and human behaviour. Electroencephalogr Clin Neurophysiol 34:45–52.

Talairach J, Tournoux P. (1988). Co-planar Stereotaxic Atlas of the Human Brain:Three-Dimensional Proportional System; An Approach to Cerebral Imaging. Translated by Mark Rayport. New York: Thieme Medical Publishers.

Tatemichi TK, Desmond DW, Prohovnik I, et al. (1992). Confusion and memory loss from capsular genu infarction: a thalamocortical disconnection syndrome? Neurology 42:196–1979.

Tench CR, Morgan PS, Wilson M, Blumhardt LD. (2002). White matter mapping using diffusion tensor MRI. Magnetic Resonance in Medicine 47:967–972.

Terada S, Ishizu H, Yokota O, et al. (2004). An autopsy case of hereditary diffuse leukoencephalopathy with spheroids, clinically suspected of Alzheimer's disease. Acta Neuropathol 108:538–45.

Thomas HM, Keen WW. (1896). A successful case of removal of a large brain tumor. Am J Med Sci, Phila, n.s. 122:503–522 (Quoted in Barker 1899, p. 1071).

Tian B, Reser D, Durham A, Kustov A, Rauschecker JP. (2001). Functional specialization in rhesus monkey auditory cortex. Science 292:290–293.

Todd RB. (1845). The Descriptive Anatomy and Physiological Anatomy of the Brain, Spinal Cord, and Ganglions and of Their Coverings. Adapted for the Use of Students. London: Sherwood, Gilbert, and Piper.

Tomasch J. (1954). Size, distribution, and number of fibres in the human corpus callosum. Anat Rec 119:119–135.

Tourtellotte WG, Van Hoesen GW. (1992). Computer-aided two-dimensional high-resolution axon tracing: an application using the anterograde tracer Phaseolus vulgaris leucoagglutinin (PHAL). J Neurosci Methods 41: 101–112.

Tranel D, Brady DR, Van Hoesen GW, Damasio AR. (1988). Parahippocampal projections to posterior auditory association cortex (area Tpt) in Old-World monkeys. Exp Brain Res 70:406–416.

Trapp BD, Peterson J, Ransohoff RM, Rudick R, Mork S, Bo L. (1998). Axonal transection in the lesions of multiple sclerosis. N Engl J Med 338:278–285.

Trevarthen C. (1965). Functional interactions between the cerebral hemispheres of the split-brain monkey. In: Ettlinger EG, ed. Functions of the Corpus Callosum, Ciba Foundation Study Group, No. 20, pp. 24–41. Boston, Little, Brown & Co.

Trolard. (1905). Au sujet de l'avant-mur. Rev Neurol 13:1068–1071.

Trolard P. (1906). Le faisceau longitudinal inférieur du cerveau. Rev Neurol 14:440–446.

Tuch DS, Salat DH, Wisco JJ, Zaleta AK, Hevelone ND, Rosas HD. (2005). Choice reaction time performance correlates with diffusion anisotropy in white matter pathways supporting visuospatial attention. Proc Natl Acad Sci USA 102:12212–12217.

Tupler LA, Coffey CE, Logue PE, Djang WT, Fagan SM. (1992). Neuropsychological importance of subcortical white matter hyperintensity. Arch Neurol 49:1248–1252.

Türck L. (1849). Mikroskopischer Befund des Rückenmarkes eines paraplegischen Weibes. Zeitschrift der kais kön Gesellschaft der Aertze zu Wien 5:173–176. Also in Jahrbücher für Psychiatrie und Neurologie 1910; 31: 30–33. Also in Neuburger, 1910, pp. 30–33.

Türck L. (1850). Ueber ein bisher unbekanntes Verhalten des Rückenmarkes bei Hemiplegie. Zeitschrift der kais kön Gesellschaft der Aertze zu Wien 6: 6–8. Also in Jahrbücher für Psychiatrie und Neurologie 1910; 31: 37–39. Also in Neuburger, 1910, pp. 37–30.

Türck L. (1851). Über sekundäre Erkrankung einzelner Rückenmarksstränge und ihrer Fortsetzungen zum Gehirne. Sitzungsberichte der mathematisch-naturwissenschaftlichen Classe der kaiserlichen Akademie der Wissenschaften (Wien), 6, 288–312. Also in Zeitschrift der kais kön Gesellschaft der Aerzte zu Wien, 1852, 8:511–534. Also in Jahrbücher für Psychiatrie und Neurologie 1910;31:64–85. Also in Neuburger, 1910, pp. 64–85.

Türe U, Yasargil MG, Friedman AH, Al-Mefty O. (2000). Fiber dissection technique: lateral aspect of the brain. Neurosurgery 47:417–426.

Türe U, Yasargil MG, Pait TG. (1997). Is there a superior occipitofrontal fasciculus? A microsurgical anatomic study. Neurosurgery 40:1226–1232.

Turner MA, Moran NF, Kopelman MD. (2002). Subcortical dementia. Br J Psychiatry 180:148–151.

Tusa RJ, Ungerleider LG. (1985). The inferior longitudinal fasciculus: a reexamination in humans and monkeys. Ann Neurol 18:583–591.

Tusa RJ, Ungerleider LG. (1988). Fiber pathways of cortical areas mediating smooth pursuit eye movements in monkeys. Ann Neurol 23:174–183.

Ugolini G, Kuypers HG, Simmons A. (1987). Retrograde transneuronal transfer of herpes simplex virus type 1 (HSV 1) from motoneurones. Brain Res 422:242–56.

Ungerleider LG, Desimone R. (1986). Cortical connections of visual area MT in the macaque. J Comp Neurol 248:190–222.

Ungerleider LG, Gaffan D, Pelak VS. (1989). Projections from inferior temporal cortex to prefrontal cortex via the uncinate fascicle in rhesus monkeys. Exp Brain Res 76:473–484.

Ungerleider LG, Mishkin M. (1982). Two cortical visual systems. In: Ingle DJ, Goodale MA, Mansfield RJW, eds. Analysis of Visual Behavior, pp. 549–586. Cambridge, Mass.: MIT Press.

Urquhart AR. (1880). Case of congenital absence of the corpus callosum. Brain 3:408–412.

Vaadia E, Benson DA, Hienz RD, Goldstein MH Jr. (1986). Unit study of monkey frontal cortex: active localization of auditory and of visual stimuli. Neurophysiology 56:934–952.

Van Essen DC, Newsome WT, Maunsell JH, Bixby JL. (1986). The projections from striate cortex (V1) to areas V2 and V3 in the macaque monkey: asymmetries, areal boundaries, and patchy connections. J Comp Neurol 244:451–480.

Van Gehuchten A. (1897). Anatomie du système nerveux de l'homme, 2nd ed. Louvain: A. Uystpruyst-Dieudonné.

Van Valkenberg . (1911). The origin of the fibres of the corpus callosum and the psalterium. Royal Academy of Amsterdam. Referenced in Tomasch (1954).

Van Wagenen WP, Herren RY. (1940). Surgical division of commissural pathways in the corpus callosum. Relation to spread of an epileptic attack. Arch Neurol Psychiat 44:740–759.

Varolio C. (1573). De neruis opticis nonnullisq; aliis praeter communem opinionem in humano capite obseruatis. Ad Hieronymvm Mercvrialem. Patauij, Apud Paulum & Antonium Meiettos fratres.

Veenman CL, Reiner A, Honig MG. (1992). Biotinylated dextran amine as an anterograde tracer for single- and double-labeling studies. J Neurosci Methods 41:239–254.

Vesalius A. (1543). De humani corporis fabrica. Basil: Johann Oporinus.

Vialet. (1893). Les centres cérébraux de la vision et l'appareil nerveux visuel intra-cérébral. Paris: Félix Alcan.

Vicq D'Azyr F. (1786). Traité d'anatomie et de physiologie, avec des planches coloriées. Représentant au naturel les divers organes de l'homme et des animaux. Tome premier. Paris: De l'imprimerie de Franç. Amb. Didot l'âiné.

Vieussens, R. (1684–1685). Neurographia universalis:hoc est, omnium corporis humani nervorum, simul & cerebri, medullaeque spinalis descriptio anatomica: cum ipsorum actione et usu, physico discursu explicatis. Editio nova. Lugduni: Apud Joannem Certe.

Vilensky JA, van Hoesen GW. (1981). Corticopontine projections from the cingulate cortex in the rhesus monkey. Brain Res 205:391–395.

Vogt BA, Gabriel M, eds. (1993). Neurobiology of Cingulate Cortex and Limbic Thalamus. Boston: Birkhäuser.

Vogt BA, Pandya DN. (1987). Cingulate cortex of the rhesus monkey: II. Cortical afferents. J Comp Neurol 262:271–289.

Vogt BA, Pandya DN, Rosene DL. (1987). Cingulate cortex of the rhesus monkey: I. Cytoarchitecture and thalamic afferents. J Comp Neurol 262:256–270.

Vogt BA, Rosene DL, Pandya DN. (1979). Thalamic and cortical afferents differentiate anterior from posterior cingulate cortex in the monkey. Science 204:205–207.

Vogt C, Vogt O. (1919). Allgemeinere Ergebnisse unserer Hirnforschung. J Psych Neurol 24:279–462.

Vogt O. (1895). Ueber Fasersysteme in den mittleren und caudalen Balkenabschnitten. Neuro Centralbl 14:208.

Vonsattel JP, Myers RH, Hedley-Whyte ET, Ropper AH, Bird ED, Richardson EP Jr. (1991). Cerebral amyloid angiopathy without and with cerebral hemorrhages: a comparative histological study. Ann Neurol 30:637–649.

Wada JA. (1991). Transhemispheric horizontal channels for transmission of epileptic information. Jpn J Psychiatry Neurol 45:235–242.

Wahlsten D, Ozaki HS. (1994). Defects of the fetal forebrain in acallosal mice. In: Lassonde M, Jeeves MA, eds. Callosal Agenesis, pp. 125–133. New York: Plenum.

Waldeyer W. (1891). Ueber einige neuere Forschungen im Gebiete der Anatomie des Centralnervensystems. Deutsche Medizinische Wochenschrift 17:1213–1218; 1244–1246; 1287–1289; 1331–1332; 1352–1356.

Walker EA. (1938). The Primate Thalamus. Chicago: University of Chicago Press.

Ward AA Jr. (1948). The anterior cingulate gyrus and personality. Res Publ Ass Nerv Ment Dis 27:438.

Watson RT, Heilman KM, Cauthien JC, King FA. (1973). Neglect after cingulectomy. Neurology 23:1003–1007.

Watson RT, Miller B, Heilman KM. (1978). Nonsensory neglect. Ann Neurol 3:505–508.

Weigert C. (1884). Ausführliche Beschreibung der in No. 2 dieser Zeitschrift erwähnten neuen Färbungsmethode für das Centralnervensystem. Fortschritte der Medicin (Berlin) 2:190–191.

Weller RE, Kaas JH. (1983). Retinotopic patterns of connections of area 17 with visual areas V-II and MT in macaque monkeys. J Comp Neurol 220:253–279.

Weller RE, Kaas JH. (1987). Subdivisions and connections of inferior temporal cortex in owl monkeys. J Comp Neurol 256:137–172.

Wenzelburger R, Kopper F, Frenzel A, et al. (2005). Hand coordination following capsular stroke. Brain 128:64–74.

Wernicke C. (1874). Der aphasische Symptomencomplex. Eine psychologische Studie auf anatomischer Basis. Breslau: Cohn.

Wernicke C. (1897). Photographischer Atlas de Gehirns. Schniktte durch das menschliche Gehirn in photographischen Originalen. Abteilung I–32 Frontalschnitte durch eine Grosshirnhemisphäre. Schletter'schen Buchhandlung (Franck & Weigert). Breslau. Abteilung II–20 Horizontalschnitte durch eine Grosshirnhemisphäre. Verlag der psychiatrischen Klinik. Breslau 1900. Abteilung III–21 Sagittalschnitte durch eine Grosshirnhemisphäre. Verlag der psychiatrischen Klinik. Breslau 1903.

Wernicke C. (1908). The symptom complex of aphasia. In: Church ED, ed. Modern Clinical Medicine: Diseases of the Nervous System. New York: Appleton-Century-Crofts.

Wethered FJ. (1888). On a new method of staining sections of the central nervous system. Br Med J 1:510.

Whitlock DG, Nauta WJH. (1956). Sub-cortical projections fom the temporal neocortex in *Macaca mulatta*. J Comp Neurol 106:183–212.

Whitman GT, Tang Y, Lin A, Baloh RW. (2001). A prospective study of cerebral white matter abnormalities in older people with gait dysfunction. Neurology 57:990–004.

Wiitanen JT. (1969). Selective silver impregnation of degenerating axons and axon terminals in the central nervous system of the monkey (*Macaca mulatta*). Brain Res 14:546–548.

Willis T. (1664). Cerebri anatome: cui accessit nervorum descriptio et usus. Londini, typ. J. Flesher, imp. J. Martyn & J. Allestry.

Wise RJ, Scott SK, Blank SC, Mummery CJ, Murphy K, Warburton EA. (2001). Separate neural subsystems within "Wernicke's area." Brain 124:83–95.

Witelson SF. (1985). The brain connection: the corpus callosum is larger in left-handers. Science 229:665–668.

Witelson SF. (1989). Hand and sex differences in the isthmus and genu of the human corpus callosum. A postmortem morphological study. Brain 112:799–835.

Witelson SF, Nowakowski RS. (1991). Left out axons make men right: a hypothesis for the origin of handedness and functional asymmetry. Neuropsychologia 29:327–333.

Woodward WR, Chiaia N, Teyler TJ, Leong L, Coull BM. (1990). Organization of cortical afferent and efferent pathways in the white matter of the rat visual system. Neuroscience 36:393–401.

Woodward WR, Coull BM. (1984). Localization and organization of geniculocortical and corticofugal fiber tracts within the subcortical white matter. Neuroscience 12:1089–1099.

Yakovlev PI, Locke S. (1961a). Corticocortical connections of the anterior cingulate gyrus; the cingulum and subcallosal bundle. Trans Am Neurol Assoc 86:252–256.

Yakovlev PI, Locke S. (1961b). Limbic nuclei of thalamus and connections of limbic cortex. III. Corticocortical connections of the anterior cingulate gyrus, the cingulum, and the subcallosal bundle in monkey. Arch Neurol 5:364–400.

Yakovlev PI, Locke S, Koskoff YD, Patton RA. (1960). Organization of the projections of the anterior group of nuclei and of the midline nuclei of the thalamus to the anterior cingulate gyrus and hippocampal rudiment in the monkey. Arch Neurol 3:620–641.

Yazawa S, Ikeda A, Kunieda T, et al. (2000). Human presupplementary motor area is active before voluntary movement: subdural recording of Bereitschaftspotential from medial frontal cortex. Exp Brain Res 131: 165–177.

Yeterian EH, Pandya DN. (1985). Corticothalamic connections of the posterior parietal cortex in the rhesus monkey. J Comp Neurol 237:408–426.

Yeterian EH, Pandya DN. (1988). Corticothalamic connections of paralimbic regions in the rhesus monkey. J Comp Neurol 269:130–146.

Yeterian EH, Pandya DN. (1991). Prefrontostriatal connections in relation to cortical architectonic oganization in rhesus monkeys. J Comp Neurol 312:43–67.

Yeterian EH, Pandya DN. (1993). Striatal connections of the parietal association cortices in rhesus monkeys. J Comp Neurol 332:175–197.

Yeterian EH, Pandya DN. (1995). Corticostriatal connections of extrastriate visual areas in rhesus monkeys. J Comp Neurol 352:436–457.

Yeterian EH, Pandya DN. (1997). Corticothalamic connections of extrastriate visual areas in rhesus monkeys. J Comp Neurol 378:562–585.

Yeterian EH, Pandya DN. (1998). Corticostriatal connections of the superior temporal region in rhesus monkeys. J Comp Neurol 399:384–402.

Yeterian EH, Van Hoesen GW. (1978). Cortico-striate projections in the rhesus monkey: the organization of certain cortico-caudate connections. Brain Res 139:43–63.

Yin TC, Mountcastle VB. (1978). Mechanisms of neural integration in the parietal lobe for visual attention. Fed Proc 37:2251–2257.

Zeki SM. (1973). Comparison of the cortical degeneration in the visual regions of the temporal lobe of the monkey following section of the anterior commissure and the splenium. J Comp Neurol 148:167–176.

Index